HUMAN SEXUAL BEHAVIOR

William Griffitt
KANSAS STATE UNIVERSITY

Elaine Hatfield
UNIVERSITY OF HAWAII

SCOTT, FORESMAN AND COMPANY
GLENVIEW, ILLINOIS
LONDON, ENGLAND

Cover Photos
Top left: Mike Mazzaschi/Stock, Boston
Top center: Brent Jones
Top right: Scott, Foresman
Bottom left: Jim Brandenburg
Bottom center: Steve Lissau
Bottom right: Rick Browne/Picture Group
Background: Paul Thompson/FPG

Credit lines for copyrighted materials appearing
in this work are placed in the "Acknowledgments"
section at the end of the book. These pages are to be
considered an extension of the copyright page.

Library of Congress Cataloging in Publication Data

Griffitt, William.
   Human sexual behavior.

   Bibliography: p.
   Includes index.
   1. Sex.   I. Hatfield, Elaine.   II. Title.
HQ21.G679   1985   612′.6   84-10684
ISBN 0-673-15057-7

Preface

One of the most important responsibilities of teaching is the selection of textual material that meets the needs both of students and of instructors. Like many others who teach courses dealing with human sexuality, we have been frustrated in our efforts to find a satisfactory text. This book was partly motivated by and is partly a product of that frustration.

Human Sexual Behavior is a comprehensive text written for undergraduate courses in human sexuality regardless of the specific disciplines in which the courses are taught. Recognizing the diversity among students who enroll in such courses, we wrote the book so that no prerequisites in psychology, sociology, anthropology, or biology are necessary. Nevertheless, the complexity of human sexuality requires that contributions and perspectives from all these disciplines be marshaled in its understanding. By approaching the many facets of sexuality from biological and psychosocial perspectives, this book does so.

Our emphasis is decidedly scientific, with a major goal that the content must be as accurate as the limits of current scientific knowledge allow. Empirical evidence and theoretical interpretations are examined in some detail and an overview of the scientific perspective and scientific methodology is presented in Chapter 1. Science has not and cannot, however, provide answers to all the important questions concerning sexuality. Scientific evidence is sometimes weak, ambiguous, contradictory, or even nonexistent regarding many issues and we have noted these limitations in "data" presented wherever appropriate. Science simply cannot answer moral and ethical questions—facts to which we give full recognition in our consideration of religious and legal issues in Chapter 16 and in other contexts as well.

The seventeen chapters of the book are grouped into seven major sections. Part 1 (Introduction) discusses the scientific study of sexuality and provides a conceptual perspective for understanding human sexuality. Part 2 (Sexual

Structures, Functions, and Responses) presents basic information concerning sexual anatomy and physiology and reproductive processes, and in addition discusses the origins and characteristics of sexual arousal. Part 3 (Sexual Identities) considers gender identities and gender roles as important elements of human sexual existence. Part 4 (Sexual Behaviors) includes five chapters that explore major as well as variant forms of sexual expression. Part 5 (Problems in Sexuality) examines some of the ways in which sex can become troublesome. Part 6 (The Interpersonal and Social Contexts of Sexuality) places particular emphasis on the personal relationships that characterize much of sexual functioning and on the ways in which sexuality is molded by cultural, religious, and legal concerns. Part 7 (Conclusions) includes a final chapter in which we speculate, rather guardedly, about possible future trends and issues in sexuality.

We have attempted a more scholarly approach in *Human Sexual Behavior* than do many other texts. This is reflected in at least two ways. First, even though we focus on research findings, we have been very selective in our choice of research to discuss. We have not simply presented a "smorgasbord" of scientific evidence for readers to wade through and attempt to integrate or memorize. Instead, where scientific evidence is weak or nonexistent, we have pointed this out. Where the evidence is somewhat ambiguous or contradictory we have noted that firm conclusions cannot yet be reached. Second, we have carefully avoided taking a judgmental stance regarding human sexuality. Sex means many different things to different people, as we emphasize throughout. Societal attitudes towards various aspects of sexuality are constantly in flux and what is "in" this year may be "out" next year. Our approach concerning most topics is to leave personal decisions about sexual matters to our readers. All of this does not mean that *Human Sexual Behavior* is more "difficult" than other texts. We think not. We do think, however, that it is more valuable as a scholarly, research-based textbook for undergraduates than most others.

Acknowledgments

No book is solely the product of those whose names appear on the cover. We owe special thanks to four reviewers who provided detailed comments and suggestions concerning the entire manuscript: Ellen A. Berscheid, University of Minnesota; Shirley Feldman-Summers, University of Washington; Mary Lou MacVean, State University of New York at Albany; and Kevin L. Murtaugh, State University of New York at Albany. Many other important contributions were made by three anonymous reviewers of early drafts and by the comments and suggestions of Luis T. Garcia, Richard Rapson, and Gerdi Weidner. In addition, we owe thanks to nearly one hundred professors around the country who took time to complete a lengthy questionnaire concerning their needs in a human sexuality text.

We have been provided excellent editorial support and assistance by those at Scott, Foresman. For their extraordinary skill and patience in transforming sometimes illegible scribbles into superbly typed manuscript pages we express our thanks to a number of people: Dora Gruber, Rose Korte, Sheryl Nakahara, Irene Sakoda, Carolyn Tessendorf, Dolores Thorne, and Marilyn Whitaker.

Without their invaluable assistance the project would have remained as a collection of yellow and white legal pad pages. Special gratitude is extended to Judy Bleicher, our copy editor, who played a key role in making this book readable.

Though frustrating at times, writing this text has also been enjoyable. We hope that those of you who learn from it, teach from it, or simply read it find it enjoyable and valuable.

William Griffitt
Elaine Hatfield

Overview

Contents

PART 1

INTRODUCTION

CHAPTER OUTLINE

PIONEERS IN SEX RESEARCH
Richard von Krafft-Ebing
Sigmund Freud
Henry Havelock Ellis

METHODS AND ISSUES IN SEX RESEARCH
Evaluating Sex Research
Methods of Sex Research
Ethical Issues in Sex Research

MODERN SEX RESEARCH
Survey Research
Laboratory Studies Using Direct Observations

A CONCEPTUAL PERSPECTIVE
Dimensions of Sexual Existence
Levels of Sexual Existence

CHAPTER 1

SEX RESEARCH AND KNOWLEDGE

Few dimensions of human experience equal sexual behavior and sexuality in their potentials as sources of joy and pleasure, and paradoxically, of agony, misery, and fear. In many ways sexual behavior and sexuality permeate most aspects of our lives, and most of us would like to have as much accurate knowledge about these topics as possible. Unfortunately, until relatively recently, accurate sex knowledge has been difficult to obtain. In part, this is because culturally and religiously based taboos (discussed more fully in Chapter 16) have inhibited both the acquisition and transmission of accurate information about sexual behavior and sexuality.

Before the twentieth century, views of sexuality were expressed almost exclusively in the context of religion and morality. Indeed, our Puritan and Victorian heritage was such that, in some quarters, it was necessary to cover piano legs for the sake of propriety. Sex "knowledge" consisted mostly of religious perspectives on what was "right" and "wrong" sexual behavior and of religiously influenced medical views on what was "normal" and "abnormal" sexual behavior. The religious taboos surrounding it were such that sexuality was not seen as a proper subject of scientific inquiry. The efforts of the few nineteenth-century pioneers who did attempt to apply some of the methods of science to sex were widely regarded as sacrilegious (Bullough & Bullough, 1977).

The taboos surrounding sexuality were sufficiently powerful that their inhibiting influence on scientific investigation continued well into the twentieth century and is felt even by contemporary scientists. A major breakthrough occurred, however, when Alfred Kinsey and his associates (Kinsey, Pomeroy, & Martin, 1948; Kinsey, Pomeroy, Martin, & Gebhard, 1953) began large-scale investigations of the sexual activities of American men and women. With the publication of the "Kinsey Reports," scientific perspectives on sexuality gained footholds that continue to be strengthened by the work of contemporary scientists. But even the Kinsey work

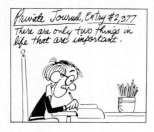

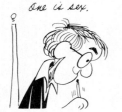

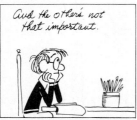

Despite the pervasive influence of sexual behavior and sexuality, it is only in recent years that accurate information about this subject has become widely available.

SOURCE: From *Non-Being and Somethingness: Selections from the Comic Strip Inside Woody Allen,* by Woody Allen, drawn by Stuart Hample. Copyright © 1978 by IWA Enterprises, Inc. and Hackenbush Productions, Inc. Reprinted by permission of Random House, Inc.

and that of William H. Masters and Virginia E. Johnson (1966) that followed were viewed in some quarters as an attack on the Judeo-Christian tradition of sexual morality (Bullough & Bullough, 1977; Gebhard, 1976).

Religious and moral taboos have blocked not only the scientific acquisition of sex knowledge but also its transmission. Until relatively recently, the most common channels of information transmission have been closed to sex knowledge. That is, although parents and educational systems play important roles in transmitting such knowledge as how to read, write, drive a car, and so on, they have played rather minor roles when it comes to specific sex information. Parents continue to be somewhat inadequate sources of sex knowledge, and systematic sex education in the public schools is fraught with controversy (Gagnon & Simon, 1973).

In the early parts of this century, "sex education" in the schools consisted mostly of moral and religious proscriptions against such activities as masturbation (Foster, 1914). Today, although sex education in the elementary and secondary schools has been freed from earlier moralistic restraints, it is limited mostly to information concerning reproduction and the basics of sexual "plumbing" (Alan Guttmacher Institute, 1981). Since the mid-1960s, however, the scene has changed dramatically, at least at the college level. In addition to the biological processes involved in sexual behavior, its psychological and social origins are now the subject of study. Indeed, the course for which this book is intended was unheard of even in the late '50s and early '60s. Though such courses are now rather common, there are those who suggest that they should be more widely available at the secondary or even elementary school level (Alan Guttmacher Institute, 1981).

This book focuses on human sexual behavior and sexuality from the perspective of scientific research. Though we fully acknowledge the existence and value of religious, ideological, and philosophical perspectives, we believe that the methods of science are uniquely suited to obtaining and evaluating sex knowledge in a way that can be *relatively* free from the sometimes distorting biases of those other perspectives. In this chapter we provide a brief overview of some of the major methods and issues involved in sex research.

PIONEERS IN SEX RESEARCH

As we noted above, the idea that the methods of science might be applied to the study of human sexuality is relatively modern. Nineteenth-century thinking was dominated by religious and Victorian views concerning the morality and propriety of various forms of sexual conduct. There were, however, a few bold individuals who took tentative steps toward examining sexuality from a somewhat different perspective—that of science and research. In part because their findings and interpretations sometimes challenged prevailing views, these pioneers were often subject to scorn, disdain, and even threat of criminal prosecution (Bullough & Bullough, 1977). Nonetheless, some of their ideas have had a powerful impact on thinking about sexuality.

Who were the major figures in early sex research and what were their contributions? At least three generalities stand out. First, most were formally educated as physicians and based their findings on observations of their patients. Second, none were immune to the sometimes biasing influences of the religious and social views

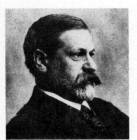

Sigmund Freud.

of their time. Third, in spite of the latter, each challenged many of the prevailing views and, in doing so, shocked and angered many of their contemporaries. Let us briefly review the contributions of a select few of these pioneers in sex research.

Richard von Krafft-Ebing

Richard von Krafft-Ebing (1840–1902) was a German physician who specialized in neurology and psychiatry. Krafft-Ebing's major interest was in what were regarded as "abnormal" or "perverted" forms of sexuality. Based in part on his own psychiatric practice, in 1886 he published the first edition of *Psychopathia Sexualis*, a textbook dealing with sexual disorders. This volume presented in lurid detail over two hundred case histories of individuals showing various forms of "sexual aberrations." The case histories were originally published in Latin in an attempt by the author to limit the work to medical and scientific readers. It has since been translated into many languages.

Krafft-Ebing was one of the earliest proponents of the view that sexual "perversions" were due to disease or "degeneration" of the nervous system. At the same time, though, he was very much influenced by the moral and social forces of his age. He condemned all forms of sexual expression other than heterosexual intercourse as both "sick" and immoral. He regarded sex as an instinct that was powerful and dangerous in men but rather weak or nonexistent in women. He also came to believe that masturbation was a symptom of and an important contributing factor in the development of sexual abnormalities. In spite of his moralistic views and some of his erroneous conclusions, Krafft-Ebing was a major force in bringing psychiatry into the study of sexuality. Indeed, some of his classifications of sexual disorders are in wide use even today.

Sigmund Freud

Sigmund Freud (1856–1939) was one of the most controversial figures of the late nineteenth and early twentieth centuries. Even after his death his ideas continue to be controversial and influential in such diverse areas as psychology, medicine, history, philosophy, sociology, and art. Best known as the founder of psychoanalysis, Freud was an Austrian physician and an accomplished physiologist and neurologist. His interests in psychological processes had many origins but were strongly influenced by Jean Charcot, who introduced Freud to the use of hypnosis as a treatment for psychological disorders. This and other experiences fully convinced Freud of the importance of unconscious processes as controllers of mental and emotional life.

His classic work, *Three Essays on the Theory of Sexuality*, was first published in 1905 and has had a profound and continuing influence on thinking about sexuality. Freud thought of sex as an inborn drive (sometimes with an unconscious quality) that continually strives for expression. He viewed the sex drive as present at birth and as a force that could be channeled and rechanneled in many directions. His theory of infantile sexuality was the foundation for his views that the adult personality (neurotic or normal) could be traced to childhood sexual experiences.

Though Freud's theories about sexuality were shocking to some, in many ways they bolstered some of the then-current Victorian views. For example, although he thought of heterosexual intercourse as the normal mode of sexual expression, he regarded masturbation, oral sex, and anal sex as immature. Homosexuality was described as an "abnormal" outgrowth of disturbed psychosexual development. He viewed women as less "sexual" than men; as he saw it, a strong sex drive was masculine, and women with active sex interests were inappropriately masculine or sexually disturbed. Freud has had no shortage of critics, but his views have had an enormous impact on thinking about sexuality. We elaborate on many of these views throughout this book.

Henry Havelock Ellis

Henry Havelock Ellis (1858–1939) was a contemporary of Freud's. Ellis was an English physician who, like Krafft-Ebing and Freud, relied heavily on case histories of his own and others' patients for his views of sexuality. More than Krafft-Ebing and Freud, however, his interests were primarily in the normal range of sexual variations found in all societies rather than in sexual pathology. Ellis sought to base a science of sexuality on the study of "normal" people rather than of sex criminals or deeply disturbed people in psychiatric therapy.

Originally published in six volumes between 1897 and 1910, *Studies in the Psychology of Sex* established Ellis as an important pioneer of sex research. His views of many aspects of sexuality have a surprisingly modern ring. For example, unlike both Krafft-Ebing and Freud, Ellis thought of masturbation as a basically normal, harmless, and widespread form of sexual expression practiced by both men and women. He held the then-unpopular view that the sexual capacities and needs of women were equal to those of men. In addition, he maintained that homosexuality was a variation in sexuality that did not always involve pathology. Though these and other of Ellis' views were not received favorably in Victorian England, they were forerunners of many modern opinions (Bullough & Bullough, 1977).

We owe much to these and other early pioneers in sex research. Their theories, ideas, and opinions have had a pervasive influence on thinking about sexual matters. But, in light of contemporary scientific knowledge, we know now that some of their most socially important and influential ideas about sexuality were erroneous. This was due in part to the influences of the moral and social biases that they brought to their work. Equally important, however, was the fact that the sciences of human behavior (psychology, psychiatry, sociology, anthropology) were in their embryonic stages of development. Yet to emerge were many modern scientific principles and methods that aid in the reduction of bias and error in the study of behavior. In the next section we briefly examine some of the major methods and issues involved in the scientific study of sexual behavior.

METHODS AND ISSUES IN SEX RESEARCH

A substantial amount of what we know (or think we know) about sexual behavior and sexuality has been learned through the scientific research efforts of the twentieth century. Most people who are not directly involved in it, however, find science and scientific research a bit puzzling:

For most people, "science" evokes images of men in white jackets surrounded by gleaming equipment or memories of biology labs in which the "experiments" never quite worked out the way the lab manual said they should. To some, whatever scientists do seems incomprehensible and somewhat frightening, like the activities of a powerful secret society. (Byrne, 1974, p. 3).

But scientific research is not really very mysterious. Scientific research in sexual behavior simply involves the use of a few procedures by which scientists attempt to obtain and evaluate information with the goals of improving our abilities to understand, predict, and possibly exert some degree of control over sexual behavior. How can we judge how adequate their attempts are?

Evaluating Sex Research

In all methods of sex research with humans, scientists obtain information from or about people and attempt to reach accurate conclusions or draw accurate inferences about sexual behavior from this information. The type of conclusions and inferences that may be reached and their accuracy depend on from *whom* and *how* the information is obtained (Bentler & Abramson, 1981).

Sampling.   In most sex research the goals are to achieve accurate descriptions of the sexual behaviors of a population and to describe the relations between these behaviors and other attributes of the members of that population such as, for example, personality characteristics or religious background. Another frequent goal is to learn the relations between sexual behaviors and the events or objects to which people are exposed (for instance, genital stimulation, pornography, people of the opposite or same sex). In several ways the accuracy of the descriptions obtained and conclusions reached depends on *who* is studied.

In most research it is impossible to study all the people in the population of interest (for example, all American men and women, all married couples over sixty-five, all homosexuals). Instead, scientists must study smaller *samples* of people and attempt to generalize the sample findings to the larger population. For example, many investigators have sought to estimate the percentages of American men and women who engage in heterosexual intercourse before marriage by studying only limited numbers of men and women from the American population.

It should be apparent that in such investigations, who is studied—the composition of the samples—has an important bearing on what is found and on the accuracy of the generalizations that may be made regarding the larger population. A *representative* sample of adequate *size* is needed for accurate generalization. Representativeness is the degree of match between the sample and the larger population in such characteristics as religion, liberalness, educational level, and other important variables. For instance, if the sample contains more liberals than does the population as a whole and if liberals tend to have more premarital intercourse than conservatives, population estimates of the prevalence of premarital intercourse will be too high. Sample size is important because the accuracy of statistical estimates tends to increase as the sample size increases. An enormous sample size cannot "make up" for the limited accuracy of a nonrepresentative sample. A sample that is too small for accurate estimates can, however, seriously weaken a study with a representative sample.

Even if a large and representative sample is initially selected, another problem remains. Because of the sensitive nature of the topics of interest, some people refuse to participate in sex research. For example, in the Playboy Foundation–sponsored survey (Hunt, 1974) only 20 percent of those people asked to participate actually did so. The problem is that volunteers for sex research may be very different from those who refuse to participate, and the conclusions reached from volunteer data may therefore be inaccurate.

Research Procedures.   As stated, who sex information is obtained from is an important consideration in judging the extent to which findings may be taken as applicable to people other than those sampled. Also important is *how* the information is obtained. There are many possible ways to obtain sex information about people, and each has its advantages and disadvantages. One approach is simply to ask people to report on their sexual behavior through interviews or questionnaires. A major issue here is the extent to which *self-reports* are accurate reflections of people's actual sexual behavior. Respondents may underreport, overreport, or do both when responding to sex interviews or questionnaires.

Underreporting may occur for at least two reasons. First, people may have engaged in certain sexual activities that they wish to conceal because of guilt, fear of censure, or fear of disrupting their marriages, social standing, or careers. This is most likely when information concerning taboo topics such as homosexual or extramarital heterosexual involvements is requested. For this reason it is important that respondents be assured of the privacy and anonymity of their responses. Second, people's memories may fail them. They may simply forget about sexual experiences or be unable to recall accurately how often they engaged in certain activities at certain times in their lives.

Overreporting may occur when people seek to bolster their sexual image by claiming experiences they have never had. They may be embarrassed because they lack sexual experience and simply expand a sexual history to more fully coincide with what they think is "normal" or desirable. Both under- and overreporting may occur when, for example, a person conceals homosexual involvement and exaggerates heterosexual accomplishments. Such problems may be minimized when

One of the difficulties of conducting psychological research is that subjects frequently underreport or overreport information about themselves.

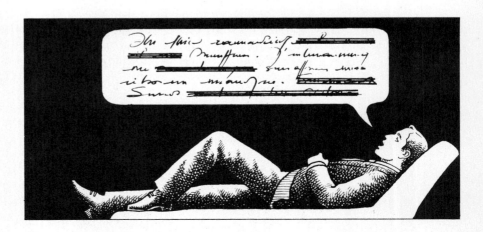

investigators communicate to respondents full assurance that all experiences are equally valued and that honesty is important. Furthermore, questionnaires and interviews can be and often are designed with built-in checks for accuracy such as the repetition of questions.

Information may also be obtained through *direct observations* of behavior as in Masters and Johnson's (1966) investigations of physiological responses to sexual stimulation or the observational work of Hooker (1965a) in the gay community. Although observational studies are more difficult and time consuming than self-report studies, they minimize some of the problems of obtaining data distorted by respondents' self-interests. Still, the mere presence of observers may influence the behavior of respondents in unknown ways. Are peoples' sexual responses the same when they are knowingly being watched as when they are in the privacy of their bedrooms? Do homosexuals behave the same when they are being observed by a "straight" investigator as when they are alone? A second issue in observational studies concerns the ability of observers to accurately record what they observe. The use of sophisticated recording instruments can in some cases minimize inaccuracies, but such equipment is often not accessible or appropriate. Most often observers must either commit observations to a possibly faulty memory for later recording or unobtrusively take notes at the time the behavior is taking place. Observer bias, another problem, occurs when the observers' own attitudes influence their interpretations and reports of observed events. Others may simply not "see" the same thing.

Though these are only some of the methodological issues involved in sex research, they are important considerations in assessing the quality of research and interpreting research findings. We hope that readers adopt the habit of considering such issues in their evaluations not only of the research discussed in this book but also of the tremendous amount of sex "information" and advice found in almost every issue of daily newspapers and popular magazines.

Methods of Sex Research

Scientists use a variety of methods to obtain information about sexual behavior and sexuality. Each method has its own advantages and disadvantages. Let us briefly examine the most common of these methods.

Case Study Methods. Much early sex research involved intensive in-depth studies of the lives of individuals or small groups of individuals. In one common type of case study, for instance, an individual's life is explored extensively. From the quantities of information thus collected, the investigator can learn much about the sexual preferences, experiences, conflicts, desires, and aversions of that individual. In addition, the patterns of meanings associated with the individual's sexuality and the circumstances surrounding his or her sexual development can be examined in great detail. Usually such studies are unstructured and open-ended with respect to the topics covered, and far more information about the individual is obtained than in survey or experimental investigations.

The work of Irving Bieber and his colleagues (1962) is representative of the case study method. The investigators, all psychoanalysts, compiled and compared the case histories of 106 male homosexuals and 100 male heterosexuals. All research participants were patients undergoing psychoanalytic therapy. By comparing the cases, the investigators derived several far-reaching conclusions about the nature and origins of male homosexuality. The following excerpts are illustrative of the detailed life history obtained from each patient:

The patient entered psychoanalysis with a female analyst at age thirty-five. . . . His homosexual practices began with mutual masturbation at the age of seventeen with a partner of the same age. During the following years he participated in homoerotic activities of all types, with mutual fellatio predominating. (Bieber et al., 1962, p. 58)

The patient described his mother as an extremely nervous woman who was overprotective, seductive, and close-binding—intimate. . . . The mother stated that she would raise the child without the father's help. . . . Between the ages of four and seven the patient had a minor intestinal condition and his mother kept him in bed most of the time. Her daily ritual was to rub his back, then pat his buttocks and kiss them. When he was seven years old he had an erection while his mother was such engaged. He was completely terrified and was desperately frightened that she would notice it. (p. 59)

He attempted heterosexual intercourse for the first time at age twenty-eight and failed. . . . He attempted intercourse with another woman and failed again. Following his three failures he gave up heterosexuality entirely. (p. 60)

The ability of the investigator to explore many facets of a person's life in great detail is the primary advantage of the case study method. There are, however, many drawbacks to studying single cases. First, it is risky to generalize findings obtained from a single person or relatively few people to a larger population. The difficulty of generalizing findings is increased by the fact that most such studies are made of persons who are undergoing therapy or treatment for some medical or psychological disturbance. The investigators are usually therapists and gather their information during the course of diagnosis and treatment of respondents who are actually "patients." A sample size of one person or a few people who are atypical by virtue of being in therapy provides little or no basis for accurate generalization to "people in general" or even to "patients in general."

A second problem is the manner in which information is gathered in case studies. It is usually gathered by an investigator with a particular theoretical viewpoint concerning the nature of sexuality, and this viewpoint may well bias the observations and inferences that are drawn. For example, those who view homosexual behavior as indicative of psychopathology will tend to look for evidence of pathology in the lives of their homosexual patients.

Though case study methods are beset with a number of difficulties, they are often quite valuable in generating testable hypotheses or ideas about certain types of sexual behavior. For example, the case studies of Bieber and his colleagues have stimulated a tremendous amount of research concerning the nature and origins of homosexuality.

Survey Methods.   Though case study methods obtain a great deal of information about a small number of people, survey methods typically acquire a relatively small amount of information from a large number of people. Because of this, there is the *potential* for both the representativeness and the size of survey samples to be more adequate for generalization to larger groups of people. As we noted earlier, however, large sample sizes provide no guarantees of representativeness. For example, even though the large-scale questionnaire studies conducted by *Redbook* magazine (Tavris, 1978a, 1978b; Tavris & Sadd, 1977) obtained responses from over 100,000 women and 40,000 men, the samples were underrepresented by those over the age of fifty, those with limited educations, and nonwhites. Similarly, the widely acclaimed and monumental studies of Kinsey and his colleagues (1948, 1953) involved interviews with a sample of nearly 12,000 people that, for reasons to be discussed later, could not be considered representative of the population of American men and women.

A second potential advantage of survey methods is that the procedures used for gathering data are usually fairly well standardized and the method of questioning is more or less consistent from one respondent to another. That is, there may well be less potential for error in recording responses than there is in case studies. Whatever their shortcomings, survey methods can provide quite useful information concerning the prevalence of certain sexual activities, sexual attitudes, and the relationship among these variables and other characteristics of respondents.

Experimental Methods.   One of the important shortcomings of both case study and survey methods is that it is virtually impossible to make causal interpretations of observed relationships between or among variables.

For example, in a study of male and female college students, Griffitt (1975) found that those with a great deal of sexual experience were more erotically responsive to photographs of explicit sexual activities than were those with limited sexual experience. How might this finding be interpreted? At least three possibilities exist. First, it might be that as a result of increasing degrees of sexual experience people become more sexually responsive. Second, the reverse could be true, people who are most sexually responsive might be more inclined to become sexually active. Still another possibility is that some third factor such as sexual liberalness accounts for the relationship between experience and responsiveness. Those who are most sexually liberal acquire more sexual experience and are more responsive to erotic stimuli than are the sexually conservative. Without some method of identifying which of these three variables (experience, responsiveness, or liberalness) controls the other two and any additional potentially important variables, there is no way to determine cause and effect relationships among them.

The primary advantage of experimental methods is that they involve procedures in which substantial control may be exerted over the critical variables of interest allowing for the possibility of drawing causal inferences. For example, in their experimental investigations of male and female sexual response cycles, Masters and Johnson (1966) were able to demonstrate the effects of orgasm on the physiological release of sexual tension. When women who were highly sexually aroused were allowed to reach orgasm, the many physiological "symptoms" of sexual arousal, such as tissue engorgement with blood and muscular tension, dissipated much more rapidly than when the women were not allowed to reach climax. Thus, orgasm was shown to play an important causal role in the resolution of sexual tension.

A disadvantage of many experimental studies, however, is that they obtain data using relatively small samples of respondents whose behavior may or may not be generalized to larger populations. For example, Masters and Johnson (1966) studied comparatively few people and only those who were able to respond and perform sexually while attached to various recording instruments and being observed and filmed. The extent to which the findings may be generalized accurately to people who would not be "caught dead" in such circumstances is open to debate. Similarly, much experimental sex research is conducted using college freshmen and sophomores as subjects, and it is unclear how accurately investigators may generalize from such samples to the larger population of interest.

These, then, are the major methods used in sex research. Most other methods discussed in this book (for instance, cross-cultural and participant observation) are variations of the case study, survey, or experimental approaches. Each approach has its advantages and disadvantages, and ideally, of course, all three would be used in any investigation of a particular form of sexual behavior (for example, masturbation) to capitalize on the unique merits of each.

Ethical Issues in Sex Research

In their pursuit of knowledge about human sexual behavior, scientists must not only be concerned with obtaining accurate and useful information about people but also with guarding the rights and welfare of those whom they study. The ethical responsibilities of researchers are formally recognized and codified by professional organizations such as the American Psychological Association and the American Sociological Association and the human research arms of the federal government such as the National Institute of Mental Health. The ethical responsibilities of those who conduct human research involve obligations to ensure that research participation is based upon informed consent and that subjects are not harmed by their participation in the research.

Informed Consent.   The principle of informed consent requires that research subjects be fully informed of the potential risks and harm associated with participating in the research, the general type of information to be obtained in the research, and the manner in which their own information will be used. They must understand that they are free not to participate and that they may withdraw at any time even if they do agree to participate. When minors are involved, their parents or guardians must provide informed consent.

Protection from Harm.   According to the ethical principle of protection from harm, participants must suffer no harm from the research, or the likelihood and degree of possible harm must be outweighed by the benefits of the research to the participants or the larger society. How might participants in sex research be harmed? First, some of the behaviors (for example, homosexual acts, oral-genital contacts, and extramarital intercourse) are illegal in many states or at least considered socially undesirable by many people. For this reason, the *anonymity* of research participants must be carefully guarded. Leakage of the fact that a person has engaged in any of these acts may lead to legal prosecution, marital disruption, professional ruin, or other negative consequences.

Second, most sex research focuses on topics that some people may find emotionally distressing. For example, even though childhood homosexual experiences are rather common, adults who are asked to recall and discuss such experiences may react with guilt, shame, or embarrassment. For this reason, researchers must attempt to use procedures that minimize such stressful reactions in any way that is feasible.

These, then, are some of the major methods and issues involved in sex research. For more detailed discussions of methodological issues, interested readers should refer to the work of Bentler and Abramson (1981). A thorough examination of ethical issues is provided by Masters, Johnson, and Kolodny (1977). Let us now turn to a brief overview of some of the major studies of human sexual behavior.

MODERN SEX RESEARCH

What may be regarded as the modern era of sex research began with the monumental surveys of Alfred Kinsey and his associates (1948, 1953). Since the appearance of the "Kinsey Reports," the quantity of research devoted to human sexual behavior has shown steady growth. Much of this research is cited throughout this book; in this section we highlight some of the major and most frequently discussed studies. As we do so, we will note some of the strong and not-so-strong features of each.

Survey Research

Numerous surveys of relatively large numbers of people are a major source of the information we have about sexual behavior and sexuality. As we noted earlier, the accuracy of the information is influenced by the samples and research procedures used in the various studies.

The Kinsey Reports (1948, 1953). The two most widely cited and highly respected surveys of human sexual behavior were conducted and reported by Alfred Kinsey and his associates at the Indiana University Institute for Sex Research. The two volumes resulting from the surveys, *Sexual Behavior in the Human Male* and *Sexual Behavior in the Human Female,* described the sexual practices of nearly 12,000 American males and females. The information was obtained by use of interviews.

The samples for the two studies were 5300 white men and 5940 white women. Those studied ranged in age from two to ninety and were drawn from all forty-eight states in existence at the time, from all educational and occupational levels, from several religions, and from rural and urban areas. In spite of the variety and rather large number of people in the samples, they were not representative of the general American male and female populations. For example, no blacks were in either of the samples. In addition, the well educated, college students, Protestants, urban residents, residents of Indiana and the Northeast, and young people were overrepresented in the samples. Underrepresented were laborers, rural residents and those from the West, less well-educated people, the elderly, Catholics, and Jews.

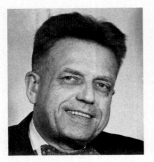

Alfred Kinsey.

Kinsey and his colleagues were fully aware that their samples were not representative. They were, however, convinced that no sample truly representative of the American population could be obtained for a sex survey. They were probably correct in assuming that refusal rates would be so high that attempts at random sampling would be futile. To compensate for weaknesses in the male sample, statistical adjustments were made in an effort to improve the accuracy of generalizations to the general population of American males. Nevertheless, a study committee of the American Statistical Association was highly critical of the Kinsey samples (Cochran, Mosteller, & Tukey, 1954).

Although weaknesses in the Kinsey samples make generalizations to the population risky, the research procedures used with the obtained samples are praiseworthy. The basic interview consisted of 350 questions and required about ninety minutes to conduct. The interviewers memorized all the questions and recorded respondents' answers in a code known only to themselves. Moreover, they developed techniques for putting respondents at ease and keeping them at ease as sensitive topics were raised. Their approach was nonjudgmental; all reported sexual experiences were recorded with acceptance. Questions were asked directly and the interviewers were adept at and free to adjust their language to that favored or most easily understood by the respondents (Pomeroy, 1972).

All of these and the many other interviewing procedures employed were designed to obtain as accurate information as possible. Also included were built-in checks and crosschecks to detect fabrications. The data obtained by the various interviewers were compared. Some respondents were interviewed twice, and the answers of wives and husbands were often compared for agreement. Thus, it was determined that incidence data (responses that indicated whether or not respondents had ever engaged in certain behaviors) and vital statistics data (age, occupation, and so on) were fairly accurate. On the other hand, frequency data (how many times people had engaged in sexual acts) were less accurate, perhaps because respondents' memories failed them.

In short, even though the sampling procedures were relatively poor, the excellent interview procedures seem to have produced fairly accurate information from those actually studied (Cochran, Mosteller, & Tukey, 1954). The Kinsey Reports stand out as monumental pieces of work in the field of sex research.

Morton Hunt (1974).   In 1972, Research Guild, Inc., a Chicago-based independent market-survey and behavioral research organization, surveyed American sexual behavior under the commission of the Playboy Foundation. The data were analyzed and presented by Morton Hunt, a professional writer, in *Sexual Behavior in the 1970s* (Hunt, 1974). Most of the data were obtained with written questionnaires but were supplemented by interviews with an additional 100 men and 100 women.

The final sample consisted of 982 males and 1044 females. These respondents were selected from the phone books of twenty-four cities around the country. Potential respondents were contacted by phone and asked to take part in small groups to discuss sexual behavior. No mention of a questionnaire to be completed was made. About 20 percent of those contacted agreed to participate (an 80 percent refusal rate). Because names were selected from the phone book, young people were underrepresented in the original sample; to correct this, several hundred young people were added by individual solicitations. But again because of the selection method, several other groups such as prison inmates, illiterates, and the very poor were either underrepresented or passed over entirely.

According to Hunt, the final sample closely matched the general population eighteen years old and over in age, occupational status, education, urban-rural background, and attitudes on a number of different issues. No empirical evidence for these claims is presented, however. Even if it were, the fact that 80 percent of the initially randomly selected sample refused to participate raises serious questions about how representative the sample actually was. Were those who refused less sexually experienced, less open about sex, less interested in sex, or more easily embarrassed by sex than the participants? We do not know. Hunt acknowledged that the sample was not perfectly representative of the American adult society. But his belief that it was "reasonably good" (p. 16) led him to draw inferences that were frequently phrased as if they were accurate generalizations to the population as a whole.

Two procedures were used to obtain information. The actual data were collected using four different versions of a questionnaire. The one completed by a given respondent depended on the participant's sex and marital status. The questionnaires contained between 1000 and 1200 questions. Even if some could be skipped, this is a formidable number of questions to ask. Boredom, fatigue, lack of attention, and other factors may have resulted in many inaccurate replies. The questionnaire data were supplemented by interviews with 100 men and 100 women. Excerpts from the interviews are sprinkled throughout the book as illustrations of some of the conclusions drawn.

The Hite Reports (1976, 1981).   In 1976 Shere Hite published *The Hite Report,* an analysis of female sexuality based on the responses of women to questionnaires prepared by the author. Partly because of its controversial conclusions and a tremendous amount of media promotion, the book received wide public attention. In 1981 the same author published a companion book titled *The Hite Report on Male Sexuality.* Both books have been highly controversial, drawing praise from some but severe criticism from others on sampling and procedural grounds.

The female report recorded and presented some summary statistics of the responses of about 3000 women who returned questionnaires sent to over 100,000 women. The women who returned questionnaires were from many parts of the country, ranged in age from fourteen to seventy-eight, and represented a variety of religious, educational, and professional backgrounds. In spite of this, however, the sample was definitely not representative of the general population of American women. The 97 percent refusal rate virtually guarantees this. In addition, the questionnaires were distributed with assistance from many women's groups (such as the National Organization for Women) with decidedly feminist memberships and from publications such as *Ms.* and the *Village Voice. Oui* magazine published the entire questionnaire. Because of the low response rate and the manner in which questionnaires were distributed, it is likely that the final sample of women was considerably more sexually liberal than the general population and perhaps different from it in many other ways as well.

For the male report, 119,000 questionnaires were distributed and 7239 returned—a 6 percent return rate. The questionnaire distribution method was

similar to the earlier study and included reprinting the questions in such magazines as *Penthouse*. Even though its exact characteristics are difficult to determine
from the book, the final sample is not representative of American men. Among
other differences, the sample appears to be more sexually liberal and more
economically and educationally advantaged than the general population (Robinson, 1981).

In short, the sampling methods for both reports leave much to be desired if
one is seeking representativeness. The author, however, did not attempt to generalize her findings to the general population. They are presented mainly as insights
into the sexuality of some American women and men.

Both reports rely mostly on open-ended questions in which respondents were
asked to elaborate on their experience with and feelings about various sexual
activities. The female questionnaires included about 60 such questions and the
male questionnaires 183. Many of the questions required lengthy replies, and
respondents were encouraged to omit questions if they wished. Some questions
were rather bluntly and, for some respondents, possibly offensively phrased ("How
do you masturbate?" "Do you like rectal penetration?") or even leading ("Are most
of your partners sensitive to the stimulation you want?"). Many questions undoubtedly went unanswered; one must wonder how those who answered certain questions differed from those who did not. Though they cannot be regarded as accurate
barometers of the sexuality of American females and males, the detailed statements
of the respondents are a rich supply of information about the sexual concerns of at
least some people.

Beyond the Male Myth (1977).   Shortly after the appearance of the *Hite Report*
on female sexuality, Anthony Pietropinto, a psychiatrist, and Jacqueline Simenauer,

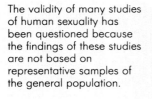

The validity of many studies
of human sexuality has
been questioned because
the findings of these studies
are not based on
representative samples of
the general population.

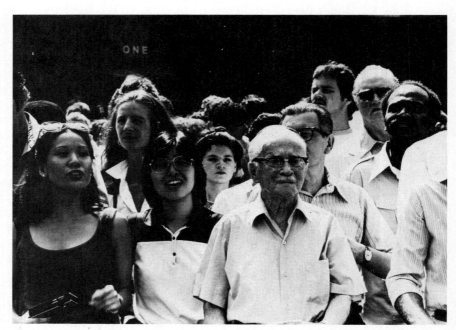

a medical writer, published a report on the responses of over 4000 American men to a sex questionnaire.

Crossley Surveys, Inc., contacted about 8000 men at various sites in eighteen different states and Washington, D.C. The sites included shopping centers and malls, office complexes, tennis clubs, college campuses, airports, and bus depots. Of those contacted, 4066 men agreed to complete the forty-item multiple-choice questionnaire. They also completed four additional open-ended questions in which they described in detail various aspects of their sexual experiences. The response rate of around 50 percent is relatively good, and respondents represented a variety of ages, occupations, educational, and income levels. Though the sample thus appears to have been fairly representative for such studies, Pietropinto and Simenauer did not analyze it with reference to national census data to see how well it reflected the general population. One must wonder whether selecting men from college campuses, tennis clubs, airports, and shopping centers produces a sample that is better educated, wealthier, or more mobile than a truly representative sample. Moreover, did those 50 percent who refused to participate differ in some important way from those who agreed?

The questionnaires were relatively short and required about twenty minutes to complete. A few of the multiple-choice questions violated some of the basic principles of response format and may have influenced the accuracy of answers. In the report, more attention was devoted to answers to the open-ended questions as expressions of the men's opinions and feelings about sexual activities, women, and themselves than to the answers to the multiple-choice questions. In addition, the interpretations of respondents' answers have been severely criticized by well-known sex therapists Wardell Pomeroy and Leah Schaefer (1978). Their criticism focuses on what they regard as a strong psychoanalytic bias in the authors' analyses. Pietropinto and Simenauer are, indeed, highly critical of Shere Hite's earlier work, which they view as seriously biased by a feminist perspective. In fact, both reports appear to reach rather extreme (and opposing) conclusions regarding male sexuality. The "truth" is likely to fall between these two extremes.

Magazine Surveys—*Psychology Today, Redbook.* Although several popular magazines have surveyed their readers' sexual attitudes and experiences, surveys conducted and reported by *Psychology Today* and by *Redbook* have received the most attention and publicity.

Over 20,000 people responded to a 100-item sex questionnaire included in the July 1969 issue of *Psychology Today*, and an analysis of the results was reported in the July 1970 issue (Athanasiou, Shaver, & Tavris, 1970). *Redbook* printed a questionnaire about female sexuality in its October 1974 issue and responses were received from over 100,000 women. In June 1977 a questionnaire about male sexuality appeared for women to distribute to male friends, lovers, or husbands and over 40,000 replies were received. The female data were reported and analyzed in book form by Tavris and Sadd (1977) and the male data were presented in the February and March 1978 issues of *Redbook* (Tavris 1978a, 1978b).

None of these large samples may be considered representative of the American population. For one thing, all respondents were *Redbook* readers, acquaintances of *Redbook* readers, or readers of *Psychology Today*. The young, the well educated, those with middle to high incomes, sexual liberals, and whites were overrepresented. Furthermore, it is likely that only those who were most comfortable in reporting on their sexuality actually returned the questionnaires. Thus, the findings of these large surveys cannot be considered representative of the American population. Nevertheless, the questionnaires were fairly well designed and provide information of value concerning those who did reply.

Homosexualities (Bell & Weinberg, 1978).   Continuing somewhat the traditions of the original Kinsey studies, Alan P. Bell and Martin S. Weinberg began a large scale interview survey of American homosexuals in 1970 and reported their findings in 1978. In 1981 a further analysis of the data was published as an exploration of the origins of homosexuality (Bell, Weinberg, & Hammersmith, 1981).

The homosexual samples included 575 white males, 111 black males, 229 white females, and 64 black females recruited in the San Francisco Bay area. Respondents were recruited through public advertisements, in gay bars and clubs, through personal contacts, in gay baths, in gay organizations, through mailing lists, and in public places. The homosexual respondents were compared with 284 white male, 53 black male, 101 white female, and 39 black female heterosexuals selected to match the homosexual sample in race, sex, age, and education. Neither sample can be considered representative of the American male and female population, in part, of course, because all were residents of the San Francisco Bay area.

The interview was a lengthy one, containing 528 questions that were asked of the heterosexual respondents and about two thirds that number asked of the homosexual respondents. It normally required two to five hours to complete with the homosexual and one to three hours with the heterosexual respondents. Interviews were conducted in private, mostly by graduate students recruited from local universities. Several checks on the accuracy and consistency of answers were made and both appeared to be adequate.

Overall, the samples and procedures used are probably as good and the basic findings as accurate as one can expect from this type of study. We discuss some of these in Chapter 11. The authors, however, were admittedly sympathetic to the gay movement, and Harold Lief, in his review of the work (1978), suggested that these sympathies may have slanted some of their interpretations of the data. For example, in emphasizing the similarities of the homosexual and heterosexual respondents, they glossed over glaring differences such as the extremely high level of sexual activity of the homosexual males. Nevertheless, the study is valuable for the large amount of data it offers and the impetus it should provide for further investigations.

Surveys can be valuable in the acquisition of knowledge about sexuality if the samples are adequate and if the self-reports obtained from the sample of respondents are accurate. Truly representative samples, however, are extremely difficult to design and are in actuality rarely, if ever, obtained in studies of sexuality. From any single study, then, generalizations to larger populations concerning the prevalence or frequency of sexual activities such as masturbation and premarital intercourse or of particular attitudes about sex should be viewed as *potentially* inaccurate. Comparisons within a single study are likely to be more accurate. For example, we can be fairly confident that differences found between men and women on some variable are accurate *for the sample* since sampling errors should affect the sexes similarly. Finally, within a sample, relationships between variables such as sex attitudes and sex behavior are usually not seriously affected by minor sample inadequacies.

Even if adequate samples are obtained, interview or questionnaire self-reports are potentially subject to errors of overreporting, underreporting, or memory failure. For this reason some investigators turn to direct observations of sexual activities to reduce self-report errors. Let us briefly examine the major laboratory studies that have used direct observations.

Laboratory Studies Using Direct Observations

Earlier we discussed some of the potential advantages of observing sexual behavior directly rather than relying exclusively on respondents' self-reports. Among those advantages are reductions in the likelihood of bias introduced by respondents' self-interests. In addition, sophisticated measuring and recording devices may be employed to obtain accurate and permanent records of behaviors. Potential disadvantages include the unwillingness of many people to allow their sexual behavior to be observed, the possibility that the presence of observers or recording devices might alter the behavior being observed, and the sometimes prohibitive costs involved.

Though it was not widely publicized, the Kinsey research team used direct observations of sexual activity in compiling knowledge about the physiological aspects of sexual responses (Pomeroy, 1972). Their preliminary findings were reported in the 1953 volume dealing with female sexual behavior. But it was the research team of William Masters and Virginia Johnson that first brought to national and worldwide attention the use of direct observation of sexual activity in the laboratory as a major research method.

Masters and Johnson (1966, 1979).   In *Human Sexual Response* (1966), Masters and Johnson summarized several years of research concerning the physiological changes that take place in humans in response to sexual stimulation and during sexual activity. Their major findings are discussed in detail in Chapter 5 of this text. Though their initial reports (1966) concerned physiological responses in heterosexuals during masturbation and heterosexual activity, they later confirmed that responses during homosexual activity and in homosexuals are virtually identical. Their findings for homosexuals are reported in *Homosexuality in Perspective* (1979).

The 1966 report is based upon observations of 382 women and 312 men as they engaged in sexual activity in a laboratory setting. The sample is not representative of the general population of American women and men. The women ranged in age from eighteen to seventy-eight and the men from twenty-one to eighty-nine. The final sample consisted of 276 married couples, 108 unmarried women, and 36 unmarried men. Most participants were associated with the Washington University of St. Louis community and were selected only if their sexual anatomy was normal, if they could respond sexually in a laboratory setting, and if they were able to describe in detail their sexual reactions. They were mostly white, well-educated urban dwellers of above average socioeconomic level. Most important, however, they were willing to perform sexually while being observed, photographed, and attached to physiological recording equipment. Even though the sample was not a representative one, there is little reason to suspect that the recorded physiological reactions of the respondents differ dramatically from those of other people.

The second observational study included a sample of 94 male and 82 female homosexuals who were compared with two heterosexual groups. The first heterosexual group consisted of 57 male and 57 female heterosexuals selected specifically for the new study. The second group was formed from 286 male and 281 female heterosexuals who took part in the original study. The homosexual participants were recruited from various parts of the country but it is unlikely that they were a representative sample of American homosexuals. Their educational level was higher than average, they were more likely to have a committed stable relationship with one person than most gays, their ages were concentrated in the twenty to forty range, and they were specifically selected for a history of easily reaching orgasm in a variety of ways. Nearly all were white. Furthermore, there are many difficulties involved in designating persons as heterosexual or homosexual (see Chapter 11). Some critics have argued that Masters and Johnson's selection of their homosexual participants was seriously flawed by their failure to adequately consider such problems (Zilbergeld & Evans, 1980).

Many of the same procedures were used to gather data in both of the studies. Participants were interviewed concerning their sexual histories and given medical exams. As in the original study, participants were observed in a variety of sexual activities. These included masturbation, manual stimulation by partners, fellatio, cunnilingus, coitus, and anal intercourse. Visual observations, film, and recording instruments were used to record body changes during sexual activity. Cardiovascular reactions, muscle reactions, skin reactions, and respiratory reactions were recorded. A special artificial plastic penis that contained a light source and photo-

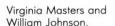

Virginia Masters and
William Johnson.

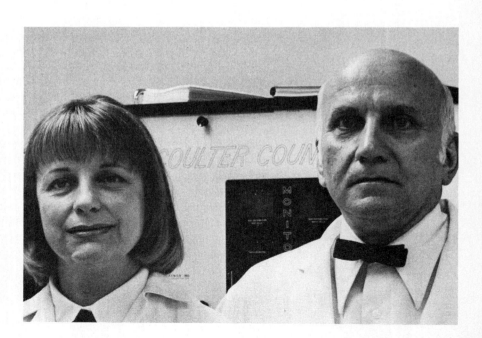

graphic equipment was used to record vaginal, cervical, and uterine changes during sexual responses. Participants were interviewed after their sexual activities.

The Masters and Johnson work is important but not without its flaws. Many of their most important conclusions and interpretations are based not on their physiological data but on rather vaguely supported impressions gathered from the interview material. Their statistical breakdowns are confusing and difficult to interpret and other researchers would benefit from more complete descriptions of their study participants, particularly those participants who received treatment for their sexual problems (Zilbergeld & Evans, 1980).

Masters and Johnson were the first to use direct physiological recordings on a large scale in the study of sexual reactions. Now, however, the use of sophisticated instruments to record sexual responses is rather common. We discuss research based on these techniques in several places in this book.

A CONCEPTUAL PERSPECTIVE

Our existence as sexual beings is but one dimension of being human. But our sexual existence is itself complex and multidimensional. We conclude this chapter with an overview of a conceptual perspective that we think is useful in capturing some of the complexity of human sexual existence. At the same time this perspective brings some order to what could simply be an overwhelming and chaotic collection of "facts" concerning seemingly unrelated aspects of sexual existence.

Dimensions of Sexual Existence

What are we sexually? *Who* are we sexually? *How* do we function sexually? These three questions highlight the most salient dimensions of human sexual existence.

What Are We Sexually?   Ultimately our sexual existence is traceable to the fact that we are one of many species of animals that reproduce sexually. Thus, we consist, in part, of a number of anatomical structures and physiological processes that define our biological sex and determine our potential roles in reproducing others of our own species. A human female has ovaries, a uterus, a vagina, and other sexual structures that allow her to become impregnated and bear offspring. A human male has testes, a penis, and related reproductive ducts that allow him to impregnate a female.

As obvious as they may seem, these elementary facts concerning the "what" of sexual existence are of tremendous importance in shaping who we are sexually and how we function sexually. An adequate understanding of human sexual existence, then, requires some basic knowledge of our sexual "equipment," how it functions, and the role it plays in the "who" and "how" dimensions of human sexuality. The basic anatomic and physiological aspects of human sexual existence have been thoroughly investigated and are discussed in some detail in Chapter 2 of this book. Chapter 2 provides the basic foundation for understanding what we are sexually, and we repeatedly return to this foundation as we explore sexual identities (Chapters 6 and 7), sexual stimulation, arousal, and orgasm (Chapters 4 and 5), conception, pregnancy, and birth control (Chapter 3), and many other topics.

Who Are We Sexually?   There is a remarkable degree of similarity between humans and other mammals in basic sexual equipment (Beach, 1969). A major difference between humans and other mammals, however, is that humans form identities of themselves as sexual beings and actors and adopt roles that are related to these identities. That is, most of us have rather deep-seated conceptions of ourselves as males and females, which are referred to as our "gender identities." Furthermore, we tend to create social conventions concerning how males and females should behave and to acquire gender roles (private self-views and public behaviors) that reflect these social conventions. That is, we think of ourselves and behave in ways that reflect our socially defined "masculinity" or "femininity." Finally, on the basis of sexual preferences or behaviors, we form identities of ourselves as sexual "actors." That is, we view ourselves as heterosexuals, homosexuals, bisexuals, or even asexuals.

All of these identities are part of the "who" dimension of sexual existence. Who we are sexually influences and is influenced by what we are and how we function sexually. Our basic sexual equipment influences our conceptions of ourselves as male or female and as masculine or feminine. At the same time, gender identities that are at variance with biological sex may lead to alterations of what we are sexually, as in the case of transsexual sex reassignment surgery. Our gender identities and roles dictate to some extent how we function sexually in the sense that "masculine males" and "feminine females" are expected to engage in different types and "styles" of sexual behavior. In addition, our identities as sexual actors influence our selections of the sex of those we interact with sexually and these selections "feed back" to strengthen or modify our heterosexual or homosexual identities.

Who we are sexually is the specific focus of Chapters 6 and 7, where we discuss gender identities and gender roles. This "who" issue continually resurfaces, however, as we examine the types of cues to which we react sexually (Chapters 4 and 15), the emergence of homosexual identities (Chapter 11), and the origins and consequences of sexual dysfunctions (Chapter 13).

How We Function Sexually.   Among others, Beach (1977, p. 191) and Masters and Johnson (1966) have characterized sexual functioning as consisting of three phases of activity: (1) the *stimulation* and arousal of sexual desire, (2) the *behaviors* motivated by sexual arousal that further intensify sexual excitement, and (3) the culmination or gratification of sexual desire through *orgasm*. These three phases of sexual functioning have been the subject of a substantial amount of research during the last several decades and they are the major focus of this book.

Thus, in Chapter 4 we consider in detail the types of stimuli that evoke sexual arousal and in Chapter 5 we discuss the physiological and anatomic reactions that accompany sexual arousal. Aroused sexual needs may find behavioral expression in a multitude of ways. Sexual stimulation may lead to autosexual behaviors (Chapter 8), a variety of heterosexual behaviors (Chapters 9 and 10) with the potential for pregnancy and childbirth unless birth control methods dictate otherwise (Chapter 3), homosexual behaviors (Chapter 11), and a number of variant forms of sexual expression that are widely regarded as socially undesirable (Chapter 12). Furthermore, sexual functioning may be disrupted at the stimulation, behavior, or orgasm phase (Chapter 13).

Levels of Sexual Existence

What we are, who we are, and how we function sexually may be considered on at least two levels. At the *biological level* our sexual existence may be analyzed in terms of the influences of genetic, hormonal, and neural processes. At the *psychosocial level* we may examine the roles of learning, imagination, and emotional processes in our sexual existence.

The Biological Level.   At the biological level we must consider the roles played by genetic, hormonal, and neural processes in shaping sexual existence. The greatest influence of biological processes is in determining what we are sexually. That is, the structure and function of our sexual equipment is largely determined by our genetic sex and the patterns of hormone secretion during our prenatal existence that are associated with our genetic sex (Chapters 2 and 6).

Who we are sexually is influenced to some extent by genetic, hormonal, and neural processes. Genetic and hormonal influences are largely indirect. That is, our gender identities and roles appear to be shaped mostly by the treatment and rearing we receive following birth when our parents and others label us as male or female on the basis of the appearance of our external genital anatomy. It has been suggested, however, that neural processes may play a more direct role in predisposing us to develop male or female gender identities and masculine or feminine gender roles (Money & Ehrhardt, 1972). This rather controversial issue is discussed in Chapters 6 and 7.

To what extent do biological processes influence how we function sexually? There is general agreement that patterns of sexual functioning among nonhuman mammals are in many ways "programmed" by genetic and hormonal processes. That is, the cues that are sexually stimulating to some animals seem to be genetically fixed and many animals respond to sexual cues only when they are hormonally primed to do so. In contrast, few if any stimuli are "automatically" arousing to humans and our readiness to respond sexually is not tightly controlled by our hormonal state (Beach, 1969). The biological processes involved in the stimulation phase of sexual functioning are discussed in Chapter 4.

The sexual behaviors of nonhuman animals tend to be rather rigid and unvarying from one occasion to another. The penis is inserted into the vagina and a series of movements that insure genital friction follow. Little variety is involved, suggesting the operation of biologically based programs for sexual behavior at least among some animals. In contrast, sexually aroused humans may engage in a tremendous variety of sexual acts including, but not limited to, penile-vaginal insertion. In short, human sexual behavior appears to be relatively liberated from the rigid controls imposed by biological processes (Beach, 1969).

Because the sexual acts of nonhuman mammals are mostly limited to vaginal intercourse, orgasm is usually limited to the ejaculation of sperm by the male into the vagina of the female. Sexual acts are linked closely to the biological processes of reproduction. But much of what humans do sexually is independent of biological urges for reproduction. Genital friction and orgasm resulting from masturbation, oral-genital contacts, and homosexual acts do not lead to fertilization. Furthermore, humans often take deliberate steps to prevent fertilization even when coitus takes place (Chapter 3).

To be sure, how we function sexually is at least indirectly influenced by biological processes. A man has a penis and a woman does not. A woman can become pregnant and a man cannot. Sexual arousal and response in both sexes are dependent on the existence of a functional sexual anatomy. But, in comparison with other animals, what we react to sexually, how we behave sexually, and how (or if) we have orgasms seem to be relatively free of the strict controls of biological processes. The various ways in which biological processes may shape our sexual functioning are discussed throughout this book.

The Psychosocial Level. The three dimensions of sexual existence discussed earlier—the "what," "who," and "how" of human sexuality—are influenced in many ways by the psychosocial processes of learning, imagination, and emotions. In comparison with that of other animals, our sexual existence is shaped in important ways by our ability to learn. With respect to what we are sexually, this means that we are capable of learning the functions of and acquiring labels for our sexual anatomy. We can teach others these functions and labels and increase their understanding of what they are sexually through sex education. Such education may function to transmit accurate sexual information. Sometimes, however, inaccurate and distorted sexual facts that, in turn, affect other dimensions of our sexual existence are taught and learned. Learning also contributes greatly to our formation of gender identities and gender roles. Though biological processes may play some role, our conceptions of who we are sexually are mostly acquired through learning.

In terms of sexual functioning, our ability to learn has meant that almost any stimulus can through experience be associated with sexual arousal and as a result of conditioning become capable of producing sexual arousal. Thus, rather than being fully biologically programmed to respond only to the opposite sex, we can learn to respond erotically to a variety of stimuli, including people of our own sex, places, particular smells, sights, sounds, tastes, and touches, articles of clothing such as, say, shoes or raincoats, and even physical abuse. Similarly, we learn that many sexual acts other than penile-vaginal penetration are capable of producing genital friction. The variability in human sexual behavior is largely traceable to our abilities to learn alternate modes of sexual expression. This, of course, means that sequences of sexual functioning do not always culminate with ejaculation in the vagina and that human sexual behavior is not invariably tied to reproduction.

Our ability to symbolize experiences—that is, represent them mentally—makes it possible for us to shape in imagination our own sexual existence. In terms of what we are sexually, for example, we can imagine ourselves as possessing more attractive genitals or more physical sexual appeal than we really do. Who we are sexually can be altered in imagination so that we may create images of ourselves as more or less masculine or feminine than we really are. Or, in fantasy, we may even imagine ourselves as someone of the opposite sex.

The products of our imagination, our fantasies, can be potent sources of sexual arousal or, conversely, they can inhibit or interfere with our abilities to respond sexually and reach orgasm. In our fantasies we may symbolize and imagine engaging in a variety of sexual acts that might find expression in actual behavior. Fantasies may also serve as substitutes for the performance of forbidden or otherwise unacceptable behaviors. Further, fantasies may also provide mental rehearsals or practice for actual behavior we may engage in.

Humans not only learn and symbolize many aspects of their sexual existence but also react emotionally to their sexuality. We all have attitudes and feelings about what we are sexually, who we are sexually, and how we function sexually. For example, we respond positively or negatively to the sexual aspects of our bodies, and these emotional reactions influence the ways we use our bodies when we function sexually. In some cases dissatisfaction with our bodies may lead to attempts to alter them hormonally and surgically.

Who we are sexually is also of emotional importance to most of us. Experiences that confirm our gender identities and gender roles evoke positive emotional reactions, and those that lead us to question our sexual self-images evoke unpleasant feelings.

Emotional processes exert important influences on the ways we react to sexual stimuli and whether we regard sexual arousal as something that should be sought out or avoided. The types of sexual behaviors we engage in and consider acceptable and pleasurable depend to a large extent on learned emotional reactions. Furthermore, emotional processes influence whether or not we ever have orgasms, the frequency of our orgasms, whether we experience orgasms as positive or negative, and the behavioral contexts (oral-genital sex, masturbation, coitus, anal intercourse, and so on) within which we consider orgasms acceptable or unacceptable.

In summary, our sexual existence may be considered in terms of what we are, who we are, and how we function sexually. These dimensions of sexual existence are shaped jointly by biological and psychosocial processes.

SUMMARY

Until relatively recently, religious and cultural taboos inhibited both the acquisition and transmission of accurate sex knowledge. The scientific perspective on sexuality did not gain a strong foothold until around the middle of the twentieth century. Nineteenth-century pioneers in sex research such as Krafft-Ebing, Freud, and Ellis provided a foundation for later research with their case history studies.

Although other potentially useful approaches might be adopted, this book considers human sexual behavior and sexuality from the perspective of scientific research. The usefulness of sex research depends on who is studied and how studies are conducted. Because it is impossible for scientists to study the sexual behaviors or sexuality of all people, they must rely on samples of research participants from whom they hope to obtain information that can be generalized to larger populations of interest.

Representative samples of adequate size are required for valid generalization. How sex information is obtained plays an important role in determining how accurate that information will be. When sex reports are obtained, the problems of underreporting or overreporting must be minimized. Observational methods are difficult and time consuming but potentially less subject to the effects of distortion due to respondents' self-interests. Observers, however, may influence the behavior of respondents simply by their presence, and they may have difficulty recording information accurately.

Several procedures for obtaining sexual information are used by scientists, including case study methods, survey methods, and experimental methods. Each method has its own advantages and disadvantages.

Ethical considerations obligate scientists to insure that the participation of their research subjects is based upon informed consent and that subjects are not harmed by participation in the research. These ethical principles are sometimes more difficult to follow in practice than in theory.

The monumental survey studies of Alfred Kinsey and his associates launched the modern era of sex research. Kinsey's research and the many relatively large-scale studies that followed are all limited to some extent by sampling and procedural problems. Even so, most studies contribute something of value to our knowledge about sexuality.

Human sexual existence is complex and multifaceted. What we are sexually, who we are sexually, and how we function sexually are basic dimensions of our sexual existence. These dimensions of sexual existence are jointly shaped by biological and psychosocial processes.

SUGGESTED READINGS

Beach, F. A. (Ed.) (1977). *Human sexuality in four perspectives.* Baltimore: Johns Hopkins University Press.

Bermant, G., & Davidson, J. M. (1974). *Biological bases of sexual behavior.* New York: Harper & Row. (See especially chapter 8.)

Bullough, V. L. (1975). Sex and the medical model. *Journal of Sex Research, 11,* 291–303.

Bullough, V. L., & Bullough, B. (1977). *Sin, sickness, and sanity.* New York: Garland Publishing.

PART 2

SEXUAL STRUCTURES, FUNCTIONS, AND RESPONSES

CHAPTER OUTLINE

PRENATAL SEXUAL DIFFERENTIATION AND DEVELOPMENT
Genetic Factors
Hormonal Factors

POSTNATAL SEXUAL DEVELOPMENT AND PUBERTY
Birth to Puberty
Puberty

ADULT SEXUAL ANATOMY AND PHYSIOLOGY
Female Sexual Anatomy and Physiology
Male Sexual Anatomy and Physiology

CHAPTER 2

SEXUAL ANATOMY AND PHYSIOLOGY

Through his famous dictum "Anatomy is destiny," Sigmund Freud (1927) expressed his view that virtually all significant aspects of human experience (conscious and unconscious) could be understood in terms of the structure and functioning of the sexual organs. A man has a penis and a woman does not. Freud thought that most of the psychological differences between men and women could be traced to these basic anatomical facts. That is, men fear loss of their penis ("castration anxiety") and women grieve over their lack of a penis ("penis envy").

Although few scientists still adhere to Freud's extreme views, most agree (Bermant & Davidson, 1974; Masters & Johnson, 1966) that full comprehension of human sexual expression requires a basic understanding of both the anatomy (structure) and physiology (functioning) of human sexual systems. This is not to say, of course, that most of us are unable to perform basic sexual acts without formal knowledge of sexual anatomy and physiology. Thousands of years of reproductive "success" among humans provide striking evidence to the contrary. But, just as racing drivers' performances are enhanced by at least rudimentary knowledge of the various parts and workings of their automobiles, knowledge concerning the parts and workings of one's "sexual equipment" can be of benefit in the sexual arena.

In this chapter we will consider some of the "basics" of sexual anatomy and physiology. First we will examine what is known concerning the **prenatal** (before birth) *differentiation and development* of male and female systems. Next, we will turn our attention to the growth and development of sexual systems that occur **postnatally** (following birth). We will devote particular attention to the transformations associated with *puberty*. Finally, we will describe the anatomy and physiology of the sexual systems of *adults* as well as some of the changes associated with aging.

PRENATAL SEXUAL DIFFERENTIATION AND DEVELOPMENT

Barring unusual circumstances such as disease, nutritional deficiencies, injury, or surgical intervention, *genetic* and *hormonal* factors shape people's sexual anatomy and physiology. Much of this influence is exerted prenatally (prior to birth). In this section we will outline what takes place in the emergence of human sexual systems from the time of fertilization to the time of birth. This span of time is generally subdivided into two periods—the period of the **embryo** (first two months following conception) and the period of the **fetus** (final seven months of pregnancy). First, we will examine the critical importance of genetic factors in early development. Then, we will turn our attention to hormones and their effects on the differentiation of internal and external genital systems into male and female forms. Our focus will be on the "normal" course of events in which the outcomes are clearly formed and properly functioning female and male sexual systems. In Chapter 6 we will discuss rare instances in which the sexual systems are incomplete or ambiguous and function is impaired.

Genetic Factors

With one important exception, all of the cells of any given individual contain twenty-three pairs of **chromosomes** (a total of forty-six per cell). Chromosomes contain the **genes** that constitute the genetic stamp of the individual. There are twenty-two pairs of chromosomes that shape the individual's nonsexual hereditary characteristics and one pair of **sex chromosomes** that determine the genetic sex of the person. The exception to this rule occurs in **germ cells**, or reproductive cells. Germ cells are referred to as **ova** (singular, *ovum*) in females and as **sperm** in males. Both types of cells contain twenty-three *single* chromosomes rather than twenty-three pairs of chromosomes. Of these, twenty-two are nonsexual and one is a sex chromosome. All ova contain only a single type of sex chromosome, designated X, while two types are carried by sperm, designated, respectively, as X or Y.

Fertilization (conception) takes place when a single sperm carrying either an X or Y sex chromosome contacts and unites with an ovum. If an ovum, with its X chromosome, is fertilized by a sperm bearing an X chromosome, the combination of two X chromosomes (XX) leads to the differentiation and development of a female child. If an ovum is fertilized by a Y-bearing sperm, the XY combination leads to male differentiation. Thus, the XX sex chromosome pattern is used to designate a chromosomal female and the XY pattern a chromosomal male. At least two points are of importance here. First, the sex of a child is totally determined by whether an X or Y sperm fertilizes the ovum. Second, the chromosomal sex of an individual is forever fixed at the time of fertilization, and no surgical, hormonal, or other factor can ever change a chromosomal female to a chromosomal male or vice versa.

Until about the sixth or seventh week after conception, the internal and external sexual systems of the developing embryo are *undifferentiated*. That is, females and males are identical in terms of the appearance of their internal and external genitals (see Figures 2–1 and 2–2). At this time the internal genital systems of each sex consist of two **gonads** (sex glands), each of which is connected to two pairs of primitive genital ducts, the **Wolffian ducts** and the **Müllerian ducts**. In normal male (XY) development, the Wolffian ducts are the precursors of the ducts for sperm transport (epididymes, vasa deferentia, seminal vesicles). In normal female (XX) development, the Müllerian ducts are the forerunners of the uterus, fallopian tubes, and upper portion of the vagina (see Figures 2–1, 2–8, and 2–12).

If the chromosomal sex of the embryo is male (XY), the indifferent gonads begin a transformation around the sixth or seventh week of pregnancy. The inner cores *(medulla)* of the gonads grow and the outer layers *(cortex)* regress or degenerate. Under the influence of the XY code, these inner portions of each gonad develop into the paired male *testes* and remain in the abdominal cavity until around the seventh month of pregnancy. At this time they descend through the inguinal canals into the scrotum. In the chromosomal female (XX), little change in the structure of the gonads is apparent until around the eleventh or twelfth week of prenatal existence. At this time, however, the paired *ovaries*, the glands that produce ova, begin to differentiate from the outer portions of the gonads, which grow rapidly while the inner portions degenerate. Ovarian development is completed around the sixth month of pregnancy. Though the mechanisms by which the X and Y chromosomes regulate gonadal differentiation are not fully understood (Diamond, 1977; Money & Ehrhardt, 1972), it is clear that the XY code programs the gonads to differentiate into testes and the XX code programs their differentiation into ovaries. Following testicular or ovarian differentiation, the sex chromosomes have no known direct effect on sexual differentiation (Money & Ehrhardt, 1972).

Hormonal Factors

After the genetically programmed transformation of the indifferent gonads into testes or ovaries, further sexual differentiation of the organism is, under normal circumstances, determined fully by the nature of the gonads themselves. In addition to their roles in producing germ cells (sperm by the testes and ova by the ovaries), the differentiated gonads also function as **endocrine glands**. Endocrine glands are organs that secrete chemical substances called hormones directly into the bloodstream. In turn, the hormones exert specific effects on other organs. The fetal testes produce a group of hormones called **androgen** (the "male" sex hormones), the most important of which is **testosterone**, and the fetal ovaries produce a group of hormones called **estrogen** (the "female" sex hormones).

In the genetic male fetus, at least two secretions from the testes are responsible for the further development of male internal and external genitals and for the degeneration of the precursors of internal female genitals (Müllerian ducts). The secretion responsible for suppressing and degenerating the Müllerian ducts is simply called the **Müllerian inhibiting substance** since its chemical composition is unknown. The second secretions are the androgens. Androgens induce growth and differentiation of the Wolffian ducts into the internal male genitals. If, for some reason, functioning testes fail to develop in the genetic male, or if their effects are somehow blocked, female rather than male differentiation will occur. That is, the Wolffian structures will degenerate and the Müllerian structures will differentiate into uterus, fallopian tubes, and the upper portion of the vagina.

Figure 2–1.

Differentiation of the
internal male and female
genitals.

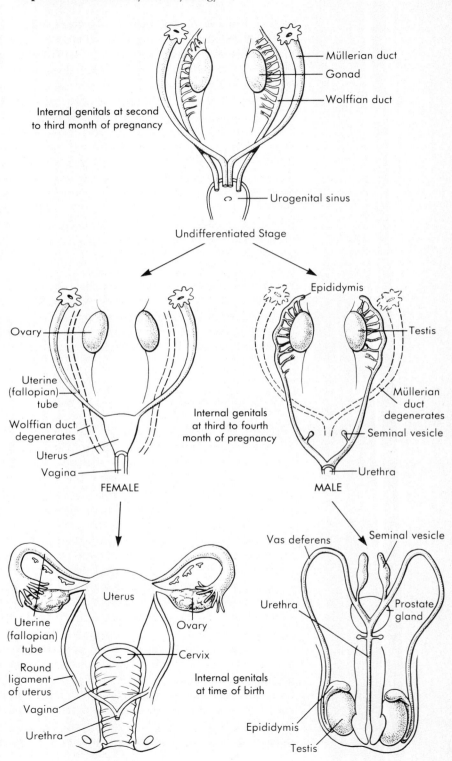

Internal genitals at second
to third month of pregnancy

Müllerian duct
Gonad
Wolffian duct

Urogenital sinus

Undifferentiated Stage

Ovary
Uterine
(fallopian)
tube
Wolffian duct
degenerates
Uterus
Vagina

FEMALE

Internal genitals
at third to fourth
month of pregnancy

Epididymis
Testis
Müllerian
duct
degenerates
Seminal vesicle
Urethra

MALE

Uterus
Uterine
(fallopian)
tube
Ovary
Round
ligament
of uterus
Cervix
Vagina
Urethra

Internal genitals
at time of birth

Vas deferens
Seminal vesicle
Urethra
Prostate
gland
Epididymis
Testis

In the female fetus, the female pattern of development occurs even in the absence of functioning ovaries. That is, no gonadal hormonal influence is necessary for female development. It appears, then, that the *female pattern of development is the basic one and that in order for male development to occur something must be added.* The addition of the Müllerian inhibitor and androgens in the male leads to masculine internal development. These substances disrupt or interfere with the primary tendency in both sexes to develop in the female pattern. Even though the Müllerian inhibitor plays no known role in the differentiation of external genitals, the presence (or addition) of androgen in the fetal male is necessary for male external development. A lack or blockage of androgen in the male during the third and fourth months of fetal development results in the external development of clitoris, clitoral hood, labia minora, and labia major rather than penis, scrotum, and foreskin. Similarly, late in pregnancy the presence of excess androgen in the female fetus resulting from a malfunctioning adrenal cortex or from drugs given to the mother during pregnancy may lead to partial or complete masculinization of the external female genitals.

Differentiation of the Internal Genitals. As we noted above, after the chromosomally coded differentiation of the indifferent gonads into the male testes or the female ovaries, further differentiation of the internal genitals is determined by the presence or absence of testicular secretions. The sequential progress of this differentiation is shown in Figure 2–1. Between the second and third month of pregnancy, the indifferent gonads differentiate into either testes or ovaries. In the male pattern of development, testicular secretions then promote both the degeneration of the female (Müllerian) structures and the growth and development of the male (Wolffian) structures into the male internal sex organs (epididymes, vasa deferentia, and seminal vesicles). Under the continued influence of testicular androgens, the testes descend from the abdominal cavity into the scrotum, and the accessory organs complete their structural development. At the time of birth all of the male internal sexual structures are present (see Figures 2–1 and 2–12).

In the basic female pattern of development, the Wolffian structures degenerate while the Müllerian ducts evolve into the female internal sex organs (uterus, fallopian tubes, and upper vagina). The ovaries, unlike the male testes, remain in the abdominal cavity near the uterus and fallopian tubes, while the accessory organs continue to grow until the time of birth, when all female internal structures are present (see Figures 2–1, 2–8, and 2–9).

Differentiation of the External Genitals. The differentiation of the external genitals is similar to that of the internal genitals. There is, however, at least one major difference. The external genitals of both sexes evolve from only one set of structures, while the internal genitals differentiate from two separate sets of structures (the Müllerian and Wolffian ducts). Until around the seventh or eighth week of prenatal existence, the precursors of male and female external genitals are identical and have the potential to develop in either the male or female direction. By the seventh or eighth week these primitive undifferentiated structures have developed to include a phallus-like **genital tubercle** above a **urogenital slit**, or groove, that is flanked on both sides, first by the **urethral folds** and then by the **labioscrotal swellings** (see Figure 2–2).

During the third and fourth months following conception, these primitive structures rapidly differentiate into either the male or female external genitals (see Figures 2–5, 2–12, and 2–13). The direction of differentiation is determined by the presence or absence of androgen. The presence of androgen leads to the evolution of male structures while its absence leads to female differentiation. Under the influence of androgen, the genital tubercle grows rapidly to form the corpora cavernosa of the penis. The urethral folds fuse to form the corpora spongiosum of the penis and enclose the urethral tube. The labioscrotal swellings fuse at the midline to form the scrotum. Around the seventh month of pregnancy, the testes descend to fill the scrotal pouch. In the female pattern of development, the genital tubercle forms the body and glans of the clitoris. The urethral folds remain separate. They form the labia minora flanking the urogenital groove, which deepens to fashion the vestibule surrounding, and including, the urethral meatus (opening) and vaginal opening. In the female, the labioscrotal swellings do not fuse but become the labia majora and mons pubis. At the time of birth, all external male and female genital structures are present (see Figure 2–2).

POSTNATAL SEXUAL DEVELOPMENT AND PUBERTY

With some exceptions, the external genitals of the newborn are clearly distinguishable as male or female (see Figure 2–2). For the most part, genital appearance is the only gross visual method of distinguishing infant males from infant females. Between birth and adulthood, however, very significant changes in the genital and reproductive systems of both sexes occur.

Birth to Puberty

From the time of birth to the onset of puberty, changes in the genitals and reproductive systems of both sexes are mostly confined to structural growth. The growth pattern of the reproductive systems of both sexes parallels, but lags behind, general body growth. That is, by the age of two, the bodies of both males and females have attained nearly 25 percent of their adult size but their reproductive structures (gonads, penis, uterus) are only around 5 percent of their size at adulthood. By the age of ten, general body growth is 50 percent complete but reproductive systems have reached only 10 percent of adult size (Tanner, 1967). This relatively slow reproductive development is due at least in part to the fact that, until the onset of puberty, androgen and estrogen, the hormones primarily responsible for male and female growth, are present in only about 10 percent of the amounts that characterize adult males and females, respectively (Kinsey, Pomeroy, Martin, & Gebhard, 1953).

Even before puberty, however, anatomical and physiological differences in the growth and functioning of males and females are apparent. Until around the age of four, boys grow faster and, between the ages of six and nine, develop greater muscular capacities than do girls. Around the age of six, the bodies of both sexes begin to show early signs of characteristics that differentiate adult males from females. That is, boys' shoulders are broader than their hips and their chests are longer and broader than those of girls. The skin and fat layer in girls is approx-

Figure 2–2.

Differentiation of the external male and female genitals.

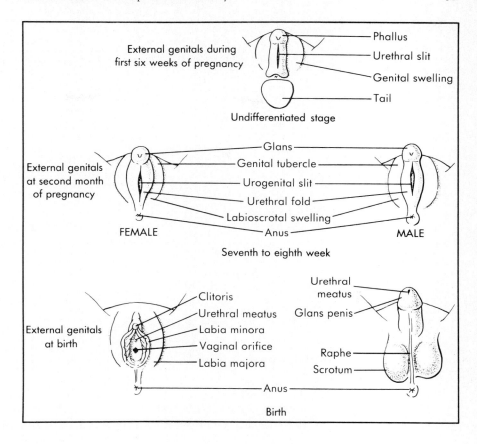

imately 50 percent thicker than it is in boys and is distributed mostly around the hips and buttocks. Even at this age, most girls have broader hips than most boys (Diamond, 1977). All of these differences are, of course, forerunners of more dramatic differences that are found after the completion of puberty.

Puberty

Sometime between the ages of eight and eleven in the average boy and girl, the **pituitary gland**, located in the base of the brain, increases its output of a number of different hormones. Two of these hormones, called **gonadotropins**, are of particular importance since they exert direct effects upon the gonads (testes, ovaries). In females, the **follicle-stimulating hormone (FSH)** stimulates the ovaries (Figure 2–9) to manufacture and secrete estrogen and initiates the maturation of ova (oogenesis). In males, FSH stimulates the seminiferous tubules of the testes (Figure 2–15) to begin the manufacture of sperm (spermatogenesis). The **luteinizing hormone (LH)** in females produces ovulation, the release of mature eggs from the ovaries. LH also leads to the manufacture and release of progesterone from the **corpus luteum**, which develops in the ovarian cavity (follicle) previously occupied by the developing egg. In males, LH is referred to as **interstitial-cell-stimulating hormone (ICSH)** because it stimulates the interstitial cells of the

Figure 2–3.

Schematic representation
of the hormonal relation-
ships among the hypo-
thalamus, anterior
pituitary, and gonads.

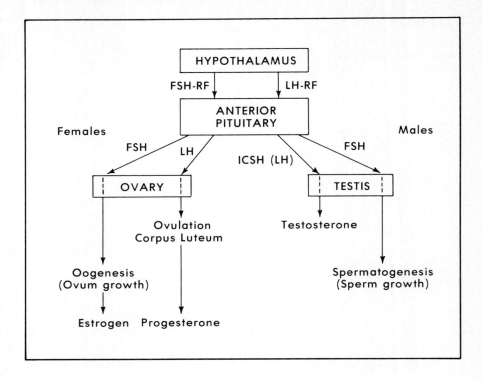

testes to produce and release the male hormone *testosterone*. The pituitary release
of FSH and LH (ICSH) is, in turn, regulated by the **hypothalamus**, which in many
ways, acts as a control center for the pituitary gland. The cells of the hypothalamus
secrete, among others, two chemicals of importance to reproductive functions. The
follicle-stimulating hormone-releasing factor (FSH-RF), as the name
implies, stimulates the pituitary to release FSH and the **luteinizing hormone-
releasing factor (LH-RF)** prompts the pituitary to release LH. The relationships
among the hypothalamus, pituitary, and gonads are shown in simplified form in
Figure 2–3.

These dramatic increases in pituitary secretion of FSH and LH (ICSH) lead to
equally dramatic increases in the ovarian production of estrogen and in the
testicular production of testosterone. In turn, the elevated levels of estrogen and
testosterone exert profound influences on the bodies of girls and boys, respectively. Increases in estrogen and testosterone initiate the transformations of puberty. **Puberty** may be roughly defined as the sudden growth and maturation of
the gonads, other genitals, and secondary sexual characteristics that lead to full
reproductive capacity (Tanner, 1967). But, what controls the onset of puberty? The
answer to this question has been elusive. It is generally thought, however, that the
hypothalamus acts as a sort of "biological clock" that is somehow set to increase its
secretions of FSH-RF and LH-RF at a certain stage of maturity. It is unclear whether
the setting of this hypothetical clock is based on body weight, age, disinhibition of
hypothalamic cells, or some other factors (Frisch & Renelle, 1970).

Puberty in Females. The first outward signs of puberty in females begin to appear between the ages of nine and twelve, some eighteen months to two years before pubertal changes are evident in males (National Center for Health Statistics, 1976). Between ten and eleven, breast growth first begins with the appearance of breast buds. Under the influence of estrogen, the *areolae* (pigmented areas around the nipples) become elevated and the nipples begin to protrude. As puberty progresses, the breasts continue to grow and swell as a result of the development of ducts in the nipple area and of connective and fatty tissues in the breast mass itself (see Figure 2–4).

The primary purpose of the female breasts is, of course, the production of milk. During pregnancy the milk glands of the breasts enlarge, and shortly before or after childbirth the breasts are capable of secreting milk.

The size and shape of female breasts are of great psychosocial importance to females and males in our culture. They are the most obvious visible distinctions between the sexes and are of substantial erotic significance. As noted in several places throughout this book, however, neither the size nor the shape of the female breasts is related to erotic responsiveness in women.

Shortly following the appearance of breast buds, pubic hair begins to appear in the average eleven-year-old girl. This hair is initially soft and rather colorless but, with development, becomes coarse, curly, darker, and eventually grows downward into the pubic area in the shape of an inverted triangle. Pubic hair growth in girls is

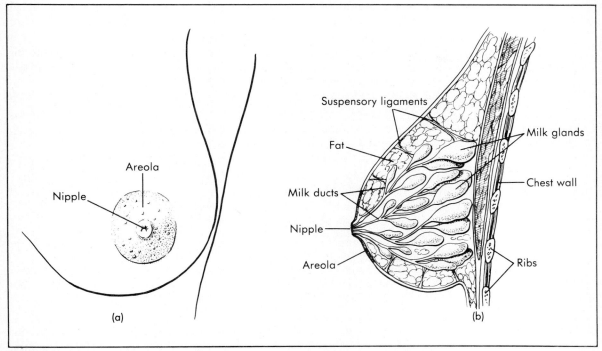

Figure 2–4.

External (a) and internal (b) anatomy of the female breast.

prompted by estrogen as well as by some androgen secreted by the adrenal glands. Stimulated by adrenal androgen, **axillary hair** (underarm) does not appear until around the age of thirteen. At about the same time as pubic hair first appears, the shape and size of a girl's body begin to undergo dramatic change. These changes are jointly produced by estrogen, adrenal androgen, and pituitary growth hormones. Between the ages of eleven and sixteen, girls rapidly grow taller and larger and reach an average height of 161 centimeters (5 feet, 4.5 inches) and weight of 55 kilograms (123 pounds) by the age of eighteen (National Center for Health Statistics, 1976). Accompanying this period of rapid *body growth* is continued broadening of the pelvis and development of the fatty tissue in the hips, buttocks, thighs, and back, which distinguish the adult female body contour from that of the average male.

Prompted by the pituitary gonadotropins, a girl's ovaries begin increased production of estrogen when she is around the age of ten. The estrogen, in turn, stimulates rapid growth of the *ovaries* themselves, as well as other *genital structures*, both internal and external. Internally, the fallopian tubes, uterus, cervix, and vagina all mature quickly under the influence of high levels of estrogen. The uterine muscular wall enlarges and the lining of the vagina becomes substantially thicker. Externally, the fatty layer of tissue underlying the mons pubis thickens. The labia minora grow and the labia majora thicken and become more fleshy so that they meet at the middle of the **vestibule** (the area surrounding the urethral and vaginal openings) and cover the widening vaginal entrance. At the same time, the clitoris increases in size and sensitivity, but under the influence of andrenal androgen rather than ovarian estrogen. These structures are described in more detail in the section on female sexual anatomy.

As we have seen, increased levels of estrogen secretion are responsible for many of the physical changes of puberty in females. Estrogen secretions not only increase at puberty but also assume a pattern of cyclical variation between relatively high and low levels of secretion that continues throughout the reproductive life of a woman (puberty to menopause). One consequence of the cyclic variations in estrogen secretion is the occurrence of **menstrual cycles**—cyclic changes in the lining of the uterus, including the periodic shedding of the outer portions of this lining (blood, tissue) during the **menstrual period** (also called menstruation or menses). In the average girl, the first menstruation **(menarche)** occurs between the ages of twelve and thirteen and may come as somewhat of a surprise if she has not been adequately informed concerning its occurrence.

In adult women, menstrual cycles and **ovarian cycles** (including ovulation) are closely tied but, for the first year or two following the menarche, the pubescent girl's menstrual cycles are irregular and ovulation does not occur in each cycle. Thus, even though *pregnancy is possible shortly following (before in unusual cases) the menarche*, most girls are relatively infertile for some time after their first period. Note, however, that fertility at this time does occur in some instances and pregnancy may be possible.

The cyclic pattern of ovarian hormone secretion is regulated by cyclic variations in secretions of FSH and LH by the pituitary gland. The pituitary cycles are, in turn, controlled by cyclic variations in hypothalamic secretions of FSH-RF and LH-RF (Figure 2–3). Thus, hormonal cycling in females is ultimately controlled by a brain structure—the hypothalamus. In contrast to the female cyclic pattern, gonadal hormones in males (testosterone) are secreted on a rather steady (tonic) basis and, under normal circumstances, testosterone levels in males remain *relatively* constant following puberty. As is true in the case of prenatal sexual differentiation, research findings (summarized by Bermant & Davidson, 1974; Money & Ehrhardt, 1972; and others) have suggested that the female (cyclic) pattern is the basic one. The male (tonic) pattern develops only under the masculinizing effects of androgen during prenatal development. That is, the addition of prenatal androgen exerts a masculinizing effect on the brain structure (hypothalamus) responsible for regulation of gonadal hormone secretions later in life. Androgen disrupts the basic female cyclic pattern of secretion, and imposes the tonic pattern characteristic of adult males. It has also been suggested that the prenatal hormonal environment exerts important feminizing or masculinizing effects on the brain which are manifest in a variety of overt sexual behaviors (Diamond, 1977; Money & Ehrhardt, 1972).

Puberty in Males.   Generally, puberty begins later and extends over a longer period of time in boys than in girls. Some eighteen months to two years later than the average girl, the average boy (between the ages of eleven and thirteen) begins to show the first outward signs of physical change associated with puberty (National Center for Health Statistics, 1976). These changes are, of course, prompted by FSH and LH (called ICSH in males), the same hormones that initiate puberty in females. Distributed through the bloodstream, ICSH reaches the testes and stimulates the interstitial cells to begin the manufacture and secretion of testosterone. Testosterone is responsible for virtually all the changes of puberty in males.

First (between the ages of eleven and twelve), the testes and scrotum begin to grow under the influence of testosterone produced by the testes, themselves. Around the same time, there begins a minor, but noticeable, enlargement of the penis which, prior to puberty, averages about 3.75 centimeters (1.5 inches) long in the relaxed state and less than 7.5 centimeters (3 inches) in erection (Katchadourian & Lunde, 1975). Between the ages of twelve and thirteen, fine straight pubic hair appears at the base of the penis.

The physical changes of male puberty occur at a substantially more rapid rate between the ages of thirteen and fourteen. By this time the testes have more than doubled in size, and their capacity to produce testosterone has increased remarkably. These high levels of testosterone now prompt accelerated growth of the testes themselves, the penis, the prostate, the seminal vesicles, and Cowper's glands, all of which are described in the section on male sexual anatomy. Under the influence of testosterone and pituitary growth hormone, the boy's "growth spurt" begins between the ages of thirteen and fourteen, trailing the average girl by up to two years. According to data from the National Center for Health Statistics (1976), his weight and height rapidly increase until age eighteen, at which time the average American male is 174 centimeters (5 feet, 9.5 inches) tall and weighs around 67.5 kilograms (150 pounds) (National Center for Health Statistics, 1976). Body growth in the average male may continue for up to seven more years, until the ages of twenty or twenty-one. Male growth is characterized by increases of bone and muscle volume, decreases in subcutaneous fat, and broadening of shoulders and chest, which combine to produce a body shape and size distinctly different from that of the usual female.

Axillary, body, and facial hair do not appear on most boys until they are about fourteen years old. At first, facial hair is rather soft and colorless ("peach fuzz") and confined to the upper lip. The more coarse, dark, and widely distributed adult "beard" does not develop in the average boy until he is about seventeen. Around the age of fourteen, the voice begins to deepen in most boys as a result of growth of the larynx or "voice box." Larynx growth is stimulated by testosterone and produces the Adam's apple that distinguishes males from females.

Full reproductive capacity is attained in males when mature sperm are produced by the testes. By the age of thirteen or fourteen, the prostate gland produces sufficient seminal fluid for ejaculation to occur, but the ejaculate at this time usually contains no mature sperm. As in females, where it stimulates maturation of ova, FSH is necessary in males for the production of mature sperm. FSH, in combination with other hormones, prompts the differentiation and maturation of the germ cells that line the seminiferous tubules of the testes. This maturation process (spermatogenesis) cannot be completed unless testicular temperature is 2° to 3°C lower than normal body temperature. Thus, complete spermatogenesis cannot occur in testes which have not descended from the abdominal cavity into the scrotal pouch.

As we noted earlier, hormonal activity in males follows a tonic rather than a cyclic pattern, presumably due to the masculinizing effects of prenatal androgen on the hypothalamus. From the time of puberty onward, testosterone and sperm production in males is relatively constant.

It should be emphasized that our consideration of the physical developments of puberty has focused on the most usual course of events. We have described puberty as it occurs in the "average" boy and girl, and it must be recognized that variations around these averages are the rule rather than the exception. For example, although it begins earlier in most girls than it does in most boys, some boys complete puberty by the age of thirteen while some girls at the same age show no signs of the beginnings of puberty. As with other aspects of sexuality, there are no rigidly fixed rules for puberty that apply to all males or all females. Average ages for the various changes of puberty are summarized in Table 2–1.

Table 2–1.

Average ages of various pubertal changes in females and males.
The ages shown are only averages and it is normal for each of the changes to appear from two years earlier to two years later.

Females		Males	
Average Ages		**Average Ages**	
11–12	Puberty begins Breast buds appear Pubic hair appears Growth spurt begins	12–13	Puberty begins Growth of testes and scrotum Pubic hair appears
12–13	Axillary hair appears First menstruation (menarche)	13–14	Growth spurt begins Rapid growth of penis
		14–15	Body, facial, and axillary hair appears Larynx enlarges First ejaculation (thorarche)

ADULT SEXUAL ANATOMY AND PHYSIOLOGY

From the perspectives of anatomy and physiology, the completion of puberty marks the beginning of sexual adulthood in both sexes. Though not always adults in the social or legal sense, postpubescent males and females possess all of the physical "equipment" necessary to function biologically as sexual adults. In this final section we will examine the structure (anatomy) and functioning (physiology) of adult female and male sexual systems.

Female Sexual Anatomy and Physiology

As noted, the sexual systems of both sexes consist of external and internal genital structures. First, we will consider the external genitals of females.

Female External Genitals.　The external genitals of females are collectively referred to as the **vulva** and consist of the mons pubis, the labia majora, the labia minora, the clitoris, and the vaginal opening, as diagrammed in Figure 2–5.

　　The **mons pubis** (or simply mons) is the soft, thick, and fatty elevation of tissue that lies over the pubic symphysis (joining of the pubic bones). Covered with pubic hair in adult women, the mons is richly endowed with nerve endings and highly erotically responsive to tactile stimulation. Because of its sensitivity, the mons is often stroked and rubbed during female masturbation and, during sexual interac-

Figure 2–5.

The female external genitals (vulva).

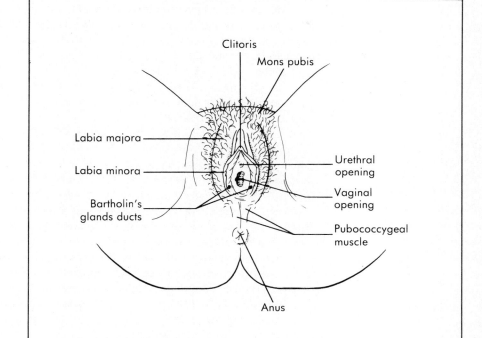

tion, many women endeavor to press and rub the mons against the bodies of their partners.

Flaring out and down from the mons pubis are the **labia majora** (major or outer lips). They flatten out and merge just above the anus to form the outer boundaries of the vulva. The labia majora are folds of skin containing fatty as well as smooth muscular tissue, sweat and sebaceous glands, and ample supplies of nerve endings and blood vessels. Their outer surfaces are rather darkly colored and covered by pubic hair. When not sexually stimulated, and in nonparous women (those who have never given birth), they often meet at the vulvar midline and cover the minor labia, the vaginal opening, and the urethral meatus. During sexual stimulation, the labia majora swell markedly and separate, exposing the underlying structures.

Within the cleft formed by the labia majora are the **labia minora** (minor or inner lips), which are paired folds of reddish (darker in women who have given birth), hairless, skin. The labia minora surround the vaginal **vestibule**, into which open the urethral and vaginal outlets as well as the ducts of the Bartholin's glands (described below). The upper portions of the labia minora merge to form a fold of skin over the clitoris called the **prepuce** (hood or foreskin) of the clitoris. Below the clitoris, the labia minora join to form the **frenulum** of the clitoris. Richly endowed with nerve endings, blood vessels, and sebaceous glands, the labia minora are highly responsive to sexual stimulation. During sexual arousal they increase dramatically in thickness and in length. At high levels of sexual arousal they undergo vivid color changes and may protrude through the separated and flattened labia majora.

Flanking the vaginal entrance and exiting through the lower portions of the labia majora are the ducts of the paired **Bartholin's glands**. During the plateau phase of sexual arousal, these glands secrete minute quantities of a mucoid substance. The function of this secretion is unclear since too small a quantity is released to aid in vaginal lubrication.

The **clitoris** is a small (usually less than three centimeters long) cylindrical structure located at the top of the vestibule and just below the mons. This small organ consists of the **shaft**, which is covered by the upper portions of the labia minora (prepuce), and the rounded **glans**, which projects just beyond the prepuce. In anatomical origin, the clitoris corresponds to the glans of the male penis and, like the penis, is composed mainly of erectile tissue in the form of two *corpora cavernosa* (cavernous bodies), which fill with blood and swell during sexual arousal. The glans, in particular, is amply supplied with nerves and highly erotically sensitive. The clitoris functions as a receiver and transmitter of sexual stimuli (Masters & Johnson, 1966). It is unique because no other male or female organ has sexual sensation as its sole function. Even though the clitoris is similar in origin to the male penis, the urethra does not pass through it as it does through the penis. Instead, the urethra exits at the urethral meatus (opening), which lies between the clitoris and the vaginal opening (see Figure 2–5).

The *vaginal opening* lies just below the urethral meatus and normally is visible only when the minor labia are separated. The **hymen** is a thin membrane of connective tissue that rings or partially covers the vaginal opening. The most common type, the *annular* hymen, surrounds and narrows the vaginal opening. The less common *septate* and *cribriform* hymens block more of the vaginal orifice,

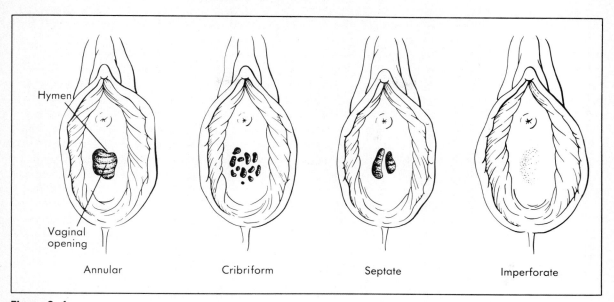

Figure 2–6.

Types of hymens.

as Figure 2–6 illustrates. Quite rare is the *imperforate* hymen, which completely blocks the opening and must be surgically altered to permit passage of menstrual fluids. Traditionally, the presence of an intact hymen has been regarded as evidence of virginity. If intact at the time of first intercourse, the hymen usually ruptures or tears. Often, however, the hymen may be ruptured long before first intercourse through a variety of activities. Alternately, some hymens are so flexible that they can withstand multiple acts of intercourse without rupturing. Thus, neither the presence nor the absence of an intact hymen is firm evidence of virginity or nonvirginity. Some common variations in the appearance of the female genitals are shown in Figure 2–7.

Female Internal Genitals. The internal genital structures of females consist of paired sets of *ovaries* and *uterine,* or *fallopian, tubes,* the *uterus,* the *cervix,* and the *vagina* (see Figure 2–8).

The two **ovaries** are the primary sex glands (gonads) of the female and perform two functions—the production of *ova* (eggs) and of the sex hormones *estrogen* and **progesterone**. Flanking the uterus and attached to it by the **ovarian ligaments**, the ovaries are small almond-shaped organs measuring around 2.5 centimeters (1 inch) in length and 3.75 centimeters (1.5 inches) in diameter in adult women. Each ovary contains a number of round capsules called *follicles,* each of which contains one ovum. At any one time, the ova are widely varied with respect to the state of maturity they have attained. The follicles are located in the outer portions of the ovary while the inner core consists primarily of soft tissue and blood vessels. Ova production begins during prenatal development. At birth each ovary contains between 200,000 and 400,000 follicles housing immature ova. It is

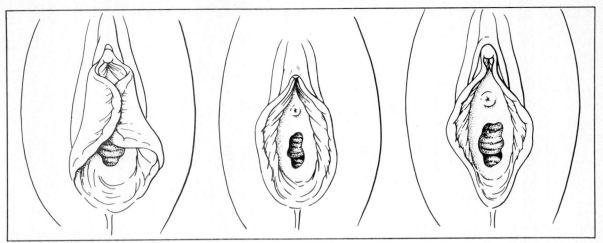

Figure 2–7.

Common variations in the appearance of the female genitals.

generally thought that no new ova are produced throughout the remainder of a woman's life.

At puberty some of these ova begin to mature and each month one follicle ruptures, discharging one ovum into the bodily cavity. By an unknown process, the discharged ovum finds its way to the entrance of the uterine, or **fallopian tube**, adjacent to the ovary from which the ovum was discharged. The two fallopian tubes are around 10 centimeters (4 inches) in length and extend from each side of the uterus to the vicinity of the ovaries. The fallopian tubes are not attached to the ovaries but small projections **(fimbriae)** from the end portion (infundibulum) of each fallopian tube may reach or even surround the ovary near it, (as shown in Figure 2–9).

Including the *infundibulum*, or end portion, the fallopian tubes consist of three sections. The *ampulla* is an enlarged funnel-shaped portion that leads from the infundibulum to the more narrow *isthmus*, which, in turn, enters the uterus. The tubes are lined with tiny hairlike protrusions *(cilia)* that slowly propel the discharged ovum toward the uterus. If intercourse has taken place and fertilization is to occur, it usually happens in the ampullar portion of the fallopian tubes. Coitally ejaculated sperm make their way through the cervix, uterus, and tubes to meet the slowly moving ovum. The fertilized ovum is then transported by the tubal cilia to the uterus, where it becomes implanted in the uterine wall. Movement of the ovum through the tubes to the uterus normally takes between three and four days. In rare cases, the fertilized ovum becomes implanted in the wall of the fallopian tube itself. This form of out-of-place, or **ectopic pregnancy** ultimately leads to the death of the embryo and in some cases rupture of the tube with potentially dangerous complications for the woman. Surgical intervention is often necessary under such circumstances.

Because of their roles in fertilization and ova transport, the fallopian tubes are the most frequent targets for female sterilization. **Tubal ligation** is a surgical

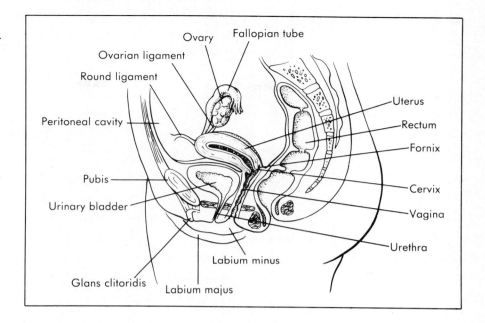

procedure in which both tubes are tied or severed, preventing sperm and ovum
contact and, thus, fertilization. This procedure results in no alteration of hormone
production, sexual characteristics, desire, or responsiveness.

The **uterus**, or womb, is a hollow pear-shaped organ lying in the body cavity
between the bladder and rectum (see Figures 2–8 and 2–9). Heavily muscled, the
uterus is normally between 5 and 7.5 centimeters (2 and 3 inches) long and varies
in diameter from 5 to 6.25 centimeters (2 to 2.5 inches) at the **fundus** to 2.5
centimeters (1 inch) at the **cervix**, which extends into the vagina about 1.25
centimeters (.5 inch). This organ houses and nourishes the fertilized ovum
(embryo, fetus) and is capable of remarkable expansion during pregnancy.

The wall of the uterus is composed of a thin outer layer of connective tissue
(perimetrium), a thick muscular middle layer **(myometrium)**, and an inner
layer composed of numerous glands and blood vessels **(endometrium)**. The
perimetrium is simply the external cover of the uterus. The myometrium is a thick
network of smooth muscles running in numerous directions. These muscles are
capable of powerful contractions at the time of birth and also contract less vigorously during orgasm. It is in the endometrium that a fertilized ovum implants and
is housed and nourished during pregnancy. The structure of the endometrial lining
varies in response to fluctuations in the levels of circulating hormones. During her
reproductive years (puberty to menopause) and when she is not pregnant, a
woman's uterine lining changes in a cyclic manner and is periodically shed (every
twenty-eight days or so) in response to cyclic variations in ovarian production of
estrogen and progesterone. These changes are collectively referred to as the
menstrual cycle, which we will discuss more fully later in the chapter.

The **vagina** is a muscular tube extending from just behind the cervix to the
vulva or external genital structures (see Figure 2–8). During coitus the vagina

Figure 2–9.

Ovaries, fallopian (uterine) tubes, and uterus.

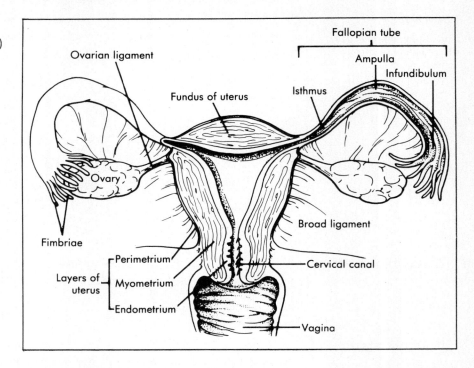

receives the penis and serves as the depository for semen. It also serves as a passageway for the discharge of menstrual fluids and for the baby at the time of birth. In the absence of sexual stimulation the anterior (front) and posterior (back) walls of the vaginal canal are, respectively, about 7.5 and 10 centimeters (3 and 4 inches) long and collapsed together. During sexual stimulation, however, this "potential space" becomes a "real space" as the vagina widens and lengthens (Masters & Johnson, 1966).

Much thinner than the uterine wall, the vaginal wall is composed of three layers. The outer layer *(fibrous coat)* is a thin covering membrane which also connects the vagina to other bodily tissues. The middle layer *(muscular coat)* consists of smooth involuntary muscles that contract during sexual arousal. The inner lining **(mucosa)** is a heavily convoluted layer of moist mucous membrane containing no glands. During sexual stimulation, however, vaginal lubricating fluids seep from the mucosa as a result of engorgement of the surrounding tissues with blood (Masters & Johnson, 1966). The vaginal mucosa is highly sensitive to estrogen levels. Following the estrogen withdrawal associated with menopause, the internal vaginal walls thin, dry somewhat, and lose some of their convoluted appearance.

Surrounding the vaginal opening are the **vestibular bulbs**, which are composed of erectile tissue. During sexual arousal these bulbs swell, producing the vaginal platform prior to orgasm (Masters & Johnson, 1966). The vestibular bulbs are, in turn, encircled by the pubococcygeal muscles. These muscles can be developed by exercise. By repeatedly contracting and then relaxing them in much the same way that she contracts and relaxes the urethral sphincter to control urination, a woman can gain increased control over the tightness of her vaginal opening. This sometimes results in increased coital pleasure for her as well as her sexual partner (Hartman & Fithian, 1974). The area around the vaginal opening is highly responsive to sexual stimulation but the vaginal walls are poorly supplied with nerve endings and, thus, rather insensitive.

Hormonal Cycles.   Hormonal activity in females from puberty until menopause is cyclic. That is, there are recurring variations in the amounts of the hormones estrogen and progesterone circulating in a woman's bloodstream at any given time. These recurring variations or cycles are coordinated by the joint actions of the hypothalamus and the pituitary gland. Recall that, through its secretions of FSH-RF and LH-RF, the hypothalamus prompts the pituitary gland to secrete the gonadotropic hormones FSH and LH. Reaching the ovaries through the bloodstream, FSH and LH, in turn, are responsible for triggering the maturation and release of ova as well as ovarian production of high levels of estrogen and progesterone (see Figure 2–3). The increased levels of circulating estrogen and progesterone then act to "turn off" hypothalamic secretions of FSH-RF and LH-RF. Cutbacks in the production of these secretions then turn off ovarian production of estrogen and progesterone.

Thus, through a complex set of feedback mechanisms, the hypothalamus, the pituitary gland, and the ovaries constantly interact to produce cyclic changes in a woman's reproductive and hormonal status. Although it should be understood that they are ultimately regulated by the hypothalamus, the ovarian cycle and the resulting menstrual cycle are of primary interest to our present discussion.

Ovarian Cycle.   The term **ovarian cycle** refers to a series of changes that recur in the ovaries roughly every twenty-eight days in the average woman. These ovarian changes, in turn, trigger recurring alterations in the inner lining of the uterus (endometrium) which are collectively referred to as the **menstrual cycle**. Let us now examine these two cycles and their interrelationships by tracing the usual sequence of events involved in each cycle.

At puberty, each of the ovaries contains between 200,000 and 300,000 immature ova, each of which is encapsulated within a *primary follicle*. Complete ovarian cycles begin shortly after puberty when increased secretions of FSH from the pituitary gland stimulate growth in a few of the primary follicles. Thereafter (until menopause), a few of the remaining follicles begin development roughly each month (each ovarian cycle), although only one follicle per month normally completes the developmental process and releases a mature ovum. This process of development and release of ova (ovulation) usually alternates between the two ovaries each month. Throughout a woman's thirty to forty reproductive years, only about four hundred of her thousands of primary follicles ever reach maturity. The remaining follicles regress and degenerate.

As shown in Figure 2–10, maturation of the primary follicle is characterized by rapid growth of the ovum and proliferation of cells *(follicular cells)* within the follicle itself. During the latter part of the first week of this development, the follicle, under the combined influences of relatively high levels of FSH and small amounts of LH, begins to produce and secrete substantial quantities of estrogen. Through a negative feedback mechanism, the rising estrogen content of the blood then leads to a decline in pituitary FSH production (see Figure 2–11). The follicle continues to grow, fills with fluid, and moves toward the surface of the ovary. At the end of this phase of the cycle (known variously as the *follicular, proliferative,* or *preovulatory phase*), approximately fourteen days after it began to grow, the follicle reaches maturity and is referred to as a *Graafian follicle*. A sharp, but brief, rise in estrogen output then stimulates a sudden surge of LH from the pituitary as well as a less dramatic brief increase in FSH production (Figure 2–11). This surge in LH production marks the end of the follicular phase and stimulates the Graafian follicle to rupture and release the mature ovum into the bodily cavity **(ovulation)**. Thus, in the average twenty-eight-day ovarian cycle, ovulation occurs roughly at the midpoint, or on the fourteenth day.

Following ovulation, LH is the dominant gonadotropin and causes the ruptured follicle to collapse and heal, forming the **corpus luteum** (Figure 2–10). Under the influence of LH, the corpus luteum begins to secrete a substantial quantity of progesterone and lesser amounts of estrogen. This *luteal,* or *secretory, phase* consumes the second half of the average twenty-eight-day cycle, which is characterized by the dominance of the gonadotropin LH and of the hormone progesterone (Figure 2–11). Unless the released ovum is fertilized, the relatively high levels of progesterone and estrogen lead to a decline in both FSH and LH production during the fourth week of the cycle. The corpus luteum begins to degenerate

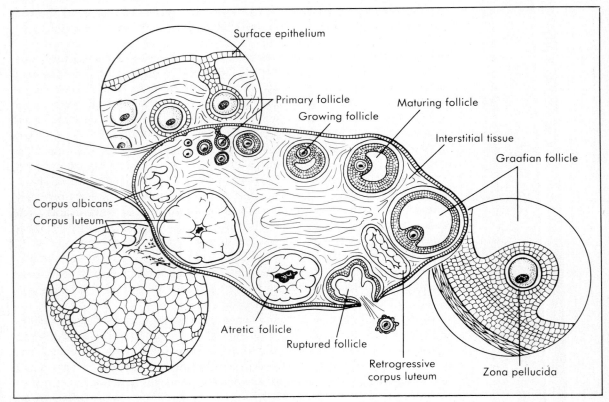

Figure 2–10.

Cross section of the ovary, showing the several stages of development of the ova.

and ceases production of progesterone and estrogen. This, in turn, triggers menstruation as well as the pituitary release of FSH. The FSH stimulates new follicle growth, and the entire cycle begins anew. The regressed corpus luteum is replaced by connective tissue and appears as a small scar, the corpus albicans (see Figure 2–10).

If fertilization has occurred, however, ovarian cycling is disrupted and ceases throughout the period of pregnancy. For the first two to three months following fertilization, the corpus luteum continues to function, secreting the progesterone and estrogen necessary to maintain the uterine endometrium which houses and nourishes the developing embryo. It is thought that the corpus luteum is sustained during this period by **human chorionic gonadotropin (HCG)**, a hormone secreted by the **chorion**, a membrane that develops around the embryo. For the final six months of pregnancy the hormone-secreting function of the corpus luteum is taken over by the **placenta**. Progesterone and estrogen secretions continue to increase and the corpus luteum gradually degenerates (see Figure 2–11).

Menstrual Cycle.   Intimately connected to and, in fact, controlled by the events of the ovarian cycle are changes that take place in the inner lining of the uterus (the endometrium). The ovarian cycle involves the development and release of an ovum followed by the formation of a corpus luteum and its degeneration if fertilization does not occur. In the uterus, these ovarian events correspond to the buildup of endometrial tissue, blood supply, and fluids in preparation for the fertilized ovum and the breakdown and loss of these substances during menstruation if the ovum is not fertilized. Collectively, these changes in the uterine lining are referred to as the *menstrual cycle*.

By convention, the beginning of a menstrual cycle is marked by the onset of uterine bleeding, or *menstruation*, since it is easier to detect than the other events of the cycle. Menstruation involves the discharge of the endometrial blood, tissue, and fluids of the previous cycle and typically lasts from three to seven days. This breakdown and shedding of the endometrium is prompted by the rather abrupt declines in progesterone and estrogen that occur in the final day(s) of the ovarian cycle when the corpus luteum rapidly degenerates. The actual menstrual flow, however, corresponds to the early days of the follicular phase of the ovarian cycle in which a primary follicle begins to mature under the influence of FSH from the pituitary. The endometrial tissue continues to degenerate and shed until the growing follicle secretes substantial quantities of estrogen. The renewed estrogen supply then stimulates regrowth of the endometrium in preparation for the ovum following its release at ovulation roughly fourteen days after the *beginning* of menstruation in the average twenty-eight-day cycle.

Following ovulation, the corpus luteum secretes mostly progesterone and some estrogen. The combined influence of these hormones stimulates further growth and development of the endometrium and prompts the endometrial glands to secrete substances required to nourish the ovum if it is fertilized. This period of endometrial growth corresponds to the luteal, or secretory, phase of the ovarian cycle. If fertilization does not occur, the corpus luteum regresses and ceases progesterone and estrogen production. The uterine endometrium then degenerates. Some of its blood vessels rupture and some of its tissue breaks away and is

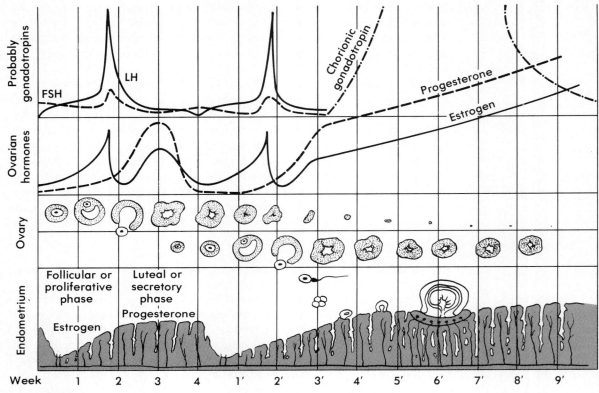

Figure 2–11.

Composite representation of changes in pituitary gonadotropins, ovarian hormones and follicle (ovarian cycle), and uterine endometrium (menstrual cycle). First cycle (weeks 1-4) is without fertilization but second cycle is shown with fertilization and early stages of pregnancy (week 1'-9').

SOURCE: Adapted from Landau, 1976.

shed during menstruation. The amount of menstrual discharge varies greatly from woman to woman and even from period to period within the same woman. The average woman, however, loses only about 60 milliliters (2 ounces) of blood during each menstrual period.

Most commonly, menstrual fluid is absorbed by sanitary napkins, which are worn externally, or by tampons, which are inserted and worn inside the vagina. In 1980, **toxic shock syndrome (TSS)**, a disorder caused by an abnormal growth of the bacterium *Staphylococcus aureus* was reported to be associated with tampon use. The symptoms of TSS include high fever, vomiting, diarrhea, and headache, and the disorder sometimes results in death. It is thought that tampon use may encourage the abnormal bacterial growth. Though TSS sometimes occurs in men as well as women, 85 percent of all cases reported in 1980 occurred in women during their menstrual flow and 98 percent of these women were tampon users (Centers for Disease Control, 1982). It is now recommended that women who experience TSS symptoms during their menstrual period immediately discontinue tampon use and consult a physician. Furthermore, frequent changes of tampons are recommended and women are encouraged not to use tampons continuously throughout their menstrual periods (Price, 1981).

The decrease of estrogen and progesterone that triggers menstruation also stimulates the pituitary to renew its secretion of FSH. This, of course, starts the process all over again with the growth of another follicle and the beginning of new ovarian and menstrual cycles. If the ovum is fertilized, however, the endometrial lining is not shed; it remains to receive the fertilized ovum, which it maintains and nourishes throughout pregnancy under the influence of estrogen and progesterone supplied first by the corpus luteum and then by the placenta (see Figure 2–11).

Our description of ovarian and menstrual cycles has focused on those of average duration for the adult human female. Cycle length is determined by the number of days that pass from the first day of one menstrual flow to the first day of the next menstrual flow. For most women this will be between twenty-one and thirty-five days, with an average of around twenty-eight days. As suggested by these figures, cycle lengths may vary substantially from one woman to the next. Furthermore, rather wide variations in the length of cycles within the same woman are not uncommon. This is particularly true for the first year or two following menarche, the first menstrual flow. During this time most girls are quite irregular and an interval of several months may pass between the first and second periods in some girls. Typically, cycle length is somewhat longer (thirty-one days) and more variable in teenage girls than in women in their late thirties and early forties (twenty-eight days) (Chiazze, Brayer, Macisco, Parker, & Duffy, 1968).

As we have previously noted, reproductive cycling in females is ultimately controlled by the hypothalamus, a brain structure. Thus, it is not surprising that emotional factors may influence cycle regularity. For example, many women imprisoned in German concentration camps during World War II ceased menstruating for the duration of their imprisonment. The emotional stress associated with college attendance disrupts the regularity of some girls, whose cycles then become regular again during their summer months at home. Following intercourse, unmarried women who fear pregnancy may have "late" periods, presumably due to fear-related emotional stress (Katchadourian & Lunde, 1975). As a further example, McClintock (1971) has found that college roommates sometimes tend to develop parallel and synchronous cycles, perhaps due to olfactory cues or to unknown social cues. All of these observations point to the important role of psychosocial influences on hormonal activities.

Premenstrual Syndrome and Dysmenorrhea.　Considering the tremendous alterations in body chemistry associated with ovarian and menstrual cycles, it is not surprising that many women (perhaps all at some time or another) experience some degree of fluctuation in physical or emotional well-being associated with various phases of their cycles. Several decades of research (summarized by Melges & Hamburg, 1977, and Parlee, 1973) have verified the occurrence of such fluctuations even though attempts to link them to specific hormonal processes have met with some difficulty and the strength of whatever links exist is unclear (Parlee, 1973).

Most commonly observed are physical, emotional, and sometimes behavioral phenomena associated with menstruation and the few days preceding the menstrual flow. Three or four days prior to the onset of menstrual bleeding, many

RESEARCH HIGHLIGHT

Menstruation, Stress, and Performance

Among the many beliefs concerning menstruation's "side effects," there is the greatest amount of research support for the observation that, for many women, it is accompanied by varying degrees of physical and emotional distress. Less clearly supported (Parlee, 1973) is the frequently cited assertion that, during their monthly "distress," menstruating women are subject to diminished capacity to concentrate, ability to withstand stress, and performance levels. In spite of the fact that most studies (Bernstein, 1977; Golub, 1976) reveal no such effects associated with menstruation, the argument is often encoun-

tered that, because of their recurring biological cycles, women are less suited than men for positions of importance that require concentration, stability, and the ability to maintain high levels of performance under stress. They might "fold" during their periods, it is claimed.

Judith Rodin (1976), however, suggested that just the opposite might occur. Her hypothesis, derived from attribution theory, was that menstruating women who normally experience rather strong distress symptoms during their periods would perform better under stress than would menstruating

women with no symptoms and nonmenstruating women. Her reasoning was that menstruating strong-symptom women would tend to attribute any task-produced stress to the fact that they were menstruating but that no-symptom and nonmenstruating women would perceive the stress as originating in the task itself. Strong-symptom women should, thus, be better able to disregard and overcome the interfering effects of stress while the performance of no-symptom and nonmenstruating women should be adversely affected by induced stress.

In order to test these predictions, three groups

of female subjects were chosen. One group consisted of menstruating women who typically experienced relatively strong symptoms of distress during their periods. A second group was composed of menstruating women who reported no symptoms from menstruation. Finally, a third group of nonmenstruating women was selected. All subjects were told that they were going to perform a series of tasks that were to be timed and that required rapid, accurate performance. They were also told that the tasks were very good indicators of intelligence and that one task would involve receiving painful

women experience what is often referred to as the **premenstrual syndrome**. The premenstrual syndrome consists of a loosely defined collection of physical and emotional symptoms associated with the period of time immediately preceding menstruation. The physical symptoms include pain in the lower back and abdomen, headache, fatigue, and sensations of pelvic heaviness or swelling. Emotional manifestations include feelings of irritability, depression, anxiety, tension, low self-esteem, and hostility (Bardwick, 1971; Dalton, 1964, 1969; Williams, 1977). The intensity of distress experienced from these symptoms varies dramatically from one woman to another. Some are severely affected and others experience little or no disturbance. Furthermore, it has been reported that women are more prone to crimes of violence, suicide, accidents, and psychiatric disorder during the premenstrual period than at any other time (Dalton, 1964).

Hormonal activity is sometimes suggested as the "cause" of the premenstrual syndrome. For example, it has been variously suggested that estrogen withdrawal, progesterone withdrawal, estrogen *and* progesterone withdrawal, estrogen-

shock. These instructions were designed to produce stress-related arousal, and empirical checks revealed that they were successful in doing so.

On three of four tasks that the women actually performed, it was found that, as predicted, the strong-symptom subjects obtained higher scores than did either the no-symptom or nonmenstruating subjects. The results are summarized in the table below. Two of the tasks (digit symbol substitution and anagrams solutions) require sustained and intense concentration and are typically disrupted by stress. The third task (an unsolvable puzzle) was chosen as a measure of tolerance for frustration, with high scores indicating high tolerance.

Thus, it is clear that distressing menstrual symptoms do not inevitably handicap a woman in terms of her intellectual and emotional performance under stress. In fact, women who are "used" to such distress may simply assume that their stress-produced symptoms are merely menstrual symptoms and be less affected by the stress than women who have no symptoms or who are not menstruating. There is, obviously, no justification for employment discrimination on the basis of sex in these findings.

Average performance scores under stress for menstruating women who experience strong symptoms, no symptoms, and who are not menstruating. SOURCE: Data from Rodin, 1976.

| | Task | | |
Group	Digit Symbol Substitution (Number Correct)	Anagrams (Number Correct)	Unsolvable Puzzle (Number of Attempts Made)
Menstruating/ strong-symptom	40.0	1.32	14.7
Menstruating/ no-symptom	32.8	0.92	9.6
Nonmenstruating	31.4	1.01	5.0

progesterone imbalances, altered adrenal functioning, and so on precipitate the symptoms described (Melges & Hamburg, 1977). It should be understood, however, that clear causal connections between hormones (or cycles) and symptoms have not yet been established. This is due in part to the fact that, with over 150 symptoms associated with it at one time or another, the syndrome is not well defined (Moos, 1969). A second difficulty is that many investigators have been somewhat imprecise in determining cycle phases (Parlee, 1973) and that actual hormone secretion patterns within cycles vary somewhat from woman to woman (Whalen, 1975). Finally, it is clear that the amount of distress associated with the premenstrual period is also influenced by a number of nonhormonal factors such as a woman's attitudes toward menstruation, sex, and the feminine role (Paige, 1973).

Perhaps 50 percent or more of women experience discomfort at some time in their lives during the first few days of the actual menstrual flow (Williams, 1977). **Dysmenorrhea** (painful menstruation) is pain in the pelvic area usually experienced as "cramps." Cramps are thought to be caused by spasmodic contractions of the uterus during the early stages of menstruation. They occur in cycles that include ovulation and thus are relatively rare in a girl's first few periods, which are typically anovulatory (without ovulation). Dysmenorrhea occurs most frequently in relatively young women, usually disappearing by the age of twenty-five, and is almost always terminated by childbirth. The mechanism underlying "childbirth cures" of menstrual cramping is unknown (Lennane & Lennane, 1973). For some women who experience it, menstrual pain is relatively mild and may be relieved by aspirin or other analgesics. These women are usually able to continue their daily activities with little disturbance. Some women, however, have such severe cramps, backache, and nausea, that they are functionally disabled for a day or more during each menstrual period. Even among these women, though, menstrual cramping and pain usually last only through the first or second day of menstruation.

One of the reported benefits of combined oral contraceptive pills (those that contain estrogen and progesterone) is reduction of some of the symptoms associated with menstruation and the premenstrual period (Moos, 1968). Combination pills act in various ways (suppressing ovulation, FSH, LH, and so on) to reduce hormonal variations and "level out" a woman's body chemistry throughout her cycle. In some women, this leveling reduces or eliminates cyclic distress.

Centuries of mythology to the contrary, menstrual blood has no special fire extinguishing qualities, does not ruin crops, break violin strings, stop clocks, ruin wine, or kill men (DeLora & Warren, 1977; Paige, 1973). Nor are there any inherent reasons for menstruating women to refrain from bathing, swimming, strenuous work, or any of their other usual activities. Similarly, even though it is somewhat taboo in virtually all societies, there are no medical or physiological reasons for avoiding coitus during menstruation. Nevertheless, many couples rarely or never have intercourse during the menstrual flow, primarily because of widely shared attitudes that the menstruating woman is "unclean" or polluted (Paige, 1973). But there is some evidence that orgasm during menstruation may be of potential benefit to women who suffer from painful menstrual cramping. Masters and Johnson (1966) reported that orgasm during the early stages of menstrual flow markedly reduces uterine and pelvic congestion as well as produces rapid expulsion of menstrual fluids from the uterus. Many women report that orgasm at this time dramatically reduces the severity of their menstrual pains.

Climacterium and Menopause.   Sometime between the ages of forty-five and fifty, the reproductive life of the average woman slowly comes to an end. For unknown reasons, her ovaries gradually begin a decline in function and no longer respond to the pituitary gonadotropin FSH. This cessation of ovarian functioning is referred to as the **climacterium**. Ovarian cycling becomes less regular and little by little, as the ovaries become less sensitive to the gonadotropic hormones, less estrogen and progesterone are secreted. Because of these changes, menstrual cycling is disrupted, uterine endometrial growth is slowed, and menstruation becomes irregular. The ultimate cessation of menstruation that follows is known as **menopause**. Accompanying menopause are various changes in the vagina, external genitals, and breasts, which are supported by estrogen. The vaginal wall thins and decreases its lubricating capacity, the labia thin and lose some of their softness, and the breasts shrink somewhat and begin to sag.

In part because of estrogen withdrawal, a number of distressful symptoms are commonly associated with menopause. The most widely recognized of these symptoms is the so-called "hot flush," or "hot flash," which is experienced as a sudden wave of heat spreading over the body and is sometimes accompanied by reddening of the skin and perspiration. Flushes may occur several times in a single day and may last from only a few seconds to several minutes. Some women are very discomforted and embarrassed by the flushing reaction and some report no disturbance at all. Other physical symptoms sometimes associated with menopause include chills, breast pains, back pains, headache, dizziness, and heart palpitations (Bardwick, 1971; Neugarten & Kraines, 1965). These symptoms, of course, vary in intensity from one woman to another and it has been estimated that no more than 10 percent of all women suffer from menopausal distress that is severely disturbing (Melges & Hamburg, 1977).

Because many of these symptoms may dissipate in response to estrogen, estrogen-replacement therapy for menopausal women has gained many followers since the mid-1960s (Wilson, 1966). More recently, alarming suggestions that long-term administration of estrogen increases the risk of uterine cancer have led to some tempering of the initial excitement generated by exaggerated claims concerning the benefits of estrogen (Ziel & Finkle, 1975). Recent evidence, however, suggests that combining estrogen with progesterone may actually lessen the risk of uterine cancer (Hulka, Chambless, Kaufman, Fowler, and Greenberg, 1982).

Along with the physical symptoms of menopause, some women report depression, anxiety, irritability, inability to concentrate, and confusion (Neugarten & Kraines, 1965). It is difficult to determine whether these distressing experiences are due to hormonal, psychosocial, or both influences. Certainly the psychosocial significance of aging and menopause cannot be ignored. Menopause provides a clear signal that a woman's reproductive life has ended. Her children have probably all left home or are soon to do so and for those women whose self-concepts are defined by their maternal roles, the apparent termination of those roles can be somewhat disturbing. Other "facts of life" she must face at this time include her possible perceptions of her declining physical attractiveness, the prospect of a less active sex life, her probable widowhood, since she will normally outlive her husband, and her own eventual death.

But menopause is not a traumatic period for all women. For some, it signals the beginning of a new, less anxiety laden, and more exciting sex life because fears of pregnancy have ended. Many women are relieved by the termination of their monthly menstrual cycles. Others enjoy the relative freedom from childrearing chores and responsibilities that usually comes around the age at which menopause occurs. In any case, as we noted earlier, the majority of women are not severely disturbed either by physical or emotional symptoms during menopause (Neugarten & Kraines, 1965).

Male Sexual Anatomy and Physiology

Although they appear to be radically different, male and female genitals are, in fact, similar in two important ways. Some structures are similar in origin **(homologous)**, having evolved from the same embryonic tissue. For example, the male scrotum and female labia majora are homologous structures since both evolve from the primitive labioscrotal swelling (see Figure 2–2). Some, like the penis and vagina, both organs of copulation, are similar in function **(analogous)** but not in origin. Still others, like the testes and ovaries, are both homologous and analogous, having similar origins and functions. Like those of the female, the genitals of the male consist of structures found inside as well as outside the body cavity. We will begin our examination of the male sexual system with the external genitals.

Male External Genitals.   The external genitals of males consist of the penis and the scrotum (see Figure 2–12). The testes, or testicles, are suspended within the scrotum and not usually regarded as part of the external genitals.

Shown in side section in Figure 2–12 and in longitudinal and cross section in Figure 2–13, the **penis** is a cylindrical organ composed primarily of three sponge-like bodies. On top are the two larger of these, the **corpora cavernosa**. Running the length of the underside of the penis is the third, the smaller **corpus spongiosum**, through which the urethra passes. As shown in Figure 2–13, each of these bodies is enclosed by a separate sheet of connective tissue (fascia) and all three are enclosed by a single common sheet of connective tissue. The cavernous and spongy bodies consist of a network of cavities much like a sponge. They are richly supplied by nerves, arteries, and veins. Erection of the penis occurs when the rate of arterial blood flow to these tissues increases and venous outflow decreases. The corpora cavernosa and corpus spongiosum become engorged with blood and, because they are constricted by their fibrous wrappings, the penis swells, stiffens, and hardens. When venous outflow of blood once again increases and inflow from the arteries decreases, the erectile tissue drains and the penis returns to its flaccid state.

The two corpora cavernosa separate at the root of the penis, and their tips *(crura)* attach to the pubic bones. The corpus spongiosum does not attach to any bone but extends beyond the base of the penis to form the *penile bulb.* Together, the crura and bulb form the root of the penis. At the outer end of the penis the corpus spongiosum expands and flares to form the **glans** of the penis. The male counterpart of the female clitoral glans, the glans penis is richly endowed with nerve endings and extremely sensitive to tactile stimulation. It is shaped much like a cone or acorn, with a crownlike ridge **(corona)** at its back edge that slightly overhangs the narrower neck of the penis. At the underside of the glans is a thin strip of skin, the **frenulum**, connecting the glans to the prepuce, or **foreskin**, of the penis. Both the frenulum and corona are highly erotically sensitive, as is the rest of the glans.

Emerging from the tip of the glans is the **urethral meatus**, or opening of the penile urethra that runs through the corpus spongiosum (see Figures 2–12 and 2–13). The shaft of the penis is relatively free of nerve endings and thus far less erotically sensitive than the glans. Penile skin is hairless and loose, permitting free movement and expansion of the body of the penis during erection. At the neck near the corona, the skin is attached to the penis, but a portion of it is loose and extends over and partially covers the glans, forming the prepuce, or foreskin.

In a procedure known as circumcision, a portion of the foreskin is often removed surgically shortly after birth, leaving the glans totally exposed. Circumcision is performed for hygienic, medical, esthetic, and religious reasons. Bordering the neck and corona of the penis are small glands that secrete a cheeselike substance (smegma) with a characteristic odor. The function of this substance is

Figure 2–12.

Side-sectional representation of the male reproductive system.

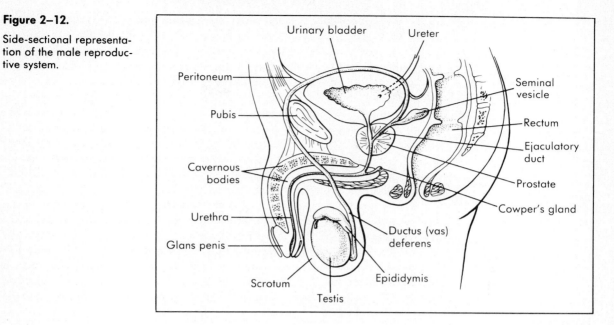

unknown but if trapped under the foreskin, it can lead to painful infection and irritation. Circumcision decreases the possibility of such infections and simplifies cleansing the penis. In some cases the foreskin is tight and unretractable or attached to the glans by connective tissue (phimosis), and surgical removal is the treatment of choice. There is no difference in erotic sensitivity between the circumcised and the noncircumcised penis (Masters & Johnson, 1966). Even though more than 80 percent of American boys are circumcised shortly after birth, the American Academy of Pediatrics (AAP) has raised doubts about the necessity of routinely performing such surgery. The AAP argues that careful hygiene provides the same medical benefits of circumcision without the pain and hazards of surgery (Paige, 1978).

There are no bones or muscles in the human penis. The root (crura and bulb) of the penis are, however, surrounded by muscles that allow voluntary, but slight and jerky, movements of the penis. The primary function of these muscles is to aid in ejecting urine through the urethra during urination and semen through the urethra during ejaculation.

When flaccid, the average adult penis is between 7.5 and 10 centimeters (3 and 4 inches) long and about 3 centimeters (slightly over 1 inch) in diameter. Erection increases the average penis to a length of around 15 centimeters (6 inches) and to a diameter of 3.8 centimeters (1.5 inches). These are, of course, average figures around which substantial variations occur from man to man. In spite of widespread concern by males and females alike over penis dimensions, a man's virility, potency, and ability to give or receive sexual pleasure during coitus are, except in cases involving extreme variations, generally unrelated to the size of his penis (Masters & Johnson, 1966). As Figure 2–14 illustrates, there is substantial variation in the appearance of the male external genitals.

The **scrotum** is a loose-hanging outpocket of the abdominal cavity consisting of an outer layer of dark skin and two internal muscle groups. Scrotal skin contains many sweat glands and is lightly covered with hair. Beneath the skin is the **tunica dartos**, a layer of connective tissue and smooth (involuntary) muscle that contracts and tightens the scrotal skin around the testes in response to cold, sexual stimulation, and other conditions. The **cremasteric muscles** and their connective tissue attach not only to the scrotum but also to the spermatic cords. The cremasters are striated muscles and under some degree of voluntary control. In response to sexual stimulation, these muscles lift and draw the testes toward the body cavity. Involuntary contraction of the cremasters in response to stroking of the inner thighs is called the *cremasteric reflex*. Together, the dartos and cremaster muscles assist in regulation of scrotal temperature by tensing and relaxing the scrotal skin and by varying the closeness of the testes to the body.

Within the scrotum are two separate capsules, each of which houses one testicle and the lower section of its **spermatic cord**. The spermatic cords consist of cremasteric musculature as well as blood vessels and nerves. Also within the spermatic cords are the **vasa deferentia** (sing., **vas deferens**), which transport sperm from the testes. The spermatic cords pass into the abdominal cavity through the **inguinal canal**, through which the testes descend during prenatal development. Normally the inguinal canal is sealed off by connective tissue following

Figure 2–13.

Longitudinal and cross-sectional representations of the penis.

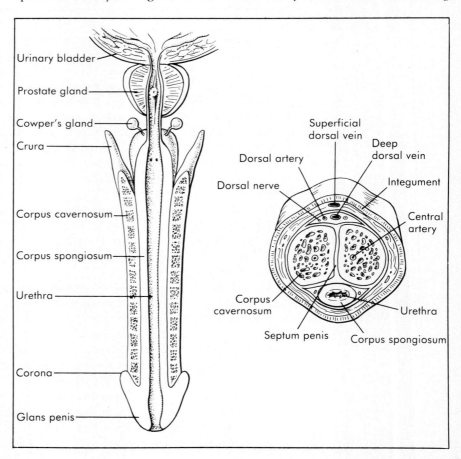

Figure 2–14.

Some normal variations in the appearance of the male genitals.

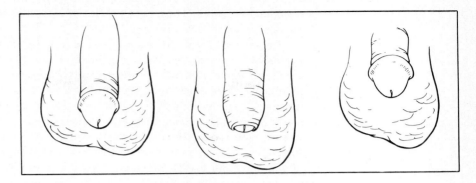

descent of the testes. Failure of one or both of the testes to descend prior to birth occurs in less than 10 percent of males and seriously interferes with sperm maturation due to the high temperatures within the body (see earlier discussion). Sometimes the inguinal canal fails to close and part of the intestinal tract protrudes into the scrotum producing an *inguinal hernia*, which can be treated by surgery.

Male Internal Genitals.   The **testes**, or testicles, are both homologous and analogous to the ovaries in the female. That is, they are the gonads and serve the dual purpose of germ cell production and hormone manufacture and secretion. The testes are paired glands about 4 centimeters (1.5 inches) long and 2.5 centimeters (1 inch) in diameter that are suspended within the scrotum, usually with the left one hanging a bit lower than the right one. Each testicle is sheathed by a dense fibrous sheet. At the top and back of each testicle this covering penetrates the organ with many protrusions *(septa)* that divide it into hundreds of chambers.

As noted, germ cell production is one of the testes' two functions. It occurs in the following manner. Within each chamber are the highly coiled **seminiferous tubules** (see Figure 2–15), each of which, when uncoiled, measures 0.3 to 1.0 meters (1 to 3 feet) long to produce a combined length from both testes of several hundred meters.

Within the seminiferous tubules, the process of **spermatogenesis** takes place. Under the stimulus of FSH from the pituitary, primitive cells *(spermatogonia)* in the lining of the seminiferous tubules begin to mature shortly following puberty. Development from spermatogonia to mature sperm cells *(spermatozoa)* requires about seventy days, and several hundred million sperm reach maturity each day in the average adult male. A mature human sperm averages about sixty micrometers in length (one micrometer equals only 1/25,000 inch) and consists of a head, neck, body, and tail. The head contains the chromosomes and the acrosome, which secretes an enzyme allowing the sperm to penetrate the ovum. The body of the sperm processes sugars and fats for energy required for the whiplike movements of the tail as the sperm swims.

Moved by ciliary action and perhaps by peristalsis (wavelike muscle contractions), mature sperm migrate from the seminiferous tubules to the **epididymes**, paired tubes attached to the testes which, although around six meters (twenty feet) long, are so coiled and convoluted that they appear not much longer than the testes themselves (see Figure 2-15). The sperm are transported through the epididymes (head to tail) over a period of between two and six weeks, during which time they continue to mature. Thus, the epididymes serve the three functions of sperm storage, transport, and ripening.

The second function of the testes—the manufacture of hormones—is carried out in the cells between the seminiferous tubules. In response to the pituitary gonadotropin ICSH (LH), the **interstitial cells** secrete testosterone as well as small amounts of other androgen hormones and some estrogen. Unlike its counterpart (LH) in females, ICSH is continuously rather than cyclically released in males. There is, however, a negative feedback relationship between testosterone and ICSH secretion. That is, as testosterone levels in the bloodstream increase, secretions of LH-RF from the hypothalamus and consequently of ICSH from the pituitary are temporarily decreased. Thus, the testes slow testosterone production, which prompts the hypothalamus to once again step up LH-RF secretions and, consequently, causes testosterone production to increase again. Although hormone production and spermatogenesis are relatively tonic or acyclic processes in males, they are not completely devoid of rhythms. Recently, for example, complex daily as well as annual variations in patterns of gonadotropin and hormone secretion have been observed in males (Reinberg & Lagoguey, 1978). Considerably more research is required for a complete understanding of the nature and significance of these rhythms.

The paired *vasa deferentia* serve to transport as well as to store mature sperm. As shown in Figures 2–12 and 2–15, each *vas deferens* passes from the tail portion of each epididymis upward into the abdominal cavity, where it continues over and around the urinary bladder. Sperm passage through the vasa deferentia is accomplished in part by ciliary action and by wave-like muscle contractions (peristalsis) of the ducts themselves. The terminal portion of each of these 46-centimeter (18-inch) long ducts broadens to form an enlarged portion called the *ampulla* and narrows once again to join the duct of one seminal vesicle. Each vas deferens joins the duct of the adjacent seminal vesicle to form an **ejaculatory duct**. The ejaculatory ducts enter and pass a short distance through the prostate before opening into the prostatic portion of the urethra.

The vasa deferentia are the most frequent targets for male sterilization. In **vasectomy**, both ducts are simply cut or tied through small incisions in the scrotum. The passage of sperm is thus prevented and the man is sterile. There is, however, no alteration of hormonal functioning, sex drive, potency, or sexual pleasure. He will continue to have orgasms and ejaculate but the semen will contain no sperm. Sperm will continue to be produced but will be absorbed by the body. Rarely, the vasa may be surgically reconnected and fertility restored. For practical purposes, however, a vasectomy should be considered irreversible.

The **seminal vesicles** are two sacs about 5 centimeters (2 inches) long, each of which lies adjacent to one of the vas deferens. The ducts of these two structures combine to form the ejaculatory duct. Once thought to function primarily as storage depots for sperm, the seminal vesicles (each of which holds 2 to 3 cubic centimeters of fluid) supply fluids and substances that energize and contribute to the motility of sperm. Accounting for the major portion of the seminal fluid (Mann, 1970), the contents of the seminal vesicles are discharged into the ejaculatory ducts during the first (emission) stage of ejaculation (Masters & Johnson, 1966).

The **prostate** is a partially glandular, partially muscular organ about the size of a chestnut located with its base at the bottom of the urinary bladder. Through the

Figure 2–15.

Representation of a
testicle.

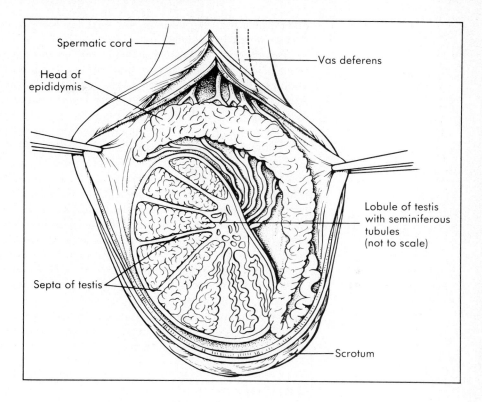

Spermatic cord

Vas deferens

Head of
epididymis

Lobule of testis
with seminiferous
tubules
(not to scale)

Septa of testis

Scrotum

prostate pass the ejaculatory ducts and a portion (prostatic) of the urethra. Near the
area where the ejaculatory ducts join the urethra are a number of sieve-like ducts
through which pass a number of prostatic secretions that further contribute to the
volume of semen. These prostatic fluids are released during the emission stage of
ejaculation. During ejaculation a sphincter muscle at the neck of the urinary
bladder is closed, preventing urine from flowing into the urethra and mixing with
the seminal fluid (Masters & Johnson, 1966).

The prostate usually shrinks with age but sometimes becomes enlarged or
hardened. This often results in discomfort as well as interferes with urination.
Under such circumstances, part or all of the prostate may be removed by surgery.
Prostate surgery sometimes interferes with the function of the urethral sphincter
and during ejaculation semen may be forced into the bladder rather than out of the
urethra (retrograde ejaculation). Orgasmic sensations are still present but the
semen does not leave the body until urination.

Located immediately below the prostate and flanking the second (membranous) portion of the urethra are the paired bulbourethral, or **Cowper's, glands**.
These pea-sized glands secrete a small quantity of clear, sticky fluid (pre-ejaculatory
emission) that appears at the tip of the penis during sexual arousal. Although the
precise function of this secretion is unknown (too little is secreted to aid significantly in coital lubrication), its alkaline composition is thought to neutralize acidity
in the urethra, facilitating sperm survival. Those practicing the "withdrawal
method" of contraception should be aware that this preejaculatory emission some-

times contains a few active sperm. Thus, *pregnancy can sometimes result from coitus without ejaculation*.

The urethra continues through the penis and terminates at the urethral meatus in the glans. In the second (expulsion, or ejaculation proper) stage of ejaculation, semen is forced through the penile urethra by powerful contractions of the muscles surrounding the penile bulb. The bulb is repeatedly compressed by these muscles at the rate of once every 0.8 seconds, forcefully expelling semen from the urethral meatus in spurts. These contractions during ejaculation constitute a central part of the experience of orgasm in males.

Since they have no uterus, men, of course do not go through menopause. Similarly, there is no male equivalent to the female climacterium. Unlike the ovaries in women, the testes do not abruptly cease functioning, either in terms of hormone production or spermatogenesis. As men age, however, the rates of testosterone and sperm production gradually decline due to the gradual shrinkage of the testes. These declines begin in late adolescence. The aging male is slower to erect and ejaculate in response to sexual stimulation and some of his physiological responses at orgasm are less intense.

Some men do experience depression, irritability, anxiety, and other distressing emotions as they grow older. These feelings are, however, not related to any known hormonal changes but due, for the most part, to the prospect of forced retirement, less physical vigor, a less interesting and exciting life in general, loss of youthful attractiveness, and death.

SUMMARY

Full comprehension of human sexual expression includes a basic understanding of the anatomy (structure) and physiology (functioning) of sexual systems. Sexual anatomy and physiology are shaped by the combined influences of genetic and hormonal factors. At the time of conception the genetic sex of an individual is determined by whether a sperm cell carrying an X (female) chromosome or one carrying a Y (male) chromosome fertilizes an ovum (egg), which always carries only an X chromosome. An XX sperm-ovum combination produces a female and an XY combination produces a male embryo. Until around the sixth or seventh week following fertilization the internal and external sexual systems of chromosomal (XX) females and chromosomal (XY) males are indistinguishable or undifferentiated. If the sex is male (XY), previously undifferentiated gonads then evolve into testes, while a female (XX) code produces differentiation of the gonads into ovaries.

The male testes secrete hormones known as androgens that prompt development of male internal and external genital structures. Ovaries secrete hormones known as estrogens but the presence of estrogen is not necessary for female genital development. The female pattern of development is basic. Female genital systems always develop in the absence of androgens but androgens must be added to the system in order to produce male development. At birth, males and females both possess all of their basic genital structures.

Between birth and puberty, genital development is limited to structural growth although some physical differences between the sexes such as muscle and fat distribution appear by the age of four. Complete physical maturation of male and female genital systems begins at puberty, which is initiated between the ages of eleven and twelve in females and a year or two later in males. In females, increases in the concentration of estrogens are responsible for most of the changes of puberty. Increased testosterone production stimulates pubertal changes in males. At the completion of puberty, both sexes possess all of the physical equipment necessary to function biologically as sexual adults.

The external genitals of females are collectively referred to as the vulva and consist of the mons pubis, labia majora, labia minora, clitoris, and vaginal opening. Together, the ovaries, fallopian tubes, uterus, cervix, and vagina make up the female internal genitals. Reproductive and hormonal functioning in females is cyclic. Circulating levels of the hormones estrogen and progesterone undergo recurrent changes roughly every twenty-eight days. These cyclic fluctuations are associated with recurring changes in the activities of the ovaries (ovarian cycles) and related recurring alterations in the structure of the lining of the uterus (menstrual cycles). In some women the few days preceding menstruation are associated with physical and emotional stress (premenstrual syndrome). Some also experience pelvic pains and cramps (dysmenorrhea) during the actual menstrual bleeding.

Ovarian and menstrual cycling continues during periods of nonpregnancy from shortly after puberty until the climacterium and menopause, which begin between the ages of forty-five and fifty in the average woman. Climacterium refers to the cessation of ovarian functioning and menopause to the cessation of menstruation which follows. In part, due to estrogen withdrawal and, in part, because of the psychosocial effects of aging, some women experience considerable physical and emotional distress during menopausal years.

The penis and scrotum constitute the male external genitals and the testes, epididymes, vasa deferentia, seminal vesicles, and prostate the internal genitals. Hormonal and reproductive functioning in males is tonic rather than cyclic. That is, the production of sperm and testosterone by the testes is continuous. Slight daily and annual variations in hormone levels have been detected in males but their significance is as yet unknown. Males do not undergo a climacterium but there is a gradual decline in sperm and testosterone production as men age.

SUGGESTED READINGS

Diamond, M. (1977). Human sexual development: Biological foundations for social development. In F. A. Beach (Ed.), *Human sexuality in four perspectives*. Baltimore: Johns Hopkins University Press.

Landau, B. R. (1976). *Essential human anatomy and physiology*. Glenview, IL: Scott, Foresman and Company. (See Chapters 30, 31.)

Melges, F. T., & Hamburg, D. A. (1977). Psychological effects of hormonal changes in women. In F. A. Beach (Ed.), *Human sexuality in four perspectives*. Baltimore: Johns Hopkins University Press.

Money, J., & Ehrhardt, A. A. (1972). *Man and woman, boy and girl*. Baltimore: Johns Hopkins University Press. (See Chapters 1–4, 10.)

CHAPTER OUTLINE

CONCEPTION, PREGNANCY, AND CHILDBIRTH
Conception
Pregnancy
Childbirth

BIRTH CONTROL
Contraception
Hormonal Contraceptives
Nonhormonal Methods of Contraception
Sterilization
Induced Abortion

CHAPTER 3

CONCEPTION, PREGNANCY, CHILDBIRTH, AND BIRTH CONTROL

One of the potential consequences of coitus between fertile individuals is pregnancy. For some people this is an occasion for joyous celebration while in others it provokes crisis. In spite of the tremendous responsibilities associated with parenting a child, relatively few people know very much about the details of how a child is conceived, the nature of pregnancy, the process of childbirth, or how conception, pregnancy, and childbirth may be controlled. In this chapter we will provide a brief overview of each of these topics.

CONCEPTION, PREGNANCY, AND CHILDBIRTH

The basis for understanding the essentials of conception was established in Chapter 2, where we discussed the anatomy and physiology of the male and female reproductive systems. In the following sections we will provide a brief overview of the processes of conception, pregnancy, and childbirth. More detailed discussion may be found in several books devoted exclusively to these topics (for example, Pritchard & MacDonald, 1976; Rugh & Shettles, 1971).

Conception

Conception (fertilization) occurs when a sperm unites with an ovum. An ovum remains viable for only about twelve hours after ovulation and sperm live only around forty-eight hours in the female reproductive tract. Thus, in order for conception to occur, sperm must be introduced into the female tract close to the time of ovulation (between forty-eight hours before and twelve hours afterward).

Upon its release from the ovary, an ovum enters the fallopian tube, where it is slowly (over a two- to three-day period) transported through the tube toward the uterus (see Chapter 2). The ejaculate of a healthy male adult contains between 150 and 600 million sperm but only about 1000 to 2000 reach the vicinity of a fallopian tube following ejaculation in the vagina. Movement of sperm from the region of the cervix to the upper third (ampullar region) of the fallopian tubes, where fertilization usually occurs, takes from an hour to an hour and a half (Katchadourian & Lunde, 1980). There, one sperm, of the millions ejaculated, penetrates the outer layer of the ovum (zona pellucida) and completes the process of fertilization.

While continuing its two- to three-day migration through the fallopian tube, the fertilized egg (zygote) undergoes several cell divisions and becomes, by the time it reaches the uterine cavity, a fluid-filled ball of cells known as a **blastocyst**. Six or seven days following conception, after further cell divisions, the blastocyst implants in the uterine lining (endometrium). With implantation completed, a thin membrane **(chorion)** develops around the entire egg and combines with the endometrial tissue ultimately to form the **placenta**, which serves as the organ of nutritional

Figure 3–1.

Fertilization and implantation of an ovum.

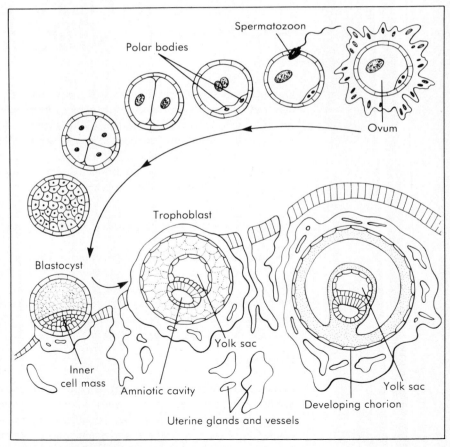

SOURCE: Adapted from Landau, 1976.

and waste exchange between the embryo and the mother. The **amniotic membrane** (sac) forms within the chorion, creating a fluid-filled cavity within which the embryo is suspended (see Figure 3–1). The fluid serves as a cushion and protective covering for the embryo (Landau, 1976). The pregnancy is now established.

Our discussion of conception has focused only on the most usual type of fertilization—that which results from intravaginal ejaculation during coitus. But at least two other means of fertilization should be mentioned. The first, **artificial insemination**, has been used successfully in animals for centuries, and in humans for several decades. In this process, viable sperm are inserted into a woman's vagina or cervix shortly before ovulation is expected and conception takes place as usual. Artificial insemination in humans is often performed when a man's sperm count is so low as to make him functionally sterile. Several ejaculates may be collected from the man, frozen, and stored until enough sperm are available to successfully impregnate his wife. Alternatively, the semen from an anonymous donor is sometimes used. Some men who obtain a vasectomy (surgical sterilization) first store semen samples for use in artificial insemination should they later desire to father a child. It should be emphasized, however, that semen storage methods have not been perfected (Goldstein, 1976). By one estimate, over 250,000 artificial insemination pregnancies are produced each year in the United States (McCary, 1978).

The second method, **ovum transplantation**, was first accomplished in England in July 1978. A near full-term baby girl was successfully delivered in that instance. Success with ovum transplantation was first achieved in the United States in 1981. In this procedure an ovum is first removed from a woman's ovary and transplanted to a culture dish containing supportive nutrients and viable sperm. When fertilized, the zygote begins the process of cell division in the culture dish, where it remains until it reaches the blastocyst stage (see above). It is then placed in the uterus for normal implantation (Clark & Gastel, 1978). Though the technique is far from perfected, it may prove useful for those women who ovulate but whose fallopian tubes are blocked, scarred, or severed as a result of disease, injury, or even sterilization (discussed later in this chapter).

Pregnancy

The first and most commonly recognized sign of pregnancy is a missed menstrual period. Other indicants include nausea and vomiting ("morning sickness"), breast enlargement and tenderness, frequent urination, and fatigue. All of these changes suggest that a woman may be pregnant but, since such symptoms may arise from other sources, a medical examination is necessary for verification of pregnancy in its early stages.

Two clinical procedures are commonly used to diagnose pregnancy. The first involves *laboratory tests* designed to detect the presence of the hormone *human chorionic gonadotropin* (HCG), which is secreted by the chorionic membrane (see above and Chapter 2) surrounding the embryo. In the past, the most common test of this sort was one in which a sample of urine from a woman was injected into an immature female laboratory animal such as a rat or rabbit. Since the presence of HCG stimulates the production of eggs by the animal's ovaries, pregnancy is detected by destroying the animal and examining the ovaries (Goldstein, 1976)

Such tests take several days, however, and are now rarely used. In a more common procedure, a urine sample is combined with a substance (on a slide or in a test tube) and the mixture is observed for **agglutination** (coagulation). Depending on the particular type of test used, the presence of HCG either inhibits or causes coagulation of the mixture. The slide tests require only two minutes to perform but do not become reliable (95 to 98 percent accuracy) until forty-one days after the first day of the last menstrual period **(LMP)**. The "test tube" test requires two hours but is reliable thirty-eight days LMP. A recently developed blood test is extremely sensitive to HCG and may be used to detect pregnancy with 99 percent accuracy within eight days of ovulation and before a woman is late for her next menstrual period. This procedure, which requires costly and complicated equipment, is not yet widely available. In 1978, "do-it-yourself" pregnancy testing kits for home use became available, but they have not yet been thoroughly evaluated for accuracy. Early indications, however, are that nearly 20 percent of the time these "early pregnancy tests" fail to detect a pregnancy when it actually exists (Carpenter, 1979).

In addition to the laboratory tests described above, a *pelvic exam* is also used to diagnose pregnancy. After about six weeks of pregnancy the cervix becomes softer and darkens in color. The uterus softens and may bulge, providing physical as well as chemical evidence of pregnancy (Boston Women's Health Book Collective, 1976).

The average length of pregnancy is around 270 days but variations from 240 to 300 days are not abnormal. The nine-month period of pregnancy is often divided into three-month segments known as **trimesters**.

During the *first trimester* (through the twelfth week) the fetus reaches a length of between 3.8 and 10 centimeters (1.5 and 4 inches) and attains a weight of nearly 28 grams (1 ounce). It is clearly recognizable as human, with distinguishable fingers, toes, ears, nose, closed eyes, and some well-developed organ systems (Katchadourian & Lunde, 1980). For the mother, some of the early symptoms of pregnancy such as mild nausea, intermittent "spotting" (uterine blood discharge), and general fatigue may continue. This is a time during which most women begin to "come to terms" with their pregnancy, and the feelings of many are ambivalent (Boston Women's Health Book Collective, 1976). In part because of the discomforts associated with the early symptoms of pregnancy, the sexual desire and responsiveness of up to a third of women decreases during the first trimester. About half experience no change in sexual interest and some even report increased sexual desire and activity (Kenny, 1973; Masters & Johnson, 1966; Tolor & DiGrazia, 1976).

Although the growth rate of the fetus decreases during the *second trimester* (the beginning of the 13th to the end of the 24th week), it increases in weight from about 28 grams (1 ounce) to 1 kilogram (2 pounds) and in length from about 10 to 35 centimeters (4 to 14 inches). Figure 3–2 illustrates embryonic and fetal development through the 15th week. Fetal movement and heartbeat can be detected, and the fetus is sensitive to sound and light during this trimester. The mother becomes increasingly aware of her pregnancy as fetal movements become more apparent, and because of increases in the size of her abdomen, waist, and breasts, the pregnancy begins to "show" (see Figure 3–3). Many of the discomforting symptoms of the first trimester begin to fade but may be replaced by others such as constipation and **edema** (fluid retention and swelling). Coitus may, and usually does, continue, though at a lower frequency than before. For some women, sexual interest increases during the second trimester, presumably due to the partial disappearance of the distresses of early pregnancy (Masters & Johnson, 1966). Male superior coital positions are (and should be) used less frequently, and female superior, side, and rear-entry positions are used more frequently (Wagner & Solberg, 1974).

During the *third trimester* (25th through 36th week), fetal changes consist primarily of growth and maturation since all of the major organ systems have developed by the seventh month. During the final month, the fetus, which has assumed a head-down position, is said to "drop" as its head settles into the lower portions of the mother's pelvis. At birth the average full-term baby weighs 3.5 kilograms (7.5 pounds) and is 50 centimeters (20 inches) long. Often the mother becomes increasingly uncomfortable near the end of pregnancy because of crowd-

Figure 3–2.

Embryonic and fetal sizes from 2 to 15 weeks following conception.

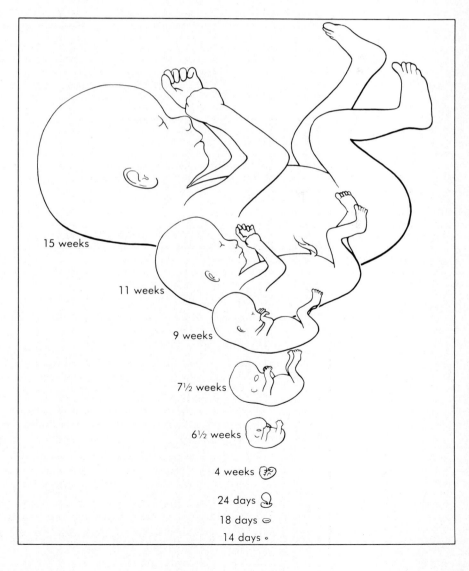

15 weeks

11 weeks

9 weeks

7½ weeks

6½ weeks

4 weeks

24 days

18 days

14 days

Figure 3–3.

Uterine and abdominal size and position during pregnancy.

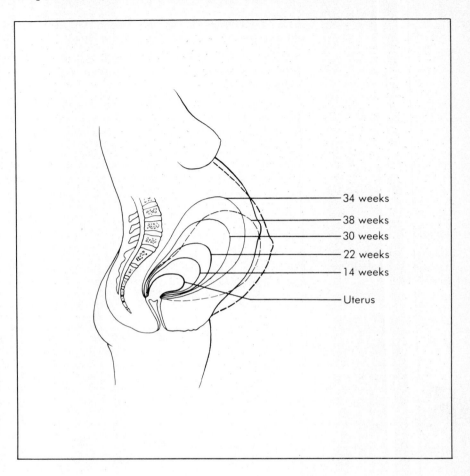

34 weeks
38 weeks
30 weeks
22 weeks
14 weeks
Uterus

ing of her stomach and other internal organs, and she may experience a frequent need to urinate. Sitting and standing are both more difficult because of the size and weight of the third-trimester fetus.

During the ninth month of pregnancy, coital frequency decreases for most women and over half discontinue coitus altogether (Wagner & Solberg, 1974). Medical opinion varies concerning the advisability of coitus during the final weeks of pregnancy. Masters and Johnson (1966) assert that, during a healthy normal pregnancy, coitus may be continued until at least the final four weeks. Others suggest that, in the absence of particular contraindicators such as uterine bleeding or ruptured membranes, intercourse may continue up until labor begins. It is, of course, up to a couple, in consultation with the physician, to make a judgment on whether or not coitus may involve risk to the fetus. If coitus is medically prohibited, a couple may use other forms of sexual interaction such as manual or oral-genital stimulation. No air, however, should ever be blown into the vagina; there is a remote possibility that air forced into the placenta and the mother's or fetus's bloodstream could cause a fatal air embolism (Masters & Johnson, 1966). Following birth, coitus may be resumed within two to three weeks or as soon as it is comfortable for the woman, providing there are no postpartum complications (Masters & Johnson, 1966).

Childbirth

Throughout pregnancy, a woman's uterus contracts (sometimes imperceptibly) at irregular intervals. As the end of pregnancy nears, these irregular contractions become stronger and stronger, thus providing one signal that the birth of the child is near. These irregular (Braxton-Hicks) contractions, however, are not the contractions of labor and are sometimes referred to as *false labor*. They may precede labor by up to three weeks and serve to strengthen the uterus for the actual labor of childbirth. After the fetus has "dropped" (see above), the cervix begins to dilate and soften and shortly before labor begins a mucus plug, which has obstructed the cervical opening to prevent infection during pregnancy, is discharged *(bloody show)*. In some 10 percent of women the membranes surrounding the fetus and containing the amniotic fluid burst, releasing the fluid. Labor usually begins within twenty-four hours after this occurs (Katchadourian & Lunde, 1980).

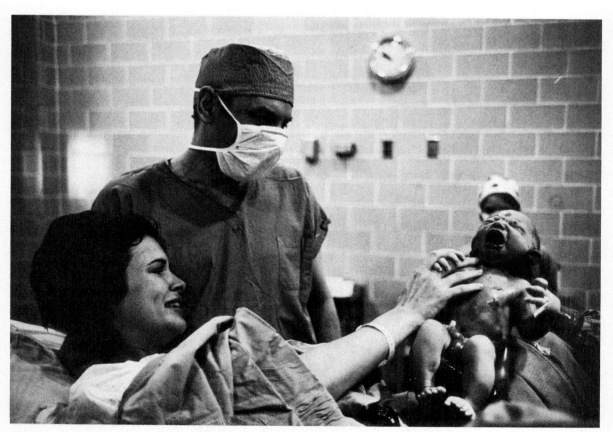

A husband and wife share the experience of their son's birth.

The process of childbirth, or **parturition**, consists of three stages of what is often referred to as *labor*. *First-stage labor* may be as short as two hours or as long as fifteen hours but averages around twelve hours for a woman's first pregnancy. Strong, regular uterine contractions lasting between forty-five seconds and one minute and spaced ten to twenty minutes apart mark the beginning of first-stage labor. These contractions serve to produce *effacement* (thinning) and *dilation* (opening) of the cervix (to about 10 centimeters, or 4 inches, in diameter) so that the baby may be passed from the uterus. There are three substages of first-stage labor: early, late, and transition.

In *early first-stage labor* the uterine contractions are relatively mild, widely spaced (fifteen to twenty minutes apart), and produce little in the way of discomfort for the woman. The cervix dilates to about 4 centimeters during this stage. In *late first-stage labor* the contractions become more intense, painful, and more frequent. Most physicians advise a woman to go to the hospital when contractions are coming four or five minutes apart. Cervical dilation reaches a diameter of 5 to 8 centimeters (2 to 3 inches) during this stage. The *transition stage* involves final dilation of the cervix from 8 to 10 centimeters and, though shorter than the first two stages, is usually experienced as more exhausting and painful due to the intensity of the uterine contractions (Boston Women's Health Book Collective, 1976).

Second-stage labor begins when the cervix is fully dilated and the baby's body moves into and through the vagina (see Figure 3–4). This is the actual birth of the baby during which voluntary "pushes" by the mother may assist in delivery. Second-stage labor may last from only a few minutes to more than two hours (Katchadourian & Lunde, 1980).

Third-stage labor is simply delivery of the placenta. Like delivery of the baby, placental ("*afterbirth*") delivery involves uterine contractions that expel the placental tissue from the uterus and may require from a few minutes to an hour (Katchadourian & Lunde, 1980).

BIRTH CONTROL

It has been estimated that, of every one thousand acts of coitus, only one is performed with pregnancy as a desired outcome (Jones, Shainberg, & Byer, 1977). At the same time, even though the probability of pregnancy resulting from a single act of coitus is less than 4 percent (Tietze, 1960), within one year ninety out of one hundred sexually active and fertile women will become pregnant if no steps are taken to prevent it (Hatcher, Stewart, Stewart, Guest, Stratton, & Wright, 1980).

Aside from the fact that most coital acts are motivated by pleasure rather than procreation, there are a number of sensible reasons for attempting to exert some control over birth. Among the most obvious are (1) curbing the alarming increase in world population growth; (2) avoiding unwanted pregnancies and, thus, unwanted children; (3) spacing pregnancies to reduce health risks to women; (4) limiting family size for social or economic reasons; and (5) avoiding births of children with birth defects or genetically transmitted diseases.

For a number of legal, ethical, moral, and technological reasons, highly effective methods of birth control (short of total coital abstinence) were not made widely available in the United States until the mid-1960s. In the following sections,

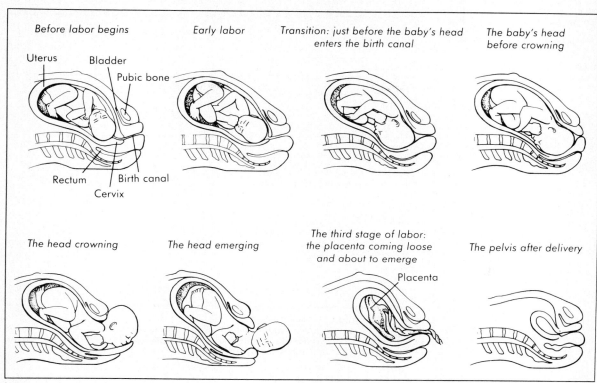

Before labor begins

Uterus
Bladder
Pubic bone

Rectum
Birth canal
Cervix

Early labor

Transition: just before the baby's head enters the birth canal

The baby's head before crowning

The head crowning

The head emerging

The third stage of labor: the placenta coming loose and about to emerge

Placenta

The pelvis after delivery

Figure 3–4.

The process at birth.

we will discuss *contraception, sterilization*, and *abortion* as methods of birth control. Total coital abstinence is neither a feasible nor an attractive birth control method for a majority of people and for this reason will not be considered.

Contraception

Contraception is defined here as any *birth control method or device permitting coitus between a fertile male and fertile female that prevents conception and pregnancy* (McCary, 1978). A number of contraceptive methods or devices are now available, and our discussion will include consideration of how each works and its effectiveness, advantages, and disadvantages. Before we begin, however, some comment on the concept of contraceptive effectiveness is necessary. Estimates of *contraceptive effectiveness* are usually based on the percentage of coitally active women who become pregnant within one year while using a particular method. That is, if during a year of use of Method X, five out of one hundred women become pregnant, the *effectiveness* of Method X is 95 percent. Conversely, the *failure rate* of Method X is 5 percent. Our discussion will focus on two types of failure rates. First, there is the *theoretical failure rate*, which is the percentage of failures that would occur if the method were used perfectly. The second is the *actual failure rate*, which is the empirically estimated percentage of failures that

Table 3–1.

Theoretical and actual failure rates of various methods of birth control.

Method	Theoretical Failure Rate[1]	Actual Failure Rate[2]
Total abstinence	0.00	?
Abortion	0.00	0.00+
Sterilization		
Tubal ligation	0.04	0.04
Vasectomy	0.15	0.15+
Contraception		
Combined oral contraceptive	0.34	4–10
Progestin-only pills (mini-pill)	1.0–1.5	5–10
Long-acting progesterone injections	0.25	5–10
IUD	1.0–3.0	5.0
Diaphragm and spermicide	3.0	17.0
Spermicidal foam	3.0	22.0
Douche	?	40.0
Condom	3.0	10.0
Condom and spermicide	Less than 1.0	5.0
Withdrawal	9.0	20–25
Rhythm (calendar)	13.0	21.0
Chance (no method)	90.0	90.0

SOURCE: Adapted from Hatcher et al., 1980.
[1]Percentage of failures that would occur if the method were used perfectly.
[2]Empirically estimated percentage of failures that occur among all users, including those who use the method inconsistently or fail to follow all directions for its use.

occur among all users, including those who use the method inconsistently or fail to follow all directions for its use. Table 3–1 summarizes recent estimates of theoretical and actual failure rates of various birth control methods including contraceptives.

Hormonal Contraceptives

Fairly substantial gains in understanding the complex relationships among hormones and fertility and in biochemistry during the 1930s and 1940s made possible the development in the 1950s of orally administered hormones capable of altering female fertility. It is estimated that throughout the world nearly 100 million women, including some 15 million in the United States, now use the *Pill* as a method of contraception (Hatcher et al., 1980).

The Pill may, in fact, be one of several different types of hormonal tablets available by medical prescription for contraceptive use. All birth control pills function by disrupting one or more aspects of the natural ovarian or menstrual cycles. Recall from our discussion in Chapter 2 that ovarian and menstrual cycles consist of sequential changes in the ovaries and uterine lining associated with varying circulating levels of the hormones estrogen and progesterone. During the first half (menstrual and follicular phases) of the ovarian cycle, low levels of estrogen stimulate the pituitary gland to secrete FSH, prompting the growth and development of an ovum. Circulating levels of progesterone are relatively low at this time, allowing the pituitary to secrete substantial amounts of LH as estrogen levels peak around midcycle (fourteen days after the beginning of menstruation in the average twenty-eight-day cycle). Ovulation is triggered by the sharp rise in LH. During the second half (secretory, or luteal, phase) of the cycle, estrogen and progesterone secreted by the corpus luteum prepare the uterine lining for implantation of the fertilized ovum if fertilization has taken place.

Combination Pills.   The most widely used Pill is the *combination birth control pill*, which contains both *estrogen* and **progestin** (a synthetic progesterone) in dosages far in excess of normal circulating levels. Starting on the fifth day of her menstrual period a woman takes one pill per day for twenty-one days, then takes no pill (or inactive placebo pills) for seven days, and then resumes the cycle. Combination pills act as contraceptives in several ways but most importantly by preventing ovum growth and ovulation. The high levels of estrogen and progestin contained in the pills inhibit pituitary secretions of FSH and LH, both of which are necessary for ovulation. In addition, high levels of progestin change the mucus secretions of the cervix, creating a "hostile environment" for sperm and making the mucus so thick that sperm movement is hampered or blocked. Further, the uterine lining is altered by progestin so that even if fertilization occurs, implantation of the egg is inhibited. Withdrawal of estrogen and progestin when the pills are stopped after day 21 results in *withdrawal bleeding* resembling menstruation but usually briefer and lighter since full endometrium development has been inhibited. So that users will not have to continually "watch the calendar," most manufacturers include seven placebo pills for the seven days when no contraceptively active pills are taken (Hatcher et al., 1980).

The hormonal effects of combination pills are in many ways similar to the hormonal changes associated with pregnancy when estrogen and progesterone levels are elevated, preventing ovulation and menstruation (see Figure 2–11). Since the pattern of taking pills is designed to overtly mimic but physiologically short-circuit ovarian and menstrual cycles, timing and consistency are extremely important if the Pill is to be effective.

The first pill in the series of twenty-one should be taken on the fifth day of the menstrual cycle and no later than the sixth day or ovulation might occur. Thereafter, one pill per day is taken until the twenty-one-day supply is expended. Consistency is important since missing even one pill slightly increases the probability of ovulation. If a woman misses one pill, she should take two the following day (the one she missed plus the regular pill for that day). If she misses two pills in a row, she should immediately take those two and two more on the following day. Since missing two pills increases the chances of ovulation, an additional means of contraception such as condoms or foam should be used along with the Pill throughout the remainder of the cycle. If three pills are missed, ovulation is likely and the woman should discard the pills remaining in the packet and immediately use another method of birth control. Since the Pill is not reliable during the first cycle of its use, a second method of birth control should be used until the beginning of the second cycle (Hatcher et al., 1980).

Theoretically and in actual practice, combination pills are exceeded in effectiveness as a birth control method only by total abstinence, sterilization, and abortion, as indicated in Table 3–1. The theoretical failure rate is less than 1 percent, meaning that less than 1 percent of women who use the Pill perfectly, exactly according to instructions, and without error, become pregnant during a year of Pill use. In actual use the failure rate is from 4 to 10 percent, with most failures occurring as a result of forgetting to take a pill for two or more days (Hatcher et al., 1980).

Hormones are powerful systemic agents affecting nearly all of the body's major organ systems. It is not surprising, then, that the use of oral contraceptives is associated with a number of noncontraceptive side effects, some of which are desirable and some undesirable. Although the undesirable side effects of the Pill have received the greatest amount of media publicity, beneficial effects have also been reported. Pill use minimizes premenstrual tension and menstrual cramping, reduces the number of days of menstrual flow and amount of blood loss, and eliminates midcycle pain associated with ovulation. Contraceptive pills are sometimes prescribed to inhibit growth of ovarian cysts and nonmalignant breast growths, for relief of endometriosis (abnormal growth of uterine tissue), and to postpone menstruation. Pill users experience a lower incidence of iron deficiency anemia and sometimes report relief from acne. The increased breast size associated with Pill use is sometimes also perceived as beneficial (Boston Women's Health Book Collective, 1976; Hatcher et al., 1980; Royal College of General Practitioners, 1974).

The effects of contraceptive pill use on sexual behavior are unclear. Some couples report more pleasurable and spontaneous coitus because the risk of pregnancy is virtually absent and the contraceptive method is not used at the time of coitus (DeLora & Warren, 1977). Both married (Udry, Morris, & Waller, 1973) and unmarried (Spitz, Gold, & Adams, 1975) women using contraceptive pills engage in coitus more frequently than do women using other types of contraceptives. The question of whether or not female sexual responsiveness is modified by contraceptive pills is, at this time, unanswered (Bragonier, 1976).

The undesirable side effects and complications resulting from Pill use range in seriousness from "fairly minor" to "life threatening" (Hatcher et al., 1980). Around 40 percent of those who use the Pill experience at least minor undesirable side effects while taking it, although many of those side effects disappear after two or three cycles or after users switch to different brands. Minor side effects include nausea, weight gain, mild headaches, spotting (bleeding) between periods, missed periods, increased problems with vaginal yeast infections, and chloasma (the "mask of pregnancy") in which the facial skin darkens (Hatcher et al., 1980). Another 1 percent experience serious or life-threatening complications such as hypertension, gallbladder disease, diabetes, and increased susceptibility to gonorrhea (Boston Women's Health Book Collective, 1976; Hatcher et al., 1980).

More rare, but potentially life threatening, is a slight increase in the probability of blood clotting (thromboembolic) and related cardiovascular disorders. The late 1960s and early 1970s witnessed a rash of alarming (and alarmist) reports of the dangerous consequences of using contraceptive pills. Although it is difficult to interpret some of the claims concerning complications resulting from the Pill, it is estimated that very few women actually die from Pill-related complications. The death rate due to blood clots and cardiovascular disorders linked to Pill use has been rather consistently estimated at between 0.3 and 3 per 100,000 (Boston Women's Health Book Collective, 1976; Hatcher et al., 1980), although a recent British study suggested the death rate is much higher, 20 per 100,000 (Hatcher et al., 1980). In comparison, however, it should be noted that the death rate due to complications associated with pregnancy and childbirth is estimated at 9.4 per 100,000 women, or at least three times as high as that reported in most studies of Pill use ("Annual Summary," December 7, 1978). There is no clear evidence linking use of the Pill to cancer.

Substantially more research is needed to accurately define the medical risks associated with contraceptive pills. It does seem clear, however, that the risks of clotting disorders and death are considerably higher among Pill users over age forty and among smokers. Because of the above-mentioned and other potential side effects, some women should *definitely not* use estrogen-containing (combination) contraceptive pills. Such women include those with clotting or circulatory disorders, those with liver diseases, those with reproductive system or breast cancer, and those who are pregnant. Other strong contraindications include migraine headaches, hypertension, diabetes, gallbladder disease, acute mononucleosis, sickle cell disease, and age over forty coupled with obesity, heavy smoking, or high cholesterol levels (Hatcher et al., 1980).

All of this may seem a bit frightening. It is not meant to be so. But one should be aware that combination pills do have some serious potential dangers for high-risk individuals. At the same time, however, the Pill is a highly effective contraceptive that poses little or no danger to *most* users. All Pill users should have regular and thorough medical examinations and should *never borrow pills* from a friend since prescriptions are tailored to medical needs and tolerances on an individual basis. If a woman runs out of pills, she should use some other birth control method (Hatcher et al., 1980).

Progestin-Only Pills.   Most of the undesirable side effects associated with combination pills are estrogen-related. In part because of this, *progestin-only pills* (the **Mini-Pill**) were introduced in the United States in January 1973. These pills contain low dosages of progestin and no estrogen. Progestin-only pills are taken continuously and their contraceptive action is thought to result from inhibition of sperm transport and motility, of ovum transport, and of implantation in the event an egg is fertilized. Ovulation may or may not be inhibited. The theoretical (1 to 1.5 percent) and actual (5 to 10 percent) failure rates of Mini-Pills are higher than those for combination pills, but most failures occur during the first six months of use. The major side effects of the Mini-Pill are irregular menstrual bleeding, spotting, and amenorrhea (failure to menstruate). Thromboembolic disorders have not been linked to the Mini-Pill, but women with histories of blood clotting should avoid all hormonal contraceptives (Hatcher et al., 1980).

Diethylstilbestrol (DES) Tablets.   In 1973 the synthetic estrogen **diethylstilbestrol (DES)** was granted approval by the FDA for emergency use following unprotected coitus at midcycle. This so-called **morning-after pill** is reserved for use following such emergencies as rape or incest and should not be used as a regular method of birth control. Within seventy-two (preferably twenty-four) hours of unprotected intercourse, the woman begins a five-day regimen of taking two daily massive doses (25 milligrams per tablet) of DES. These high doses of estrogen are thought to inhibit implantation of a fertilized egg if fertilization has occurred. The failure rate of the morning-after pill has been reported to be less than 1 percent, but some pregnancies do occur resulting from excessive time lapse between coitus and DES ingestion, inadequate dosages of DES, and regurgitation of the ingested dosage. One of the most frequent side effects of the morning-after pill that sometimes causes failure is severe nausea and vomiting. If pregnancy does occur, abortion should be seriously considered since DES may harm the fetus. *Possible effects* include vaginal cancer in female offspring and testicular abnormalities in male offspring (Hatcher et al., 1980).

Other Hormonal Contraceptives. A variety of other hormonal contraceptive methods are currently under investigation for safety and effectiveness, including long-acting progesterone injections (the Shot) for contraceptive protection lasting up to three months. Although very effective and currently marketed in sixty-four countries, because of serious side effects associated with it, in mid-1978 the FDA rejected one form of the Shot (Depo Provera) for use as a long-acting contraceptive in the United States (Hatcher et al., 1980). Yet another drug, called **RU–486**, has been developed in France and is currently undergoing testing. RU-486 is an "antiprogesterone" drug that blocks the action of progesterone and prevents implantation of a fertilized ovum or dislodges an already implanted ovum from the uterine walls. The drug seems to be relatively free of negative side effects (Clark, Nater, & Witherspoon, 1982).

Other devices undergoing development include under-the-skin implants that slowly release hormones, vaginal rings that gradually release estrogen or progestin or both, and hormonal contraceptives for use by men. Many of these methods may not be available for several years, although the Chinese claimed in 1979 to have developed an effective contraceptive pill for men with few undesirable side effects. Receiving FDA approval in 1976 was a progesterone impregnated intrauterine device (IUD), the Progestasert–T (Hatcher et al., 1980).

Nonhormonal Methods of Contraception

Though many of the hormonal contraceptives discussed above are quite effective, for many people they are not the method of choice for any number of different reasons. There are, however, several contraceptive methods that do not rely on hormones for their effect. In this section we discuss the most common of these.

Intrauterine Devices (IUDs). Modern **intrauterine devices** are small, sometimes oddly shaped pieces of plastic that are placed in the uterus for contraceptive purposes. Although widely used in the United States for scarcely more than two decades (Hatcher et al., 1980), various types of foreign objects have been placed in uteri for many purposes for over two thousand years. Some of these objects have been made of wool, wood, silver, gold, ivory, and even diamond-studded platinum. Arab and Turkish camel drivers have, for centuries, placed small stones in the uterus of each camel to prevent pregnancy on long desert trips (DeLora & Warren, 1977). After years of investigation in Britain, Germany, and Japan, IUDs were finally developed for use in the United States in 1959. Some 15 million women throughout the world, including over 3 million in the United States, were using IUDs in 1978 (Hatcher et al., 1980).

The types of IUDs approved for use by the FDA and marketed in 1976 are shown in actual size in Figure 3–5. The Dalkon Shield, once a widely used IUD, was recalled from the market by the manufacturer in 1974 because of the high rates of

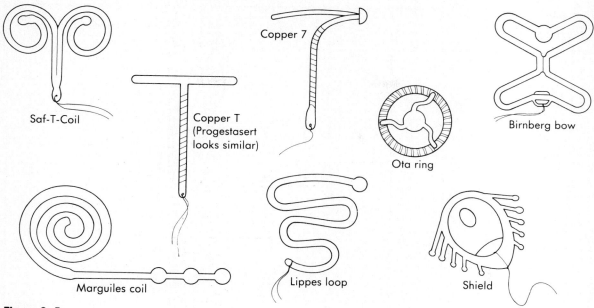

Figure 3–5.

Types of IUDs (actual sizes).

infection and other complications it caused (Boston Women's Health Book Collective, 1976). Two of the devices shown (the Copper 7 and Copper T) are wrapped with copper wire and one (the Progestasert T) is impregnated with progesterone.

Although the mechanisms by which IUDs work are not definitely established, current thought is that they provoke a mild inflammatory reaction in the uterus, thus rendering the uterine walls resistant to implantation of a fertilized egg. The copper devices release small amounts of copper, which is thought to further increase the inhospitality of the uterus to the egg. The Progestasert T releases tiny quantities of progesterone into the uterus, adding a hormonal contraceptive effect to the physical effects of the device itself (Boston Women's Health Book Collective, 1976; Hatcher et al., 1980).

IUDs may be inserted rather simply, quickly, and painlessly in most cases. As shown in Figure 3–6, for example, the Lippes Loop (like the other devices) is stretched into linear form and placed into the uterus through a small plastic tube (3 to 6 millimeters in diameter), which is inserted in the cervical opening. The tiny plastic or nylon threads attached to the devices protrude 2 to 5 centimeters (an inch or two) into the vagina so that the woman, her sexual partner, or her physician may easily determine if the IUD is in place, or has been expelled. If the plastic end of the IUD itself is protruding from the cervix, it is ineffective; a backup birth control method must be used and a physician consulted.

The theoretical (1 to 3 percent) and actual (1 to 8 percent, depending on the device) failure rates, though somewhat higher than those for combination pills, are nevertheless excellent. Most of the failures actually occur during the first three months of use, when expulsions are most likely to occur. In addition to being

Figure 3–6.

IUD insertion.

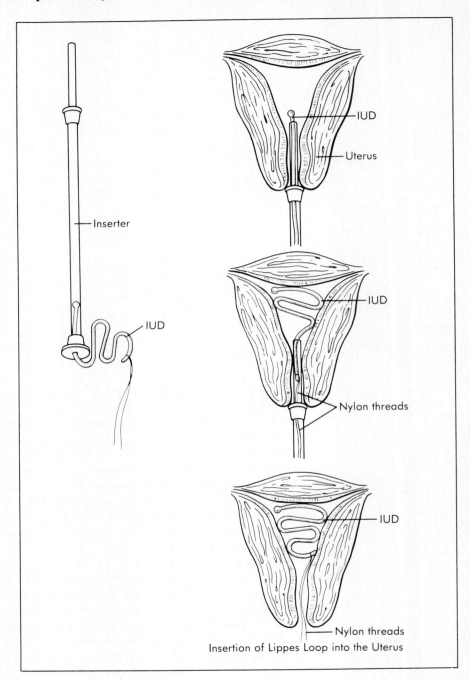

Inserter

IUD

IUD

Uterus

IUD

Nylon threads

IUD

Nylon threads

Insertion of Lippes Loop into the Uterus

highly effective, IUDs offer a number of other advantages. First, like the Pill, an IUD does not interfere in any way with coitus. Once inserted, it is left in the uterus until the woman desires to become pregnant or has it removed for other reasons. One advantage of an IUD over pills is that the woman does not have to remember to use it. All she needs to remember is to check the strings periodically to make sure it is in place. Finally, unlike the Pill, IUDs exert no known systemic effects; the liver, heart, breasts, and other major organ systems are unaffected by them.

There are, however, some potential disadvantages to IUD use. Some women experience considerable pain during and immediately following insertion of an IUD. Others (10 to 20 percent) experience painful cramping and heavy bleeding during the first two or three menstrual periods following insertion. Two more serious complications may arise from faulty insertion practices. When nonsterile devices or insertion techniques are used, there is a high probability of pelvic infections. When infections occur, the IUD should be removed and the infection treated before the IUD is replaced. In rare instances (less than 1 per 100,000 users), death may result from serious infections. Faulty insertion techniques may (1 in 1000 to 10,000 cases) result in perforation of the uterus and escape of the IUD into the abdominal cavity. The IUD must then be surgically removed and the woman treated for the very real possibility of serious infection (Katchadourian & Lunde, 1980).

In those relatively rare instances in which pregnancy occurs during IUD use, the chances of spontaneous abortion are about 50 percent if the IUD is left in place. Removal of the IUD induces abortion in around 25 percent of the cases. There is some evidence that use of IUDs increases the incidence of ectopic pregnancy (see page 44). Finally, the expulsion rate of IUDs is fairly high. Depending on the type and size of device used, expulsion occurs in between 3 and 12 percent of the women fitted, most frequently during the first three months after insertion and during menstruation. As noted earlier, users should periodically check their IUDs, particularly after menstruation (Hatcher et al., 1980). There is no reliable evidence linking IUD use to cancer.

Because of possible side effects, a number of women should not use IUDs. These include those who are pregnant and those who have endometriosis, venereal diseases, pelvic inflammatory disease, cardiac disease, anemia, sickle cell disease, uterine abnormalities, or vaginal and uterine infections. Also included are those who experience heavy menstrual flows or cramping, those with a very small uterus, and young teenagers (Boston Women's Health Book Collective, 1976).

Diaphragms.   The **diaphragm** is a thin dome-shaped rubber cup stretched over a rubber-covered flexible circular rim. Prior to coitus, it is inserted to fit snugly in the vagina with its posterior (back) rim resting behind the cervix and the anterior (front) rim wedged behind the pubic bone. Spermicidal (sperm-killing) cream or jelly is placed in the cup and around the rim of the diaphragm prior to insertion. As a contraceptive, the diaphragm works in two ways. First, the diaphragm itself seals off the entrance to the uterus (cervix) and acts as a physical barrier to sperm penetration. Second, the spermicidal cream or jelly inactivates or kills any sperm that circumvent the diaphragm or remain in the vaginal barrel. *To be effective, the diaphragm must be used with a spermicidal.*

Since women differ in the size and muscular tone of their vaginas, diaphragms also differ in rim diameter (50 to 105 millimeters) and must be individually fitted by a physician. It is important that a woman be fitted with the largest diaphragm that she can comfortably tolerate. Vaginal depth, angulation, and muscle tone all change during sexual arousal, and the movements and positions (particularly woman above) of coitus may dislodge an undersize diaphragm, rendering it virtually useless. If a woman experiences pregnancy, abortion, pelvic surgery, or weight changes of more than ten pounds, she should have her diaphragm refitted because of possible changes in her vaginal dimensions. In any event, she should be refitted with a new diaphragm at least every two years as a precaution against possible deterioration of the device. A diaphragm cannot be fitted if the hymen is intact, and, since her vaginal characteristics will change with coitus, a virgin should be fitted only after a few coital experiences using another type of birth control (Boston Women's Health Book Collective, 1976; Hatcher et al., 1980). Since proper fit is critical to the effectiveness of a diaphragm, the importance of never borrowing one from another woman should be apparent.

A diaphragm may be filled and rimmed with spermicidal and inserted up to two hours prior to coitus. If inserted more than two hours before coitus, additional spermicidal should be inserted in front of the diaphragm with an applicator before any penile-vaginal penetration occurs. Following coitus, the diaphragm should be left in place for six to eight hours so that the spermicidal may fully inactivate all sperm. A new application of spermicidal is necessary *before* penile-vaginal penetration *each time* coitus occurs during the six hours the diaphragm must stay in place. The diaphragm should be removed within at least twenty-four hours to avoid unpleasant odors. When removed (no sooner than six hours after intercourse), it should be washed with warm water and a mild soap, dried carefully with a towel, and stored in its plastic container. It may be dusted lightly with cornstarch but *not with talcum powder or perfumed powder*, since the latter two products may destroy the diaphragm. Similarly, *Vaseline should not be used* in association with a diaphragm (or condom) because it causes the rubber to deteriorate. A diaphragm should be inspected for holes before each use by holding it up to a light or filling it with water and looking for leaks (Boston Women's Health Book Collective, 1976; Hatcher et al., 1980).

Diaphragms are easily inserted (Figure 3–7), and a woman's physician or nurse should provide instruction when the device is fitted. Some couples integrate diaphragm insertion into their foreplay—they may put it in together or the man may insert it.

When used properly, the diaphragm can be an extremely effective means of birth control. Its theoretical failure rate is 3 percent, and in actual use failures occur in from 2 to 17 percent of users, depending on the particular study consulted (Hatcher et al., 1980). Most failures result from improper use, such as failing to apply or reapply spermicidal or taking the diaphragm out too soon. Obviously, a diaphragm simply does not work if it is left in a purse or dresser drawer (DeLora & Warren, 1977).

Other than the possibility that the spermicidal cream or jelly may irritate the vagina or the penis, there are virtually no side effects from use of a diaphragm. Irritation may be remedied by switching to another brand of spermicidal. Some *potential* disadvantages do exist, however. Since its insertion must closely precede coitus, those who insist on total spontaneity in their sexual relationship will be disappointed with the diaphragm. To be effective, it must be used every time and a

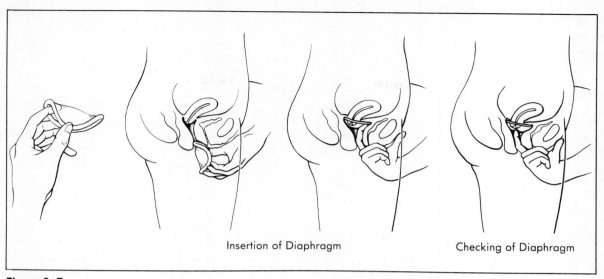

Insertion of Diaphragm   Checking of Diaphragm

Figure 3–7.

Inserting and checking the placement of a diaphragm.

woman must remember to have it and a supply of spermicide with her whenever intercourse might take place. For some women who are averse to touching their genitals, a diaphragm is not the preferred birth control method. Finally, some women may dislike the leakage of the cream or jelly following coitus and others may experience declines in sexual arousal if diaphragm insertion interrupts foreplay (Vonderheide & Mosher, 1981).

For many, however, these potential disadvantages are outweighed by the positive aspects of the diaphragm, including its reliability, its freedom from major side effects, and complete return to fertility as soon as it is removed. The diaphragm is a good choice for the woman who has coitus infrequently and neither needs nor desires continuous infertility. Finally, for those who wish to have coitus during the woman's menstrual period, the diaphragm may be inserted for a few hours to hold the menstrual flow.

Somewhat similar in function to the diaphragm is a device called a *cervical cap* that is custom-molded to fit over and cover a woman's cervix blocking the passage of sperm. A one-way valve allows menstrual fluids and cervical secretions to flow outward but keeps out sperm. The device may be left in place up to a full year and is currently undergoing testing.

Vaginal Spermicides.   Vaginal **spermicides** are foam, cream, or jelly substances placed in the vagina prior to coitus for the dual purpose of (1) mechanically blocking the cervical opening and so preventing the entry of sperm and (2) chemically immobilizing and killing sperm. Contraceptive foams (Delfen, Emko) are available in aerosol cans along with plastic applicators that are filled from the cans. The filled applicator is inserted into the vagina and the foam is then pushed out of the applicator near the cervix with a plunger. Spermicidal creams and jellies are packaged in tubes but inserted into the vagina in much the same way as are foams (see Figure 3–8).

Figure 3–8.

Insertion of vaginal spermicides.

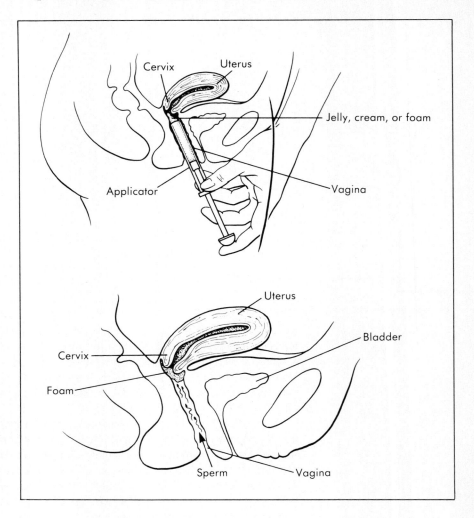

Spermicides must be placed in the vagina before (but not more than thirty minutes before) coitus takes place, left in for at least eight hours after, and to be effective, must be reapplied before each act of coitus that takes place within this time period. If a woman wants to douche (flush the vagina with a liquid), she should wait until at least eight hours have elapsed (Hatcher et al., 1980).

Spermicidal creams and jellies are not as effective as foams since they do not distribute as well within the vagina. Thus, one influential source (Hatcher et al., 1980) does not recommend their use without a diaphragm. Theoretically, with perfect use, foams have a failure rate of 3 percent. In actual use, however, failure rates as high as 29 percent have been reported. Failures occur not so much because of the limitations of the method itself as to careless use. Often, women use too little foam, fail to reapply foam before each act of coitus, douche too soon, fail to shake the foam container thoroughly, or simply run out of foam and "take their chances" (Hatcher et al., 1980).

The major advantage to vaginal spermicides is that they are readily available without prescription in a drugstore and may be used as a backup contraceptive method if no more effective method is available at the time. Furthermore, it appears that foam exerts a slight inhibiting effect on the transmission of gonorrhea.

Vaginal spermicides are, however, not very effective and should not be used as the primary means of birth control. Some couples find them a bit messy and do not appreciate interrupting lovemaking to apply them. Their taste is generally very unpleasant and thus interferes with cunnilingus (oral-genital stimulation of the female). Some irritate the vagina or penis but switching brands often eliminates this problem. Because of their relatively high failure rates, spermicides should be used primarily as a temporary substitute or supplement for other more reliable methods—with a new IUD, immediately following a vasectomy, or when a woman has missed a pill.

Recently a new product, the Encore Oval, which is a spermicidal vaginal suppository that melts and then foams in the presence of vaginal warmth and moisture, has been marketed in the United States. In limited studies, very low failure rates (less than 1 percent) have been reported for the Oval, but until more thorough and adequate research has been conducted, it should be considered no more effective than foam. Development is currently underway on condoms designed to dissolve during coitus, releasing a spermicidal agent (Hatcher et al., 1980). Approved and entering the market in 1983 was the *contraceptive sponge*, a spermicidally treated foam rubber device that combines a sperm blockage and spermicidal approach to contraception. Requiring no prescription, the device is vaginally inserted to cover the cervix and may be left in place several days.

Douches.   Some women believe that using **douches** (liquid flushed into the vagina) of water, cola, vinegar, or some commercially available solution is an effective contraceptive. Actually, the only way for douching to be contraceptively effective is for a woman to skip intercourse and douche instead. The basic idea behind douching involves an attempt to flush semen from the vagina before sperm are able to enter the uterus. Generally, though, sperm can swim to the uterus faster than a woman can run to the bathroom. Even if a woman is able to win the race, the douche itself may force some sperm *into* the uterus (Boston Women's Health Book Collective, 1976). About 40 percent of those women who rely exclusively on douching for contraception become pregnant within one year (Hatcher et al., 1980). It is *not effective* as a contraceptive method. In addition, frequent douching can remove some of the beneficial bacteria that reside in a healthy vagina, increasing susceptibility to vaginal infection (DeLora & Warren, 1977).

Condoms.   The **condom** ("rubber," "safe," "prophylactic") is a thin sheath made of latex ("rubber") or the intestinal tissue of lambs ("skins") that fits over the erect penis and acts as a physical barrier to the transmission of semen into the vagina. Upon ejaculation, it catches the semen and holds it until the condom is removed. Although the history of condoms may be traced to the Egyptian practice of wearing decorative covers over their penises as early as 1350 B.C., their widespread use as contraceptives awaited Goodyear's development of a vulcanization process for rubber in the mid-1800s (Hatcher et al., 1980).

Most condoms come rolled up in a small packet and are simply unrolled over the erect penis before it enters the vagina. Condoms are about 19 centimeters (7.5 inches) long, and the open ends are fitted with a soft rubber ring approximately 3 centimeters (1⅜ inches) in diameter that help keep them on the penis (see Figure 3–9). Two condom designs are available. Some have protruding nipplelike tips that act as reservoirs for semen. Others have rounded or "plain" ends; when these are put on, about one half inch of air-free space should be left at the tip to hold semen and help prevent the condom from bursting during ejaculation. Some condoms are lubricated but, if needed to ease penetration, additional lubricant may be added. *Petroleum jelly should not be used* because it will cause the rubber to deteriorate. Contraceptive foams, creams, jellies, and saliva may all be used.

Although all condoms sold in the United States must meet minimal government standards, those that are available in gasoline stations, pool halls, and taverns are of rather poor quality and should be avoided if possible. High-quality condoms are readily available in most drugstores and from a variety of mail-order firms (which ship in unmarked packages). High-quality condoms remain effective for about two years if stored in dark sealed containers away from heat. They deteriorate quickly when carried in wallets, pockets, or glove compartments of cars. If used for contraceptive purposes only (and not VD protection), they may be reused a few times if they are washed in warm soapy water, carefully dried, powdered with cornstarch, tested for leaks (by filling them with water or blowing them up like balloons), and stored properly after each use. Those used for disease protection should be used only once and discarded (Hatcher et al., 1980).

To be effective, condoms must be put on before the penis nears, touches, or penetrates the vagina, since before orgasm a small amount of sperm-containing secretion often escapes from the penis (see Chapters 2 and 5). Following ejaculation, the man or his partner must hold onto the condom near the base of the penis as it is withdrawn in order to prevent spillage of any semen into the vagina. Withdrawal should occur shortly after ejaculation for, as the erection is lost, the condom may slip, allowing semen to escape.

When used properly, condoms are quite effective as contraceptives. The theoretical failure rate is around 3 percent. In use, however, failure rates as high as 15 to 20 percent have been reported in some studies. Failure rates of less than 1 percent may be achieved by combining contraceptive foams or diaphragms with condom use. Most failures result from improper use, such as putting the condom on after a period of penetration but before ejaculation, failure to withdraw carefully, or inconsistent use—leaving the condom in its package.

Many couples object to condoms because they must be put on after the penis is erect and thus interrupt sex play. Some, however, integrate this into their sex play, with the woman putting the condom on her partner's penis. Many men complain that condoms reduce glans sensitivity and the pleasures of coitus ("It's like taking a shower with a raincoat on"). This problem may be partially overcome through the use of natural "skin" condoms, which provide more effective heat transfer. In recent years, manufacturers have developed very thin condoms and condoms that are "preshaped" in forms that grip more tightly just behind the glans of the penis. There have been other innovations designed to increase the attractiveness of condoms as contraceptives as well. Condoms may be transparent, decoratively colored ("sunset red," "siesta green," "midnight black," "dawn gold"), scented

Figure 3–9.

Putting on a condom.

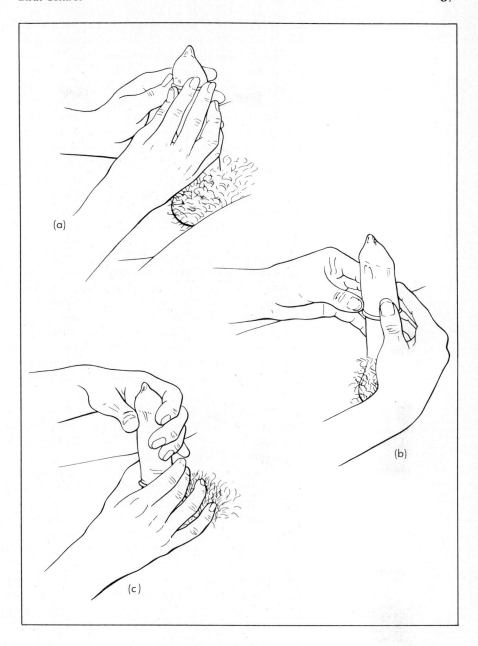

(a)

(b)

(c)

(musk, strawberry, banana, lime), textured with raised ribs or dots on the outside to increase stimulation of the woman, and even capable of glowing in the dark. A recent catalogue from a well-known distributor (Adam & Eve) devotes over ten pages to various types of condoms.

In addition to their contraceptive value, condoms may help prevent premature ejaculation, are readily available, are relatively simple to use, and provide significant (but not total) protection against the spread of venereal diseases.

Withdrawal.   The **withdrawal** ("coitus interruptus," "pulling out," "being care-ful") method of birth control allows a couple to engage in coitus any time they wish but requires the man to withdraw his penis from the vagina prior to ejaculation so that semen is prevented from entering the uterus. Ejaculation must, however, occur as far from the vulva as possible since sperm that contact the warm moist labia may be able to work their way to the uterus. Withdrawal is the oldest known method of birth control and has probably been practiced since humans first recognized a connection between ejaculation in the vagina and conception.

Although some couples rely on withdrawal with success for many years, it is not a very effective means of birth control. It has a theoretical effectiveness rate of 10 to 15 percent; if one hundred couples use withdrawal perfectly for one year, ten to fifteen pregnancies will result. In practice the actual failure rate is between 20 and 30 percent (Hatcher et al., 1980). Failures occur for many reasons, the most important of which is the failure of the man to withdraw in time. Some men do not experience the sensation of "coming" during the emission stage of ejaculation preceding the actual expulsion of semen from the penis (see Chapter 5). Thus, they are unable to accurately anticipate ejaculation. Many men are able to withdraw prior to ejaculation only with great difficulty. The most usual impulse for men as ejaculation nears or begins is to thrust the penis deeply into the vagina and hold it there as orgasm takes place (Chapter 5)—an impulse that is directly counter to that which is required for withdrawal. Furthermore, even if a man withdraws prior to ejaculation, some semen may escape the penis with the preejaculatory secretion from the Cowper's glands (see Chapters 2 and 5). Finally, following ejaculation, some couples resume coitus with semen and sperm that may escape remaining in the penile urethra.

Because of the necessity for withdrawal, some couples find that this method detracts from relaxed enjoyment of coitus, since the man's attention and efforts are partly diverted to monitoring his own level of arousal and anticipating ejaculation. It is sometimes suggested that long-term use of withdrawal leads to premature ejaculation in men or orgasmic dysfunction in women (Boston Women's Health Book Collective, 1976). Although there is little direct evidence for these effects, it is possible that if the man withdraws before his partner has reached orgasm, she *may* be left with genitals swollen from sexual arousal (see Chapters 2 and 5) and some discomfort. There are, of course, many other avenues to orgasm (manual and oral) open for women as well as men.

Rhythm Methods.   A woman's reproductive capabilities vary rhythmically, shift-ing between periods of fertility and infertility. The basis for the **rhythm method** of birth control is abstinence from coitus during the fertile period of a woman's cycle. The major difficulty with this method is determining precisely when a woman is fertile and when she is not. At least three methods of calculating periods of fertility have been devised. Each is based on at least two assumptions: (1) that sperm remain viable and capable of fertilizing a viable ovum for two to three days; and (2) that an ovum survives for twenty-four hours following ovulation. Using the "calendar method" of calculation described below requires the additional assump-tion that ovulation occurs fourteen (plus or minus two) days *prior* to the onset of a menstrual period.

The *calendar method* allows a woman to roughly calculate the beginning and

Table 3–2.

Calculating fertility intervals using the calendar rhythm method. To determine her fertile period a woman should find the length of her shortest cycle in Column 1 and her first fertile day following the onset of menstruation in Column 2. Her last day of fertility following the onset of menstruation will be shown in Column 4 adjacent to the number of days corresponding to her longest menstrual cycle. She is fertile and should abstain from unprotected coitus between the days calculated from Columns 2 and 4.

Length of Shortest Cycle	First Fertile (Unsafe) Day	Length of Longest Cycle	Last Fertile (Unsafe) Day
21 days	3rd day	21 days	10th day
22	4th	22	11th
23	5th	23	12th
24	6th	24	13th
25	7th	25	14th
26	8th	26	15th
27	9th	27	16th
28	10th	28	17th
29	11th	29	18th
30	12th	30	19th
31	13th	31	20th
32	14th	32	21st
33	15th	33	22nd
34	16th	34	23rd
35	17th	35	24th

SOURCE: Adapted from Hatcher et al., 1980.

end of her fertile period—that time during which a viable egg is available for fertilization by viable sperm. The woman first must determine the degree of variability in the length of her menstrual cycles. (Length of cycle is the number of days from the first day of one menstrual period up to the first day of the following menstrual period.) Although the "model" menstrual cycle is twenty-eight days in length, there are substantial variations from one woman to another in cycle length and, in some women (particularly the young and those who have just given birth, had abortions, or are nearing menopause), from one cycle to the next. Thus, the woman must keep records of her cycle for eight to twelve months to determine the lengths of her shortest and her longest cycles. From this information she may then calculate the earliest day prior to ovulation on which she is *likely* to be fertile by subtracting eighteen days from the number of days in her shortest cycle. To estimate the latest day in a cycle on which she is likely to be fertile she subtracts eleven days from the length of her longest cycle. These two numbers represent the *possible* beginning and end of her fertile period in any given menstrual cycle during which she must abstain from coitus or use another method of birth control (Hatcher et al., 1980).

Periods of fertility for various combinations of shortest and longest cycles are shown in Table 3–2. As Table 3–2 indicates, women with very regular cycles have fewer days of fertility and required abstinence than do those with highly irregular cycles. For example, a woman with regular twenty-eight-day cycles need abstain only from day 10 to day 17 (eight days) following the first day of menstruation. In contrast, a woman whose cycles vary from twenty-five to thirty-three days must compensate for this irregularity by abstaining from day 7 through day 22 (sixteen).

A more accurate method for determining the time of ovulation, but one which *can pinpoint fertile days only after ovulation*, is the *basal body temperature (BBT) method*. This method is based upon the fact that during menstruation and prior to ovulation, a healthy woman's lowest daily body temperature (measured in the morning just after waking and before rising, eating, smoking, drinking, going to the bathroom, or having sex) will occur during menstruation and prior to ovulation.

Immediately preceding ovulation, her BBT will drop slightly and then rise sharply following ovulation and remain elevated until the next menstrual period. Thus, the sharp rise in BBT indicates that ovulation has occurred and she should abstain from coitus during the next three days.

In a *model twenty-eight-day menstrual cycle*, a chart of BBT readings would look like that shown in Figure 3–10. Figure 3–10 also depicts a liberal allowance of "safe days" for unprotected coitus. It should be understood, however, that the BBT method is unable to determine preovulatory fertility, and perfect use of this method alone would require total coital abstinence until three days after ovulation. Since ovulation sometimes occurs as early as day 7 of a cycle, a woman using the BBT method should totally avoid coitus or use some other method of birth control from day 3 until three days after ovulation if she truly wishes to prevent pregnancy. Ovulation virtually never occurs during menstruation, however, and unprotected coitus may take place fairly safely during the first two days of bleeding (Hatcher et al., 1980). Body temperature fluctuations due to infection, disease, emotional factors, medications, use of electric blankets, and so forth may interfere with the BBT method.

A third method of estimating time of ovulation depends on examination of *cervical mucus* secretions. These secretions change both in quantity and quality throughout the menstrual cycle. For a few days following menstruation there is generally a "dry period" during which no mucus is secreted, creating a sensation of

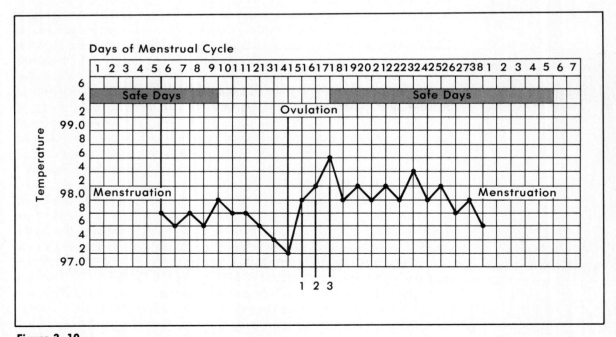

Figure 3–10.

Basal body temperature (BBT) variations during a model 28-day menstrual cycle.
SOURCE: From Hatcher et al., 1980.

vaginal dryness. This is a period of relative safety followed by the appearance of a thick yellowish preovulatory mucus. Around ovulation the secretion increases in quantity and immediately before ovulation becomes a sticky clear discharge resembling a raw egg white. There are two *peak days* of the clear discharge, and ovulation occurs within twenty-four hours after the last peak day. Coitus should be avoided from the appearance of the first discharge until four days after the peak days, at which time the mucus, if present, once again becomes cloudy or yellowish and coitus is safe (Hatcher et al., 1980).

It is often jokingly said that "Those who use the rhythm method are called parents." In fact, in actual use, rhythm methods of birth control result in failure in 15 to 40 percent of couples who use them. When the calendar method is used in combination with the BBT or cervical mucus method or both, however, lower failure rates are sometimes achieved (Hatcher et al., 1980). There are two major reasons for such high failure rates. First, less than 10 percent of women of childbearing age have regular menstrual cycles, which are necessary for accurately pinpointing the time of ovulation. Second, the rhythm method sometimes requires rather long periods of coital abstinence and some couples simply do not "follow the rules." The use of noncoital techniques of sexual expression can help alleviate this problem for many couples. The primary advantage of the rhythm method is that it is the only form of birth control approved by the Roman Catholic Church.

Sterilization

Sterilization is a term referring collectively to a number of surgical procedures wherein a man or a woman is rendered permanently incapable of reproduction (sterile or infertile). In part because it is a highly effective, permanent method which need be used only once, the popularity of sterilization as a birth control procedure has increased substantially in recent years. It is the most common method used worldwide (McCary, 1978) and it is estimated that the number of sterilized adults in the United States is nearly 10 million. In the late 1970s around 1.5 million adults in the United States were being voluntarily sterilized per year. These sterilizations were evenly split between men and women (Hatcher et al., 1980).

Because of well-known abuses of sterilization in Nazi Germany and in some parts of the United States (Boston Women's Health Book Collective, 1976), the spectre of involuntary sterilization imposed by governments or cruelly used by racist physicians is a very real one for many people. Even with voluntary sterilization, however, most physicians are relatively conservative. Recognizing the virtual finality of the procedures and the important roles of the abilities to impregnate and become pregnant in our conceptions of "manliness" and "womanliness," most physicians who perform sterilizations go to great lengths to be sure their patients are fully informed of the implications of permanent sterility. This involves explaining the procedures in some detail, emphasizing the irreversibility of sterilization, detailing the attendant risks, and discussing possible alternatives (Hatcher et al., 1980). Only after careful consideration of all these factors should a person make a decision concerning sterilization. Let us now examine the procedures involved in the surgical sterilization of males and females.

RESEARCH HIGHLIGHT

Teenagers, Sex, and Contraception

Although unwanted pregnancy and illegitimacy rates have shown a decline among women over twenty during the last several years, the trend has been just the opposite among teenage women. An obvious question is "Why so many unwanted teenage pregnancies when contraceptives are increasingly available and effective?" The equally obvious answer is that, even though sexually active, many teenagers are not making effective use of the available contraceptives. Melvin Zelnik and John Kantner (1977) reported that over 25 percent of sexually active teenage women never use contraceptive precautions, nearly 45 percent take precautions inconsistently, and only 30 percent always do so. Researchers have found that several conditions must be met before at least one member of a couple wishing to prevent pregnancy will take effective steps to do so (Byrne, Jazwinski, DeNinno, & Fisher (1977):

Condition 1. The relationship between coitus and pregnancy must be recognized.

Problems: (a) Only 40 percent of sexually active teenage women correctly perceive that the greatest risk of pregnancy occurs during the middle of the menstrual cycle. Taking a sex education course improves this rate to only 45 percent (Zelnik & Kanter, 1977). (b) Over 70 percent of sexually active teenage girls who do not use contraceptives do not think that they can become pregnant, because of the infrequency of their coitus, because of vague notions concerning coitus at certain times during the "menstrual month," or because of unfounded beliefs that they are sterile (Cvetkovitch, Grote, Bjorseth, & Sarkissian, 1975; Shah, Zelnik, & Kantner, 1975). (c) The guilt and generally negative attitudes our culture promotes concerning sexual matters interfere with acquisition of knowledge concerning conception (Schwartz, 1973).

Condition 2. At least one member of a potentially sexually active couple must acknowledge that coitus might occur.

Problem: In spite of its increasing prevalence, premarital coitus among teenagers is widely regarded as unacceptable unless it takes place spontaneously and in the context of love (see Chapters 9 and 10). The premeditation that is necessary for use of the most effective contraceptives is highly aversive to those who are generally guilty about their sexual activity (Allgeier, Przybyla, & Thompson, 1978).

Condition 3. At least one member of a sexually active couple must acquire knowledge of possible means of effective contraception.

Problem: Many teenagers have only superficial knowledge of contraceptive methods or devices. Some think that contraceptives are "dangerous" (Shah et al., 1975), and others have no knowledge whatsoever concerning methods for preventing pregnancy (Furstenberg, 1976).

Again, it is the sexually guilty who are least likely to obtain contraceptive knowledge (Schwartz, 1973).

Condition 4. At least one member of a sexually active couple must take the necessary actions to obtain contraceptive devices or medical services.

Problems: (a) Contraceptives requiring a medical prescription are not readily available to many teenagers (Zelnik & Kantner, 1977), and over 30 percent of sexually active teenage women who do not use contraceptives cite unavailability as their major reason (Shah et al., 1975). (b) Obtaining contraceptives can be an embarrassing experience for teenagers. This is particularly true for those who feel guilty concerning their sexuality (Fisher, Fisher, & Byrne, 1977).

Condition 5. At least one member of a sexually active couple must actually use a contraceptive method or device.

Problems: (a) Use of some contraceptives requires a medical prescription, a problem discussed above. Contraceptive pill use requires scheduled ingestion, which may be problematic for those of limited knowledge or intelligence (Shah et al., 1975). (b) Guilt and negative feelings about sexuality inhibit proper use of contraceptives for many. Those who think that sex should be spontaneous and impulsive are unlikely to interrupt sex play to insert a diaphragm, put on a condom, or insert spermicides. High-guilt individuals find contraceptive methods that require genital manipulation (condoms, diaphragms, spermicides, checking an IUD string) aversive (Byrne, 1977).

It may be seen that the odds are, in many ways, "stacked against" effective contraceptive use among unmarried teenagers. Assuming that trends toward an increasing incidence of coitus among teenagers will not be reversed, what are some of the possible solutions? First, it seems clear that earlier and more effective sex education focusing on the details of conception and its probability as a consequence of coitus at specific times during the menstrual cycle is essential. Also essential is sex education involving detailed information about contraception (Cvetkovitch, et al., 1975; Furstenberg, 1976). But knowledge alone is not the only answer. Contraceptives must be made more widely available to sexually active teenagers and in a way that minimizes the problems of embarrassment, shame, and fear of detection (Fisher et al., 1977; Zelnik & Kantner, 1977). Finally, the emotional barriers to contraceptive use must be weakened (Griffitt, 1983).

The idea that contraception can and should be an integral part of sex for those who wish to avoid pregnancy must somehow replace the notion that intercourse is pleasurable and acceptable only if it occurs "unintentionally," "spontaneously," "impulsively," or "in a moment of uncontrolled passion." That is, through sex education, contraceptive advertising, media representations of sex, or other means (Byrne, 1977), the attitude must be created that pleasurable, acceptable, rational, and responsible sex is that in which contraceptive practices appropriate to the situation are used (Fisher, Byrne, Edmunds, Miller, Kelley, & White, 1979).

Male Sterilization.   The primary method of male sterilization is the **vasectomy**, which involves severing the *vasa deferentia*, the two large ducts which transport sperm from the testes to the remaining reproductive structures and ducts (see Chapter 2). Vasectomy is a relatively minor surgical procedure requiring fifteen to twenty minutes, which can be performed in a physician's office.

Under local anesthesia, a small incision is made on one side of the scrotum, the vas on that side is located, cut, clamped or tied off, and, in some cases, cauterized. The incision is sewn up with absorbable sutures and the procedure is repeated on the other side (see Figure 3–11). Following a few minutes for recovery the man can then return home but should keep an ice pack on the scrotum for a few hours to reduce swelling, bleeding, and discomfort. He should wear a scrotal support for a period of time to prevent pulling the incision, remain relatively inactive for a couple of days, and avoid strenuous exercise or hard physical exertion for at least a week. Coitus may be resumed in from two to three days if it is not extremely uncomfortable (Hatcher et al., 1980).

Vasectomy does not confer instant sterility upon a man since some viable sperm remain in the ducts beyond the point where they are severed. Following at least ten ejaculations, the man brings a semen specimen to the laboratory for a sperm count. A second sperm count is taken around a month later; following *two negative sperm*

Figure 3–11.

Schematic representation of vasectomy.

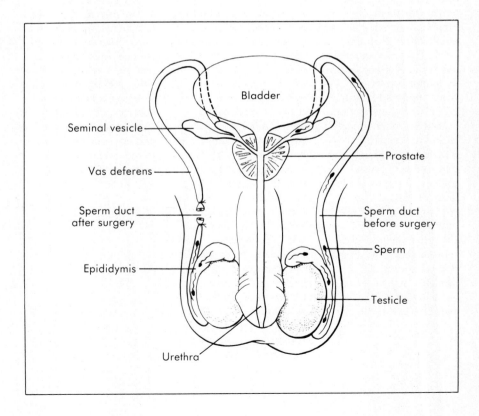

counts, the man may consider himself sterile. Until sterility is confirmed, some other method of birth control should be used. Vasectomy is virtually 100 percent effective, although failures do occur in around 0.15 percent of the cases. The few pregnancies that occur following vasectomy are mostly due to resumption of unprotected coitus prior to voiding the reproductive tract of viable sperm. In extremely rare cases a third, undetected vas exists or the severed ends of a vas grow back together (Hatcher et al., 1980). It is important to realize that failures sometimes do occur (though rarely) and a man may retain his capability of impregnation after vasectomy. Ignorance of this possibility understandably results in severe discord between a couple if the woman becomes pregnant after the man has had a vasectomy (McCary, 1978).

Medical complications arising from vasectomies are rare and affect less than 5 percent of men. Most of these complications are rather minor, such as infections of the vas, which are easily treatable. Shortly following surgery, some pain, swelling, and discoloration in the scrotal region are not uncommon (Hatcher et al., 1980). Up to one third of men who have vasectomies may experience some discomfort when they first resume intercourse, and in around 10 percent this discomfort remains for up to a year (Freund & Davis, 1973). Such discomfort is due primarily to the pulling effect of testicular and scrotal elevation which accompanies sexual arousal (Chapter 5). In spite of these rather minor discomforts, over 98 percent of all men interviewed in one study indicated that, if they had it to do over, they would again have a vasectomy (Maschhoff, Fanshier, & Hansen, 1976).

Vasectomy should be considered a *permanent and irreversible* method of birth control. Although some success in reversing the effects of vasectomy through sophisticated microsurgical techniques has been reported, effective reversal depends heavily on the type of surgery initially used. Important variables include the length of vas removed, the placement of the incisions, the use of electrical current in cauterization, and the type of ligature employed to tie off each vas. Around a half to two thirds of men develop antibodies to their own sperm following vasectomy, further reducing the prospects for successful reversal (Hatcher et al., 1980). Thus, no man who thinks he might want to father a child (or more children) should undergo vasectomy under the assumption that its effects are readily reversible.

Very few men, however, "change their minds" or regret their decision to have vasectomies (Maschhoff et al., 1976). To be sure, some men, equating fertility with masculinity, experience doubts about their "manliness" or virility following vasectomy, and some even begin to experience difficulties with erection or ejaculation (Ziegler, 1971). It should be understood that if such difficulties occur they are psychosocially rather than biologically rooted. Vasectomy interferes with sperm transport only and disrupts neither hormonal production nor distribution, which is accomplished by the bloodstream. Furthermore, since sperm and other testicular products constitute less than 10 percent of semen, ejaculation continues as usual.

Vasectomy should not be confused with or equated with **castration**—surgical removal of the testes. Although castration does insure sterility, it also removes the major source of the male sex hormone androgen. Generally, such a drastic reduction of androgen leads to a gradual loss of sexual desire and loss of male secondary sex characteristics (see Chapters 2 and 4). Fortunately, castration is rarely performed for purposes of sterilization alone.

Several studies have revealed that the majority of men report complete satisfaction with their vasectomies. In many cases, sexual satisfaction increases for the man as well as his sexual partner. For example, few men report any postvasectomy decreases in their ability to obtain a strong erection, in the time required to ejaculate, or in the strength of their ejaculation (Freund & Davis, 1973). Those changes that do occur are most often positive ones, such as increased desire for, pleasure during, satisfaction with, and frequency of coitus (Freund & Davis, 1973; Maschhoff et al., 1976). Wives of men with vasectomies generally experience increased feelings of freedom to initiate and play an active role in intercourse, and they evaluate intercourse as more pleasurable than prior to vasectomy. Both men and women freely attribute such improvement in their sex lives to the vasectomy, which relieves both partners from fears of unwanted pregnancy (Freund & Davis, 1973; Maschhoff et al., 1976).

Female Sterilization.   The basic principle behind the primary methods of sterilization of women is the same as that for males—to permanently eliminate fertility by blocking reproductive system ducts so that male (sperm) and female (ova) germ cells cannot meet. In the case of females, the target ducts are the fallopian (uterine) tubes, which transport ova from the ovaries to the uterus (see Chapter 2). The generic name for the surgical procedures involved is **tubal ligation** (popularly called "tying the tubes"). By any one of various means the fallopian tubes are severed or blocked (with silastic bands or clips), preventing egg and sperm contact (see Figure 3–12).

Figure 3–12.

Schematic representation of female sterilization.

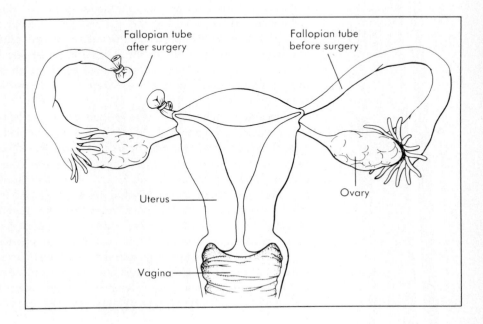

Methods of tubal ligation differ primarily in terms of the type of procedures used in locating and blocking the fallopian tubes and in the path of entry. All of the procedures are usually performed under general anesthesia and require at least a minimal hospital stay. In the procedure known as **laparotomy**, the tubes are visually located through a small (2 to 3 centimeter) incision in the lower abdomen. A small segment of each tube is surgically removed and the ends are tied off. Alternatively, the tubes are sometimes cauterized (burned). In a **culpotomy**, access to the tubes is gained via an incision at the end (cul de sac) of the vagina past the cervix. The tubes are visually located through the incision and cut and tied as in the laparotomy.

Laparoscopy and culdoscopy are variants of the general technique of **endoscopic sterilization**, in which a slender, self-contained, heatless light source (endoscope) is inserted into the abdominal cavity and used to locate the fallopian tubes. When the tubes can be seen through the instrument, a cauterizing device is inserted through the same puncture or through a second puncture and each of the tubes are burned through (cauterized) in one or more places. In **laparoscopy**, entrance is gained through a small puncture in the abdomen (often the navel) after the abdominal cavity has been inflated with carbon dioxide gas to separate the internal organs. After laparoscopy the gas is allowed to escape. Laparoscopy is sometimes called "belly-button" or "Band-Aid" surgery since the only bandage required is a small adhesive strip. Laparoscopic sterilization is sometimes performed under local anesthesia and an overnight hospital stay is not required. Though it is not a trivial surgical procedure, serious complications such as intestine damage or hemorrhage occur in fewer than 5 out of 1000 cases. The death rate is lower than 3 per 100,000 (Hatcher et al., 1980).

Culdoscopy is performed through the vaginal cul de sac and requires more skill and training than laparoscopic procedures. For this reason culdoscopy is seldom performed (Hatcher et al., 1980).

Like vasectomy, tubal ligation procedures have very low failure rates (less than 1 percent). The few failures that do occur result from undetected preexisting pregnancies, physician error in cutting something other than a fallopian tube, or a rare rejoining of the severed ends of the tubes (Hatcher et al., 1980). The procedures should be considered irreversible although if tissue damage is minimal (more likely in laparotomy and culpotomy than in the endoscopic techniques), microsurgical reversals are sometimes successful.

Until recently, **hysterectomy** was a popular method of sterilizing women. In the simplest form of hysterectomy, a woman's entire uterus is removed. Because it is a major surgical procedure with a relatively high complication rate (Hatcher et al., 1980) and because removal of the "womb" often has a strong negative psychological impact on a woman, hysterectomy is not frequently performed solely for birth control purposes. **Ophorectomy** is surgical removal of the ovaries, which, of course, permanently halts ovulation. Ovary removal (castration) is not often advised as a birth control method since the ovaries are the primary source of the hormones estrogen and progesterone, which are vital to the maintenance of female secondary sex characteristics as well as to other functions of the female body.

Induced Abortion

Induced abortion is the deliberate termination of pregnancy by the removal of the embryo or fetus from a pregnant woman's uterus early in pregnancy before the fetus is able to survive on its own (DeLora & Warren, 1977). Although methods for inducing abortion have been known for over four thousand years (McCary, 1978), the use of abortion as a means of birth control is one of the most hotly debated ethical, moral, legal, and political issues of our time (Fraker et al., 1978). The questions and arguments are multiple (Tietze, 1974), and the conclusions reached by some will undoubtedly meet strong resistance from others (Hatcher et al., 1980):

Questions about abortion rage on in spite of the more than 1 million abortions performed each year in the United States. Is abortion murder? Is abortion any different than infanticide? When does an embryo or a fetus become a human being? When does the soul enter the body? Why do so many teenagers become pregnant and then turn to abortion? To what extent does the father have rights when abortion decisions are being made? To what extent is it appropriate for the physician or counselor to try to influence abortion decisions? If contraceptive services were adequate, would abortions be necessary? And last, but certainly not least, who speaks for the fetus?

These important questions concern women choosing to have abortions. They concern family planners. They concern clinicians performing abortions and counselors in abortion clinics. These questions have concerned thoughtful individuals for the past several thousand years. They continue to be raised today, and they will undoubtedly be raised for generations to come. (Hatcher et al., 1980, p. 111)

In January 1973, the Supreme Court of the United States granted, in a limited way, the abortion decision prerogative to women. In effect, the ruling was that during the first trimester (twelve weeks) of pregnancy, the abortion decision must be left to the pregnant woman and her physician; during the second trimester, the states may choose to regulate abortion decisions in ways that are reasonably related to the health of the woman; and once the fetus is considered viable—able to live on its own (twenty-four to twenty-six weeks)—the states may, if they choose, regulate and even proscribe abortion except where necessary, in appropriate medical judgment, to preserve the life or health of the pregnant woman (Hatcher et al., 1980). In subsequent decisions the Court has ruled that abortion veto power cannot be exercised by a spouse or parent (1976), that the government is not obliged to pay for abortions (1977), that physicians may not be forced by states to use an abortion technique most likely to save a fetus's life, and that a physician may not be punished for performing an abortion when a fetus has only a marginal chance of living (1979).

Debate, protest, and violence surround this issue and will undoubtedly continue to do so. Many who oppose abortion as a birth control procedure have turned to legislative efforts to restrict its use. Among these efforts are attempts to legally define the moment of conception as the beginning of human life. Abortion would, therefore, constitute murder. Other proposals are to amend the Constitution so as to prohibit abortion or to give the states and Congress increased power to restrict abortion and remove the authority of the courts to do so. In the following sections we describe the major techniques of abortion and briefly examine some of the consequences of abortions.

Vacuum Methods.   In vacuum methods of abortion ("suction abortion"), a small hollow tube is inserted through the cervical opening into the uterus, and the contents of the uterus, including a fertilized ovum or any fetal tissue, are simply sucked out. Although vacuum methods may be performed during the first trimester (twelve weeks) of pregnancy and even up to twenty weeks from the beginning of the last menstrual period (LMP), the procedures vary somewhat at different stages of pregnancy (Hatcher et al., 1980).

   Endometrial aspiration (sometimes called "menstrual regulation," "preemptive abortion," or "menstrual extraction") is a technique performed within the first few weeks after a late menstrual period (four to six weeks after LMP) when there is some suspicion of pregnancy but before it can be confirmed by laboratory tests. Without cervical dilation and usually without anesthesia, a thin flexible tube is inserted through the cervix and the endometrial lining of the uterus is evacuated. If a fertilized ovum is present, it is removed as well. The entire procedure requires no more than a few minutes and may be performed in a clinic or physician's office. The side effects of the technique sometimes include minor cramping, intermittent menstrual bleeding for a few days, and rarely, scarring or perforation of the uterus.

   To decrease risk of infection, the woman is advised to abstain from coitus for at least one week and to have intercourse during the second week only if her partner wears a condom. Since ovulation may occur and conception is possible, she should use some form of birth control. Fetal tissue at this stage is tiny and difficult to detect and she should have a pregnancy test. If menstruation does not resume within four or five weeks she should consult a physician to insure that no products of conception remain in the uterus and that there is no ectopic pregnancy (Boston Women's Health Book Collective, 1976; Hatcher et al., 1980).

   Early abortion ("early uterine evacuation," "mini-abortion") is identical in procedure to endometrial aspiration but occurs after pregnancy has been positively confirmed. The method may be used up to eight weeks following LMP. Since no cervical dilation is required and a flexible tube is used, the side effects and risks are the same as those for endometrial aspiration. The potential psychological impact on the woman may be greater, however, since there is no question that she is pregnant and that the procedure is abortive. (This sometimes remains unconfirmed with endometrial aspiration.)

   After the eighth week of pregnancy, the fetal tissue is too large for removal through the small flexible tubes described above. The **vacuum curettage** method (used up to the twelfth week of pregnancy) is similar but the tube (vacurette) is both larger and rigid and the suction used is stronger. The cervix must be slightly dilated to allow insertion of the larger tube. Dilation is accomplished gradually by inserting dilating rods of increasingly larger diameters into the cervical opening under local anesthesia applied to the cervical area. Alternatively, a **laminaria** may be inserted into the cervix from six to twenty-four hours before the abortion. A laminaria is a stick-shaped mass of seaweed that slowly expands as it absorbs cervical and uterine moisture, causing the cervix to dilate painlessly.

The plastic suction tube (between 6 and 12 millimeters in diameter) is inserted into the uterus until it contacts the fetus, as shown in Figure 3–13. Suction is then applied and in less than a minute the fetus is broken up and evacuated into a container. Some physicians then use a sharp curette (see below) to scrape the uterine walls to insure complete removal of the fetus and any placental material. Menstrual-like cramps during and a few hours following the procedure are not unusual. Menstrual-like bleeding may be expected for a few days. Coitus and douching should be avoided for at least a week to reduce the chance of infection and, since ovulation will occur within a month, birth control methods should be used when coitus is resumed. The possible complications associated with vacuum curettage are similar to those associated with other vacuum methods. Less than 10 percent of women who obtain vacuum abortions experience serious complications such as infections, uterine perforations, or severe bleeding (Hatcher et al., 1980).

Dilation and evacuation (D&E) is a vacuum procedure that is most appropriate for the early weeks (13–16) of the second trimester of pregnancy but may also be used from eight to twenty weeks LMP. The fetus is too large for the simpler vacuum curettage and must usually be broken up with surgical instruments prior to evacuation with a large-diameter vacurette. Substantial cervical dilation is required and some physicians administer a uterine contracting agent (oxytocin) to assist in expulsion of fetal and placental material, thus reducing blood loss. The precautions, side effects, and complications associated with D&E are similar to those with other vacuum methods (Hatcher et al., 1980).

Dilation and Curettage.   From the eighth through the fifteenth week of pregnancy the **dilation and curettage (D&C)** method of abortion may be used. Prior to development of the vacuum methods discussed above, it was the most frequently used first trimester technique. It is similar to the D&E but, instead of a vacuum curette, uses a sharp metal loop-shaped cutting curette to scrape out the uterine contents. D&C procedures require general anesthesia (thus, a hospital stay), are generally more painful, cause greater blood loss, result in less complete uterine evacuation, and are associated with more complications (infection, uterine perforation) and deaths than are the vacuum methods. The primary advantage of D&C is that for physicians it is a standard and familiar gynecological technique used for treatment of infertility and menstrual problems (Hatcher et al., 1980).

Chemical Induction of Labor.   Although the D&E procedure has been shown to be safer during the early and middle parts of the second trimester of pregnancy, in the late parts (weeks 20 through 24) abortion is usually performed by inducing labor through chemical means. In a **saline abortion** a long thin needle is inserted through the abdomen and uterine wall and a hypertonic saline (salt) solution is injected into the amniotic sac surrounding the fetus. The saline kills the fetus by halting the production of pregnancy-supporting hormones. Within six to forty-eight

Figure 3–13.

Abortion by vacuum
curettage.

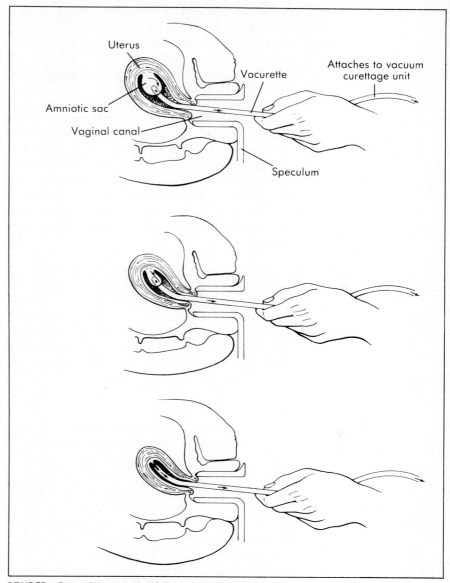

SOURCE: Boston Women's Health Book Collective, 1976, p. 230.

hours contractions of the uterus begin, the cervix dilates, and the fetus and placenta are expelled as in a natural birth.

In part because of the complexities and side effects of the method itself, but also because it is more frequently used late in pregnancy, the risk of various complications associated with saline abortion is from two to thirty times higher than that from D&E. In addition, the mortality rate (18 deaths per 100,000 procedures) is nearly nine times higher than for D&E and, as reported by the Center for Disease Control (1977) and the former U.S. Department of Health, Education and Welfare ("Annual Summary," 1978), exceeds that for pregnancy-related deaths (9.4 per 100,000 live births). Recently developed variations of this procedure involve the uterine administration of *prostaglandins* or *urea*, both of which induce labor and cause abortion (Hatcher et al., 1980). Because each of these methods resembles normal childbirth and involves the actual delivery of a fetus (sometimes alive when prostaglandins are used), induced abortions may be emotionally difficult for the woman and for the medical staff. Clearly, earlier termination is much more desirable.

Hysterotomy.   An infrequently used procedure, **hysterotomy**, is actually a small Caesarean section in which the fetus and placenta are removed through incisions made in the abdominal and uterine walls. It is a major surgical procedure with a high (43 per 100,000) death rate (Center for Disease Control, 1977). Complications are frequent and since it is not performed until late (around twenty-four weeks) into pregnancy, the fetus is sometimes alive and may move or cry before it dies (DeLora & Warren, 1977). Due to such circumstances, hysterotomy is, of all the methods of abortion discussed here, the one most likely to provoke public moral outrage.

Risk.   How safe is abortion? The answer to this question depends on two important variables: (1) how early in pregnancy the abortion is performed and (2) the type of procedure used. Of course, since the type of procedure used depends in part on the stage of pregnancy, these two variables are not totally independent. If we use the 9.4 maternal deaths that occur per 100,000 live births ("Annual Summary," 1978) as a comparison point, it is clear that abortion is safer than childbirth. In a study of nearly 3 million legal abortions performed in the United States between 1972 and 1975, the Center for Disease Control (1977) reported an overall abortion death rate of 3.7 per 100,000 procedures. But this is somewhat misleading because the abortion death rate increases substantially from the first (2.2) to the second (16.7) trimester. Up to eight weeks of pregnancy it is less than 1 and beyond twenty weeks it is nearly 23 per 100,000. Statistics from the Center for Disease Control (1977) indicate that vacuum techniques have the lowest death rate (1.9 per 100,000), followed by D&C (2.6), chemically induced abortions (17.7), and hysterotomy (42.6). Thus, it is clear that early abortion by vacuum or D&C is safer to a woman than is childbirth. Fortunately, 85 percent of all abortions are during the first trimester and vacuum methods and D&C account for 90 percent of all abortions (Center for Disease Control, 1977).

Nearly two thirds of all abortions are performed on women who are between the ages of fifteen and twenty-four and half of these (33 percent of the total) on teenagers. Most of the rest are performed on women between twenty-five and forty. Although the absolute number of abortions performed on women under fifteen (about 13,000) is low, it exceeds the number of live births (12,600) for women at this age (Center for Disease Control, 1977; "Teenage Childbearing," 1977). Similarly, women over forty have relatively few abortions, but for every 1000 live births, there are 600 abortions in this age group (Center for Disease Control, 1977).

Although it is sometimes argued that women who seek abortion are psychologically disturbed, few data support this assertion (Simon & Senturia, 1966). The major difference between those sexually active women who become pregnant and seek abortions and those who are pregnant and do not is the abortion group's failure to use contraceptives effectively (Gerrard, 1977; Zimmerman, 1977). Generally speaking, these are people who are relatively conservative and poorly informed concerning sexual matters (Gerrard, 1977; Mirande & Hammer, 1976). Their lack of information regarding and reluctance to utilize effective means of birth control result in unwanted pregnancies which, for a variety of reasons (Bogen, 1974), are terminated with abortion.

In part because of countless motion pictures depicting the sordid and often tragic results of illegal "back-alley" abortions, it is widely believed that women are emotionally scarred for life by the experience of abortion. Although some women are undoubtedly emotionally distressed following abortions, the available evidence indicates that the incidence of serious psychological distress is quite low. A number of studies, for example, have found that the primary feeling experienced by women following abortion is relief (Bogen, 1974; Zimmerman, 1977). The majority are pleased that their pregnancy has been terminated and that they are able to "get on with life" once again. Nearly 90 percent report no feelings of guilt or shame and those who do are often somewhat disturbed and lacking in social support from friends or family prior to the abortion (Belsey, Greer, Lal, Lewis, & Beard, 1977; Freeman, 1978). Indeed, most research (e.g., Athanasiou, Oppel, Michelson, Unger, & Yager, 1973) suggests that unwanted childbirth is the origin of more psychosocial problems than is abortion.

SUMMARY

Among the potential consequences of coitus are conception and pregnancy. Conception, which may also result from artificial insemination or ovum transplantation, occurs when a sperm penetrates and unites with an ovum. Pregnancy is established when the fertilized ovum (zygote) implants and begins to develop in the wall of the uterus. Missed menstrual periods and other symptoms such as nausea or breast tenderness suggest pregnancy but verification through various laboratory tests designed to detect the presence of human chorionic gonadotropin, a pregnancy-related hormone, is required.

The average duration of pregnancy is around nine months and is often divided into three-month trimesters. During the first trimester the fetus reaches a weight of 28 grams and a length of approximately 10 centimeters; the mother experiences various discomforting "symptoms" such as nausea, fatigue, and a frequent need to urinate. In the second trimester the fetus acquires a distinctly human appearance, begins to move, and reaches a weight of 1 kilogram and a length of 35 centimeters. The mother begins to "show" the pregnancy but many of the uncomfortable first-trimester symptoms disappear. Third-trimester fetal changes consist primarily of growth; at birth the average baby weighs 3.5 kilograms and is 50 centimeters long. Due to the size and weight of the fetus, the mother becomes increasingly uncomfortable until the fetus "drops" a few weeks before birth.

The impending birth of the child is signaled by increasingly powerful but irregular uterine contractions and discharge of the cervical mucus plug. Actual labor is divided into three stages. In first-stage labor regular uterine contractions dilate and thin the cervix to allow for passage of the fetus from the uterus. In second-stage labor the baby passes through and out of the vagina and child delivery is complete. In third-stage labor, the placenta (afterbirth) is delivered.

Relatively few acts of coitus are performed for the explicit purpose of producing pregnancy, and various methods exist for controlling birth. *Contraception* is any birth control method permitting coitus between fertile partners that prevents conception or pregnancy. There are many contraceptive methods and devices including hormonal controls (the Pill), which inhibit ovulation or implantation; intrauterine devices (IUDs), which inhibit implantation; diaphragms, which, when used with spermicides, physically block cervical entry by sperm and kill sperm; spermicides alone; condoms, which physically block vaginal and uterine entry by sperm; douching intended to flush sperm from the vagina; penis withdrawal prior to ejaculation; and the rhythm method of coital abstinence during periods of female fertility. In spite of the wide availability of effective contraceptives, pregnancy rates among unmarried teenagers are soaring. Possible solutions include earlier and better sex education, greater availability of contraceptive devices, and breaking down emotional barriers to contraceptive use.

Sterilization refers to several surgical techniques for permanently rendering a man or woman infertile. In *vasectomy*, the most frequent form of male sterilization, each vas deferens is severed, blocking sperm transport from the testes to other reproductive structures. The generic term for female sterilization, *tubal ligation*, refers to any of various procedures in which the fallopian tubes are severed, preventing passage of ova from the ovaries to the uterus. Sterilization does not affect sex drive or ability in either sex.

Induced abortion is the deliberate termination of an established pregnancy by removal of the embryo or fetus from the uterus early in pregnancy before the fetus is able to survive on its own. In vacuum methods of abortion, fetal material is sucked from the uterus through a small tube. Vacuum methods are most often used during the first trimester of pregnancy but dilation and evacuation may be used through the twentieth week LMP. In dilation and curettage, the cervix is dilated and the uterine walls are scraped removing the products of conception. During the second trimester, abortion is often performed by chemically inducing labor with amniotic injections of saline solution or uterine injections of prostaglandins or urea. Most women experience few if any negative emotional effects from abortion.

SUGGESTED READINGS

Boston Women's Health Book Collective (1976). *Our bodies, ourselves* (2nd ed.). New York: Simon & Schuster.

Cvetkovich, G., Grote, B., Bjorseth, A., & Sarkissian, J. (1975). On the psychology of adolescents' use of contraceptives. *Journal of Sex Research, 11,* 256–270.

Hatcher, R. H., Stewart, G. K., Stewart, F., Guest, F., Stratton, P., & Wright, A. H. (1980). *Contraceptive technology, 1980–1981.* New York: Irvington.

Osofsky, H., & Osofsky, J. (Eds.) (1973). *The abortion experience: Psychological and medical impact.* New York: Harper & Row.

Rugh, L., & Shettles, L. (1971). *From conception to birth: The drama of life's beginnings.* New York: Harper & Row.

CHAPTER OUTLINE

CHAPTER 4

SEXUAL STIMULATION: THE SOURCES OF SEXUAL AROUSAL

Dear Ann Landers: Concerning the woman with the oversexed husband: She said he was after her every minute. When she was doing the dishes he was right behind her "making obscene gestures." When she tried to take a nap on the couch he'd lie down right beside her, etc. You gave her the dumbest answer I have ever read—suggested he should pitch in and help her with the housework to get rid of some of that "excess energy." Your advice was "Hand 'Hot Stuff' the vacuum cleaner."

Well I tried it and what he did with that vacuum cleaner is unprintable. Now, I'm afraid to leave this man alone with the Thanksgiving turkey. —Rhode Island Reader (Ann Landers Advises, September 28, 1976)

Rhode Island Reader's dilemma highlights three major issues that we will pose as questions and discuss in this chapter. First, she seems perplexed concerning what triggers sexual arousal not only in "oversexed husbands," but in other people as well. Thus, our first question will be, *"What is sexually stimulating?"* For example, is sexual arousal programmed biologically or do psychosocial processes such as learning, thinking, and emotions play greater roles? What dimensions determine the sexual arousal value of erotic stimuli? Are men and women sexually aroused by the same kinds of stimuli?

Second, Rhode Island Reader seems to assume that people differ in their sexual responsiveness and that men are "oversexed" in comparison with women. Our second question is, *"Who is sexually stimulated?"* Do genetic and hormonal processes account for differences in sexual responsiveness? How important are personality characteristics and age as determinants of sexual responsiveness? Do men and women differ in their sexual responsiveness?

Third, Rhode Island Reader implies that states of sexual arousal demand behavioral expression whether with other people, vacuum cleaners, or Thanksgiving turkeys. We discuss this issue by asking, *"What are the effects of sexual stimulation?"* Does the sexual arousal produced by erotic stimuli lead to sex crimes? Does exposure to erotic stimuli produce changes in sexual behavior? Does erotica-produced sexual arousal influence our reactions to potential or actual sexual partners?

WHAT IS SEXUALLY STIMULATING?

It is impossible to compile a complete list of all factors that are capable of influencing human sexual arousal. It is, however, possible to view sexual arousal as a product of the combined actions of internal and external cues, which, to varying degrees, are influenced by biological and psychosocial processes.

Biological Processes

Most of the available evidence concerning biological processes in sexual stimulation has been obtained from research using animals and in many cases the meanings of this research for human sexuality are, at best, unclear. For this reason, we will discuss only those influences that have been reliably demonstrated and show promise of shedding some light on the nature of what is sexually arousing for humans.

Genetic Influences.   Very little is known about the impact of inheritance in determining what is sexually arousing. It seems clear, though, that genetic makeup plays a role in determining those stimuli to which some organisms respond sexually. Under normal circumstances, one species of animal is not sexually stimulated by the "sexual cues" associated with an animal of a different species (Blair, 1955). That is, at least some organisms seem to be genetically "primed" to respond sexually to some external stimuli and not to others. This selective priming plays an important role in preventing cross-species mating (Bermant & Davidson, 1974).

Genetic factors are less important determinants of sexual responses among animals classified higher on the evolutionary scale (Beach, 1969). Thus, although strong genetic effects on what cues are sexually stimulating are found in many subprimates, few, if any, such effects are evident in mammals, including humans. For example, captive apes, gorillas, chimpanzees, monkeys, and other animals have been observed to respond sexually to animals of several different species. There are reliable records of gorillas responding sexually to dogs and humans, of monkeys responding to humans, dogs, and cats, of chimpanzees to baboons and orangutans, and even of porpoises to turtles and sharks (Ford & Beach, 1951).

The diversity among humans in the scope and variety of sexually arousing stimuli defies any simple genetic explanation. Our genetic makeup does not prevent us from becoming sexually aroused by animals of different species (Kinsey, Pomeroy, & Martin, 1948; Kinsey, Pomeroy, Martin, & Gebhard, 1953). Nor does it prevent some people from responding sexually to shoes, garter belts, the taste of clam dip, the smell of aftershave lotions and perfumes, or the music of the Rolling Stones.

Of equal importance is the fact that our genetic makeup does not *compel* us to respond to any particular stimulus. Thus, the fact that one's genetic sex may be either male or female does not prevent sexual responses to other people of either sex (Money & Ehrhardt, 1972; Pritchard, 1962). In short, there is no reliable evidence that humans are genetically programmed to respond sexually to some stimuli and not to others (Beach, 1965).

Hormonal Influences.   From shortly after conception until death, hormones are intimately involved in the sexuality of all mammals, including humans. Their profound influence on the differentiation, development, and functioning of the sexual apparatus throughout the life-span was described in Chapter 2. In addition, sex hormones play an important role in shaping the sexual *activities* of mammals.

Research using both animals and humans has revealed two important ways in which hormones may influence sexuality. First, exposure to hormones during critical periods in development may *organize*, or "program," the sexual response tendencies of an organism later in its life. Second, during adulthood, circulating hormones may *activate* sexual responses to external erotic cues. Let us first consider the organizational role of hormones.

Androgen from the fetal gonads is the critical hormone involved in organizing, or programming, the prenatal physical development of reproductive structures in both males and females. A number of investigators have explored the possibility that prenatal androgen levels might organize patterns of sexual activity as well as patterns of sexual anatomy (Gerall, 1973; Young, Goy, & Phoenix, 1965; Money & Ehrhardt, 1972). The sexual responses of female rats are profoundly influenced by exposure to large doses of androgen shortly before or after birth. As adults, they fail to respond sexually when approached by males and, if stimulated by additional androgen, sexually mount other females and display typical male copulatory movements. In short, their sexual activities are organized in a masculine rather than feminine pattern. Male rats deprived of androgen by castration shortly before or after birth display distinctly feminine styles of sexual behavior, including sexual responses to other males rather than females during adulthood. In lower mammals, then, the presence or absence of androgen during brief and critical periods of development plays a crucial role in organizing adult erotic response and sexual activity patterns.

In primates, the organizing influence of prenatal androgen is reflected primarily in the "masculinity" or "femininity" of nonsexual behavior patterns. Anke Ehrhardt (1973) compared girls with the adrenogenital syndrome (AGS), in which a hyperactive adrenal gland produces an overabundance of androgen, with normal girls. Generally, the AGS girls seemed to be somewhat more "masculine" in behavior and attitudes than the normal girls. There was no evidence, however, that the AGS girls' sexual preferences or erotic responses differed significantly from those of normal females.

Thus, although hormones present during critical stages of development seem to shape an erotic template for the adult sexual patterns of some lower mammals, their effects appear to be rather minimal in higher mammals, including humans. The available evidence does suggest, however, that the expression of some behaviors that are traditionally regarded as masculine or feminine may be hormonally influenced even in humans (Ehrhardt, 1979).

The activating, or priming, effects of circulating hormones have been extensively studied. It is generally agreed that sexual arousal in mammals is a joint function of the influence of internal cues arising from hormonal processes and external cues associated with a sex object. If the proper hormonal state is present, the organism is primed to respond to the external cues when they appear. What is the "proper hormonal state" and how does it influence response to external sexual cues?

The reproductive capacities of all mammalian females are rhythmic and controlled by cyclic ovarian secretions of estrogen and progesterone. Periods of fertility in mammals occur in three stages: (1) the ovaries step up their secretion of estrogen; (2) as the concentration of estrogen reaches a peak, ovulation, the release of a fertile egg from one of the ovaries, occurs; and (3) the level of circulating estrogen declines while progesterone concentration reaches a peak and then drops (see Chapter 2). In some animals (including humans) fertility periods cycle continuously throughout the year while in others (horses, sheep) such periods occur only during a restricted season of the year. Some animals (bears, deer) have only one period of fertility per year.

When she is sexually receptive, a female mammal is said to be "in heat" or "in **estrus**" (from Greek and Latin meaning "mad desire or frenzy"). In many species, periods of estrus occur in cycles that coincide with periods of fertility so that maximum receptiveness occurs immediately before or at the time of ovulation. Both estrus and ovulation are triggered by cyclic changes in ovarian secretions of estrogen. The estrogen peak that occurs soon before ovulation also creates and maintains a state of sexual receptiveness in many species. For the most part, sexual receptiveness in lower mammalian females (cats, dogs, goats) is totally dependent on the presence of high levels of circulating estrogen.

The estrus cycles of some of the lower mammals should not be confused with the menstrual cycles that occur in humans as well as in some species of monkeys and apes. The two types of cycles are defined differently. Estrus cycles are defined behaviorally in terms of sexual receptivity, whereas menstrual cycles refer to changes in the walls of the uterus accompanied by periodic discharges of blood. Such periodic bleeding appears only in higher mammals, including humans (Bermant & Davidson, 1974). Like lower mammals, female monkeys and apes generally show clear rhythms of sexual responsiveness. Even though some will permit copulation during other portions of their menstrual cycles (Ford & Beach, 1951), they are most eager for sexual contact and most attractive to males during the middle phase. This is when high concentrations of estrogen are circulating and when ovulation occurs (Michael & Zumpe, 1970; Czaja & Bielert, 1975).

Although the reproductive cycle phases of human females bear a striking resemblance to those of chimpanzees and rhesus monkeys, the hormonal states producing heat in the latter animals are of little importance in humans. Adult women are hormonally "ready" to respond sexually and engage in sexual activities during all phases of their menstrual cycles. Several studies, however, have detected slight variations in sexual responsiveness and frequency of sexual activity that correspond to phases of the cycle (Davis, 1929; Udry & Morris, 1968; Moos, Kopell, Melges, Yalom, Lunde, Clayton, & Hamberg, 1969). Although the results of these studies have been somewhat contradictory, at least two different patterns have been observed.

Udry and Morris (1968) found peaks of sexual activity in women occurring during the ovulatory and premenstruation periods of the menstrual cycle. Peaks of sexual responsiveness to erotic stimuli at midcycle (ovulation) have also been reported by Moos and colleagues (1969) and Luschen and Pierce (1972). Heightened sexual activity and responsiveness around the time of ovulation at least suggests the possibility of an estrogen influence on female sexual arousal resembling that in subhumans.

Others, however, report two periods of heightened sex interest—one immediately before and one immediately after menstruation (Kinsey et al., 1953; Davis, 1929). These two periods correspond to no recognized hormonal events thought to influence sexual desire in other mammals. Clellan Ford and Frank Beach (1951) have suggested that the premenstrual peak in desire reflects the effects of anticipated sexual deprivation during the menstrual flow. The second rise following menstrual bleeding may result from several days of enforced sexual abstinence. This interpretation is based on the fact that the majority of societies, including our own, regard sexual intercourse during menstruation as taboo and expect a sexual "time out" during this period.

Which of these apparently contradictory patterns is the "correct" one? The answer probably is that both of these and many more are correct depending on which women are studied. Many women simply do not recognize rhythms of sexual interest or receptiveness (Kinsey et al., 1953), and the various studies of women who do recognize such rhythms typically find little agreement as to when peaks of interest or responsiveness occur during their menstrual cycles. One study concerning this issue found no relationship between phases of the menstrual cycle and how sexually aroused a woman becomes in response to erotic photographs (Griffith & Walker, 1975). These findings, coupled with those showing little if any alteration of sexual responsiveness in women whose ovaries have been removed (Bremer, 1959) or in postmenopausal women (Masters & Johnson, 1966), suggest that ovarian hormones play minor roles as primers of sexual receptivity in human females.

There is some evidence, however, that estrogen influences a female's sexual attractiveness to males. Sexual receptivity in rhesus monkeys whose ovaries have been removed may be restored by injections of small amounts of androgen (see below). Androgen administration alone, however, restores only the female's interest in sex. She seems eager for sexual contact but males do not find her sexually very inviting. Estrogen replacement restores her attractiveness to males (Michael & Keverne, 1970). High levels of estrogen produce various changes in the appearance and odor of the external genitals of most higher mammals. In the rhesus monkey it is the distinctive odor of the vaginal secretions accompanying the estrogen peak that arouses the male's interest. Michael, Keverne, and Bonsall (1971) isolated an odoriferous substance (named copulin) from the vaginal secretions of female rhesus monkeys that is a potent sex attractant **(pheromone)** to males. This substance is present at its highest level during the estrogen peak and ovulation.

The interesting possibility that sexually excited human females secrete substances which might be sexual attractants to males is suggested by the results of at least one study. Sokolov, Harris, and Hecker (1976) collected and analyzed samples of vaginal secretions from sexually aroused human females. They were successful in isolating a substance similar to the rhesus monkey pheromone previously discovered by Michael and coworkers (Michael et al., 1971). Whether this substance has a sexually stimulating effect on human males or not remains to be determined. For an excellent review of research in this general area see Rogel (1978), who concludes, along with White (1981), that there is no convincing evidence that any "smells" are natural attractants for humans.

Although the ovarian hormones (estrogen and progesterone) seem to have little influence on the sexual responsiveness of women, there is some evidence that androgen (the "male hormone") has more. In mammalian females the cortex of the adrenal gland is the primary source of androgen (Baird, Horton, Longcope, & Taite, 1968). Radical treatments for breast cancer in women sometimes involve ovary as well as adrenal gland removal. Waxenberg (1963) studied women undergoing such surgery and found that only after the adrenal glands as well as the ovaries were removed did their sexual responsiveness decline. Others have reported that women who receive androgenic hormones for medical reasons report heightened sexual interest and responsiveness (Money, 1961).

These findings suggest that androgen from the adrenal glands, rather than estrogen, is the hormone that normally controls women's eroticism. It is unclear whether the androgen effects are due to heightened responsiveness to external sex cues, heightened clitoral sensitivity, increased feelings of "well-being," or to some combination of these factors (Luttge, 1971). Androgen doses far in excess of normal physiological levels, however, produce a number of unpleasant side effects in women. These include beard growth, clitoral enlargement, deepening of the voice, and other indications of masculinization. Thus, the regular use of androgen as a sex stimulant, or **aphrodisiac**, in women is usually not recommended.

The role of hormones in regulating the sexual responsiveness of males is more straightforward than it is for females. Only androgen, which is chiefly supplied by the testes, appears to be of major importance. Surgical removal of the testes (castration) in subhuman animals inevitably leads to a decline in sexual activity and responsiveness even though there is great individual variability in the rate and severity of the decline.

Castration has been performed on human males throughout recorded history to attain a number of objectives. Men have been castrated to supply eunuchs for harems, to supply "safe" escorts for Roman ladies, to supply boy sopranos for the medieval church, to punish criminals or captured enemies, and for religious reasons. Today castration is practiced mostly in the treatment of prostate cancer, testicular cancer, or injury, on transsexuals who wish to change their anatomies from male to female, and as a method of deterring sex criminals. Despite the long history of this operation, surprisingly little is known of its effects on sexual responsiveness and functioning (Heim & Hursch, 1979).

Though there are a number of individual exceptions reported in the clinical literature, the effects of castration on some men appear to resemble the results in subhuman males. One of the most extensive studies of this question was a follow-up study by Bremer (1959) of several hundred men who were legally castrated in Norway for a variety of sex offenses and mental disturbances. Before surgery, 157 of these men had led active sex lives. Within one year following surgery, two thirds of them had lost all interest in sex and were unresponsive to sexual stimuli. Although some sex interest was retained by the remaining one third of the men, it was generally less intense than that before the operation. Thus, total loss of sexual interest and capability does not appear to be an absolute consequence of castration. Its effects seem to be dependent on a number of factors, including the man's expectations regarding its impact and the availability of an understanding sexual partner.

Castrates, of course, are almost totally deprived of internal supplies of androgen. It is important to realize that normal day-to-day variations of androgen concentrations in noncastrated males seem to bear little relationship to sexual desires, interests, or reactions to external sex cues (Evans & Distiller, 1979; Lloyd, 1968; Raboch & Starka, 1972; Rubin, Hensen, Falvo, & High, 1979). The available data (Davidson, 1972) suggest that there is a considerable "safety factor" with respect to the androgenic control of sexual responses. Only under unusual circumstances such as castration or testicular failure will androgen levels fall so low as to affect sexual performance (Bermant & Davidson, 1974).

Aphrodisiacs. The quest for chemically active substances capable of directly stimulating or enhancing sexual desire dates to the beginnings of recorded history. This search has produced a seemingly endless list of reputed aphrodisiacs (Masters, 1962): peanuts, menstrual blood, oysters, the testicles of many animals, human flesh, mandrake plants, powdered reindeer antlers and rhinoceros horns, bananas, tulip bulbs, ground insects, and many other rather unappetizing items (Appel, 1970; Katchadourian & Lunde, 1980). Though none of these substances appears capable of exerting biologically mediated aphrodisiac effects, they may, under some circumstances, indirectly enhance sexual desires through psychological processes. For example, an individual who holds an unshakable belief in the aphrodisiac qualities of carrots, bull testicles, or chocolate-covered ants may experience at least a temporary elevation in sexual desire after consuming the item because of powerful expectations regarding its sexual potency.

Various drugs are frequently reported to possess aphrodisiac powers. The drug most widely used in connection with sexual activities is *alcohol*. Its reputed effects have been immortalized in the words of Ogden Nash, who wrote "Candy is dandy, but liquor is quicker." Perhaps a more appropriate description, however, is Shakespeare's "It provokes the desire, but takes away the performance." As suggested by Shakespeare, alcohol may have a two-pronged effect on sexual expression. As a general nervous system depressant, it will act in some people to reduce inhibitions and anxiety concerning sexual activities and, thus, enhance sexual desires. In large quantities, though, it will depress erotic responses and interfere with sexual performance and pleasure (Briddell & Wilson, 1976; Farkas & Rosen, 1976; Malatesta, Pollack, Wilbanks, & Adams, 1979; Wilson & Lawson, 1978). Men who ingest alcohol to decrease sexual inhibitions often find that their overzealous efforts lead to intoxication and resultant difficulty in achieving erection. Failure to recognize that such disappointing erections are a result of inebriation may lead to distress if men assume they are unable to function sexually and this may, in turn, lead to recurrent erectile difficulties (Masters & Johnson, 1970). Chronic alcoholism is frequently associated with sexual response impairment in both sexes (Wilson, Lawson, & Abrams, 1978). This is especially true in alcoholic men, who often experience depressed sexual desires as well as impotence during their addiction.

As alcohol acts on the central nervous system, it may first enhance sexual desire but may later impair actual performance.

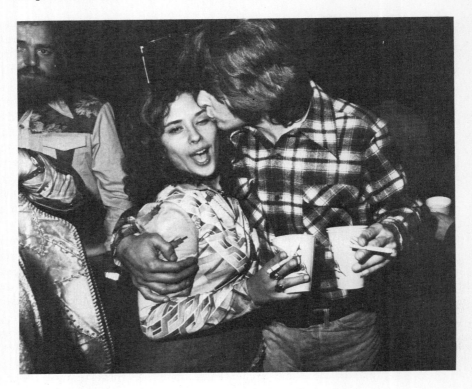

Other depressants that act on the central nervous system— tranquilizers, barbituates, and narcotics such as heroin and morphine—produce effects quite similar to those of alcohol (Kaplan, 1974).

Like the depressant alcohol, some of the central nervous system stimulants such as *amphetamines* (speed) and *cocaine* are also reported by users to increase sexual desire. In males, large doses of these drugs may produce prolonged penile erections *(priapism)* and the ability to engage in intercourse for long periods of time without ejaculation. As in the case of alcohol, barbituates, and narcotics, however, prolonged use of speed and cocaine will lead men to lose both sexual desire and erectile ability. The drugs, which originally may be used to enhance sexuality, often become more important than the sex itself. As one woman complained, "He used to shoot speed and then make love to me; now he only shoots speed" (Tinklenberg, 1971, p. 11).

The effects of LSD, marijuana, and other *hallucinogens* on sexual responses are quite varied and dependent on the individual user, the circumstances surrounding their use, and the user's expectations regarding their effects. It seems clear that they are not true aphrodisiacs but may under some circumstances enhance sexual pleasure (Athanasiou, Shaver, & Tavris, 1970; Gawin, 1978) or lead to sensations of prolonged orgasm. On the other hand, these drugs sometimes interfere with sexual responses by inducing cognitive and perceptual experiences that are incompatible with sexual responses. A "bad trip" on LSD may produce such terror and paranoia as to wipe out all interest in sexuality. More positive drug experiences may leave the user so engrossed in his or her pleasurable fantasies that sexual desires are of secondary importance (Appel, 1970).

It is popularly believed that *"Spanish fly,"* or cantharides, a drug derived from dried beetles *(Cantharis vesicatoria)* found in southern Europe, is a potent aphrodisiac. Actually, Spanish fly is a powerful and dangerous drug that, when taken in small doses, causes acute inflammation and irritation of the urinary tract and dilation of penile blood vessels. In males, erection may result even though no increase in actual sexual desire may be experienced. The drug can hardly be recommended as an aphrodisiac since one of its possible side effects is death. Its primary medical use today is in removing warts (Ferguson, 1975).

Yohimbine is a crystalline alkaloid extracted from the bark of the African Yohimbe tree. It is a diuretic that also stimulates the lower spinal neural centers controlling erection and has naturally earned a reputation as a sex stimulant. It is, however, dangerous in large doses and the erections produced by the drug are usually accompanied by little sexual desire (Masters, 1962).

In recent years the drug *amyl nitrite*, or "poppers," has gained a number of fans who claim that inhaling its vapors just before orgasm enhances erotic sensations. Most frequently, it is contained in small glass vials that are broken (popped), releasing the drug vapors. Its primary medical use is to relax the smooth muscles of the circulatory system, producing dilation of blood vessels and reduction of the pain associated with some heart conditions. The lowered blood pressure that results leads to feelings of dizziness and faintness that may account for the reported increase in orgasmic sensations. Like most of the other drugs we have considered, amyl nitrite use is accompanied by a number of potentially dangerous side effects, including, in rare cases, death (Hollister, 1974).

Despite widespread claims in the late 1960s and early 1970s attesting to the aphrodisiac properties of the drugs L-dopa and PCPA, recent research using both animals and humans has generally failed to clearly establish their efficacy as sexual stimulants. Both drugs act to counter the effects of serotonin—a naturally occurring general brain depressant. L-dopa is used in the treatment of Parkinson's disease, and early reports indicated that some male patients experienced hypersexuality after beginning L-dopa therapy. The flurry of excitement attending such reports (Appel, 1970) has been tempered somewhat by recent findings that cast doubt upon the aphrodisiac powers of this drug (Keyes, Janzik, Mayer, Eichner, & Gupta, 1976). Similarly, PCPA, which is used to treat various types of tumors and mental disturbances, has not consistently been found to produce the sexual frenzies in either animals or humans that were observed in some early investigations (Zitrin, Dement, & Barchas, 1973). Another substance—vitamin E—has been hailed as a potential aphrodisiac, but the available evidence suggests that it is of little value in this regard (Herold, Mottin, & Sabry, 1979).

The search for an effective, convenient, and safe aphrodisiac has uncovered many patently absurd and biochemically ineffective substances as well as several potent drugs with dangerous side effects. An ideal biologically active sexual stimulant has yet to be discovered, however (Gawin, 1978). The possibility of its discovery should not be dismissed even though it seems clear that "better loving through chemistry" is a dream yet to be realized.

The interest this woman arouses in these men is the result of a combination of psychosocial factors, including learning, cognitive, and emotional processes.

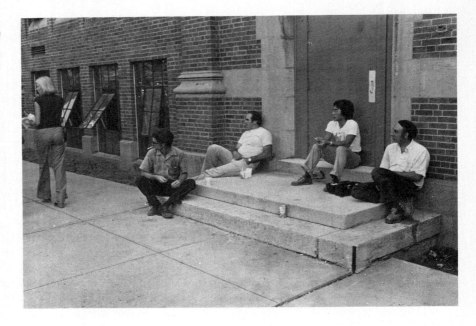

Psychosocial Processes

Although biological processes are intimately involved in shaping the sexual responses of subhuman animals, the enormous variety in what is sexually stimulating to humans precludes any simple biological explanation. Frank Beach (1969) has pointed out that hormonal and genetic processes have less and less effect on sexual responses as animals are classified higher on the evolutionary scale. At the same time, what we will refer to as psychosocial processes become more and more important. The key to this transition is found in the greater development of our brains than those of lower animals (Beach, 1969).

Because of this high degree of brain development, our species is comparatively bright and it is our brain rather than our gonads that exerts the greater influence on our sexuality. Human sexual expression is mostly a psychosocial enterprise in which our sexual responses are shaped and molded by learning, cognitive, and emotional processes.

Learning and Cognitive Processes.   In general, *learning* refers to the modification of behavior as a result of experience. It is widely agreed (Kinsey et al., 1948, 1953; Katchadourian & Lunde, 1980) that our sexual responses are greatly influenced by our ability to learn. That is, we learn to respond sexually to some things and not to others (Bandura, 1969). Conceivably any stimulus can become sexually arousing through learning.

In a simple yet convincing way, Stanley Rachman (1966) has demonstrated this in the laboratory by showing that people can learn to become sexually aroused by footwear. Men were shown a photographic slide of a black pair of women's boots followed by slides of attractive nude women. After several such sequences, the picture of the boots acquired the capacity to produce sexual arousal as indicated by a device used to measure erections. Thus, we can easily learn to become sexually aroused by stimuli which initially have little or no inherent sexual meaning.

Outside the laboratory, case history studies reveal that we can, and sometimes do, learn to respond sexually to virtually any kind of stimulus. Many of the "sexual preference variations" discussed in Chapter 12 involve instances in which people have learned, through accidental conditioning experiences, to be sexually aroused by women's dresses and undergarments, rubberized clothing, chains, whips, pain, and many other stimuli that are not usually thought of as sexual. By arranging the appropriate "relearning" conditions, sexual responses to such stimuli may be modified or eliminated (Bandura, 1969; O'Leary & Wilson, 1975).

What about responses to stimuli that are more commonly regarded as sources of sexual arousal? Even though little systematic research has been conducted concerning their origins, it seems clear that people and their nude or clothed body parts, scents of perfumes, lotions, and body odors, musical and other sounds, and the tastes of particular foods, drinks, or bodily secretions are stimuli that acquire the ability to arouse sexual desires on the basis of learning. Their erotic meaning is established through association with states of sexual arousal produced either by genital stimulation or by other stimuli that previously have themselves been conditioned to produce arousal (Kantorowitz, 1978).

Wide individual differences in what we regard as sexually stimulating result from the highly individualized details of the learning experiences we have undergone. Thus, that one person may be excited by the smell of Acme Underarm Deodorant, another by persons of his or her own sex, and yet another by people of the opposite sex is understandable. It should also be apparent that no one stimulus—whether Acme Underarm Deodorant, a same-sex person, or an opposite-sex person—is a more natural sexual stimulus than the others. If we seriously accept the possibility that most sexually arousing stimuli acquire their erotic potential through learning processes, then we must be prepared to abandon the idea that some sexual response patterns are "natural" while others are "unnatural."

That sexual response patterns can be shaped by relatively simple learning processes does not mean that we are mere sexual machines capable of being "turned on" or off capriciously by external cues to which we are conditioned. Quite the opposite is true. Our sexual responses are shaped in many important ways by our thoughts, memories, fantasies, and other *cognitive processes* and abilities (Rook & Hammen, 1977).

For example, the power of fantasy to stimulate sexual desires has been convincingly demonstrated in an experiment by Donn Byrne and John Lamberth (1971). Married couples were asked to view erotic photographs, read erotic stories, or just to imagine and think about a variety of sexual activities. They were then asked to record how sexually aroused they were by the pictures, stories, or fantasies. Those who used only their imaginations were more sexually aroused than those who actually saw or read erotic stimuli. These findings indicate that our thoughts may serve as powerful sexual stimulants. Indeed, our ability to respond sexually to several classes of external erotic stimuli—photographs, movies, stories, and musical selections, for example—is probably due to the power of the cues they contain to trigger sexual fantasies. We are able to project ourselves into them and become imaginary participants in the erotic activities they portray. In the absence of such external cues, however, we can generate and attend to our own sexual thoughts and images and, within certain limits, become sexually aroused at any time and at any place.

In most, but not all, cases (Kinsey et al., 1953) our fantasies contain elements of activities that we have personally experienced, and these memories add to the effects of otherwise fictional scenes. Memories elaborated by creative imagination may be the most arousing of all fantasies. In one study (Griffitt, 1975), college students reported on their degree of experience with various types of sexual activities. They were then shown photographic slides of people engaging in the same activities and asked to indicate how sexually arousing each picture was. As

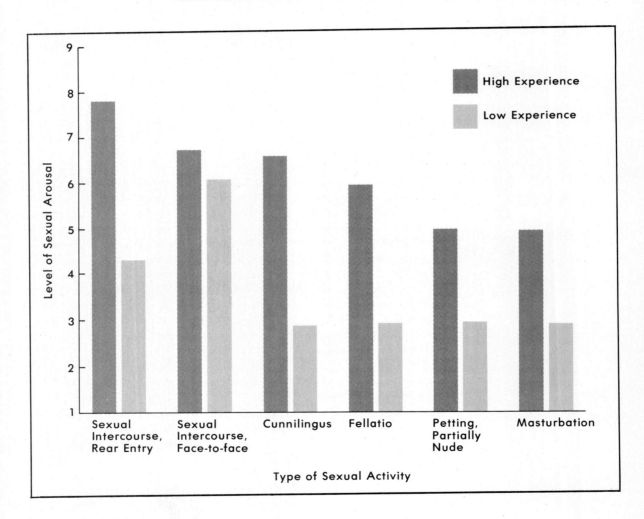

Figure 4–1.

Sexual experience as a factor in sexual arousal.
Those college students with the most experience with each of six types of sexual activity were the most sexually aroused when shown photographs depicting each activity.
SOURCE: Data from Griffitt, 1975.

Figure 4–2.

Effects of cognitive activity on sexual arousal.
While listening to an erotic story, men performed one of four types of cognitive tasks. As the complexity of the task increased, the sexual arousal produced by the erotic story decreased.

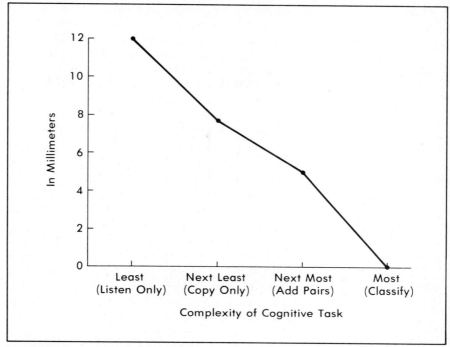

SOURCE: Adapted from Geer & Fuhr, 1976.

shown in Figure 4–1, those subjects with the most experience with a given type of activity were most aroused by a photograph depicting the same activity. Those who had had intercourse in the face-to-face position were more aroused by a photograph of such intercourse than those who had not; those who had masturbated the most were most aroused by a picture of someone of their own sex masturbating, and so forth.

In addition to stimulating and enhancing erotic responses, thoughts and images also have the capacity to interfere with or inhibit sexual desires. This has been demonstrated convincingly in a study by James Geer and Robert Fuhr (1976). While listening to an erotic tape recording, male college students were required to perform cognitive (numerical) tasks of varying complexity. Sexual arousal was measured by a **penile plethysmograph**, a device that records changes in penis size. The results are shown in Figure 4–2. As the cognitive task became increasingly complex and thus increasingly consumed the thought processes of the men, they were less and less aroused by the erotic story. More recently, similar findings have been reported for female college students (Przyblya & Byrne, 1984).

Other studies (Laws & Rubin, 1969; Henson & Rubin, 1971) indicate that people may exert conscious control over their sexual responses by generating appropriate fantasies of their own. In these experiments, men were able to voluntarily produce erections by thinking about erotic activities and to voluntarily inhibit erections while watching erotic movies by thinking about nonsexual stimuli such as lyrics to popular songs, multiplication tables, verses of poetry, or nonsexual objects in their immediate environment.

These findings indicate that cognitive processes may influence sexual responses in at least three ways. First, in the absence of external erotic cues, our fantasies may directly stimulate sexual desires. Second, our thoughts and images may intensify or enhance the sexually arousing effects of external stimuli to which we are exposed. Finally, thoughts that distract us from or are otherwise incompatible with sexual thoughts may inhibit or block erotic responses (Farkas, Sine, & Evans, 1979).

Emotional Processes.   Few dimensions of the human experience are capable of matching sexuality in the extent to which it is enmeshed in a sometimes bewildering and painful web of positive and negative emotions. The association of sexual expression with positive feelings is relatively easy to understand since the basic physical experiences of sexual arousal and orgasm are intensely pleasurable. Thus, we tend to seek out sources of sexual arousal because of their positive consequences. Somewhat paradoxically, however, for most of us, sexual arousal and those stimuli capable of triggering it also produce a variety of negative feelings. For reasons that are not entirely clear, virtually all societies have developed rules and regulations designed to strictly govern sexual expression. These regulations condone sexual responses to only a limited array of stimuli, under limited circumstances, and during only a limited portion of people's lives. At an early age the individual becomes vaguely aware of these limits and also that those who go beyond such limits are sinful, pathological, or perhaps criminal.

In our society the goal most frequently has been to teach that becoming sexually aroused by one's spouse is good but that sexual arousal to any other stimulus is bad and to be avoided. For a number of reasons, however, the teaching is seldom this precise and what is often communicated is the notion that *all* sexual desires and the stimuli capable of arousing them are somehow bad. As a result, many sexual stimuli also evoke a variety of negative feelings that we learn to label as guilt, fear, disgust, shame, and so forth.

Negative emotional responses interfere with the erotic effectiveness of stimuli to which they are attached. A number of studies demonstrate that people who are prone to experiencing guilt in association with sexuality are less aroused by erotic movies, photos, and stories than those in whom guilt responses are less intense (Mosher, 1970; Ray & Walker, 1973). Negative attitudes (feelings) regarding sexuality in general are also capable of inhibiting sexual arousal responses to a wide variety of erotic stimuli (Commission on Obscenity and Pornography, 1970).

Emotional reactions influence not only our erotic responses to sex stimuli but also whether we evaluate such stimuli as something pleasant to be pursued or something unpleasant to be avoided. Byrne, Fisher, Lamberth, and Mitchell (1974) assessed married couples' emotional reactions to various erotic stimuli as well as their attitudes regarding the public availability of such materials. Those who experienced feelings of disgust, nausea, and other negative emotions tended to label the stimuli as pornographic and to be in favor of rather strict government censorship of such materials. Those who found the materials exciting and entertaining, however, were opposed to government restriction and labeled very few of the stimuli as pornographic. Another study (Griffitt & Kaiser, 1978) suggests, moreover, that those whose emotional responses to erotica are positive actively seek sexual stimulation by intentionally exposing themselves to erotic situations. In contrast, the findings indicate, those whose emotional responses are negative tend to behave in ways that prevent encounters with sex stimuli.

Although the learning, cognitive, and emotional processes we have considered go a long way in answering questions concerning *how* responses to sexual stimuli are shaped, they tell us little about precisely *what* stimuli will be sexually arousing for any given individual. What is sexually arousing for a particular person depends on the specific learning experiences to which the person has been exposed, on the individualized thoughts and images that are evoked by erotic stimuli, and on the unique pattern of emotional reactions triggered by sexual cues and fantasies. Nevertheless, within a given culture or segment of that culture, there is enough commonality in sexual "teaching" that it is possible to determine, in general terms, what types of external sexual cues are most frequently sexually arousing.

Dimensions of Erotic Stimuli

Beyond anecdotal reports and personal experiences, the richest source of information concerning what humans find sexually exciting comes from research in which people are exposed to erotic stimuli and their degree of sex arousal is measured. Because of our intellectual development we are capable of responding to symbolic representations of objects or events in much the same way that we react to the actual objects or symbols themselves. Seeing, reading about, or hearing sexual activities or stimuli associated with sexuality produces varying degrees of sexual arousal in most people. Estimates that Americans spend approximately $600 million annually on books, photographs, magazines, and movies depicting sexual activities or stimuli (Commission on Obscenity and Pornography, 1970) attest to the erotic potential of such materials. Let us now examine the effects of such stimuli on sexual responses.

Erotic Media.   In much of the early erotica research it was simply assumed that sex stimuli presented through any medium would be sexually arousing. A rather obvious question of interest concerns whether the medium in which erotic stimuli are presented has any influence on sex arousal.

The available findings suggest that motion pictures are more arousing than audio recordings (Abel et al., 1975), still photos (Sandford, 1974), drawings, and written descriptions of sexual acts (Byrne & Lamberth, 1971; Levitt & Hinesley, 1967). However, the presence or absence of color in movies does not seem to be an important determinant of their arousal value (High, Rubin, & Henson, 1979). These findings suggest that excepting the presence or absence of color the degree of "realism" in sexual stimuli is one important determinant of their ability to turn people on.

It is possible, nonetheless, that erotic stimuli in any medium may become too realistic. Recall that Byrne and Lamberth (1971) found that fantasy alone was a more effective sexual stimulant than either photos or written passages. Our fantasies are not necessarily subject to the bounds of reality and are sometimes truly fantastic in that we are free to conjure up virtually any sexual acts, with any partner(s), and in any setting. Photographs, movies, and stories, on the other hand, supply the names, faces, bodies, or circumstances of sexual activities, and may in so doing constrain the free flow of imagery and fantasy that is critical to the arousal of sexual desires.

Odors. Because of the potential limits imposed on imagination processes by highly realistic media representations, it might be expected that rather diffuse stimuli such as odors or music would be powerful erotic cues. As we noted earlier, very little is known about the role of smell in human sexual stimulation. To date, research findings have failed to establish genital or other odors as important biologically based sources of arousal (Doty, Ford, Preti, & Huggins, 1975; Rogel, 1978). It seems clear, though, that through conditioning, many odors do acquire the ability to produce sexual excitement. Almost all people use some form of deodorant, perfume, lotion, or cleansing product that has a characteristic smell. Through association with states of erotic arousal, such smells can become capable of triggering sexual excitement. Of course, which (if any) odor is sexually meaningful to a person is determined by his or her own unique experiences.

Music. Music is associated with sexual activities in many ways. Dancers and strippers carefully select the music that accompanies their performances in order to enhance their erotic appeal. The sexual connotations within contemporary music range from the blatant sexual content of some rock lyrics to more subtle sexual meanings suggested by certain rhythmic beats (Robinson & Hirsch, 1969). From time to time, citizens and religious groups launch campaigns of protest against various forms of music on the basis of their powers of sexual stimulation. In the mid 1970s, for example, the Reverend Charles Boykin and his followers destroyed several thousand dollars worth of rock records. He explained his actions as follows:

Today's music has a tribal effect on today's youth. Just go to any rock festival and you can see the open sex, which I believe is caused by the music. The beat causes immoral sexual behavior. We felt the public burning might cause some people to reassess their morals through their music. (United Press International, Wichita Eagle, *December 6, 1975)*

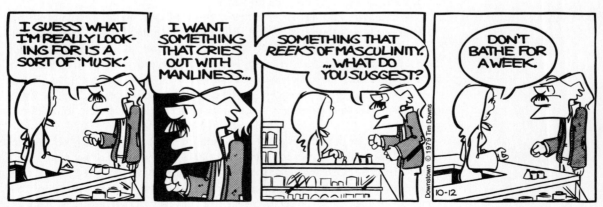

Though odors may be sexually stimulating, it is often difficult to know what odors are arousing to what people.

SOURCE: © 1979 Tim Downs.

Some people believe that the music heard at rock festivals such as the one pictured here has a powerful aphrodisiac quality; others would argue that its influence is much less powerful.

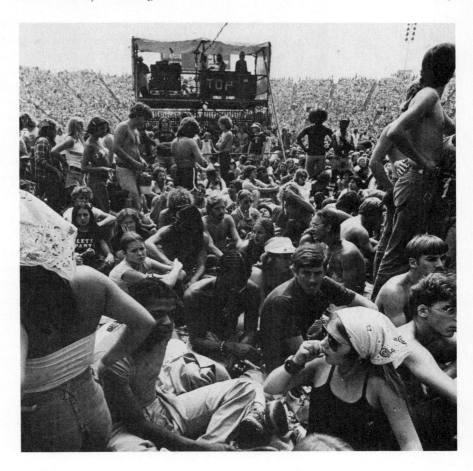

Though it is doubtful that any type of music possesses such powerful aphrodisiac qualities, the limited research findings concerning this issue do at least suggest a relationship between music and sex arousal. For example, Beardslee and Fogelson (1958) found that men and women who heard excerpts from nonvocal musical selections judged to be arousing expressed more erotic imagery in stories following the music than did those who heard nonarousing musical selections.

Even though the erotic potential of music has been examined only superficially, it does seem clear that the potential is there. Some musical selections are capable of evoking sexual imagery and thus sexual arousal. Reports suggesting that music or any other type of stimulus is overwhelming in its capacity to elicit sexual desires and acts should, however, be considered carefully. For example, the Reverend Boykin was apparently convinced of the sexual evils of music by an informal survey report that over 98 percent of a group of unmarried pregnant girls had listened to rock music during the days and nights on which they engaged in intercourse. A bit of reflection would suggest that at least 98 percent of them had also drunk a glass of water on these same days—perhaps it was the water, not the rock music, that led to their "downfall."

Erotic Themes.   What kinds of erotic messages or themes are most and least arousing? This issue has most often been examined through the use of still photos or movies that depict various sexual activities. Some sexual themes are rather consistently found to be most and least arousing across a variety of heterosexually oriented subject populations, experimental settings, and stimulus variations. From the results of a number of investigations, it is apparent that there is considerable agreement about the stimulating capacities of the erotic themes shown in Table 4–1. In general, both males and females are most aroused by pictures and movies showing nudes of the opposite sex masturbating, heterosexual genital and breast stimulation, heterosexual intercourse, and heterosexual oral-genital activities. Least arousing are depictions of sadomasochism, homosexual activities, and individuals of one's own sex. In studies of homosexually oriented individuals, however, pictures of homosexual activities among people of the subjects' own sex have been found to be most arousing (Abel et al., 1975; Freund, Langevin, Wescom, & Zajac, 1975).

At least two important factors contribute to the erotic potential of these sexual themes. First, people are generally most aroused by pictures of those activities that they might normally or, in fact, frequently have experienced. As shown in Figure 4–1, this is precisely what was found when subjects' degree of sexual experience was compared with their erotic responsiveness to photographic slides of various sexual activities (Griffitt, 1975).

A second factor appears to be the extent to which the stimuli depict sexual acts which are "elementary" or "advanced" in the degree of sexual intimacy or involve-

Table 4–1.

Most and least arousing sexual themes.
In studies using a wide variety of subject samples there is considerable agreement concerning which sexual themes are most and least sexually arousing.

Most Arousing Themes	
Males	**Females**
Sexual intercourse in various positions	Sexual intercourse in various positions
Genital petting	Genital petting
Heterosexual fellatio	Heterosexual cunnilingus
Heterosexual cunnilingus	Male stimulating female's breasts
Male stimulating female's breasts	Male masturbation
Female masturbation	
Group sex	
Nude female	

Least Arousing Themes	
Males	**Females**
Sadomasochism, male hurting female	Sadomasochism, male hurting female
Sadomasochism, female hurting male	Sadomasochism, female hurting male
Homosexual anal intercourse	Homosexual anal intercourse
Homosexual fellatio	Homosexual fellatio
Male masturbation	Homosexual cunnilingus
Nude male	Nude female

SOURCE: Based on data from Byrne & Lamberth, 1971; Griffitt, 1973, 1975; Levitt & Brady, 1965; Sanford, 1974; Sigusch et al., 1970; Steele & Walker, 1974.

ment represented. That is, among American college students at least, there appears to be a rather orderly progression in the types of sexual acts that people experience. Repertoires of sexual experience tend to expand, accumulate, and unfold along a continuum such that experience 1 is likely to occur first, followed by experience 2, then 3, and so forth. Generally, an individual who has engaged in experience 3 will also have engaged in experiences 2 and 1 but not necessarily 4, 5, or 6. It is as if the elementary acts (1 and 2) are prerequisites to more advanced acts along the continuum. Several investigators have plotted the progression of such experiences and developed scales to assess a person's degree of sex experience as it relates to the continuum (Podell & Perkins, 1957; Bentler, 1968a, 1968b). Peter Bentler's studies, for example, identified separate, but similar, orders of appearance of various sexual behaviors in males and females. The behaviors and their orders are shown in Table 4–2. It may be seen that as one moves from experience 1 (kissing) to experience 21 (mutual oral-genital contact with orgasm), the degree of intimacy and sexual involvement in the acts steadily increases.

It is possible that the advanced acts are somehow intrinsically more exciting, and also that photographs or movies that depict more advanced acts are more arousing than those that show behaviors appearing early in the experiential sequence. While the summarized findings in Table 4–1 tend to support this idea, more direct evidence is provided by a study by Fisher and Byrne (1976). Male and female college students indicated how sexually arousing they found photographic slides that depicted the same couple engaging in a variety of sexual acts. As can be seen in Figure 4–3, the sex arousal ratings of the themes are in at least rough correspondence to the sequence of the same acts in the sex experience repertoires of most college students presented in Table 4–2. Pictures of the advanced acts were rated as more sexually arousing than pictures of the elementary acts.

Familiarity and Novelty.   The saying, "Variety is the spice of life," captures the essence of observations that variety and novelty in sexual stimulation is an essential element in maintaining sexual responsiveness (Griffitt, 1981; Kinsey et al., 1948; Masters & Johnson, 1966). That is, a highly sexually arousing stimulus may become less and less arousing the more we are exposed to it.

At least some species of male animals become disinterested and unresponsive to their familiar mates following a few copulations within a relatively short period of time. They quickly regain interest and responsiveness, however, when a novel female partner becomes available (Clemens, 1967). In humans, it has been observed that married men and women who are minimally responsive to their spouses often are highly responsive with new partners (Hite, 1976; Kinsey et al., 1948; Masters & Johnson, 1966; O'Neill & O'Neill, 1972).

The notion that sexual stimuli decrease in erotic value as we become more and more familiar with them was tested with men by Howard, Reifler, and Liptzin (1971). In the experiment, men were exposed to the same set of erotic movies, photographs, magazines, and novels each day for ten days. On the eleventh day new erotic materials were provided. Sexual arousal following each session was measured by the amount of urinary acid phosphatase contained in urine samples taken from the men. This enzyme is secreted from the prostate gland and is thought to increase in amount as a result of sexual arousal (Barclay, 1971a). The results of the experiment are shown in Figure 4–4.

Table 4–2.

Sequence in which specific sexual experiences are likely to occur.
When scaled using a method that results in orderings of sexual behaviors, the sexual experiences of both male and female college students tend to progress in an orderly sequence from somewhat exciting "elementary" acts to more exciting "advanced" acts.

Order of Act	Males	Order of Act	Females
1.	One minute continuous lip kissing with female.	1.	One minute continuous lip kissing with male.
2.	Manual manipulation of clothed female breasts.	2.	Manual manipulation of your clothed breasts by male.
3.	Manual manipulation of nude female breasts.	3.	Manual manipulation of your nude breasts by male.
4.	Manual manipulation of clothed female genitals.	4.	Manual manipulation of your clothed genitals by male.
5.	Oral contact with nude female breasts.	5.	Oral contact with your nude breasts by male.
6.	Manual manipulation of nude female genitals.	6.	Manual manipulation of your nude genitals by male.
7.	Manual manipulation of your clothed genitals by female.	7.	Manual manipulation of clothed male genitals.
8.	Mutual manual manipulation of clothed genitals with female.	8.	Mutual manual manipulation of clothed genitals with male.
9.	Manual manipulation of your nude genitals by female.	9.	Manual manipulation of nude male genitals.
10.	Manual manipulation of nude female genitals to massive female genital secretions.	10.	Manual manipulation of your nude genitals by male to massive genital secretions for you.
11.	Sexual intercourse, face to face.	11.	Manual manipulation of nude male genitals to ejaculation by male.
12.	Manual manipulation of your nude genitals to ejaculation, by female.	12.	Oral contact with your nude genitals by male.
13.	Oral contact with nude female genitals.	13.	Oral contact with nude male genitals.
14.	Oral contact with your nude genitals by female.	14.	Sexual intercourse, face to face.
15.	Mutual manual manipulation of nude genitals with female to mutual orgasm.	15.	Oral *manipulation* of your nude genitals by male.
16.	Oral *manipulation* of your nude genitals by female.	16.	Oral *manipulation* of nude male genitals.
17.	Oral *manipulation* of nude female genitals.	17.	Mutual oral-genital manipulation with male.
18.	Mutual oral-genital manipulation with female.	18.	Mutual manual manipulation of nude genitals with male to mutual orgasm.
19.	Sexual intercourse, rear entry.	19.	Sexual intercourse, rear entry.
20.	Oral manipulation of your nude genitals to ejaculation by female.	20.	Oral manipulation of male genitals to ejaculation by male.
21.	Mutual oral manipulation of genitals with female to mutual orgasm.	21.	Mutual oral manipulation of genitals with male to mutual orgasm.

SOURCE: Adapted from Bentler, 1968a, 1968b.

The erotic stimuli increased phosphatase levels sharply, but continued exposure to the same stimuli produced less and less arousal as the experiment progressed. Arousal was renewed with the introduction of new erotic stimuli but it once again dropped after the first day of exposure to the novel stimuli. These findings strongly suggest that, under some circumstances, familiar sexual stimuli are less arousing to men than are novel stimuli. Similar studies of women's sexual response patterns are needed.

WHO IS SEXUALLY STIMULATED?

Up to this point our discussion has focused on general processes and principles of sexual stimulation as they are revealed by the study of a mythical person—the "average" person. The average person, as represented in most of the research we have considered, is an impossible mixture of multiple and contradictory biological and psychosocial characteristics. This creature is at once male, female, young, old,

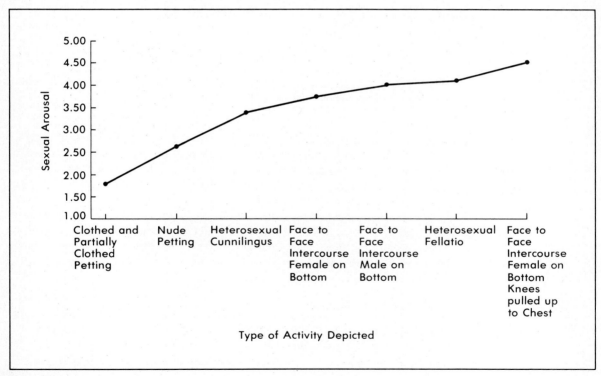

Figure 4–3.

Sexual arousal ratings by males and females combined of photographic slides depicting sexual activities that roughly correspond to selected sexual activities from the "elementary" and "advanced" portions of the sex experience sequence scales shown in Table 4-2.
SOURCE: Adapted from data from Fisher & Byrne, 1976.

Figure 4–4.

Physiological effects of exposure to erotic stimuli.

On the first day of exposure to erotic stimuli, levels of urinary acid and phosphatase increased greatly, then gradually declined over continued exposure to the same stimuli. New erotic stimuli again produced a large increase, followed by a decline with repeated exposure.

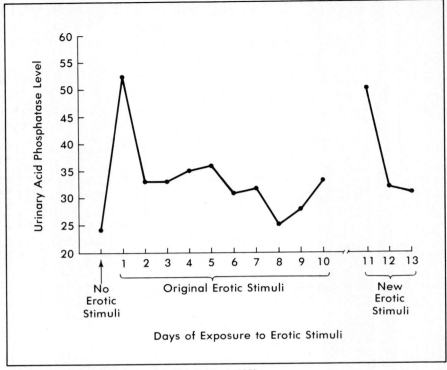

SOURCE: Adapted from Howard, Reifler, & Liptzin, 1971.

guilt-ridden, guilt-free, smart, dull, poor, wealthy, conservative, liberal, anxious, relaxed, and so forth—all rolled into a single package. Examination of this admittedly improbable being allows us to identify some of the basic processes involved in the determination of what is sexually stimulating as well as some of the more common sources of sexual arousal.

An "average-person" orientation, however, tends to obscure vast differences among people in sexual responsiveness—in what they find sexually arousing and how excited they become when exposed to various stimuli. We will now discuss how such differences are associated with various biological and psychosocial processes.

Biological Processes

Though intimately involved in the sexuality of lower mammals, biological processes play rather minor roles in determining precisely what stimuli humans find sexually arousing. The available evidence suggests a similar conclusion about the influences of biological processes on individual differences in sexual responsiveness.

Genetic Influences.   The systematic study of genetic influences on individual differences is a relatively recent trend in psychology (Hirsch, 1967). Research with several types of animals suggests that differences in sexual responsiveness are, in part, genetically determined. That is, parent animals seem to "pass on" their own high or low sexual responsiveness to their offspring (Fraser, 1968; McGill, 1965). In humans, the evidence is very sketchy but at least hints at the possibility of a weak genetic influence on sexual responsiveness (Chilton, 1972). Substantially more research is needed in the area.

Hormonal Influences. Earlier in this chapter we concluded that the sexual responsiveness of lower mammals is influenced in many important ways by levels of circulating hormones. In contrast, among humans, normal variations in steroid hormone concentrations (estrogen and progesterone in women, androgen in men) are minimally related to variations in sexual responsiveness. That is, the sexual responsiveness of women bears little direct relationship to the hormonal changes associated with the menstrual cycle, surgical removal of the ovaries, or menopause (Bremer, 1959; Griffith & Walker, 1975; Masters & Johnson, 1966). Similarly, normal testosterone variations in men are not linked to differences in responsiveness (Pirke, Kockott, & Dittmar, 1974; Rubin et al., 1979).

Psychosocial Processes

Research has generally failed to establish biological processes as important determinants of differences among people in their responses to sexual stimulation. Research focusing on psychosocial differences among people has been somewhat more enlightening. Let us now examine some of these differences.

Personality and Responses to Sexual Stimuli. A number of personality characteristics are related to how people react to sexual stimuli. For example, *sex guilt* is a general tendency for people to feel guilty when they violate sexual standards or even think about violating such standards (Mosher, 1966, 1968, 1970, 1971). A person taught that being sexually aroused by someone or something other than his or her own spouse is sinful or wrong feels guilty whenever he or she becomes aroused or anticipates becoming aroused under such circumstances. A person highly disposed to sex guilt avoids situations providing sexual temptation and experiences distress when succumbing to such temptation either in thought or in deed. In an interview during the 1976 presidential campaign, candidate Jimmy Carter expressed this notion lucidly:

I try not to commit a deliberate sin. I recognize that I'm going to do it anyhow, because I'm human and I'm tempted. . . . Christ said, "I tell you that anyone who looks on a woman with lust has in his heart already committed adultery." I've looked on a lot of women with lust. I've committed adultery in my heart many times. This is something that God recognizes I will do—and I have done it—and God forgives me for it. (Scheer & Golson, 1976, p. 86)

Research using scales to measure individual differences in sex guilt (Mosher, 1966, 1968) has shown that people who are high in sex guilt react quite differently to sexual stimuli than do people who are low in sex guilt. Three major differences have been reported.

First, when they are exposed to words with sexual meaning, photos of nudes of the opposite sex, or to photos, movies, and stories containing explicit depictions of sexual acts, those who are high in sex guilt experience fewer sexual thoughts, images, and fantasies than do those low in sex guilt (Galbraith & Mosher, 1970; Janda, 1975; Schwartz, 1975). Second, when exposed to such sexual materials, high sex-guilt people report more negative emotions such as feelings of being shocked, repelled, irritated, disgusted, embarrassed, ashamed, nauseated, angry, and depressed than do those low in sex guilt (Griffitt & Kaiser, 1978; Mosher, 1971; Mosher & Greenberg, 1969). Third, and presumably because of the first two differences, high sex-guilt people tend to be less sexually aroused by explicit sex stimuli than are low sex-guilt people (Mosher & Greenberg, 1969; Ray & Walker, 1973).

Other personality characteristics also influence reactions to sex stimuli. For example, people who psychologically avoid thoughts of sexuality, are sexually conservative, or are very traditional in their sexual attitudes experience distressing emotional reactions when exposed to erotic stimuli (Byrne & Sheffield, 1965; Griffitt, 1973; Wallace & Wehmer, 1972). These negative emotional experiences not only add elements of unpleasantness to sexual arousal, but also cause people to actively avoid situations in which exposure to sex stimuli and, thus, sexual arousal is likely (Griffitt & Kaiser, 1978; Schill & Chapin, 1972).

Age and Responses to Sexual Stimuli.   Data from a variety of sources suggest that there is a tendency for both men and women to become less and less sexually active as they grow older (Kinsey et al., 1948, 1953; Masters & Johnson, 1966). Very little research has been done concerning age differences in response to erotic stimuli. In one study, researchers interviewed a national probability sample of over two thousand adults about their experiences with and attitudes toward erotic materials (Abelson, Cohen, Heaton, & Suder, 1971). Both men and women between the ages of twenty-one and forty-nine reported being more sexually aroused by literary erotica than did those over age fifty. Additionally, experimental studies in which subjects view erotic materials generally find that 75 to 85 percent of men and women between twenty and twenty-five experience genital responses (Mosher, 1971) but only 45 to 60 percent of men and women between forty and fifty experience such responses (Mann, Sidman, & Starr, 1971). These limited findings suggest that as we become older we become less responsive to external sexual stimuli. As noted in Chapter 10, however, these declines appear to be due primarily to culturally shared expectations that erotic responsiveness decreases with age rather than to diminished capacities.

Male and Female Responses to Sexual Stimuli.   Since Victorian times, socioculturally determined beliefs concerning differences between male and female erotic responsiveness and interests have been faithfully transmitted from one generation to the next. It has been taught that males are highly driven by sexual needs, quick to respond to real or imagined sexual opportunities, aggressive in their demands on women, and highly motivated to seek sexual stimulation and outlets. Women, in contrast, are disinterested in sex, indifferent to sexual stimuli, difficult, if not impossible, to arouse sexually, and only reluctant participants in sexual activities. They tolerate and give in to male sexual demands only as a result of force, in exchange for marriage, or to become pregnant and have children of their own. Their primary interest in men is not sex but affection and security. Once a mate and offspring are acquired, sex is avoided as much as possible through deception and excuses such as feigned headaches or fatigue.

That male sexual desires are insatiable and triggered easily "like putting a quarter in a vending machine" (Comfort, 1972, p. 73) and that a husband's task in marriage is to find some way of arousing his wife so that she will at least participate in sex have been two of the central messages in the best-selling marriage manuals of the past two decades (Gordon & Shankweiler, 1971). How accurate is this picture of male and female sexual responsiveness?

Several types of evidence are, in fact, consistent with this view of male-female differences in erotic responsiveness. Females become sexually active at later ages than do males and are less likely to engage in masturbation, premarital intercourse, extramarital intercourse, and homosexual activities than are males (Kinsey et al., 1953; Hunt, 1974). Females exert less effort than males to encounter sex stimuli (Griffitt & Kaiser, 1978) and the customers of adult bookstores and pornographic movie theatres are primarily male (Nawy, 1971).

At least three major survey studies have consistently reported male-female differences in amount of exposure to erotica and degree of sexual arousal produced by such exposure. In one of these surveys (Kinsey et al., 1953) a higher proportion of males (77 percent) than females (32 percent) reported experiences of arousal when exposed to visual depictions of sexual action or of nude figures (54 percent of males, 12 percent of females). When exposed to verbal or written stories, sexual arousal was reported by 47 percent of the males and only 14 percent of the females. To the researchers, it seemed "likely that most females are indifferent to the existence of such material because it means nothing to them erotically" (Kinsey et al., 1953, p. 662). Even following dramatic societal changes in attitudes regarding sexuality, when questioned in surveys males still report more interest in and sexual arousal to erotic pictures, movies, and books than do females (Abelson et al., 1971; Berger, Gagnon, & Simon, 1971). Thus, *in surveys when people are asked to recall* their experiences with and reactions to erotic materials, males clearly exceed females in reported sexual arousal.

Only in recent years have experimenters used females in studies of responses to systematic presentations of erotica in experimental laboratory settings. The results of these studies are sharply in contrast to views of women as indifferent and unresponsive to erotic materials. Across a wide array of subject samples from Western Europe and the United States, males and females have been found to be remarkably similar in their reported levels of arousal to erotic slides, movies, and stories, as Figure 4–5 indicates.

Research using physiological measures of sexual arousal has obtained similar results. Several investigators have developed instruments to measure penile erections (Bancroft, Jones, & Pullan, 1966; Barlow, Becker, Leitenberg, & Agras, 1970; Jovanovic, 1971). These devices, the penile plethysmographs mentioned earlier, have flexible bands that are placed around the penis and stretch as the penis increases in size. A **vaginal photoplethysmograph** is a small acrylic cylinder that is placed just inside the entrance of the vagina. It records the volume of blood in the vaginal walls (Geer, Morokoff, & Greenwood, 1974; Heiman, 1975, 1977; Hoon, Wincze, & Hoon, 1976). Both devices measure blood engorgement of the genitals, which is the primary physiological response during sexual arousal. Studies using these instruments have consistently shown that both men and women are physio-

Figure 4–5.

Lack of overall male-female differences in self reports of sexual arousal following exposure to erotic photographs, movies, and written materials.

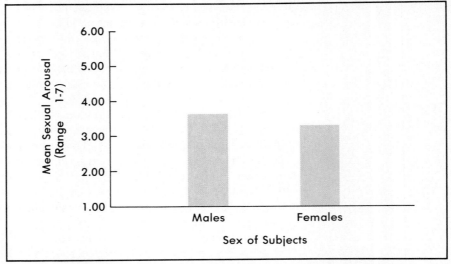

SOURCE: Data from Byrne & Lamberth, 1971, Griffitt, 1973, Sigusch et al., 1970, Schmidt & Sigusch, 1970, Schmidt, Sigusch, & Schäfer, 1973.

logically aroused when exposed to erotic materials and that their patterns of arousal are quite similar (Heiman, 1975, 1977; Wincze, Hoon, & Hoon, 1977).

In summary, it seems clear that, when they are exposed to erotic materials in laboratory studies, the sexual arousal responses of men and women are quite similar (Abramson, Perry, Rothblatt, Seeley, & Seeley, 1981; Griffitt, 1973; Hatfield, Sprecher, & Traupmann, 1978).

What might account for the differences between the survey research findings and time-honored beliefs on the one hand and the experimental findings on the other hand? One possible explanation for these differences may be found in the manner in which females are socialized with respect to sexuality. If they are taught that respectable and decent women are not interested in sex and erotic stimuli, and that actions that indicate otherwise are unacceptable, it is reasonable that they would at least outwardly accept these prohibitions. In an interview or survey, then, the majority could be expected to deny being aroused by most classes of sexual stimuli and pornography not only because of lack of exposure to erotica but also because to admit such feelings would reveal some sort of character defect or aberration. In laboratory settings, however, the experimenter is responsible for the presence of erotica, and reports of sexual arousal are legitimized by the experimental procedures (Byrne, 1976; Gebhard, 1973).

It has become fashionable in recent years to deny the existence of any differences in the sexuality of men and women (Bernard, 1972). As our earlier discussion shows, men and women are more similar in erotic responsiveness than once thought, but they are *not identical*. In virtually all of the studies discussed above females report more negative feelings after exposure to erotica than do males even when they are equally sexually aroused. After a lifetime of learning that only whores, bitches, nymphomaniacs, or easy lays are excited by such materials, this difference is understandable.

RESEARCH HIGHLIGHT

Love Versus Lust in Female Sexual Responsiveness

Among the most widely cited findings of Alfred Kinsey and his colleagues (1953) is that, although females are not very responsive to depictions of explicit sexual activities, they are aroused by movies or stories in which affectionate and loving relationships are involved. In the first experimental test of this assumption (Schmidt, Sigusch, & Schafer, 1973), male and female university students were exposed to one of two parallel stories describing the sexual activities of a young couple. In one story, the sexual activities were described very blatantly, and little, if any, affection was expressed. The other story described identical sexual activities, but in the context of a loving, tender relationship and without the use of slang expressions. Excerpts from the two stories are presented below:

Story I (Without Affection)

They walked for a long time in silence. Then he took her in his arms. . . . You're hot for me and I'm hot for you! That's all.

He shoved his cock into her. He felt his sperm spurting into her hot cunt, he arched his back, shuddered groaning, and lay down on her breathing heavily and exhausted. . . . She lay there with her hand on his cock . . . . Both of them yielded to their limpness and passivity.

Exhausted and completely satisfied, they fell apart. He turned over and reached for a cigarette. That was a good fuck, he thought.

Story II (With Affection)

They walked for a long time in silence. . . . He took her into his arms. . . . You just love me and I love you and that's all.

He thrust his member into her. He felt his sperm flow into her hot vagina. . . . Tenderly he kissed her and stroked her arms. . . . they lay there silently, enchanted by one another. . . . Both of them yielded to the pleasantness of their limpness and passivity.

. . . they lay there completely satisfied, happily exhausted. . . . "It was good, it was so good," she whispered tenderly. . . . he said nothing, only kissed her softly, lay down next to her, and pulled her close to himself. (Schmidt et al., 1973, p. 183)

After reading one or the other of the stories the students then indicated their degree of sexual arousal. It was found that both stories were equally arousing and that the females and males did not differ in their reactions to either of the stories. Thus, the presence of affection was irrelevant to the arousal of sexual desire in both females and males. Other research (e.g., Byrne, Fisher, & De Ninno, 1975; Heiman, 1977; Osborn & Pollack, 1977; Schmidt, 1975) strengthens the conclusion that female sexual responsiveness is no more dependent on elements of romance, affection, or love than is that of males.

It should be no surprise that males and females differ in how aroused they are by particular sexual themes. For example, both sexes are more aroused by nudes of the opposite sex than by nudes of their own sex (Byrne & Lamberth, 1971; Griffitt, 1973) and by movies of an opposite-sex person masturbating than of a same-sex individual masturbating (Schmidt, 1975). It is sometimes found that males are more aroused by themes of group sex and oral sex than are females (Byrne & Lamberth, 1971; Griffitt, 1973; Mosher, 1971). Sex differences in response to oral sex, however, are not found among married males and females. This convergence between the sexes would appear to be a result of increasing female experience with cunnilingus and fellatio as a result of marriage (Griffitt, 1973, 1975). Generally, it seems that sexual experience is the "great equalizer" in terms of erotic responsiveness. As males and females become more and more similar in their sexual experiences, and as attitudinal differences between the sexes fade (Hunt, 1974), we may expect to see fewer and fewer differences in erotic responsiveness.

WHAT ARE THE EFFECTS OF SEXUAL STIMULATION?

Historically, Western societies have tended to regulate strictly the extent to which people are exposed to stimuli that are potentially capable of triggering sexual arousal. One of the underlying assumptions of such regulations concerning erotica, nudity, dress codes, and public displays of sexual acts is that exposure to any sort of erotic stimulus produces changes in behavior. It is assumed that encounters with sexual stimuli rather automatically induce people to engage in sexual behavior (Commission on Obscenity and Pornography, 1970; Kronhausen & Kronhausen, 1964). Thus, it is said, in much the same way that stimuli that arouse hunger, anger, or fear lead to eating, fighting, and fleeing, stimuli that are sexually arousing lead to sexual acts. Some of the more extreme fears concerning the effects of erotica are exemplified in the following statements:

The cumulative result of pornography on a young person is practically equivalent to the sad effects felt by the victim of a child seducer. . . .

In adults—even sexually mature ones—pornography has a sexually regressive effect. It encourages sexual behavior characteristic of perverts. . . .

The regressive effect of pornography on sexual behavior brings on premature death. (Anchell, 1974, pp. 6–7)

These are potent effects. If they are true, few would disagree that pornography and other classes of sexual stimuli should be heavily regulated. What is currently known about the behavioral effects of sexual stimulation?

Sexual Stimuli and Sex Crimes

A substantial proportion of surveyed American adults believe that exposure to erotic materials leads people to commit rape (49 percent) or believe (37 percent) that it makes people "sex crazy" and presumably capable of engaging in other

Research on the effects of pornography has produced mixed results: some studies indicate that exposure to pornography increases aggression, while other studies have found that it actually leads to a decrease in sex-related crime.

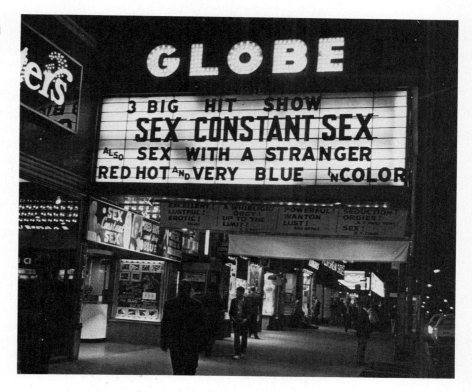

criminal sexual acts (Abelson et al., 1971). In a similar vein, it is frequently asserted that females who wear revealing clothing or otherwise display sexual cues are simply inviting sexual assaults because of the stimulating effects of those cues on men. Is it possible that the many sexual stimuli in our world produce a sufficient degree of unsatisfied sexual arousal to lead a person (usually male) to commit rape, molest children, expose his genitals to unsuspecting females, peep into windows, or engage in other forms of criminal sexual activity? At least two types of evidence are relevant to this complex question.

Several studies have been conducted in which convicted sex offenders have been compared with nonoffenders with respect to their experiences with erotica. The results of these studies have been mildly surprising. It has been found that sex offenders have *less experience* with erotica during preadolescence and adolescence than do nonoffenders (Goldstein, Kant, Judd, Rice, & Green, 1971) and the "average" sex offender first encounters such materials at a later age than does the "average" nonoffender (Commission on Obscenity and Pornography, 1970; Eysenck, 1972). Furthermore, sex offenders are no more likely to report sexual arousal or to engage in sexual behavior following exposure to erotica than are nonoffenders (Goldstein et al., 1971). In fact, the early lives of sex offenders are characterized by extremely avoiding and restrictive attitudes toward sex:

Research shows that the early social environments of sex offenders may be characterized as sexually repressive and deprived. Sex offenders frequently report family circumstances in which, for example, there is a low tolerance for nudity, an absence of sexual conversation, and punitive or indifferent parental responses to children's sexual curiosity and interest. Sex offenders' histories reveal . . . rigid sexual attitudes, and sexually conservative behavior. (Commission on Obscenity and Pornography, 1970, p. 242)

That such restrictive attitudes regarding sexuality and a relative lack of exposure to erotic stimuli might actually increase the incidence of sex crimes is suggested by a second line of evidence. In 1969, following a long period during which explicit erotic materials became increasingly available, the laws of Denmark were altered, making it possible for all forms of explicit erotic materials to be distributed and for adults to view movies and live sex shows without restrictions. When the incidence of various sex crimes was examined over a period of several years it was found that there was a dramatic *decrease* of nearly 70 percent between 1958 and 1969. That decline has continued; the frequency of rape, child molestation, peeping, exhibitionism, and all other classes of sex crimes has decreased. The decreases are not attributable to changes in law enforcement procedures, reporting methods, or public willingness to report such offenses (Commission on Obscenity and Pornography, 1970). Although such evidence is by no means conclusive, it clearly suggests that exposure to erotic stimuli does not cause sex crimes and may, in fact, have just the opposite effect.

It should be noted, however, that recent laboratory research by a number of investigators has shown that highly arousing sexual stimulation may intensify aggressive behavior in people who are already predisposed to act aggressively (Baron, 1979; Donnerstein & Hallam, 1978; White, 1979; Zillmann, 1971). Under some circumstances, exposure to erotic films leads to increases in men's and women's aggressiveness toward those of either sex. Films depicting sexual aggression against women are particularly likely to increase men's aggressiveness against women (Donnerstein & Berkowitz, 1981; Malamuth & Donnerstein, 1984). This research has, however, been conducted under artificial laboratory conditions, and its relevance to more lifelike situations is not yet clear.

Sexual Stimuli and Sexual Behavior

Does exposure to sexual stimuli increase the frequency of sexual behavior? Two types of evidence lead to the logical conclusion that exposure to erotic stimuli does increase levels of sexual activity. First, erotically stimulating materials increase levels of sexual arousal, and it might therefore be expected that increased desires would lead to increased sexual activity. Second, under certain circumstances, people imitate the behavior of models in movies, photographs, or literary works (Bandura, 1969). If the behavior portrayed is sexual, those exposed to such materials might tend to engage in similar behavior whenever possible.

More than a dozen experiments have been conducted in an attempt to determine the effects of erotic materials on overt sexual behavior. In the typical experiment, the sexual behavior patterns of subjects are ascertained, they are exposed to erotic movies, photographs, or stories, and their sexual behavior patterns are once again assessed. When compared with pre-exposure behavior or with the behavior of control groups who have not been exposed to erotic materials, changes in sexual behavior are attributed to the effects of sexual stimulation. The findings of a number of such studies are summarized in Figure 4–6. It is apparent that erotica have relatively minor effects on overt sexual behavior. Only a small percentage of people report increases in frequencies of intercourse, masturbation, or conversations about sex following exposure to sexual stimuli. The increases that do occur are in behaviors that the people have already engaged in on a regular basis. That is, increased frequency of masturbation or intercourse occurs only among those who regularly masturbate or have intercourse. Very few people report engaging in novel acts that imitate those contained in the erotic materials. Finally, the changes reported are short-lived and generally subside within twenty-four to forty-eight hours (Commission on Obscenity and Pornography, 1970).

Thus, even though erotic stimuli do produce subjective experiences and physiological reactions characteristic of sexual arousal, it is clear that such arousal does not automatically lead people to commit sexual mayhem or to seek immediate gratification of heightened sexual desires. The occurrence of intercourse, masturbation, and other overt sexual acts is determined by a variety of psychosocial factors including a lifetime accumulation of religious, social, moral, legal, and emotional influences. It would be surprising if relatively brief exposures to erotica could override the effects of these potent factors.

Figure 4–6.

Effects of exposure to erotica on reported changes in sexual behavior.
Across a number of samples of married and single males and females it has been found that exposure to erotic materials produces only temporary and slight increases in the frequencies of previously established patterns of sexual behavior in a small proportion of people tested.

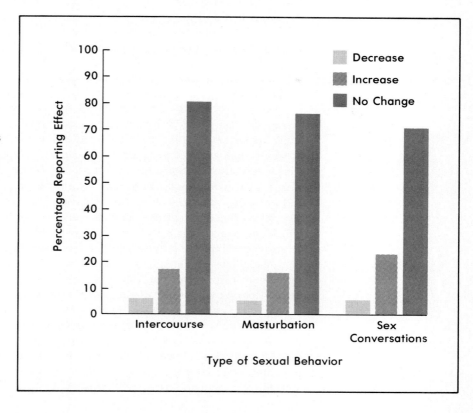

Sexual Stimuli and Sexual Perceptions

Although exposure to arousing sexual stimuli does not dramatically influence overt sexual behavior, several studies show that erotica-produced sexual arousal does affect our perceptions of and sexual attraction to potential or actual sexual partners. Two studies, for example, have shown that sexual arousal in men produced by exposure to erotica increases men's sexual attraction to attractive women (Dermer & Pyszczynski, 1978; Stephan, Berscheid, & Walster, 1971). That women's sexual attraction to attractive men is also increased when women are sexually aroused has been demonstrated by a third study (Griffitt, May, & Veitch, 1974).

There are at least two possible explanations for the effects of sexual arousal on sexual attraction. First, it may be that, when we are sexually aroused, any person who is seen as potentially capable of satisfying our sexual desires is perceived as sexually desirable and attractive (Stephan et al., 1971). This explanation suggests that, for heterosexuals, sexual arousal will increase sexual attraction to those of the opposite sex, regardless of their physical attractiveness.

A second possibility is that sexual arousal increases our perceptual sensitivity to the sexually relevant features of people and intensifies whatever positive or negative reactions we have to those features (Griffitt, 1979). This explanation suggests that, for heterosexuals, sexual arousal will increase sexual attraction to physically attractive opposite-sex persons, but decrease sexual attraction to unattractive persons of the opposite sex. This is precisely what was found in a recent study using college men and women as subjects (Istvan, Griffitt, & Weidner, 1983). Thus, it seems clear that one effect of exposure to sexually arousing stimuli is to make us more alert and reactive to the sexual characteristics of other people.

SUMMARY

Sexual stimulation in lower mammals is largely regulated by biological processes while human sexual stimulation is shaped and molded primarily by psychosocial processes. In lower animals, genetic factors play an important role in determining what is sexually stimulating. Research has failed to identify genetic determinants of what humans find sexually stimulating. Hormones may exert both organizational and activating influences on sexual responses. In lower mammals prenatal exposure to androgen organizes male patterns of sexual arousal in both males and females. In humans, the early hormonal environment exerts relatively weak effects on sexual response patterns during adulthood with the primary influence being on the "masculinity" or "femininity" of adolescent play and social interaction patterns. In subhuman mammals, the activation of sexual responses by erotic stimuli is dependent on the presence of circulating gonadal hormones. The activating function of hormones in humans is quite limited. There are no clear relationships between "normal" variations in gonadal hormone levels and sexual responsiveness in either males or females. Aphrodisiac effects have been attributed to many drugs including alcohol, amphetamines, narcotics, hallucinogens, Spanish fly, amyl nitrite, and, more recently, L-dopa and PCPA. None of these chemicals act as true aphrodisiacs and many are quite dangerous.

Human responses to erotic stimuli are shaped by a variety of psychosocial processes including learning, cognitive activities, and emotional reactions. The power of erotic cues is dependent on their acquired ability to stimulate sexual thoughts, fantasies, and memories. Most arousing to heterosexuals are those stimuli that depict or suggest heterosexual intercourse, petting, or oral-genital activities, and least arousing are those that depict sadomasochistic behaviors, people of one's own sex, and homosexual activities. Negative emotional reactions may inhibit and positive emotional reactions may enhance sexual responses to erotic stimuli.

Individual variations among humans in sexual responsiveness are largely a result of psychosocial differences. Individuals high in sex guilt tend to inhibit sexual thoughts and images, avoid erotic stimulation, and experience negative emotional reactions when exposed to sexual stimuli. The effects of aging on sexual responsiveness have not been extensively studied but the available evidence suggests that moderate declines might take place. It has generally been assumed that women are less sexually responsive than are men. Recent research findings, however, have questioned this basic assumption by demonstrating striking similarities in the responsiveness of males and females when exposed to erotic stimuli. A substantial proportion of both sexes are sexually aroused by such materials, and elements of affection or romance are not essential to the erotic reactions of either males or females. The differences that do exist seem to be based on psychosocial rather than on biological factors.

In humans, exposure to erotic stimuli results in genital reactions identical to those in actual sexual encounters but arousal does not necessarily lead to immediate sexual acts and gratification. Psychosocial constraints often require the inhibition or postponement of sexual gratification, but in most people such unsatisfied desires do not lead to criminal sexual activities. Exposure to erotic stimuli produces minor and temporary changes in the overt sexual behavior of some people. Erotica-produced sexual arousal influences our sexual attraction to potential or actual sexual partners.

SUGGESTED READINGS

Beach, F. A. (1969). It's all in your mind. *Psychology Today*, February, pp. 33–35, 60.

Bermant, G., & Davidson, J. M. (1974). *Biological bases of sexual behavior.* New York: Harper & Row.

Commission on Obscenity and Pornography (1970). *The report of the Commission on Obscenity and Pornography.* Washington, DC: U.S. Government Printing Office.

Malamuth, N., & Donnerstein, E. (Eds.) (1984). *Pornography and sexual aggression.* New York: Academic Press.

Schmidt, G., & Sigusch, V. (1973). Women's sexual arousal. In J. Zubin and J. Money (Eds.), *Contemporary sexual behavior.* Baltimore: Johns Hopkins University Press.

Zuckerman, M. (1971). Physiological measures of sexual arousal in the human. *Psychological Bulletin, 75,* 297–329.

CHAPTER OUTLINE

BIOLOGICAL PROCESSES: SEXUAL RESPONSE CYCLES
Excitement Phase
Plateau Phase
Orgasm Phase
Resolution Phase
Factors That May Alter Sexual Response Cycles

PSYCHOSOCIAL PROCESSES
Experiencing Arousal and Orgasm
Individual Differences in Arousal and Orgasm

CHAPTER 5

SEXUAL AROUSAL AND ORGASM

"Orgasms are a renewal of all my sense, an awakening of life, spring refreshing, sparkling, exciting, and complete relief of everyday boredom." . . . "They make me incredibly happy, everything on the way to orgasm is heavenly. An orgasm cancels out all rage and longing for at least forty-eight hours, and the day an orgasm bores me, I think I'll commit suicide." (Hite, 1976, p. 129)

We have seen that sexual desires, needs, and interests may be awakened or stimulated by exposure to a variety of internal or external erotic cues. All of us are exposed to a host of potentially sexually arousing stimuli on a daily basis. Whether or not we become sexually excited by such stimuli depends on a variety of factors, which were discussed in Chapter 4. Often what sexual excitement we do experience is little more than fleeting sexual longings that quickly dissolve as we go about the daily tasks of living. Sometimes, however, moderate levels of arousal lead to active sexual behavior, physical stimulation, and enhanced sexual excitement. In response to effective physical sexual stimulation our bodies undergo a series of physiological and anatomical reactions that may culminate in **orgasm**—the climactic release of accumulated sexual tensions.

Sexual arousal and orgasm are both biological and psychosocial experiences that we have only recently begun to understand. In this chapter we consider the biological and psychosocial processes associated with sexual arousal and orgasm.

BIOLOGICAL PROCESSES: SEXUAL RESPONSE CYCLES

Despite some early analyses of scattered research efforts (Kinsey et al., 1953), scientists have gained a detailed understanding of the anatomy and physiology of sexual arousal and orgasm only relatively recently. Primary credit for our current level of knowledge in this area must go to the research team of William H. Masters and Virginia E. Johnson. In 1954, they initiated a painstaking series of investigations of the sexual responses of women and men. The primary question they attempted to answer was, "What happens to the human male and female as they respond to effective sexual stimulation?" (1966, p. 10).

The subjects for the research project were 384 women and 312 men between the ages of eighteen and eighty-nine selected from the academic and nonacademic communities of St. Louis. Physically, sexually, and emotionally, the volunteers were normally functioning individuals selected only for their ability to respond sexually under laboratory conditions. As a group, the people were from higher socioeconomic and educational levels than is the general population, although individuals from virtually all backgrounds were represented in the samples. Both married and unmarried individuals of both sexes were included.

During almost a decade of research, over 7500 female and 2500 male sexual response cycles culminating in orgasm were observed. Using standard and specialized recording devices and motion pictures, the reactions of the body as a whole and of the genitals in particular were recorded as the individuals engaged in masturbation, sexual intercourse, or both. A special plastic "penis" device was designed so that intravaginal observations and films could be made.

Masters and Johnson divided the physiological reaction patterns of females and males into four phases (see Figure 5–1). In order of occurrence, the four phases are (1) *excitement*, (2) *plateau*, (3) *orgasm*, and (4) *resolution*. Although these phases occur in the same sequence in most people, the amount of time each phase takes varies widely from person to person and from occasion to occasion.

The four phases represent changes in level of sexual arousal. During the excitement phase, relatively low levels of arousal are created by psychogenic stimuli (erotic fantasies, visual, auditory, olfactory, or taste cues) and somatogenic (physical) stimuli. Arousal increases slowly or rapidly and then becomes nearly stabilized at relatively high levels during the plateau phase. Additional stimulation may result in the abrupt and explosive release of tension during orgasm followed by a longer resolution phase during which remaining tensions are more gradually dispersed. Of the four phases, excitement and resolution are usually the longest in duration. A person usually remains at plateau levels of arousal for only a short time and orgasm is usually completed in less than a minute. Specific times are not shown in Figure 5–1 because of the variability that exists between people and between separate cycles in a single individual. Also, specific levels of arousal are not shown since Masters and Johnson described arousal in only very general terms.

More variability in basic patterns of response is found among females than among males. Because of this, three patterns for females and only one for males are shown in Figure 5–1. The most common pattern for females (A) is one in which arousal mounts slowly, culminating in orgasm followed by the *possibility* of repeated orgasms. In the second pattern (B), the plateau and orgasmic phases are indistinguishable and the woman experiences a series of relatively rapidly occurring orgasms *(status orgasmus)* following a brief excitement phase. A long resolution phase typically follows the pattern B response. Pattern C characterizes those women who are quickly aroused and experience a sustained and intense climax followed by a rapid drop in sexual tensions. Patterns B and C are generally experienced as more intense and result in more striking physiological changes than does pattern A.

Figure 5–1.

Diagrammatic representation of the female (top) and male (bottom) sexual response cycles. The vertical axes represent degrees of sexual arousal and the horizontal axes represent time.

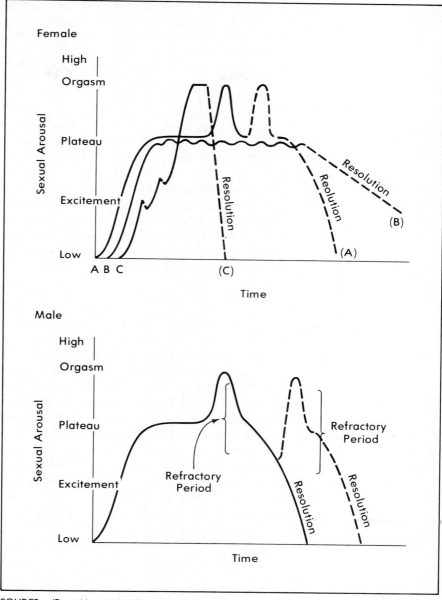

SOURCE: (From Masters & Johnson, 1965.)

The most common male pattern is one in which mounting arousal is followed by a single climactic peak at orgasm. However, following orgasm, most, but not all males (Robbins & Jensen, 1978), then enter a **refractory period**, in which they are unresponsive to further sexual stimulation; they generally must return to at least excitement levels of arousal before a second orgasmic response is possible. For many, full erection and ejaculation are impossible until the refractory period, the duration of which depends on a number of factors, terminates.

In general, sexual responses consist of vasocongestive and myotonic bodily reactions. **Vasocongestion** involves engorgement of the blood vessels of various body areas. Blood becomes "trapped" in the affected organs or structures and they become swollen, reddened, and warmed. **Myotonia** is increased muscular tension. Sexual arousal is accompanied by general as well as localized reactions in which some muscle groups become tensely and rigidly contracted while others contract and relax in regular or irregular patterns. In the following sections we will describe the physiological and anatomical response patterns accompanying the various phases of sexual response cycles in females and males.

Excitement Phase

Excitement phase levels of sexual arousal are signaled by the onset of a number of changes in the genitals as well as other body areas in both females and males. Some reactions, such as vaginal and penile responses are, of course, specific to one or the other sex, but others such as muscular and cardiovascular changes are quite similar in men and women. Let us first examine excitement phase responses in females.

Female Reactions.   The first detectable physiological response in the human female to any form of sexual stimulation is the production of lubricating fluid in the vagina. Individual droplets of moisture resembling beads of perspiration first appear throughout the folds of the vaginal wall within five to thirty seconds after the onset of sexual stimulation. As the excitement phase progresses and sex arousal levels increase, the individual droplets coalesce and coat the entire vaginal barrel with a slippery sheen of fluid. The available evidence indicates that the lubricant originates in and is forced through the vaginal walls as a result of vasocongestion of the vaginal tissues. Thus, early in the excitement phase this **sweating phenomenon** completely lubricates the vagina. As women reach their mid-fifties, vaginal lubrication becomes slower to develop and may take from one to three minutes in women over sixty. The reaction is reversible even if sexual stimulation is continued, and lubrication may be reduced or cease entirely if excitement levels of arousal are maintained for an extended period of time. The fluids already produced, however, continue to lubricate the vagina for some time.

The vaginal walls also thicken and slowly change from a purplish red to a deeper and darker purplish color during the excitement phase. Like the sweating reaction, these changes are due to engorgement of the vaginal tissues with blood. Though the neurological findings are somewhat inconclusive, it is generally thought that these vasocongestive responses are coordinated by a "reflex center" located in the sacral portion of the spinal cord (Kinsey et al., 1953).

Before the onset of sexual stimulation, the vagina is a "potential space" rather than an actual space, with the anterior (front) and posterior (back) vaginal walls in apposition, or touching (Figure 5–2). Late in the excitement phase, however, the vaginal barrel lengthens from an unstimulated 6.0 to 8.0 centimeters (2.4 to 3.2 inches) to 9.5 to 10.5 centimeters (3.7 to 4.1 inches) in depth. Near the location of the cervical entrance the vagina expands from an unstimulated width of 2.0 centimeters (.8 inches) to a width of 5.75 to 6.25 centimeters (2.3 to 2.5 inches). In addition, the corpus (body) and cervix of the uterus slowly elevate, pulling up the

Figure 5–2.

The female pelvis and clitoral structures (top) and male pelvis (bottom) before the onset of sexual stimulation.

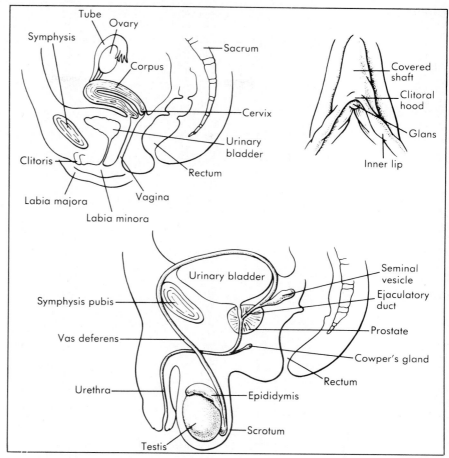

SOURCE: Based on Masters & Johnson, 1966.

anterior wall of the vagina to create a *tenting effect* and further adding to the diameter of the vagina (Figure 5–3). In the aging female, particularly following menopause, vaginal expansion is both less rapid and less extensive than in the younger woman.

Excitement phase levels of vasocongestion also produce changes in the clitoris, labia majora, and labia minora. In the unstimulated state the glans and shaft of the clitoris are partially and loosely covered by the overhanging hood (Figure 5–2), which is analogous to the foreskin of the uncircumcised penis. Late in the excitement phase blood engorgement results in **tumescence**, or swelling, of both the glans and shaft of the clitoris (Figure 5–3). Tumescence brings the glans into closer contact with the hood and surrounding tissues. This increases the probability of glans stimulation by movements of the adjacent structures (mons, minor labia). In addition to shaft and glans diameter increases, there is also lengthening of the clitoral shaft in some women. These size changes are of a rather small magnitude and the unaided eye can detect obvious glans enlargement in less than 50 percent and shaft elongation in less than 10 percent of responding women.

Figure 5–3.

The female pelvis and clitoral structures (top) and male pelvis (bottom) during the excitement phase of the sexual response cycle.

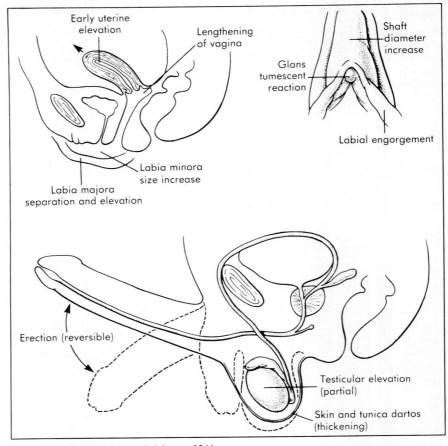

SOURCE: Based on Masters & Johnson, 1966.

The labia majora of the sexually unstimulated female normally meet and protectively enclose the labia minora, vaginal outlet, and urinary meatus (outlet). During excitement phase levels of sexual stimulation in women who have never given birth, the labia majora become thinner and "open" or are displaced away from the underlying genital structures. In women who have given birth, the lips are larger and instead of thinning become markedly congested and swollen in size.

The labia minora also begin enlarging as a result of vasocongestion during the excitement phase. By the end of this phase they may show an increase two to three times their original thickness and protrude through the expanded opening created by the labia majora. As a result of this size increase, the effective length of the vaginal barrel may be increased by 1.0 centimeter (.4 inches) or more. In women beyond the age of forty the vasocongestive changes in both the major and minor lips are markedly reduced.

The excitement phase in females also includes a number of extragenital physiological and anatomical reactions. The breasts undergo several observable changes. The first response is nipple erection produced by involuntary contractions of underlying muscle fibers. Nipple length may increase by .5 to 1 centimeter (.2 to .4 inches) and nipple diameter by .25 to .5 centimeter (.1 to .2 inches). Particularly large or small nipples increase in size less than do "average" nipples. Blood vessel engorgement increases the definition of superficial blood veins, the areolae swell, and late in the excitement phase the entire breast increases in size due to vasocongestion of deep tissues. Breast size increases due to sexual stimulation are of less magnitude in women who have breast-fed children and in women over fifty years of age.

About 25 percent of the women studied by Masters and Johnson (1966) developed a reddish **sex flush** or rashlike coloration of the skin late in the excitement phase. Due to superficial vasocongestion of skin tissues, the sex flush first appears on the lower chest and spreads upward over the breasts. During plateau levels of arousal the flush may spread to the neck, face, forehead, lower abdomen, thighs, and lower back. Relatively few women over fifty years of age develop the sex flush during any phase of the sexual response cycle. During the excitement phase, muscle tension shows a generalized but rather minimal increase and is most evident in the long muscles of the legs and arms and in abdominal muscles. Slight elevations in heart rate and blood pressure also begin during the excitement phase.

Male Reactions. The first physiological evidence of sexual excitement in the male is **erection** of the penis. Erection begins within a few (three to eight) seconds following the onset of sexual stimulation (Figure 5–3). Generally, erection occurs faster in young males than in older males and the reaction time may be two to three times longer in the fifty- to seventy-year-old man than in the twenty- to forty-year-old. Erection results from vasocongestion of the erectile tissues (corpora cavernosa and corpus spongiosum), in which the arterial blood flow into the penis greatly exceeds venous blood flow out of the penis.

Basically a reflex action, erection is coordinated by an "erection center" in the sacral portion of the lower spinal cord (Kaplan, 1974). This center receives nerve impulses triggered by tactile stimulation of the penis and adjacent tissues and, in turn, activates nerve fibers controlling penile arteries. Activation of one system of fibers leads to dilation of the arteries and, thus, increased blood flow into the penis. Loss of erection occurs when these nerves are deactivated by withdrawal of sexual stimulation or when the "opposing" nerves are activated, producing contraction of the penile arteries.

Though believed to be coordinated by the sacrally located reflex center, erection is obviously not totally controlled by physical stimulation of the genital area. A complex network of nerve fibers connects the erection center to various portions of the brain such that erection is largely directed by higher brain structures (MacLean, 1973; Masters & Johnson, 1966). Thus, erection can be stimulated by fantasies and other nontactile erotic stimuli. It may also be inhibited by various mental activities (see Chapter 4).

Although there are wide variations among men, the penis increases from an average flaccid length of 7.5 to 10 centimeters (3 to 4 inches) to approximately 15 centimeters (6 inches) and from a relaxed diameter of 3 centimeters (1.2 inches) to an erect diameter of 3.8 centimeters (1.5 inches) (Dickinson, 1949; Masters & Johnson, 1966). It must be emphasized that these are average figures. Within these average variations, neither flaccid nor erect penis size is related to a man's ability to give or receive sexual pleasure, his general body build, his "masculinity," or his race. Furthermore, erection tends to reduce differences in flaccid penis size. The smaller flaccid penis increases proportionately more in size than the large penis (Masters & Johnson, 1966).

At excitement phase levels of arousal, erections are readily lost if sexual stimulation is withdrawn or if asexual or anxiety-evoking stimuli are introduced. Reapplication of stimulation or withdrawal of intruding asexual stimuli allows for the rapid return of erection in younger (twenty- to forty-year-old) males. Men over fifty frequently experience difficulty in reachieving erection once it is lost. During excitement phases which are particularly prolonged, erection may be partially lost and regained several times even when stimulation is rather constant.

As a result of localized vasocongestion and increased muscle tension, the scrotum and testes also undergo changes during the excitement phase. Before stimulation, the thin scrotal integument, or skin, is relaxed and hangs loosely with its multiple folds and creases giving it a baggy appearance (see Figure 5–2). Stimulation produces both vasocongestive thickening and tensing of the tunica dartos layer of muscle fibers in the scrotal skin which, in effect, tightens the scrotum around the testes. Its baggy folded appearance as well as its relatively free movement are rapidly lost (see Figure 5–3).

Partial elevation of the testes from their unstimulated hanging position also occurs during the excitement phase. The musculature (cremasteric muscles) associated with the spermatic cords contracts, lifting and rotating the testes to bring them into close contact with the body. Testicular elevation is partially supported by scrotal thickening and tension and, as in the case of erection, both reactions are reversible during prolonged excitement phase levels of arousal.

Male extragenital reactions during the excitement phase essentially parallel those of females. General increases in muscle tension and moderate elevations of heart rate and blood pressure are characteristic of male excitement phase responses. Not surprisingly, however, male breast reactions are neither as evident nor as consistent as those of females. A small proportion (less than one third) of males may develop some degree of nipple erection during this phase. Vasocongestive breast size and areolar changes have not been recorded in the male, however. Sex flush reactions, which occur inconsistently in around one fourth of males, do not appear until plateau levels of arousal are reached.

Plateau Phase

As suggested by Figure 5–1, excitement phase levels of arousal are reached relatively quickly. Similarly, many of the reactions during the excitement phase are easily reversible and may be terminated quickly if stimulation is withdrawn or if asexual stimuli are introduced. If stimulation is continued, however, sexual tension levels are intensified and the individual enters the **plateau phase**, during which arousal levels reach heights from which the individual may ultimately move to orgasm. If orgasm is not reached, the tension levels achieved during this second phase of the cycle are more slowly resolved and terminated than those of the earlier excitement phase. Both females and males show specific as well as general body reactions during this phase.

Female Reactions.   Most of the vaginal changes during the excitement phase occur in the inner two thirds of the vagina; only minimal swelling and distention take place in the outer third of the barrel. During plateau phases of arousal, however, the outer third of the vaginal barrel undergoes a dramatic vasocongestive reaction (reduced in intensity by aging). Its inner diameter is actually decreased by as much as one third of that obtained during the excitement phase (see Figure 5–4).

Masters and Johnson (1966) have referred to this highly localized swelling as the **orgasmic platform**, since it constitutes the anatomic foundation for the physiological reactions of the vagina during orgasm. That is, most of the vaginal reactions during orgasm take place in this outer third, or orgasmic platform portion, of the vagina. Only minor increases in the depth and width of the inner two thirds of the vagina occur. These changes are largely produced by completion of the uterine elevation reaction, which enhances the tenting effect begun during the excitement phase. The rate of vaginal lubrication may actually be slowed during the plateau phase.

The clitoris shows an interesting reaction to sexual stimulation during the plateau phase. In virtually all women and consistently within any given woman,

Figure 5–4.

The female pelvis and clitoral structures (top) and male pelvis (bottom) during the plateau phase of the sexual response cycle.

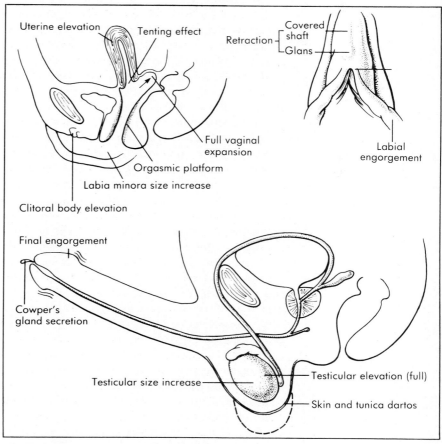

SOURCE: Based on Masters & Johnson, 1966.

both the shaft and the glans retract and withdraw from their normal position overhanging the upper vulval area. Tumescence of both the shaft and glans is maintained, but the muscles associated with the clitoral body pull the entire structure deeply beneath its protective hood (see Figure 5–4). The degree of retraction of the clitoris is directly related to intensity of sexual arousal. During the late plateau phase there may be an overall reduction of at least 50 percent in total length of the clitoris. The reaction is reversible if stimulation is withdrawn, and the clitoris may retract and reemerge several times during a prolonged plateau phase. It should be emphasized that clitoral retraction indicates increasing sexual arousal. It should not be misinterpreted as revealing loss of tension. Indeed, it has been argued (Sherfey, 1973) that the retracted clitoris is subjected to more intense stimulation by underlying and surrounding tissues than is the nonretracted organ. Thus, the retraction response may be viewed as a crucial element in the female sexual response cycle leading to orgasm.

The plateau phase reactions of the labia majora are essentially an extension of those begun during the excitement phase. The major labia become more fully distended with blood, and prolonged plateau phases may produce rather severe vasocongestion. Aside from retraction of the clitoral body, the most obvious sign of plateau phase levels of arousal in women is change in the coloration of the minor labia. In women who have never borne children, the minor labia undergo a color change from a rather light pink to bright red. In women who have borne more than one child the color change is from bright red to a deep wine color. These changes in minor labia coloration are so specific to the plateau phase, so consistent, and so predictive of impending orgasm that they have been called the *sex skin* of the sexually aroused woman. Unless the sex skin coloration appears, orgasm does not occur (Masters & Johnson, 1966).

Very small and located in each of the minor labia, the Bartholin's glands may, during the plateau phase, secrete a few drops of mucuslike material near the vaginal opening. The minute quantity of this secretion is insufficient to play an important role in vaginal barrel lubrication, although it may aid in lubrication of the vaginal opening during prolonged episodes of penile thrusting during coitus.

Extragenital manifestations of sexual arousal are intensified during the plateau phase. Already swollen breasts may enlarge to as much as 25 percent over their unstimulated state and areolar tumescence becomes so prominent that the erect nipples actually appear smaller than during the excitement phase. About 75 percent of all women sometimes show the sex flush response during the plateau phase if it was not already apparent during the earlier excitement phase. The sex flush reaches its peak of intensity late in the plateau phase and is a good indicant of degree of sexual arousal in those women who manifest the reaction.

As the sexually excited woman enters the plateau phase and moves to the brink of orgasm, her degree of sexual arousal is increasingly expressed by muscular tension, which is often evident from head to toe. As her facial muscles contract she may appear to frown, scowl, or grimace with her nostrils and mouth flaring open. Her neck muscles may become increasingly rigid and her total facial appearance is sometimes one of a person in extreme agony. Her back may become arched as a result of voluntary and involuntary contractions of abdominal and back muscles. Her buttocks are tensed and her thighs may be rigidly extended and squeezed together. Spastic contractions of involved muscles sometimes give the woman's toes and fingers a clawlike appearance **(carpopedal spasm)** and she may involuntarily clutch or grasp her sexual partner or other objects within reach. As intense levels of arousal are reached, the partially voluntary nature of many of these reactions sometimes gives way to involuntarily controlled pelvic thrusting, grasping, and other movements.

Involvement of the cardiovascular and respiratory systems in sexual responses is rather minimal during the excitement phase but becomes intense at plateau levels of arousal. Heart rate may be elevated from an unstimulated rate of 60 to 80 beats per minute to rates ranging from 100 to 175 per minute during late plateau. Late plateau arousal is also associated with rises in systolic blood pressure of 20 to 60 mm. Hg. (millimeters of mercury elevation) above the normal 120 and of 10 to 20 mm. Hg. over the normal diastolic pressure of 80. Late in the plateau phase and immediately prior to orgasm, two different patterns of respiration have been detected in responding females. The first is hyperventilation, in which the breathing rate markedly increases from an unstimulated average of 15 to as high as 30 or 40 breaths per minute (Masters & Johnson, 1966). A second pattern recorded by Fox and Fox (1969) is one in which the breathing rate immediately prior to orgasm is markedly reduced, with the woman "holding her breath" for extended periods but hyperventilating during orgasm. The available data, however, suggest that the former breathing pattern is most common (Masters & Johnson, 1966).

Male Reactions. For the most part, plateau phase reactions in the male are continuations of those responses that begin during the excitement phase. Slight increases in vasocongestion complete the erection, and the shaft of the penis becomes more rigid and hard than during excitement phase levels of arousal. In addition, the erection is somewhat more "permanent" in that minor distractions and temporary withdrawal of erotic stimulation are not as likely to result in loss of erection. The corona of the glans is the primary site of increased plateau phase tumescence (see Figure 5–4). In around 20 percent of males, the corona may undergo a color change in which a deep reddish purple color becomes evident. This color change does not consistently appear, however, and does not seem to be closely related to intensity of sex arousal. The color change has not been observed in men over sixty years old. Obviously, the penile urethra must also lengthen during erection, and plateau levels of arousal are accompanied as well by an increase in the internal diameter of the urethral passage two to three times the diameter before arousal. Late in this phase the urethral bulb located at the base of the penis undergoes a degree of rapid swelling that is predictive of imminent orgasm if stimulation is continued.

The scrotal sac completes its response to sex tension increases during the excitement phase, and no further changes are apparent until orgasm is completed. The testes, however, undergo further elevation, rotation, and swelling during the plateau phase. Prior to orgasm the testes are elevated and rotated until they are in tight contact with the perineum—the area of skin between the scrotum and anus. If tight perineal contact is not achieved, the ejaculatory pressure of orgasm is markedly reduced and complete orgasmic sensations are not experienced. In about 85 percent of males, the left testicle hangs lower in the scrotal sac than does the right testicle. As a consequence, the lower testicle must move further during elevation and frequently does not become fully elevated and rotated until immediately prior to orgasm. As a result of vasocongestion, both testicles increase in size by about 50 percent and, in some men, as much as 100 percent over their unstimulated state. Neither testicular elevation nor swelling are as marked in men over fifty years old as in younger men.

It is during plateau phase levels of arousal that some men manifest a **pre-ejaculatory emission** of a drop or two of mucuslike material that is thought to originate in the Cowper's glands (see Figure 5–4). This secretory material is not propelled from the urethra but merely appears at its opening. Preejaculatory emission does not occur in all men and its appearance is irregular even in those who do experience the reaction. The Cowper's gland secretion should not be confused with the ejaculation of semen, although it should be emphasized that *the emission sometimes contains active sperm*.

During late plateau levels of arousal, more than half of the males observed by Masters and Johnson (1966) evidenced some degree of nipple erection and in 25 percent the sex flush appeared. Nipple erection and the sex flush are less likely to occur in men than in women, and if they occur in men, they do so with less regularity.

As in females, male muscular involvement is intensified as plateau levels of arousal are reached. Identical muscle groups are involved and the contorted facial and neck musculature and tensed abdominal, back, thigh, and buttock muscles are telltale signs of high levels of arousal in most males. The grasping, clawing carpopedal spasms of the toes and fingers, if they occur, are most evident during masturbatory activity but may also appear during female-superior coitus. In the male-superior position, the man's hands and feet are usually occupied in providing body support and the clutching and grasping reactions are impossible. Late in the plateau phase, pelvic thrusting involving the abdominal, buttock, and thigh muscles becomes mostly involuntary. Such involuntary muscle spasms as well as carpopedal spasms are rarely seen in men over sixty years of age.

Heart rate, respiration rate, and blood pressure increase dramatically during plateau levels of arousal and generally parallel female reactions. From an unstimulated average range of 60 to 80 beats per minute, the heart rates of men in the plateau phase increase to rates of from 100 to 175 beats per minute. Respiration rates may climb as high as 30 to 40 breaths per minute. Systolic blood pressure may increase by 20 to 80 mm. Hg. and diastolic pressure by 10 to 40 mm. Hg. above normal readings.

Orgasm Phase

By the late plateau phase both women and men subjectively have reached heights of sexual tension that seem almost to "demand" release. Their genitals are severely congested and swollen with blood. Virtually every muscle of their bodies is tensely contracted, and some muscle groups are engaged in involuntary spasms so powerful that the responding individuals sometimes *appear* to be wracked with pain. If effective stimulative techniques are continued at this stage, both sexes will cross a hypothetical arousal threshold beyond which the accumulated sexual tensions will be climactically released during the explosive few seconds known as orgasm. Let us now examine the physiological reaction patterns of females and males during the **orgasm phase**.

Female Reactions. The physiological beginning of the orgasm is signaled by contractions of the genital organs. The orgasmic platform, created during the plateau phase by localized congestion of the outer third of the vaginal barrel, powerfully and rhythmically contracts at regular intervals during orgasmic release (see Figure 5–5). The contractions may number from a minimum of three to a maximum of fifteen during any given orgasmic experience. The first three to six contractions occur at 0.8 second intervals, with the intervals between contractions increasing in duration and their intensity decreasing as the number of contractions increase. If extremely high tension levels have been reached, the first orgasmic platform contraction may actually last from two to four seconds before resolving to the recurrent pattern of multiple contractions. These vaginal spasms are sometimes of such intensity that, subjectively, women and men may experience them as grasping and squeezing the penis during intercourse. The inner vaginal barrel does not actively participate in the orgasm but remains expanded and "tented" during the orgasmic experience.

Recent evidence suggests that the vaginal walls also undergo relatively dramatic changes in level of blood engorgement during orgasm. James Geer and Joan Quartararo (1976) recorded vaginal blood volume responses in a sample of

Figure 5–5.

The female pelvis (top) and male pelvis (bottom) during the orgasm phase of the sexual response cycle.

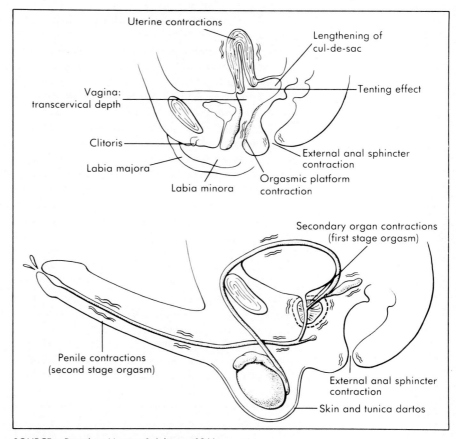

SOURCE: Based on Masters & Johnson, 1966.

women while the women masturbated to orgasm. During excitement and plateau phase approaches to orgasm, the expected increases in vaginal congestion were noted. During orgasm itself, however, a precipitous drop in vaginal blood volume occurred.

The uterus, elevated and congested during the preceding phases, also undergoes recurrent muscular contractions during orgasm. These contractions begin at the same time as those of the orgasmic platform but are less regular and distinct. The contractions originate in the upper (fundus) portion of the uterus, pass down the midzone, and terminate in the cervical region.

Intense orgasmic experiences may also be accompanied by two to five involuntary contractions of the external rectal sphincter. Such contractions do not appear consistently but when they do, their timing parallels that of the orgasmic platform contractions. Rectal-sphincter contractions typically terminate before those of the orgasmic platform. No reactions or changes in the clitoris, labia majora, labia minora, or Bartholin's glands have been recorded during orgasm.

One of the long accepted "truths" concerning female orgasm is that it is not accompanied by a fluid expulsion such as that which occurs in male ejaculation (Masters & Johnson, 1966). Recent research, however, has begun to challenge this "truth," at least in the case of some women. In 1978 Sevely and Bennett drew attention to a longstanding controversy concerning the possibility of female ejaculation. They presented evidence for the existence in women of a set of glands and ducts associated with the urethra comparable to the prostate gland and prostatic ducts in men. They argued that these structures might provide a foundation for fluid emissions from the urethra at the time of orgasm as in male ejaculation.

More recent findings have verified this possibility in some women (Belzer, 1981; Addiego et al., 1981; Perry & Whipple, 1981). These investigators described the forceful expulsion of a fluid from the urethra during orgasm in small samples of women. The fluid did not appear to be urine, and its chemical composition closely resembled that of prostate secretions. These expulsions seem to be triggered mostly by stimulation of what is known as the **Grafenberg spot**, an organ in the anterior (front) wall of the vagina about halfway between the pubic bone and the cervix. When rather vigorously stroked, the Grafenberg spot swells and expands, initially producing a sensation of having to urinate. Continued stimulation of the spot brings about feelings of erotic pleasure and in some cases orgasm that is accompanied by fluid expulsion from the urethra. The percentage of women who experience such orgasmic expulsions has not yet been determined, but these findings demonstrate that at least some do.

Although the breasts show no specific response during orgasm, rapid loss of swelling (detumescence) of the areolae surrounding the nipples begins simultaneously with the final contractions of the orgasmic platform. The areolae shrink but the nipples remain erect and firm and appear to have regained the erect stance formerly obscured by the swollen areolae. The sex flush acquires its greatest intensity and widest distribution at the point of orgasm.

Orgasmic muscular involvement is not limited to the pelvic and genital structures. The high levels of tension reached during the plateau phase reach a peak during orgasm. At the onset of an intense orgasmic experience a woman's entire body sometimes may become "frozen" and rigid, with her extremities spastically twitching and her fingers and toes curled and grasping in carpopedal spasm. Shortly after the onset of orgasm, however, rapid involuntary pelvic thrusting controlled and accompanied by powerful contractions of the abdominal, buttock, back, and thigh muscles begins in many women. The earlier rigidity is replaced by seemingly uncontrollable convulsive movements. Some women moan, groan, cry out, or sob during extremely intense orgasms, and vocalization may continue for several seconds following the termination of pelvic contractions.

Heart rate levels as high as 180 beats per minute, systolic and diastolic blood pressure increases as much as 80 mm. Hg. and 40 mm. Hg., respectively, and respiration rates that exceed 40 breaths per minute may occur during intense orgasmic episodes. As orgasmic platform contractions decrease in frequency and intensity, muscular tension levels and spasms as well as heart rate, blood pressure, and respiration rate begin to decline. This signals the end of orgasm, which may have lasted as long as fifteen to thirty seconds in some instances.

Obviously, not all orgasms are as intense as the description above implies. There are wide individual variations in orgasmic intensity among women and within individual women on different occasions. Some orgasms may be manifested in quietly subdued tones with the reactions restricted to pelvic structures and barely detectable to outside observers. In general, however, it has been observed that orgasmic intensity is frequently greater during masturbation or clitoral manipulation by a sexual partner than during intercourse (Masters & Johnson, 1966).

In comparison with *most* males, females are rather unique in their potential for multiple orgasms during a single sexual activity episode. Physiologically, many females have the capacity to return rapidly to orgasm immediately after an orgasmic experience if effective stimulation is continued or reapplied before they drop below plateau phase arousal levels (see Figure 5–1). The greatest potential for multiple orgasms occurs during masturbation, in which continuous clitoral or mons area stimulation has been noted to produce as many as one hundred orgasms within a one-hour period (Kinsey et al., 1953).

It should be noted that the physiological potential for multiple orgasms in women is just that—a *potential*. Many women never realize this potential and those who do are not multiorgasmic on every sexual occasion. Indeed, Kinsey and his associates (1953) reported that only 14 percent of the thousands of women they interviewed regularly experienced multiple orgasms during intercourse. Those women (and their sexual partners) who regard multiple female orgasm as the only satisfactory outcome of sexual activities are doomed to disappointment a large portion of the time (O'Conner, 1975). Furthermore, failure to achieve multiple orgasms should not be regarded by women as evidence of their own sexual inadequacy or by their partners as evidence of inadequacy of their sexual techniques.

Generally speaking, the orgasmic reactions of women beyond their mid-fifties parallel those of younger women but are of lesser intensity. Contractions of the orgasmic platform are less intense and numerous, rectal sphincter contractions are less likely, and uterine contractions have not been recorded in postmenopausal women due to measurement difficulties. Subjective reports obtained from older women, however, suggest their occurrence. Finally, muscular involvement is weakened in intensity, and visible signs of orgasmic experience are somewhat subdued. The potential for complete cycles of sexual response is not destroyed by the aging process. Whether or not the older woman realizes her potential is largely a psychosocial rather than a biological matter.

Male Reactions.   The cardinal characteristic of the adult male orgasm is, of course, **ejaculation**, which consists of expulsion of seminal fluid from the penis. Ejaculation is a reflex action coordinated by a center located in the lumbar portion of the spinal cord slightly above the sacrally located erection center. Triggered by neural impulses to the genital structures, the process of ejaculation, once initiated, cannot be stopped until it is completed.

Physiologically and subjectively, the ejaculatory process consists of two rather distinct stages. The initial stage, *emission*, consists of contractions of the vasa deferentia, seminal vesicles, and prostate gland (see Figure 5–5), which deliver their contents into the prostatic urethra. Simultaneously, the urethral bulb located at the base of the penile urethra swells to two to three times its size. The internal sphincter of the urinary bladder closes or remains tightly sealed, preventing the escape of urine as well as entrance of seminal fluid into the bladder. The external sphincter of the bladder then relaxes, allowing seminal fluid to flow along the prostatic urethra and enter the dilated urethral bulb. At this point many males experience a sensation of "feeling the ejaculation coming" (Masters & Johnson, 1966).

The second stage of the process, *ejaculation proper*, consists of rhythmic muscular contractions of the prostate, the penile urethra, the urethral bulb, and the muscles surrounding the base of the penis. These contractions forcefully move the **semen** along the penile urethra until it is expelled from the penis in regularly recurring spurts. The timing of the intervals between these muscular contractions is remarkably similar to the orgasmic platform contraction intervals in females. The first three or four expulsive contractions occur at 0.8-second intervals with the remaining contractions occurring with less rapidity and intensity. The initial seminal expulsion may occur with such a force that the ejaculate is propelled several inches beyond the tip of the penis. More frequently, however, it is projected barely beyond the penis, with the remaining contractions forcing semen out in weaker, more gentle spurts. The average fluid content of an ejaculation is approximately 3.0 cubic centimeters, or a teaspoonful. It amounts to less if only a short interval (a few minutes or hours) has passed since the previous ejaculation. A longer interval (several days) between ejaculations will result in a larger volume of seminal fluid ejaculated. The ejaculate itself consists of a very small volume of sperm produced by the testes and a larger volume of secretions contributed by the prostate, seminal vesicles, and Cowper's glands.

Masters and Johnson (1966) found that immediately following ejaculation most males are refractory (resistant or insensitive) to further sexual stimulation for at least a brief period of time. The duration of the refractory period varies widely among different men and within the same man from occasion to occasion. In general, however, the older the man, the longer the refractory period. Highly responsive males in their teens or early twenties may be refractory for only a brief period and, thus, be capable of several ejaculations within a short time. Men over sixty, however, may be unable to ejaculate for several hours or days following an orgasmic experience.

Recent evidence suggests that more men than originally suspected may be capable of multiple orgasms without intervening refractory periods (Robbins & Jensen, 1978). An interesting characteristic of the sexual episodes in which many of these men do have multiple orgasms is that only the last orgasm of the series is accompanied by ejaculation. The men then become refractory to further stimulation and enter the resolution phase of the sexual response cycle as described by Masters and Johnson (1966). Such men are apparently able to inhibit or control ejaculation during the early repeated orgasms. They nevertheless experience most other aspects of orgasm such as increased heart rate, muscular tension, urethral contractions, and so forth. This, of course, suggests that orgasmic and ejaculatory reactions may be separate physiological reaction patterns under the potential influence of learning (Robbins & Jensen, 1978).

Involuntary contractions of the external rectal sphincter during orgasm accompany the expulsive contractions of ejaculation. Rectal-sphincter contractions occur with the familiar 0.8-second interval, paralleling those of ejaculation, but do not recur more than three to four times and usually terminate prior to completion of the penile urethra contractions. The scrotum, testes, and breasts show no observable changes during orgasm. In those 25 percent of men who show it, the sex flush reaches its greatest intensity during orgasm.

Total body involvement in male—as in female—orgasmic expression is evidenced by high levels of muscular tension and spastic contractions in the musculature of the hands, feet, legs, back, abdomen, and face. In one potentially important way, however, males differ distinctly from females in their patterns of pelvic movement during orgasm, particularly during intercourse. We noted previously that many women tend to "freeze" and suspend all pelvic movements at the onset of orgasm only to resume extremely rapid pelvic thrusting shortly thereafter. When orgasm begins, many men also tend to halt pelvic movements but, unlike women, they do not usually resume thrusting during the orgasm itself. The differences appear to be due to variations between men and women in their preferred level of genital stimulation during orgasmic expression.

In contrast to those of men, women's orgasms may be terminated abruptly by withdrawal of genital stimulation. Thus, during masturbation, many women continue direct or indirect clitoral stimulation and the pelvic movements that facilitate such stimulation throughout the orgasmic episode. During intercourse, continual clitoral stimulation is possible only if rapid pelvic thrusting is maintained. Once initiated by the emission phase, however, orgasm in males generally cannot be terminated, and most males prefer to halt active stimulation of the penis during ejaculation. Thus, in masturbation most men cease rapid penile stroking while orgasm is occurring. In orgasm, most men attempt to achieve and maintain deep vaginal penetration rather than resume rapid pelvic thrusting during both emission and ejaculation proper. These opposing male and female tendencies may be potential stumbling blocks for those couples attempting to have simultaneous coital orgasms.

During orgasm, male heart rates may exceed 180 beats per minute, systolic and diastolic blood pressure rates may increase by as much as 100 mm. Hg. and 50 mm. Hg., respectively, and hyperventilation, with breathing rates exceeding 40 per minute, may occur. Generally shorter in duration than that of the female, the male orgasm terminates with the sixth or seventh ejaculatory contraction, and heart rates, respiration rates, blood pressure, and muscular tension levels decline rapidly.

Orgasmic reactions in older males, particularly those over sixty, are reduced in intensity in comparison with those of younger men. Perhaps because of loss of efficiency of the secondary reproductive organs (vasa deferentia, prostate, seminal vesicles), some older men may feel only ejaculation proper and not the beginning stages of ejaculation. Ejaculatory force in the aging male is reduced in intensity and fewer penile contractions may occur. Frequently, the older male does not reach orgasm as rapidly and is thus able to (or must) experience considerably longer and more intense stimulation prior to ejaculation than a younger man. In addition, as we noted above, the refractory period following orgasm tends to increase in duration with increasing age.

Resolution Phase

Of the four phases of the sexual response cycle, the orgasm phase is the briefest in both women and men. This explosive discharge of accumulated sexual tensions usually lasts only a few seconds. It quickly blends with the fourth and final resolution phase. During this phase the anatomic and physiological reactions developed during the excitement and plateau phases are completely resolved. Resolution of these reactions progresses in reverse order of their initial development such that both women and men "come down" by returning through plateau then excitement phase levels to an unstimulated state. Women *may* return to orgasm if restimulation is applied at plateau levels of arousal, and the complete resolution of sexual tensions will be delayed until the final orgasmic release occurs. Most, but not all, men are refractory to further orgasmic expression until resolution has progressed at least to excitement phase levels of arousal. Generally, if plateau levels of arousal are reached and maintained for long periods without orgasmic release, the duration of the period of resolution will be greatly increased in both sexes. Let us now examine this "coming down" or resolution process.

Female Reactions.   Following orgasm, the vaginal changes of the excitement and plateau phases resolve in reverse order of their initial appearance. The vasocongestive orgasmic platform of the outer third of the vaginal barrel dissipates rapidly and, in effect, increases the internal diameter of the outer portion of the vagina. More slowly, the tented and expanded inner two thirds of the vaginal barrel collapses in an irregular pattern, with the collapse progressing from one zone to another. Within three to four minutes the uterus and cervix descend toward the vaginal floor and the tenting effect is resolved (see Figure 5–6). The deep purplish coloration of the vaginal walls slowly resolves to the unstimulated lighter purplish red. The folding patterns of the vaginal barrel reappear. These reactions frequently require as long as ten to fifteen minutes for completion. In most cases the production of lubrication has terminated during earlier phases but, if not, it does so now.

The uterus, swollen by as much as 50 to 100 percent, returns to its unstimulated state within ten to fifteen minutes following orgasm. Uterine contractions initiated during orgasm may continue weakly for a short period during resolution. In some women, intense orgasms may be followed by a slight dilation of the cervical opening; in such cases, twenty to thirty minutes of resolution are required for constriction to occur.

Figure 5–6.

Female pelvis (top) and male pelvis (bottom) during the resolution phase of the sexual response cycle.

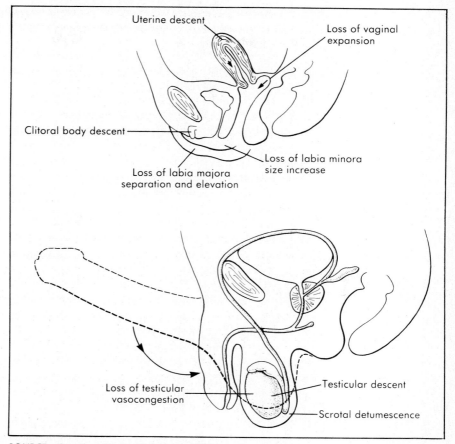

Uterine descent

Loss of vaginal expansion

Clitoral body descent

Loss of labia minora size increase

Loss of labia majora separation and elevation

Loss of testicular vasocongestion

Testicular descent

Scrotal detumescence

SOURCE: Based on Masters & Johnson, 1966.

Within five to ten seconds after orgasm the retracted clitoris returns to its normal position overhanging the upper vulval area. The swollen shaft and glans of the clitoris detumesce rather slowly, sometimes requiring five to ten minutes. Immediately following orgasm the labia minora lose the sex skin coloration. More slowly, they regain their normal thickness and return to their normal, partially closed midline positioning. Likewise, the engorged labia majora lose their swelling and return to normal position. Resolution of labia majora engorgement may require as long as two to three hours in women who have had several children.

Detumescence of the areolae of the breasts is completed rapidly while the nipples remain erect for a slightly longer period. The breasts, themselves, may remain swollen as a result of vasocongestion for as long as five to ten minutes. The sex flush reaction rapidly disappears from the breasts and the remaining body areas in reverse order of its initial appearance.

Muscular tension usually resolves rapidly (within five minutes) and heart rate, respiration rate, and blood pressure quickly return to normal levels. Finally, some women (30 to 40 percent) on some occasions develop a filmy sheen of perspiration over parts or all of their body immediately following orgasm. This *perspiratory reaction* does not result from the physical exertion involved in the sexual activity; its origin is unknown.

Male Reactions.   Loss of penile erection (see Figure 5–6) begins immediately after orgasm but occurs in two rather distinct stages. The primary stage occurs rapidly and the penis may be reduced from full erection to only 50 percent above the flaccid state in a few seconds. If arousal has been maintained at plateau levels for an extended period of time, this primary stage of detumescence may be prolonged. The secondary stage of detumescence, which returns the penis to its normal flaccid size, takes longer to occur and the penis may remain semierect for several minutes if stimulation is continued. Asexual stimuli such as extraneous conversation, walking around, or attempts to urinate will induce rapid loss of erection. In older men erection loss is a single-stage and very rapid process.

Resolution phase changes of the genitals also involve thinning and relaxation of the scrotal sac and detumescence and descent of the testes. Two distinct patterns of scrotal resolution have been noted. Seventy-five percent of men observed exhibit rapid loss of congestion and constriction of the scrotum and return of its creased baggy appearance. The remaining 25 percent manifest a more prolonged relaxation of the scrotum that may require as long as two hours for completion. This slow loss of tension increases the time required for complete testicular descent. Similarly, both rapid and slow patterns of testicular swelling loss and descent have been recorded. Generally, the longer that plateau phase levels of arousal are maintained, the slower is testicular detumescence and descent (Masters & Johnson, 1966).

In the 60 percent of men who experience nipple erection, up to an hour—and several hours in elderly men—may be required before retraction is completed. The sex flush disappears rapidly, first from the shoulders and extremities, next from the diaphragm and chest, and finally from the forehead, face, and neck. Muscular tension decreases to normal within five minutes and a perspiratory reaction develops in approximately one third of men. Heart rate, respiration rate, and blood pressure levels quickly return to normal.

It should be apparent that the bodies of both women and men undergo many dramatic changes as they progress through the four phases of the sexual response cycle. Our description has focused on the most common reactions observed by Masters and Johnson (1966). It should be borne in mind, however, that variation, both between individuals and within the same individual from one cycle to the next, is the rule rather than the exception. That is, while many commonalities may be observed, no two individuals will respond identically, and the intensity and duration of one's reactions will not be the same on every sexual occasion.

Factors That May Alter Sexual Response Cycles

Before leaving our consideration of the physiological and anatomical aspects of sexual response cycles, we should note that the reactions summarized in the preceding pages are primarily characteristic of those individuals who are relatively free of illness, physically intact, and not under the influences of various drugs. A large number of medical conditions and drugs exist that may alter one or more aspects of sexual response cycles. Although it is impossible to enumerate all of these conditions in the present context, a few prominent examples are in order.

Chronic and debilitating illnesses such as cancer, pulmonary disease, cardiac disease, and degenerative diseases or infections involving major body systems frequently interfere with sexual desire and responsiveness. Similarly, various liver diseases (cirrhosis, hepatitis, mononucleosis) and endocrine disorders (diabetes, hypothyroidism, hypopituitarism) may interfere with sexual performance in either sex. More specific diseases affecting the genitals such as localized inflammations or infections, adhesions, allergic reactions to deodorants, and skin diseases are frequent sources of pain that may inhibit genital responses. A variety of surgical procedures that damage the genitals or their nerve supply (for example, prostatectomy, spinal surgery, castration, obstetrical trauma) *are* sometimes *but not always* problematic in terms of loss of sexual desire or response. Finally, sexual functions may be impaired by neurological disorders or injuries involving central (brain, spinal cord) or peripheral structures.

We have commented previously on the role of various drugs as determinants of sexual responses (see Chapter 4). To the list of drugs that may potentially impair sexual responses we may now add those known as antiandrogens (estrogen, cortisone, ACTH), anticholinergics (atropine), and antiadrenergics (used in the treatment of hypertension and other disorders). For a more thorough and detailed discussion of the effects of various illnesses and drugs on sexual responses, the interested reader should see Helen Singer Kaplan (1974).

PSYCHOSOCIAL PROCESSES

Over two decades ago the fundamental role of biological processes in sexual arousal and orgasm was noted by Kinsey and his colleagues: "Whatever the poetry and romance of sex, and whatever the moral and social significance of human sexual behavior, sexual responses involve real and material changes in the physiologic functioning of an animal" (1953, p. 594). While our previous discussion of the biological aspects of sexual response cycles should provide convincing supportive evidence for this statement, it must be reemphasized that poetry, romance, moral, and social significance, and subjective experiences are also important aspects of sexual responses for most of us. In short, sexual arousal and orgasm are not pure biological entities; rather, they are subject to and result in a variety of psychosocial processes as well.

Sexual responses do not simply happen but are experienced subjectively. The details of the subjective experience are somewhat unique to each individual and to each sexual episode. In addition to variations in the subjective experiences accompanying sexual responses, wide individual differences in the mere occurrence of sexual arousal and orgasm are apparent to even the most casual observer. Aside from the relatively infrequent influences of physical illness and drugs mentioned previously, it is generally agreed (Masters & Johnson, 1966; Fisher, 1973; Kaplan, 1974) that variations in both the occurrence and experience of arousal and orgasm are largely a function of psychosocial processes. In the following section we will consider some of these processes involved in the experience and occurrence of sexual responses. As always, it must be remembered that distinctions between biological and psychosocial processes are somewhat artificial but nonetheless convenient aids to discussion.

Experiencing Arousal and Orgasm

The sensations associated both with the arousal of sexual tensions and with their release in orgasm are experienced by most women and men as intensely pleasurable. With the obvious exceptions of those associated specifically with anatomical structures unique to one sex or the other, the physiological reactions of women and men during the sexual response cycle are remarkably similar. Partially because of anatomical differences, however, the subjective elements vary somewhat between the sexes. In adult males, of course, orgasm is usually linked to ejaculation and its accompanying sensations while most females experience no such expulsive process.

For the most part, the physiological and anatomical reactions of both sexes during cycles of sexual response are independent of the particular form of stimulation involved. That is, in terms of physiology, arousal and orgasmic reactions are identical whether produced by autosexual, heterosexual, homosexual, or any other form of stimulation (Masters & Johnson, 1966).

To some extent, then, it is possible, particularly in the case of males, to discuss arousal and orgasmic experiences independently of the particular type of activity providing stimulation. With one important exception, which involves the "vaginal versus clitoral orgasm" controversy, the discussion that follows will focus on phenomenological experiences that accompany arousal and orgasm produced by any form of stimulation.

Female Experiences.   Although most of the phenomenological descriptions of sexual response experiences have been collected in attempts to understand orgasmic sensations, the reports of women participants in studies involving photographic, literary, and auditory erotica are informative concerning the subjective nature of lower levels of sexual arousal. A majority of women become aware of low levels of sexual excitement as vague sensations of warmth, itching, tickling, pulsating, and throbbing of the genitals. At slightly higher levels of arousal, some women also report awareness of vaginal moistness as well as poorly defined sensations in the breasts (Griffitt, 1975; Henson, Rubin, & Henson, 1979; Schmidt & Sigusch, 1973).

As arousal progresses, of course, the woman's thoughts and attention focus more and more on her sexual activity and she begins to "tune out" extraneous stimuli or objects in her environment while the sensations associated with voluntary as well as involuntary muscular tensions and spasms become increasingly salient. During the plateau levels of arousal and close to orgasm, increased feelings of warmth and tingling spreading from the pelvic region to include the thighs, abdomen, and sometimes the entire body are reported by many women (Fisher, 1973; Hite, 1976). Immediately before orgasm, sensory awareness often becomes severely restricted and may be limited to only those sensations localized in the genital area. The rapid heart rate, breathing rate, and intense levels of muscular tension that are so salient at lower levels of arousal gradually fade from awareness as the woman reaches the brink of orgasm (Hite, 1976).

On the basis of the reports of nearly five hundred women, Masters and Johnson (1966) were able to compile a composite view of women's subjective experiences of orgasm. Among these women the consensus was that orgasm progresses through at least three subjectively distinct stages. In the first stage, orgasm begins with a momentary sensation of suspension or stoppage followed immediately by intensely pleasurable feelings originating in the clitoris and radiating throughout the pelvis. These clitoral-pelvic sensations vary in intensity and are described variously as feelings of "bearing-down," "expelling," or "opening up." Some even report a sense of actual fluid emission, and, in some, an actual emission occurs. The bearing down and expelling sensations resemble those occurring during the labor of childbirth according to the reports of some women. As orgasm progresses, almost all women experience a second stage described as a "suffusion of warmth" initially localized in the pelvis but then spreading throughout the rest of the body.

The final stage of orgasmic experience is pelvic in focus and is frequently experienced in two separate phases. Initially, there is a sensation of prolonged pelvic contraction followed by feelings of throbbing concentrated in the pelvic area that soon spread throughout the body. These pulsating or throbbing sensations coincide with, but sometimes continue beyond, observable orgasmic-platform contractions until the throbs seem to blend with the beating of the heart.

Experientially, orgasm terminates as the throbbing sensations generally decrease in frequency and intensity and high levels of tension are replaced by feelings of profound relaxation, satisfaction, peacefulness, and happiness (Fisher, 1973). During intense orgasmic episodes sensory acuity and awareness sometimes becomes restricted totally to generalized sensations of pleasure. All specific sensations—pain, vision, hearing, smell, and taste—become partially numbed and some women may even lose consciousness for a few seconds (Kinsey et al., 1953; Masters & Johnson, 1966). Postorgasmic resolution involves what might be described as "reentry," in which bodily sensations and awareness of external surroundings reappear (Hite, 1976). The woman may have been so "out of contact" during orgasm that she was unaware of painful stimuli, powerful muscular spasms, and intense levels of muscular tension. In some cases, she now or later becomes aware of muscular aching and localized pains resulting from intense clitoral, labial, or breast stimulation.

Many of the subjective elements of orgasm and postorgasm are contained in the following description provided by a particularly sensitive woman studied by Seymour Fisher:

. . . completely concentrated on the feelings in my entire genital area, I reach a certain point when I know orgasm is inevitable, . . . I have absolutely no conscious thought of body movements or even of orgasm—I am only engrossed in the pleasurable sensation. The only images I have ever experienced at this time and during orgasm is fuzzy blackness with red or white muted bursts coming through it. Orgasm comes with a dizziness, a loss of self—almost as if I didn't exist as a body but I exist on as a sensation. After orgasm my body completely relaxes—goes limp for a few seconds until I am conscious of what has really happened. . . . I feel completely satisfied. . . . I feel very happy and full, . . . amazed at the fact that there is such a pleasurable experience. (Fisher, 1973, p. 207)

What words can adequately describe such an experience? While it is probably safe to say that no single word or collection of words can capture the subjective essence of orgasm, Fisher (1973) has found that women frequently use terms such as "ecstatic," "bursting," "exploding," "flooding," "flowing," "melting," "pulsating," "drunk," "dizzy," "floating," and "lightheaded," to assess their feelings during orgasm. Words such as "relaxed," "satisfied," "peaceful," "happy," "warm," and "well-being" characterize postorgasmic resolution phase feelings for many women (Hite, 1976).

It is, of course, impossible to create a subjective blueprint of sexual response experiences that is characteristic of all women or of all responses for any given woman. Tremendous variation in quality as well as intensity of experience is the rule rather than the exception, and the composite view discussed above should be considered only as a commonly observed pattern. Variations around this pattern imply nothing about the "normality" or "healthiness" of any woman's experience.

Of the many issues surrounding the nature of female sexuality, the most enduring, controversial, and, to some (Bardwick, 1971), preposterous concerns the possible existence of two or more distinct "types" of orgasm. It was first suggested by Freud (1933) that women experience two types of orgasm—"clitoral" and "vaginal." At the heart of this distinction are Freud's speculations concerning the psychosexual consequences of the anatomical differences between the genitals of females and males. The basic assumption is that in young girls the clitoris is the central focus of sexual excitement. But with psychosexual maturity (that is, puberty), so the reasoning goes, the sensual focus is transferred to the vagina. In the sexually immature girl sexual pleasure, excitement, and orgasm are derived from clitoral manipulation, but the psychosexually "mature," "adjusted," and "healthy" woman is most, if not wholly, responsive to intravaginal stimulation. In Freud's (1933, p. 161) words, "In the phallic phase of the girl, the clitoris is the dominant erotogenic zone. But it is not destined to remain so; with the change to femininity, the clitoris must give up to the vagina its sensitivity, and, with it, its importance either wholly or in part." According to this view, the ability to experience sexual excitement and orgasm from vaginal stimulation alone is a distinguishing feature of sexually mature, healthy, and feminine women.

This view of female sexuality can be and has been criticized on many grounds but it is most important to realize that current knowledge of the anatomy and physiology of female genitals and sexual response points to the biological impossibility of the clitoral-vaginal transfer proposed by Freud. The clitoris is densely packed with sensory nerve fibers and highly sensitive to touch while the inner portions of the vagina are almost totally lacking in sensory nerves and thus relatively insensitive in most women. It is extremely unlikely that any women are biologically capable of a maneuver that relocates clitoral nerve fibers in the vagina.

Masters and Johnson (1966) and Kinsey and his associates (1953) have suggested that direct or indirect clitoral stimulation is always involved in orgasm. Direct stimulation may take the form of manual or mechanical manipulation of the clitoral shaft or glans. Indirect stimulation results during intercourse from movements of the mons, labia, and clitoral hood. Masters and Johnson (1966, p. 7) note that "when any woman experiences orgasmic response to effective sexual stimulation, the vagina and clitoris react in consistent physiologic patterns. Thus, clitoral and vaginal orgasms are not separate biologic entities."

Women's subjective experience of orgasm may differ, however, depending on whether it is elicited by masturbation, manual or oral stimulation by a partner, or penile-vaginal penetration during intercourse (Bunzl & Mullen, 1974; Singer &

Singer, 1972). Some women do, in fact, report subjectively different orgasmic experiences depending on whether they occur during clitoral stimulation alone or during deep and repetitive vaginal penetration (Bentler & Peeler, 1979; Fisher, 1973; Hite, 1976; Newcomb & Bentler, 1983; Perry & Whipple, 1981).

The most extensive study of such differences was conducted by Fisher (1973) using a sample of about three hundred women residing in Syracuse, New York. When asked about the relative contributions of clitoral and vaginal stimulation to the attainment of orgasm, 64 percent of the women reported a greater contribution from clitoral manipulation than from vaginal penetration. Well over 90 percent of the women indicated a preference for at least some clitoral stimulation in their attempts to reach orgasm. When given a hypothetical choice between only clitoral or only vaginal stimulation, 64 percent of one sample (within the larger sample) selected clitoral stimulation.

The women were also asked to give their subjective impressions of clitoral and vaginal stimulation. A representative account from a woman expressing clitoral preferences follows:

Clitoral stimulation is more exciting because it tingles and makes the whole vaginal area pulsate. My body feels warm all over and as it is continued the intensity grows. Vaginal stimulation feels good but it can't make me achieve orgasm. (Fisher, 1973, p. 196)

Testimony from a vaginally oriented woman revealed quite different feelings:

Vaginal stimulation is more deep and satisfying. Clitoral stimulation takes much longer to reach an equal amount of excitement. Vaginal stimulation causes faster orgasm and is definitely more intense. (Fisher, 1973, p. 196)

Several women reported important gratifications from both forms of stimulation:

Vaginal stimulation is like a warm bath of pleasure while clitoral is a spark of pleasure. In clitoral stimulation my body is rigid with expectation of continuing pleasure. Vaginal stimulation is like a hum but clitoral is a high pitched note. (Fisher, 1973, p. 197)

Fisher, who regards the distinction between clitorally and vaginally oriented women as a psychosocial one, conducted an exhaustive analysis of the personality and social characteristics of each "type" of woman. Each woman was interviewed in depth, given an extensive battery of personality, cognitive, social, and sensory tests, and closely observed throughout her participation in the study. Most relevant to the psychoanalytic distinction between clitorally and vaginally oriented women was Fisher's findings concerning the psychological "maturity," "adjustment," and "healthiness," of the two types of women. Contrary to the psychoanalytic position, vaginally oriented women fared no better on such characteristics than did clitorally oriented women. In fact, tendencies were noted for the vaginally oriented to be somewhat more anxious, to mute and "depersonalize" body experiences more, and to experience orgasm as more controlled and less "ecstatic" than clitorally oriented women.

More recently, Peter Bentler and William Peeler (1979) have reconfirmed some of Fisher's findings. Studying female university undergraduates, they found that women's subjective experiences of orgasm from penile-vaginal penetration and from clitoral stimulation alone are distinctly different. Similar conclusions have been reached in studies by Hite (1976) and Butler (1976). Finally, Perry and Whipple (1981) report that those women who reach orgasm as a result of Grafenberg spot stimulation and expel a fluid during orgasm experience what the investigators refer to as a uterine orgasm. This is characterized by deeper sensations of uterine contractions than the clitorally triggered orgasm described by Masters and Johnson (1966). Perry and Whipple (1981) suggest that clitorally and Grafenberg spot–triggered orgasms may be based on different physiological mechanisms. This, of course, adds a new dimension to the clitoral versus vaginal orgasm controversy and leaves open to question Masters and Johnson's conclusion that, physiologically, only one kind of orgasm exists.

Male Experiences.   In contrast to the voluminous (and often contradictory) literature concerning the subjective nature of female sexual responses, relatively little in the way of detailed consideration of male experiences is available. To some extent, at least, the near universality of orgasmic response in males in comparison with many incidents of orgasmic "failure" in females accounts for this inattention (Masters & Johnson, 1966). It has also been suggested that the physiological and subjective elements of male orgasmic experiences are relatively standard with the major variations occurring in terms of intensity rather than quality (Katchadourian & Lunde, 1980). Even so, substantially different intensities of orgasm produce distinctively different subjective experiences of pleasure and other emotional responses (Zilbergeld, 1978).

It has been observed that males' subjective appreciation of sexual responses has more of a specific genital-pelvic focus than that of females (Masters & Johnson, 1966). The large difference in size of the penis in comparison with the clitoris, its female homologue, undoubtedly accounts for part of this difference in focus. Males initially become aware of growing sexual arousal on the basis of penile sensations. The initial feelings may involve mild tingling and warmth in the penis quickly followed by the beginning of erection. Erection generally occurs quite rapidly but is subjectively appreciated as occurring in a stepwise fashion by many men. As arousal progresses and as the erecting penis becomes stiffer and harder, men become increasingly aware of growing sexual tension, and their thoughts turn more and more to the pleasurable sensations associated with penile erection.

At higher levels of arousal (early plateau), men, like women, become increasingly aware of their tensing and contracting muscles, and their attention becomes focused almost entirely on their sexual activity at the expense of extraneous nonsexual elements of their environment. Late in the plateau phase, their sensory awareness usually becomes exclusively directed toward genital sensations. The salience of rapid breathing and heart rates declines as they become fully engrossed in the pleasurable feelings associated with and seemingly centered in the penis.

For the physically healthy and intact adult male, ejaculation is the experiential core of orgasm. Based on information obtained from over four hundred men, Masters and Johnson (1966) extracted a composite view of the subjective experiences associated with ejaculation. Except in men over sixty, the subjective progression through orgasm occurs in two separate stages that roughly coincide with emission and ejaculation proper. Emission is accompanied in the first stage by a deep pelvic sensation of inevitability of ejaculation. This sensation is experienced rather vaguely as a rapid swelling or expansion of the internal genital structures. Occurring two to three seconds before ejaculation proper, these feelings signal men that they can no longer delay or halt the ejaculatory process. At this point, virtually all physical movement may halt, and the man may feel as if time is momentarily suspended as he awaits the occurrence of ejaculation proper and a second-stage wave of sensations.

The second-stage sensations associated with ejaculation have two phases. First is awareness of the urethral and perineal muscular contractions that propel seminal fluid along the urethra. The first two or three contractions are felt as explosive, while the final, weaker contractions may be felt only as mild recurrent throbs and much less pleasurable than the earlier more forceful contractions. A second phase of sensation is associated with the actual passage of seminal fluid under pressure along the urethra. Generally, the greater the fluid volume, the greater is the pleasure experienced. After an extended period (several days) of sexual abstinence, a greater volume of seminal fluid is ejaculated than if ejaculations are closely spaced (a few minutes or hours apart). Thus, initial ejaculatory episodes are generally experienced as more pleasurable than are second or third orgasms spaced only a few minutes apart. This is in contrast to multiorgasmic episodes in females, in which the second or third orgasms are often reported as more pleasurable than the first orgasm. However, when male multiple orgasms occur without ejaculation until the final orgasm, the ejaculatory orgasm is usually more pleasurable (Robbins & Jensen, 1978).

The orgasmic experience ends as the sensations associated with the final contractions of the penile urethra fade from awareness. Like women, most men experience profound feelings of relaxation, satisfaction, and tranquillity following orgasm. In addition, however, men experience a refractory period during which they are temporarily unresponsive to further stimulation and may even regard additional stimulation as unpleasant or painful. The glans of the penis is frequently sensitive and painful, and mild aching may follow the intense muscular reactions that are not noticed at the peak of sexual arousal.

Individual Differences in Arousal and Orgasm

It has been apparent for a number of years (Kinsey et al., 1948, 1953) that physically healthy and intact females and males alike are physiologically capable of sexual arousal and, in some cases, orgasm at a very early age. Using trained and experienced observers, the Kinsey investigations obtained records of sexual arousal and orgasmic responses in females as young as four months and in males as young as five months of age.

Despite the early appearance of the physiological capacity to respond sexually and the fact that this capacity may continue for as long as ninety years, the degree of variation both between and within the sexes in the actual occurrence of arousal and orgasm is remarkable. Most striking to the casual observer are, of course, apparent differences between females and males. In many ways, however, within-sex variations far exceed average between-sex differences. In the following sec-

168

RESEARCH HIGHLIGHT

Sex Differences in Orgasmic Experiences

Despite the obvious differences between females and males in terms of genital anatomy, there is a remarkable degree of similarity in their physiological responses during sexual arousal and orgasm. Comparable vasocongestive, myotonic, heart rate, blood pressure, and respiratory reactions occur in both sexes regardless of the form of sexual stimulation involved. Both female and male sexual response cycles are represented by Masters and Johnson (1966) as progressing through excitement, plateau, orgasmic, and resolution phases. In spite of the physiological similarities, however, it is widely assumed that there are distinct differences between a female's and a

male's subjective experience of orgasm. While the exact nature of these assumed differences is rarely, if ever, specified, the underlying assumption seems to be that orgasm for the male is a sudden and explosive experience while female orgasms are experienced as more subdued, less violent, and more prolonged.

An interesting test of these assumptions was conducted by Ellen Vance and Nathaniel Wagner (1976) of the University of Washington. The investigators reasoned that, if such differences exist, written descriptions of orgasmic experiences should be clearly identifiable in terms of the sex

of the person providing the descriptions. Written descriptions of orgasmic sensations were obtained from twenty-four females and twenty-four males in introductory psychology courses and edited to remove any references to specific genital reactions which might serve to identify the sex of the writer. The descriptions were then randomly ordered and presented to groups of medical students, obstetrician-gynecologists, and clinical psychologists, who were asked to read each description and simply classify it as to whether it was written by a female or male.

The highest possible score was 48 and a score of 24 could be expected on the basis of chance

guessing alone. The overall average score was approximately 25, revealing that the judges were unable to accurately distinguish female from male orgasmic experiences. Only one subject performed at a level significantly better than that to be expected from chance guessing by correctly classifying thirty-three of forty-eight descriptions.

At least in terms of men's and women's abilities to provide written accounts and presumably qualified judges' ability to differentiate such accounts by sex, there appear to be few, if any, absolute differences in the orgasmic experiences of females and males.

tions we will briefly consider both types of differences in the occurrence of sexual arousal and orgasm.

Between-Sex Differences. Our earlier discussion of sex differences in response to erotica highlighted long-standing and widespread beliefs in the inherently greater capacity of males than females to respond sexually. To some extent, this belief has been laid to rest by recent findings concerning the approximately equal responsiveness of males and females to various types of erotica and by the research of Masters and Johnson (1966) revealing the equal (perhaps greater) capacity of women than men to respond to effective physical sexual stimulation.

Shown here is a sample of the descriptions used in the Vance and Wagner (1976) study. You may want to test your own ability to identify accurately the sex of the person describing each orgasmic experience. The answers are provided at the end of the chapter summary.

Sex of Orgasm Questionnaire

For each statement indicate whether you think it was written by a man (M) or woman (F).

M F 1. I really think it defies description by words. Combination of waves of very pleasurable sensations and mounting of tensions culminating in a fantastic sensation and release of tension.

M F 2. It is a pleasant, tension-relieving muscular contraction. It relieves physical tension and mental anticipation.

M F 3. It is a very pleasurable sensation. All my tensions have really built to a peak and are suddenly released. It feels like a great upheaval; like all of the organs in the stomach area have turned over. It is extremely pleasurable.

M F 4. Tension builds to an extremely high level—muscles tense, etc. There is a sudden expanding feeling in the pelvis and muscle spasms throughout the body followed by release of tension. Muscles relax and consciousness returns.

M F 5. A release of a very high level of tension, but ordinarily tension is unpleasant whereas the tension before orgasm is far from unpleasant.

M F 6. A building up of tensions—like getting ready for takeoff from a launching pad, then a sudden blossoming relief that extends all over the body.

M F 7. An orgasm is a very quick release of sexual tension which results in a kind of flash of pleasure.

M F 8. It is a great release of tension followed by a sense of electriclike tingling which takes over all control of your senses.

M F 9. An orgasm is a great release of tension with spasmodic reaction at the peak. This is exactly how it feels to me.

M F 10. A building of tension, sometimes, and frustration until the climax. A tightening inside, palpitating rhythm, explosion, and warmth and peace.

SOURCE: Vance & Wagner, 1976.

One must distinguish, however, between the capacity for and the actual occurrence of any type of response, as the data in Figure 5–7 indicate. These data show the percentages of men and women who have experienced orgasm from any source at various ages. It is apparent that, at every age beyond ten years, more men than women have actually experienced at least one orgasm. Before ten, the percentages are relatively similar for females and males but there is a marked increase for males beginning between the ages of eleven and twelve. The female curve shows only a steady increase through the late forties, at which time approximately 91 percent of the females studied by Kinsey and his colleagues (1953) had experienced orgasm. The investigators suggested that the remaining 9 percent

Figure 5–7.

Percentage of females and males who have experienced orgasm from any source relative to age.

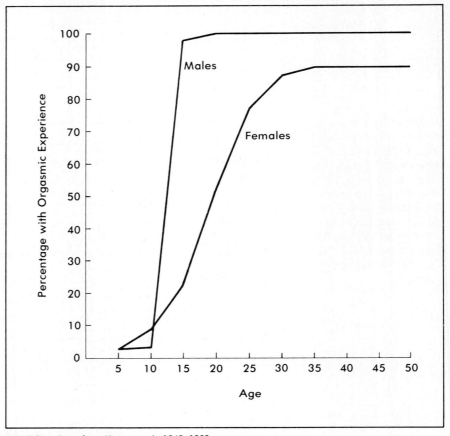

SOURCE: Data from Kinsey et al., 1948, 1953.

never have an orgasm. A comparable percentage of all males (92) have experienced ejaculation by the age of fourteen and virtually all have ejaculated by the time they are eighteen years old (Kinsey et al., 1948). Thus, despite apparently equivalent capacities, male orgasmic responses apparently occur at an earlier age than do those of females.

After experiencing their initial orgasms, men and women also differ in the frequency with which they continue orgasmic responding throughout their lifetimes. For example, the orgasmically experienced male achieves orgasm an average of over nine times per month between the onset of adolescence and fifteen years of age while his female counterpart is having an average of only two orgasms per month. Males reach and maintain their peak of a median of nine to ten orgasms per month between late adolescence and their early twenties. Females tend to peak out at a median of four to five orgasms per month between the ages of twenty-six and forty. Male orgasmic frequency continues to surpass that of females into old age, with the average male and female frequencies falling to around two and one per month, respectively, between the ages of sixty-one and sixty-five (Kinsey et al., 1948, 1953).

We previously discussed the widespread belief (Comfort, 1972) that women are slower to respond sexually than are men. Indeed, some empirical support for this belief has been obtained in research in which women and men reported on their degree of sexual arousal at various times during a one hour period of exposure to visual erotica (Kutschinsky, 1971). But what about responses to physical sexual stimulation? It has been found that in response to effective physical sexual stimulation, the average woman and the average man do not differ substantially in the speed with which they reach orgasm (Kinsey et al., 1948, 1953; Masters & Johnson, 1966). The key word in this conclusive statement is "effective." For example, during masturbation the average man takes between two and four minutes and the average female just under four minutes to reach orgasm (Kinsey et al., 1953). There are, of course, wide variations around these averages and some women and men may require as few as five to twenty seconds or as long as five to ten minutes to reach orgasm during masturbation. During intercourse, however, it is generally true that most women reach orgasm more slowly than do most men. This is largely because of the mechanics of coitus. During intercourse the clitoris is not as "effectively" stimulated as is the penis and women may tend to react more slowly than men.

The origins of the differences that exist between men and women may be found in the different psychosocial influences to which the sexes are exposed. It is generally suggested that standardized sexual behavior differences between the sexes are created by cultural expectations and demands that impose differential standards of conduct on males and females (Mead, 1935; Gagnon & Simon, 1973). It is clear that the prevailing standards of sexual conduct in Western cultures for the last several centuries have been such that female sexual expression has been discouraged, constrained, and controlled while that of males has been condoned and even actively encouraged (Staples, 1973). Coupled with beliefs in the inherent sexual response inferiority of women (Brown, 1966), severe restrictions of opportunities for female sexual expression have resulted in the types of differences between women and men described above. It is clear, however, that, as cultural expectations are gradually reshaped and women's sexual and social roles are redefined, dramatic sex differences in sexual expression fade. Indeed, the momentum of contemporary cultural change might be expected to erase (or perhaps reverse) current male-female sexual response differences in the relatively near future (Bernard, 1972; Hunt, 1974; Sherfey, 1973).

Within-Sex Differences. An inherent danger in focusing on characteristic female-male differences in the occurrence of arousal and orgasm is that the tremendous degree of variation within the sexes might be overlooked. Kinsey and his fellow researchers commented on this potential hazard:

The record will have misled the reader if he fails to note this emphasis on the range of variation, and fails to realize that he or she probably does not fit any calculated median or mean, and may in actuality depart to a considerable degree from all the averages which have been presented. . . . such averages do not adequately emphasize the individual variation which is the most persistent reality in human sexual behavior. (Kinsey et al., 1953, p. 538)

In short, the ranges of variation within females and within males far exceed the average differences between the sexes taken as separate groups. Thus, while the median age for achieving orgasm in males (13.8 years) precedes that for females (20 years) by about six years, a few individuals of each sex experience orgasm prior to their first birthdays. Similarly, there are some men whose first orgasm does not occur until the age of 24 (four years later than the average female) and some women whose first orgasm does not occur until they are over 50 years old (Kinsey et al., 1948, 1953). In terms of orgasmic frequency, there are records of males ejaculating only once in thirty years and others ejaculating more than thirty times per week over a period of thirty years. This is a difference of 46,800 ejaculations. Furthermore, average orgasmic frequencies ranging between less than one per week and twenty-nine per week have been recorded in females.

What factors might account for such dramatic differences among people? While obtained over three decades ago, the findings of Kinsey and his colleagues (1948, 1953) concerning factors associated with age at first orgasm and frequency of orgasm from any source are of interest. Among females only three personal or social characteristics were associated with age at first orgasm. First, women who married at an early age experienced orgasm earlier in their lives than those who married later. Second, those born after 1920 were much more likely to have their first orgasm at an early age than those born in the very sexually conservative years before 1900. Third, those who were least religiously devout had their first orgasm earlier in life than those who were highly religious. Among males, the only clear finding was that first ejaculatory orgasm occurred earlier in those boys who began puberty early than in those entering puberty later (Kinsey et al., 1948, 1953).

Once they initially experience orgasm, some women and men continue orgasmic responding at high frequencies and with great consistency in their sexual contacts. Others maintain low frequencies and are quite inconsistent in attaining orgasm in their sexual activities. The bulk of the research concerning orgasmic frequency and consistency has been directed toward females and variations in their responsiveness during heterosexual intercourse. Fisher (1973) conducted an exhaustive analysis of such research and summarized various characteristics that seem to differentiate consistently and frequently orgasmic women from infrequently and inconsistently orgasmic women. A brief summary of some of the most prominent of these characteristics appears in Table 5–1. Note, however, that the findings reported in Table 5–1 are most relevant to orgasm during coitus and the extent to which they apply to orgasmic responding to other sources of stimulation is somewhat unclear.

Prominent by their absence from this summary are characteristics relating to "adjustment," "body build," "femininity," "hostility," appearance, life-style, introversion or extroversion, and a variety of other personal and social attributes that are frequently suggested as important determinants of female sexual responsiveness (Fisher, 1973). Considerably more systematic research will be required before a thorough understanding of the psychosocial correlates of female orgasmic responsiveness is achieved.

While the available data are extremely sketchy, only a few personal characteristics have been identified as correlates of orgasmic frequency in males. Age is, perhaps, the single most important determinant of the frequency with which most

Table 5–1.

Summary of characteristics frequently found to empirically differentiate women who are high and low in orgasmic responsiveness during heterosexual intercourse.

In comparison with women who are infrequently and/or inconsistently orgasmic during coitus, women who are more frequently and/or consistently orgasmic have been found to be:

Better educated
Less religiously devout
From middle or upper socioeconomic levels
More sexually experienced
An only child
Happier
Less lonely
More self-confident
Less conforming
Less guilty over sexual matters
Less anxious concerning possible separation from or loss of loved persons

SOURCE: Compiled from Fisher, 1973.

males reach orgasm. As noted earlier, male orgasmic frequency is highest during the late teens and early twenties and then gradually declines with advancing age. As is true for women, religiously devout men have lower rates of orgasm than do the religiously less active, regardless of denominational affiliation (Kinsey et al., 1948).

SUMMARY

Masters and Johnson conducted the most extensive investigation of the physiological reactions of women and men as they respond to effective sexual stimulation. Female and male sexual response cycles consist of four phases (excitement, plateau, orgasm, resolution) in which progressive changes in sexual tension are expressed primarily in terms of vasocongestive and myotonic changes in genital as well as extragenital body areas. Immediately following orgasm, some females are capable of rapid returns to orgasmic responding and are thus multiorgasmic. Following orgasm, most males experience a refractory period during which they are temporarily unresponsive to additional stimulation and full erection and ejaculation are impossible.

Women frequently use terms such as "ecstatic," "bursting," and "flooding," to describe their sensations during orgasm and "relaxed" and "peaceful" as descriptive of postorgasmic feelings. Subjectively, some women report distinctly different sensations accompanying orgasms during intravaginal penile stimulation in comparison with those produced by clitoral stimulation alone. The core of the male orgasmic experience is ejaculation, which is usually appreciated as occurring in two stages. The first stage, emission, is accompanied by feelings that ejaculation is inevitable and the second stage, ejaculation proper, produces sensations in which urethral contractions and the passage of seminal fluid create intensely pleasurable feelings.

While apparently quite similar in terms of arousal and orgasmic capacity, men and women nevertheless differ substantially in their average age of first orgasmic experience and in the frequency with which they continue orgasmic responding throughout their lives. These differences are thought to result from differing psychosocial outcomes of culturally imposed standards of sexual conduct in which female sexual expression is discouraged and that of males is encouraged. In comparison with low orgasmic frequency women, high orgasmic frequency women have tentatively been characterized as better educated, less religious, happier, less guilty, and more self-confident. Male orgasmic frequency is negatively correlated with age and with degree of religiosity. Substantially more research is needed to discover the additional correlates of orgasmic response in both sexes.

Answers to Sex of Orgasm Questionnaire

1-M, 2-M, 3-F, 4-F, 5-M, 6-F, 7-M, 8-F, 9-M, 10-F.

SUGGESTED READINGS

Brecher, R., & Brecher, E. (Eds.) (1966). *An analysis of human sexual response.* New York: Signet.

Fisher, S. (1973). *The female orgasm: Psychology, physiology, fantasy.* New York: Basic Books.

Kinsey, A., Pomeroy, W., Martin, C., & Gebhard, P. (1953). *Sexual behavior in the human female.* Philadelphia: Saunders. (Particularly Chapters 14 and 15.)

Masters, W. H., & Johnson, V. E. (1966). *Human sexual response.* Boston: Little, Brown.

Sherfey, M. J. (1973). *The nature and evolution of female sexuality.* New York: Vintage.

SEXUAL IDENTITIES

CHAPTER 6

GENDER IDENTITIES AND GENDER ROLES: BIOLOGICAL CONSIDERATIONS

I was three or perhaps four years old when I realized that I had been born into the wrong body, and should really be a girl. I remember the moment well and it is the earliest memory of my life. . . . by every standard of logic I was patently a boy. I was James Humphrey Morris, male child. I had a boy's body. I wore boy's clothes. (Morris, 1974, pp. 9, 10)

To most people, the dilemma of Jan Morris (born James Humphrey Morris) is a baffling one. But it dramatically illustrates the issues of major concern in this and the following chapter. In these chapters we address two questions. First, what factors are responsible for shaping gender identities? A person's **gender identity** *is his or her personal, deep-seated sense of being male or female.* Gender identities are reflected in the labels people attach to themselves—boy or girl, man or woman, male or female. Second, what factors shape gender roles? The term **gender role** *refers to the extent that people view themselves and are viewed by others as being masculine or feminine.* Masculinity and femininity are socially defined and differ from one culture to another. By convention, certain personal characteristics, mannerisms, and behaviors are defined as masculine and some as feminine. What determines how closely people match cultural perceptions of masculinity and femininity?

Gender identity and gender role differentiation are programmed by a complex series of biological and psychosocial processes. John Money and Anke A. Ehrhardt (1972) have identified five variables that contribute to the determination of a person's gender identity and role. These variables are as follows:

1. *Chromosomal gender.* Represented under normal circumstances by sex chromosome patterns of XX in the female and XY in the male.

2. *Gonadal gender.* Represented under normal circumstances by ovaries in the female and testes in the male.

3. *Hormonal gender.* Represented under normal circumstances by the preponderance of estrogen and progesterone in females and androgens in males.

4. *Morphological gender.* Represented under normal circumstances by the presence of uterus, vagina, clitoris, and labia in the female, and prostate, seminal vesicles, penis, and scrotum in the male.

5. *Assigned gender.* The gender that an infant is declared to be at birth, based on the appearance of the external genitals. The gender in which the child is reared.

The first four of these variables may be classified as biological determinants and the last as a psychosocial determinant of gender identity and gender role. This chapter focuses primarily on the biological determinants; the psychosocial effects of assigned gender are discussed in detail in Chapter 7.

In most instances, all of the gender variables described above are in agreement in an individual. For example, as described in Chapter 2, a person will be chromosomally female (XX), have two ovaries, manufacture little or no androgen, have a uterus, vagina, and external genitals that appear female, and will be assigned and reared as female. Or, a person will be chromosomally male (XY), have two testes that produce androgen, have a prostate, seminal vesicles, and a penis, and be assigned and reared as a male. These are the normal courses of development of females and males that are discussed in detail in Chapter 2 (a brief review of Chapter 2 may be useful at this time).

What about instances in which all of the gender variables are not consistent in a person? "Errors" during prenatal sexual differentiation sometimes occur, leading to a condition known as *hermaphroditism*. In hermaphroditism, one or more of a person's gender variables disagree with the others, causing the biological gender of such a **hermaphrodite** to be ambiguous. The internal and external sexual structures may be incompletely male, incompletely female, or mixed male and female.

Hermaphroditism may result from chromosomal gender errors, hormonal gender errors, or morphological gender errors. The occurrence of such errors provides scientists with opportunities to learn something of the importance of chromosomes, hormones, and genital morphology in shaping gender identity and gender role.

SEX CHROMOSOMES, GENDER IDENTITY, AND GENDER ROLE

As we saw in Chapter 2, the chromosomal sex of an embryo is fixed at the moment of conception. Normally the chromosomal sex is female (XX) or male (XY). Two main types of sex chromosome errors have been studied—missing chromosomes and the presence of extra chromosomes (Money & Ehrhardt, 1972).

Missing Sex Chromosomes

Turner's syndrome is a condition in which either an X chromosome is missing from an XX pair or a Y chromosome is missing from an XY pair, leaving only a single X chromosome. Turner's syndrome individuals develop a female body type, incomplete or no ovaries, and are short in stature. Without ovaries, no estrogen is produced and puberty occurs only if estrogen is administered. Because their external genital appearance is female, they are usually assigned as females at birth. Barring unusual rearing conditions, they develop fully female gender identities and feminine gender roles. Thus, the presence of the normal XX sex chromosome pattern is not crucial to the development of female gender identities and feminine gender roles.

The parallel condition to Turner's syndrome is one in which an X chromosome is missing from the normal XY male pair leaving only a Y. Such a loss is always lethal. It appears that the presence of at least one X chromosome is necessary for survival.

Extra Sex Chromosomes

There are numerous possible conditions in which an individual may have more than the normal complement of two (XX or XY) sex chromosomes. On first thought it seems as though an "extra" chromosome, depending on whether it is a Y or an X chromosome, should make one either supermasculine or superfeminine, respectively. But it does not seem to work that way. An XXX pattern results in a normal female body appearance, sometimes accompanied by sterility. Mental retardation is also sometimes found in individuals with this pattern. Because their external appearance is female, they are assigned and reared as females and have female gender identities and feminine gender roles.

An XYY individual has the body type of a male and is often quite tall. In many cases, the testes do not function properly, leading to sterility. Assigned and reared as males, XYY individuals develop male gender identities and masculine gender roles. Some, however, have difficulty falling in love and establishing an enduring intimate relationship.

In **Klinefelter's syndrome**, the sex chromosome pattern is XXY. The body type is male, but with a small penis and shrunken testes. Androgen output is typically low and sterility is common. Psychopathology and mental retardation are not unusual. Gender identity and gender role disturbances sometimes, but not always, occur.

In summary, sex chromosome codes do not operate as simply or directly as might be expected. Individuals may have XX or XY patterns but other combinations are possible. If the body type allows clear assignment and rearing as male or female, gender identities and gender roles are usually consistent with assigned gender.

SEX HORMONES, GENDER IDENTITY, AND GENDER ROLE

As described in Chapter 2, sex hormones play a major role in the differentiation and development of sexual anatomy and physiology. The prenatal presence or relative lack of androgen is the most important variable affecting sexual differentiation. Whether chromosomal sex is male (XY), female (XX), or some other pattern, the presence of relatively potent concentrations of androgen will lead to a male pattern of sexual differentiation. (There is, however, at least one important exception to this rule, the androgen-insensitivity syndrome, which we will discuss later.) Similarly, the absence or relative lack of androgen allows female sexual differentiation to occur whether chromosomal sex is male, female, or ambiguous.

At least three important types of hormonal errors have been studied to discover the effects of prenatal hormones on gender identity and gender role. First are conditions in which chromosomal females are exposed to excess androgen during prenatal development. Second are Turner's syndrome individuals (described in the preceding section), whose gonads never develop and who are exposed to no significant amounts of sex hormones at all during prenatal development. Third are cases in which genetic males are exposed to deficient supplies of androgen during prenatal development or whose bodies are unresponsive to androgen (Money & Ehrhardt, 1972).

Excess Prenatal Androgen in Females

A syndrome known as **progestin-induced hermaphroditism (PIH)** was first identified in the 1950s when some pregnant women were administered a synthetic hormone, called progestin, to prevent miscarriage. The effects of this potent hormone on a female fetus are similar to those of androgen. The external genitals are masculinized in varying degrees. In most cases the clitoris is merely enlarged and the labia are partially fused. In more extreme cases, a penis and empty scrotum develop. Correct diagnosis of this syndrome leads to surgical correction of the external genitals so that they are female in appearance. Because the influence of the progestin taken by the mother ends at birth, no further treatment is needed. The girl's ovaries function normally and feminizing puberty occurs. In spite of this prenatal hormonal environment that is more characteristic of males than females, PIH girls develop female gender identities (Money & Ehrhardt, 1972).

In the female **adrenogenital syndrome (AGS)**, genetic females (XX) are exposed, at a critical stage of fetal development, to excess androgen. The androgen is produced by malfunctioning adrenal glands and enters the bloodstream as the external genitals are beginning to form. The result is varying degrees of masculinization of the external genitals similar to that found in progestin-induced hermaphroditism. A major difference, however, is that, in the adrenogenital syndrome, the androgen exposure continues after birth since the hormone is produced by the girl's own adrenal glands. Correct diagnosis is followed by surgical correction of the external genitals and treatment with cortisone to suppress production of androgen. Without continued cortisone therapy, the AGS girl will develop a masculine body build and undergo a masculinizing puberty that occurs eight to ten

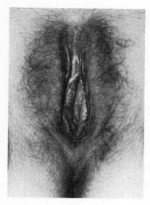

Progestin-induced hermaphroditism (PIH). This girl's (XX) hermaphroditism was induced by synthetic progestinic hormone given to her pregnant mother to prevent miscarriage. Note the incomplete masculinization of her external genitalia.

years earlier than usual (that is, at three to five instead of thirteen). Occasionally, the infant is assigned and reared as a boy. In such cases, the androgen produced by the adrenals ensures that the "boy" will develop a normal male external appearance. If AGS individuals are assigned and reared as males, they develop normal male gender identities (Money & Ehrhardt, 1972).

Lack of Prenatal Sex Hormones

Earlier we described Turner's syndrome, in which an individual has only one sex chromosome—an X. These individuals never develop gonads and thus lack sex hormones during prenatal development. In spite of the absence of hormones, a normal female external genital appearance develops, but estrogen must be administered to induce puberty. Turner's syndrome individuals are almost always reared as girls and develop female gender identities (Money & Ehrhardt, 1972).

Effect of Hormonal Errors on Girls' Gender Roles

As we have noted, if they are assigned and reared as girls, chromosomal females who are exposed to excess androgen during prenatal development nonetheless acquire female gender identities. That is, "male" sex hormones in females do not lead to male gender identities. Similarly, the absence of prenatal sex hormones does not disrupt the development of female gender identities in those assigned and reared as females. But what about gender roles? What effects do these hormonal errors have on the way these people think, feel, and act?

Money and Ehrhardt (1972) have suggested that sex hormones may have an important impact on how people think, feel, and behave. For example, scientists know that early hormonal experiences have a striking effect on rats' sexual behavior. If female rats are given an injection of androgen immediately after birth, their sexual behavior is permanently masculinized. When they confront a male, they will not wiggle their ears, hop and dart, or display *lordosis* (that is, they will not arch their backs and present their rumps) as a female rat normally would do. Even if scientists give them repeated injections of the female sex hormones at maturity, they will not behave "properly." Their male partners are understandably confused. In fact, if scientists give these female rats *male* hormones at maturity, the females will go through the whole male sexual ritual. They try to mount other rats and—undeterred by the fact that they do not have a penis—make vigorous thrusting movements (Levine, 1966).

Similarly, if scientists castrate a male rat at birth, thus making him incapable of secreting any male sex hormone, he will respond to later injections of the female hormone by behaving like a female (Young, Goy, & Phoenix, 1964; Levine, 1966).

What about people? There are some hints that prenatal hormones *may* have an effect on later gender role or sexual behavior, but the evidence is sketchy and contradictory. Again, the sparse evidence scientists do have comes from those cases in which something went wrong during fetal development. Money and Ehrhardt (1972) examined a number of different aspects of the gender roles of girls. They compared Turner's syndrome (TS) girls, progestin-induced hermaphroditism

(PIH) girls, and adrenogenital syndrome (AGS) girls with normal girls. The results of these comparisons are summarized in Table 6–1.

As can be seen from Table 6–1, the authors found that the Turner's girls were fully feminine. Neither the presence of a second X chromosome nor the absence of prenatal sex hormones seemed to be very important. All the Turner's girls day-dreamed about romance, marriage, and motherhood. They were as hesitant as other girls about sex play. In accord with cultural norms, they either avoided sex play or kept it private. If anything, Turner's girls were somewhat more likely to stick with "girls'" sports than were their normal counterparts.

The girls exposed to excess prenatal androgen (PIH and AGS) differed some-what from the normal girls. They seem to have had unusually high activity levels. Some of them liked tomboyish activities—rough and tumble sports and vigorous outdoor activities. Their liking for activity may well account for some of the other, related, differences the authors observed. For example, the AGS girls generally liked practical pants more than frilly dresses, but, when the situation was right, they liked frilly dresses too. Similarly, they preferred active "boys'" games to passive "girls'" games:

They were indifferent to dolls, or openly neglectful of them. They turned instead to cars, trucks, and guns and other toys that traditionally belong to boys. . . . Lack of interest in dolls later became lack of interest in infants. (Money & Ehrhardt, 1972, p. 101)

One third of the AGS girls did not plan to have children. In contrast, many of the control girls were enthusiastic about children, and *all* of them wanted to become mothers when they grew up. Finally, the majority of the AGS girls pre-ferred a career to marriage or wanted to try to combine both. Marriage was the normal girls' most important future goal. In adulthood, most of the differences between PIH women and normal women disappear. However, AGS women seem to display sexual and romantic interest later than do women with other psychoen-docrine syndromes or those with no psychoendocrine syndrome. In addition, their sexual interests are less heterosexual and more homosexual than those of either PIH or normal women. It appears that the effects of the adrenogenital syndrome are more long-lasting than those produced by progestin-induced hermaphroditism (Money & Mathews, 1982; Money, Schwartz, & Lewis, in press). On the basis of their findings, Money and his colleagues suggest that hormones predispose people to certain kinds of gender-linked behavior and that normal men and women may have personality traits shaped by the history, especially in fetal life, of their hormone levels.

Deficient Prenatal Androgen in Males

There are some conditions in which chromosomal males (XY) are exposed to androgen deficiencies during prenatal development (Money & Ehrhardt, 1972). In one, a rare genetic defect prevents both the adrenal glands and testes from manufacturing androgen. Both the internal and external genitals are feminized and the individual is usually assigned and reared as female, developing a female gender identity and feminine gender role.

Table 6–1.

Comparison of the gender roles of Turner's syndrome (TS), progestin-induced hermaphroditism (PIH), adrenogenital syndrome (AGS), and normal girls.

	Girls with Turner's Syndrome (TS) *vs.* Normal Girls	Girls with Progestin-Induced Hermaphroditism (PIH) *vs.* Normal Girls	Girls with Adrenogenital Syndrome (AGS) *vs.* Normal Girls
Evidence of Tomboyism			
1. The girl and her mother agree she's a tomboy.	No difference	PIH more athletic	AGS more athletic
2. She's dissatisfied with the female sex role.	No difference	No difference	AGS more dissatisfied
Expenditure of Energy in Recreation and Aggression			
3. Has athletic interests and skills.	TS less athletic	PIH more athletic	AGS more athletic
4. Prefers boys to girls as playmates.	No difference	PIH prefer boys	AGS prefer boys
5. Is aggressive and fights.	TS less aggressive	No difference	No difference
Preferred Clothing and Adornment			
6. Prefers pants to dresses.	No difference	PIH prefer pants	AGS prefer pants
7. Lack of interest in jewelry, perfume, and hairstyling.	TS more interested	No difference	No difference
Romance			
8. In childhood, has romantic fantasies.	No difference	No difference	No difference
9. At puberty, has romantic daydreams and dates the opposite sex.	No difference	No difference	No difference
10. Has homosexual daydreams and fantasies.	No difference	No difference	No difference
Childhood Sexuality			
11. Aware of genital structure.	No difference	No difference	No difference
12. Masturbates.	No difference	No difference	No difference
13. Inspects and plays with genitals.	No difference	No difference	No difference
14. Plays at intercourse.	No difference	No difference	No difference
Interest in Marriage			
15. Daydreams about getting married.	No difference	No difference	AGS dream less about marriage
16. Thinks marriage is more important than a career.	No difference	PIH prefer career	AGS prefer career
Interest in Children			
17. Prefers dolls to toy cars and guns.	No difference	PIH prefer cars and guns	AGS prefer cars and guns
18. Interested in taking care of children.	No difference	No difference	AGS less interested in children
19. Daydreams about getting pregnant and being a mother.	No difference	No difference	AGS daydream less

SOURCE: Summarized from Money & Ehrhardt, 1972.

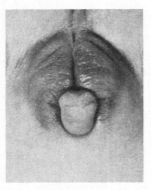

The androgen-insensitivity syndrome in a genetic male.

In the **androgen-insensitivity syndrome (AIS)**, the fetal testes of the XY male produce sufficient androgen. A genetic defect, however, causes the body cells to be insensitive to the androgen. Such individuals have undescended testes, a vagina that may or may not need dilation or surgical vaginoplasty (plastic surgery), and the external genital appearance of a female. Since the testes also produce small amounts of estrogen, a feminizing puberty occurs and the adult body form is clearly feminine.

The androgen-insensitivity syndrome is not self-correcting at birth and no amount of androgen therapy will masculinize these individuals. Correct diagnosis properly leads to assignment and rearing as female. Those who have the partial variant of the syndrome are sometimes incorrectly reared as males and develop male gender identities and masculine gender roles. The fact that their body type will always be feminine, however, produces very real adjustment problems for such individuals.

Those assigned and reared as females become women with fully female gender identities and feminine gender roles. In one study of such individuals it was found that 80 percent preferred girls' toys, 90 percent were fully content with the feminine role, 80 percent preferred to be full-time housewives, and all desired to raise a family (Money & Ehrhardt, 1972). In short, in spite of the fact that they are chromosomal males (XY) whose predominant sex hormone is androgen, AIS individuals seem comfortable in their female identities and feminine roles.

A disorder that has recently become the focus of much research attention is referred to as *pseudo-hermaphroditism* in males (Imperato-McGinley, Peterson, Gautie, & Sturla, 1979). In this disorder, the prenatal testes produce androgen but an enzyme deficiency prevents conversion of the androgen into dihydrotestosterone (DHT), the hormone particularly responsible for prenatal growth of external male genitals. The brain, however, is exposed to a form of androgen that has a masculinizing effect. At birth the external genitals of these genetic males appear to be female. At puberty, androgen production increases about tenfold and in a form that leads to the appearance of male genitals—the testes descend and the penis grows. In addition, a masculinizing puberty occurs—facial and body hair appears, the voice deepens, and male musculature develops. Thus, though the genitals of pseudo-hermaphroditic males appear to be female until this time, puberty prompts their development into complete external male genitals (Imperato-McGinley et al., 1979).

Until recently, it was difficult to diagnose this condition until puberty and many males with this disorder were assigned and reared as females and seemed to evolve female gender identities. It has now been observed, however, that, at puberty, many undergo changes in gender identity from female to male and develop male mannerisms, attitudes, and sexual attraction to females. This suggests that the prenatal androgen has a masculinizing effect on the brain that may not become manifest until androgen production increases dramatically at puberty. In at least some instances the hormonal influence seems to outweigh that of the psychosocial influences of being reared as female. Certainly, these observations raise a number of questions about often-stated conclusions (Money & Ehrhardt, 1972) that psychosocial factors are more powerful than hormonal factors in determining gender identities (Diamond, 1982). Much more research will be necessary to resolve this issue.

RESEARCH HIGHLIGHT

Sex Hormones, Gender Identity, and Gender Role— A Continuing Debate

On the basis of their studies of various hormonal errors (particularly those in which genetic females are exposed to excess prenatal androgen), Money and Ehrhardt (1972) concluded that prenatal sex hormones exert some effects on gender-linked behavior. Recently, others have conducted further research examining the effects of sex hormones on gender identities and roles that questions this conclusion (Richard Green, personal communication, 1976; Imperato-McGinley et al., 1979; Keen, 1979; Maccoby & Jacklin, 1974).

These investigators point out that the research evidence is not as clear as it once seemed. Some studies have found that prenatal hormones influence later gender-linked behavior but other studies have not. Researchers have also obtained contradictory results. For example, some have found that androgen administered prenatally produces *more active* infants while others have found that prenatally androgenized infants are *less active* (Green, 1976). At this point, scientists do not know precisely what effects, if any, prenatal hormones have on gender identities and roles.

What has been learned from these studies? Each time a study is reported, it meets with a flurry of criticism, is redone, and subjected to even more criticism. Scientists have become increasingly sophisticated about how research questions should be posed and how research should be conducted in this area. Let us briefly review some of the more important problems with the early research and some of the solutions that have been proposed.

Money and Ehrhardt simply asked children or parents to describe how the children thought of themselves and how they behaved. Critics have sharply criticized this procedure (Tavris & Offir, 1977). Hermaphroditic boys and girls and their parents *know* that they are different from other children. In the first few days or weeks of life they may have had plastic surgery to correct the appearance of their geni-tals. They may have to take hormones regularly to maintain their appearance. What effect does such knowledge have? Does it make children and their parents eager to prove that everything is normal? Or, does it make them unduly sensitive to any deviation from some perceived ideal male or female standard? These questions have not been answered.

Several guidelines for future research in this area have been offered. First, investigators must rely not only on children's, parents', or their own vague impressions of how male or female, masculine or feminine children are. Instead, they must specify objective indices of gender identity and gender role. This is more difficult than might initially be expected. What is masculine or feminine behavior? Is masculine behavior characterized by activity, aggressiveness, playing with trucks? Is feminine behavior characterized by less activity, nonaggressiveness, play-ing with dolls? Second, attention must be paid to the timing of the hormone exposure. Androgen given at one time seems to produce unusually masculine behavior. The same hormone, given at another time, generates more feminine behavior. Given at still another time, it has no effect at all. Third, the dosage or amount of hormone involved needs to be specified. Fourth, the possible differing effects of naturally occurring and exogenously (externally) supplied hormones must be determined. In subsequent research, these important factors must be controlled or understood.

GENITAL MORPHOLOGY, GENDER IDENTITY, AND GENDER ROLE

The sex chromosomes and sex hormones act to shape the morphology (structure and appearance) of the internal and external genitals. When they act in concert, as is usually the case, the chromosome patterns, the predominant hormones, and the internal and external genitals are uniformly male or female. The research discussed earlier suggests that, because it influences gender of assignment and rearing, genital appearance at birth is an important determinant of gender identity and gender role. But is the role of infant genital morphology an absolute one?

Money and Ehrhardt (1972) describe an inadvertent accident in the case of a pair of identical twin boys that addresses this question. When the boys were seven months old, the parents arranged for them to be circumcised by electrocautery. A tragic accident occurred. The electric current was too powerful, and the penis of one of the boys was accidentally burned off.

The parents were a young couple from a rural area. For some months, they shuffled from doctor to doctor, agonizing over what to do. Finally, a plastic surgeon recommended that the damaged boy be reassigned as a girl, and that his genitals be surgically altered. Thus, at the age of seventeen months, the little boy was surgically transformed into a girl and was reared from that time on as a female.

The first step in this transformation was to surgically alter the external genitals so that they resembled those of a female. This included removal of the testes, but the surgical creation of a vagina was delayed until full body growth was attained. The changes of puberty would be stimulated by administration of estrogen, which would be continued until the average age (forty-five to fifty-five) at which menopause occurs in women.

This case has become a classic. It provides a unique opportunity to compare the gender development of two boys who were genetically identical but who, because of the accident, were differentiated by their genital structures and by the way they were reared. After the surgery, the parents changed the "girl's" name, hairstyle, and clothing. The mother let her daughter's hair grow and decorated it with fancy ribbons. She started to dress her in frilly blouses and little pink slacks, or granny gowns. Not too surprisingly, the girl soon came to "adore" feminine clothing. Of course, the mother continued to dress her boy in jeans.

The mother reported that by the age of four and a half her daughter was much neater than her son:

She likes for me to wipe her face. She doesn't like to be dirty, and yet my son is quite different. I can't wash his face for anything. (Money & Ehrhardt, 1972, p. 119)

As is often the case in parental responses to children's genital play, the mother seemed willing to accept such episodes in the boy's behavior but eager to restrict them in the girl's:

In the summertime, one time I caught him—he went out and he took a leak in my flower garden in the front yard, you know. He was quite happy with himself. And I just didn't say anything. I just couldn't. I started laughing and I told daddy about it. (p. 120)

I've never had a problem with her. She did once when she was little, she took off her panties and threw them over the fence. And she didn't have no panties on. But I just, I gave her a little swat on the rear, and I told her that nice little girls didn't do that, and she should keep her pants on. . . . and she didn't take them off after that. (p. 120)

The mother encouraged her daughter to help with the housework. Soon the little girl began to copy her mother and try to help clean up the kitchen. Her brother, however, reportedly "could not care less" about such chores. At Christmas, at age six, the girl requested a doll house and doll carriage. The boy requested a toy garage complete with cars, gas pumps, and tools. By the age of twelve, the girl was reported as being fully adjusted to her female identity and role.

How are the twins faring in adolescence? We do not really know. Recently, at thirteen, the girl reported that things were going well, or at least she was "reluctant to admit she is having any difficulties" (Diamond, 1982). John Money and the girl's psychiatrists seem to agree that her adjustment is surprisingly smooth. Yet a few observers have been more pessimistic (see Diamond, 1982). Not long ago the British Broadcasting Company ran a television special on the "twin case." Some BBC psychiatrists who interviewed her concluded that she may be more ambivalent about being a girl than previous reports have suggested. The BBC reported that she has trouble making friends and is not particularly happy. She has a "masculine gait"; other children sometimes tease her about it. (They call her "cavewoman.") She says it is harder to be a girl than to be a boy. She would like to be a mechanic. Clear signs of trouble? Or just a normal teenager confronting the uncertainties of adult life? We really do not know.

Does prenatal androgen exposure predispose genetic males to evolve male gender identities? Again, more research is necessary before we will be able to sort out the roles played by chromosomes, hormones, body morphology, and psychosocial factors in shaping gender identity. Our limited understanding in this area becomes dramatically apparent with respect to the phenomenon of transsexualism.

TRANSSEXUALISM AND SEX REASSIGNMENT

Transsexualism is the condition that results when a person has developed an inappropriate gender identity. Transsexuals feel that they are "really" people of the other sex. They feel that they are imprisoned in the wrong body and possess the wrong set of genitals. The quotations that open this chapter typify the feelings of many transsexuals.

Origins of Transsexualism

No one really knows why some children—perhaps 1 in 100,000—develop confused notions as to their gender. Boys seem to have more trouble than girls developing appropriate gender identities. There are three to four times as many male-to-female transsexuals as female-to-male transsexuals (Green, 1975). Some investigators think that the origins of such confusion are genetic or hormonal (see, for example, Benjamin, 1966 or 1967). Recent data do not seem to support this contention, however. When scientists measure male and female transsexuals' hor-

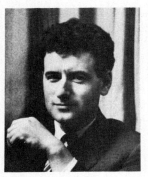

James Morris before
transsexual surgery.

monal levels, they find them within the normal range (Jones, 1974; Migeon, Rivarola, & Forest, 1968). This suggests that hormonal imbalances are *not* the problem. Other scientists think that the problem is in the way transsexual children are reared. They report that transsexual boys are often reared by domineering mothers and weak fathers or warm mothers and cold, rejecting, punitive fathers (Pauly, 1969; Stoller, 1969). Transsexual girls are reported to have weak and ineffectual mothers and strong masculine fathers (Pauly, 1974). Others suggest that transsexual children are simply encouraged to behave in inappropriate ways (Driscoll, 1971; Green, 1975).

In any case, once children have formed gender identities (some time between eighteen months and five years of age), correct or not, it is almost impossible to change them. Psychotherapy simply does not work. Although a *few* sex researchers would take issue with this conclusion (for example, Imperato-McGinley et al., 1979), transsexuals generally end therapy as they began—insisting they are "really" the man or woman they are not.

Sex Changes

Some transsexuals simply pose as members of the opposite sex. More choose to have hormone treatments or surgery to make their bodies more consistent with their gender identities. Recently, psychiatrists and physicians have become willing to help transsexuals attain this goal.

Changing Gender Role.   Changing one's sex is a long and painful process (see Green & Money, 1969, or Green, 1975). Transsexuals can obtain help in this undertaking from gender identity clinics. The first step for transsexuals when they apply for help at these clinics is a psychiatric interview and a battery of psychological tests. These are designed to screen out those candidates who have serious mental illnesses or who would not profit from treatment. Next, the transsexuals have to begin to learn the "appropriate" gender roles. They have to learn how to behave as members of the opposite sex. Generally, transsexual men and women want to learn to be the most stereotypical of men and women; they wish to look like a stereotypical male or female and have a stereotypical masculine or feminine occupation. Thus, men generally have their heavy beards removed by electrolysis, learn to use makeup, learn to talk, gesture, and walk in feminine ways, and learn to dress as women. Women learn to develop masculine skills. They have to get jobs that *they* consider are appropriate for their new gender. A professional man may choose to become a secretary, beautician, or waitress. A woman has to find "man's work." Both have to secure appropriate new birth certificates, driver's licenses, and social security cards.

Hormonal Treatment.   The male-to-female transsexual begins taking estrogen. He must continue to take estrogen throughout the rest of his life. Gradually, the man becomes more feminine. His breasts become larger; his hips begin to round. The female-to-male transsexual is given androgen. Generally he will continue to take periodic doses of androgen throughout his life. Gradually, the person's body becomes more masculine. The voice box thickens and the voice deepens. A beard may develop. The clitoris enlarges, although not, of course, to the size of a normal penis.

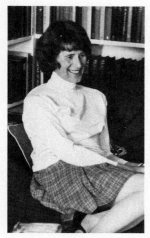

Jan Morris after transsexual surgery.

By this point, most physicians encourage their transsexual patients to begin to try living for a year or two as a member of the "opposite" gender to find out if they can adjust to the new and different life-style. This is done to be sure that they want to take the next, irrevocable, step—the operation.

Plastic Surgery. In the male-to-female transsexual, the penis and testes are removed. The plastic surgeon then reconstructs the external genitalia to look as much as possible like a woman's. Breasts may also be implanted. Next, an artificial vagina—a pouch 15 to 20 centimeters (6 to 8 inches) deep—is constructed. It is lined with the skin of the amputated penis. This provides sensory nerve endings, which allow the transsexual to respond to sexual stimulation. For about six months after the operation, the vagina must be dilated with a plastic vaginal insert to prevent it from reclosing.

The female-to-male change is more complex. First the plastic surgeon must remove the transsexual's breasts and perform a hysterectomy. Then tissues in the genital area are used to construct a penis and scrotum. Of course, this penis lacks erectile capacity. Sometimes physicians implant a silicone tube in the penis to permit patients to engage in intercourse. With such an implant the penis will always remain relatively rigid. In some cases a mechanically inflatable device will be implanted in the penis to give the person the ability to produce an "artificial" erection. So far, however, experience with the inflatable devices is limited and their use is mostly experimental.

Currently, the male-to-female operation is the better developed of the two. After surgery and hormone treatment, the male-to-female transsexual can make a fairly credible appearance and can function sexually as a woman. She cannot, of course, bear children. The female-to-male operation is far less effective. Surgeons can change the superficial appearance but are not yet able to fashion a realistic, much less a fully functional, penis.

To date, about four thousand sex change operations have been performed in this country. How effective are such operations? It depends on who is asked. So long as scientists relied on the testimony of transsexuals themselves, the answer was, "Surprisingly well." Benjamin (1967a) interviewed fifty-one male-to-female transsexuals. He concluded that the results were "good" in 33 percent of the cases. The transsexuals were accepted by their families, integrated into the world of women, and had reasonable sexual adjustments. Results were regarded as "satisfactory" in 53 percent of the cases and "doubtful" in only 10 percent. Similarly, on the basis of his study of twenty female-to-male transsexuals Benjamin concluded that "the results of either androgen therapy or operations or both have generally been decidedly satisfactory. With one doubtful exception . . . all patients under my observation . . . were benefitted" (p. 429). Similar encouraging results were reported by Randall (1969), Money (1971), and Edgerton and Meyer (1973).

Unfortunately, more carefully controlled studies cast doubt on such optimistic conclusions. Meyer and Reter (1979) interviewed one hundred men and women who contacted the gender identity clinic at Johns Hopkins University requesting sex change operations. Thirty-four of them were granted operations and sixty-six were not. In a follow-up interview, the authors attempted to determine how successful the operations had been. They measured men's and women's adjustment with respect to family relationships, work relationships, legal status, and

Postoperative appearance of genitals in (left) male-to-female and (right) female-to-male transsexual surgery.

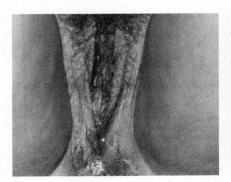

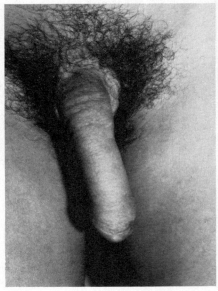

psychiatric status. The study showed that there were no significant differences in the life adjustment of the transsexuals who received surgery and that of those who did not. Meyer noted (in Motahar, 1979, p. 60): "There seems to be a period in the lives of transsexual patients, between the ages of 20 and 30, when they have an acute desire for surgery. If that time passes without surgery, they lose the intensity of this desire and frequently go on to a fair life adjustment. Psychotherapy can often help them adapt to life without surgery." At present, researchers still disagree about the best way of dealing with transsexuals who request sex change operations. For example, critics such as Fleming, Steinman, and Bocknek (1980) have attacked the way Meyer and Reter (1979) measured adjustment, pointing out that the authors ignored subjective indicants of emotional adjustment (dreams, fantasies, and family relationships) in favor of "observable and objective data" (arrest records, cohabitation with members of the "appropriate" or "inappropriate sex," psychiatric records, and employment history). Thus, as these critics have noted, someone living all alone without family or friends, would score better on the Meyer and Reter adjustment scale than someone living with a same sex roommate. Clearly, additional research is needed to help physicians advise transsexuals who request sex change operations.

SUMMARY

A person's gender identity is his or her personal, deep-seated sense of being male or female. Gender roles are people's view of themselves and others' views of them as masculine or feminine. Gender identities and gender roles are programmed by the complex interaction of biological variables (chromosomal gender, gonadal gender, hormonal gender, and morphological gender) and psychosocial variables (those linked with gender of assignment and rearing).

Studies of various types of hermaphroditism, in which one or more of the gender variables are in disagreement, have yielded valuable information concerning the relative contributions of biological and psychosocial determinants of gender identity and gender role. These studies have shown that sex chromosomes, gonads, hormones, and genital morphology all influence gender-linked behavior. Though the limits of their influence are not yet clear, the most influential factors shaping gender identity and gender role appear to be gender of assignment and rearing.

Transsexualism is a gender identity disorder in which a person's biological gender and assigned gender are in disagreement with the person's gender identity and gender role. Transsexuals feel that they are trapped in a body of the wrong sex. In recent years, numerous transsexuals have undergone surgery in an effort to make their physical appearance and body structure agree with their gender identity. The benefits of such surgery have recently been questioned.

SUGGESTED READINGS

Green, R., & Money, J. (1969). *Transsexualism and sex reassignment.* Baltimore: Johns Hopkins University.

Money, J., & Ehrhardt, A. A. (1972). *Man and woman, boy and girl.* Baltimore: Johns Hopkins University.

Morris, J. *Conundrum.* (1974). New York: Harcourt Brace Jovanovich.

Tavris, C., & Offir, C. (1977). *The longest war: Sex differences in perspective.* New York: Harcourt Brace Jovanovich.

CHAPTER OUTLINE

CHAPTER 7

GENDER IDENTITIES AND GENDER ROLES: PSYCHOSOCIAL CONSIDERATIONS

You do a girl tolerable poor, but might fool men, maybe. Bless you child, when you set out to thread a needle, don't hold the thread still and fetch the needle up to it; hold the needle still and poke the thread at it—that's the way a woman most always does; but a man always does t'other way. And when you throw at a rat or anything, hitch yourself up a tip-toe, and fetch your hand up over your head as awkward as you can, and miss your rat about six or seven foot. Throw stiff-armed from the shoulder, like there was pivot there for it to turn on—like a girl; not from the wrist and elbow with your arm out to one side, like a boy. And mind you, when a girl tries to catch anything in her lap, she throws her knees apart; she don't clap them together, the way you did when you catched the lump of lead. Why, I spotted you for a boy when you was threading the needle; and I contrived the other things just to make certain. (Mark Twain, The Adventures of Huckleberry Finn, *pp. 786–787)*

For Mark Twain things were simple. Men were men and women were women. The sexes existed in two distinct forms. Men and women thought differently, felt differently, and behaved differently. In real life, however, things are far more complicated.

Let us consider three different cultures and the sexual standards that each sets for men and women. Traditionally, the Batak boys and girls of Lake Toba in northern Sumatra move into segregated huts at puberty. Young boys are introduced to sex by an older man—they masturbate together. When a man reaches adulthood, he is expected to marry. But even after marriage, he continues to spend most of his free time in the men's hut, and to share sexual gossip with his friends. In the women's huts, girls are *not* given the same kind of explicit sexual instruction that the boys receive. A girl can gossip about love and sex, but talk is all she can do. It is considered critically important for a girl to be a virgin when she marries. Girls who are discovered having premarital sex often commit suicide. After marriage, neither men nor women are supposed to have extramarital affairs. Marriage is expected to be exclusive and permanent. That is how a "real man" and a "real woman" are expected to behave (Geertz, 1960).

Among the Marind Anim, a headhunting people of southern New Guinea, men and women live separately all of their lives—women in the women's hut, men in the men's. Couples meet briefly only when they plan a sexual excursion or have business together—and this does not happen very often. From infancy to four or five, both boys and girls stay with their mothers. Around age five, boys move in with their fathers, learning to hunt, fish, and garden. Girls always remain with their mothers, learning about housekeeping and gardening.

Children's sexual experiences begin early. When older people play with young boys and girls, they often soothe them by petting their genitals. Young boys have numerous homosexual encounters; girls do not. As soon as boys and girls reach puberty, they get married. The marriage ceremony is a lengthy one. First, the girl is escorted to a special spot where she is expected to have sexual intercourse with all of the men in her husband's clan. This is thought to increase her fertility. Only then can she embark on sexual relations with her new husband. Throughout her marriage she is expected to continue to participate in this kind of sequential group sex at regular intervals. Women regard such group sex as a duty—unpleasant, but necessary to insure their fertility.

Among the Pelaga Indians in Argentina, boys and girls' sexual experiences begin early. Until age four or five, boys and girls openly masturbate with their friends. At about five years of age, boys and girls begin playing at coitus. From then on, most of their sexual activities are with partners of the opposite sex. When boys and girls reach puberty, they experiment with a variety of sexual partners before settling down to one.

These examples, and many more that could be cited (Ford & Beach, 1951), show that gender role standards vary from culture to culture. But how are such standards passed from one generation to the next? How do people form the gender roles that are regarded as appropriate by their own culture?

GENDER ROLE FORMATION

At least three important processes are involved in gender role formation. First, children must reach a level of *cognitive development* that allows them to recognize themselves as one gender or the other. Second, once such self-recognition occurs, children *identify with and model* their own actions after important people in their lives. Third, through *reinforcement*, certain behavior patterns are strengthened and others weakened. Let us briefly consider the contributions of each of these processes to gender role formation.

Cognitive Development

Theorists such as Donald Hebb (1949), Lawrence Kohlberg (1969), Jean Piaget (1950), and Heinz Werner (1957) have pointed out that children must develop cognitively (intellectually) as well as physically. At different stages in their development, children become capable of thinking about things in radically different ways.

Lawrence Kohlberg (1969) suggests that at an early stage children are capable of comprehending only limited kinds of information about the sexes. At about age one and a half to two, children can correctly identify themselves as "boys" or "girls." It is around this age that gender identities become firmly established. To the two-year-old mind, the factors that make someone a boy or girl are very concrete. Girls are people with long hair who wear dresses. Boys have shorter hair and they wear pants. Many children at this age think that if they got a haircut or bought new clothes, they might switch their sex. No wonder, then, that toddlers sometimes become very upset if their mother wears pants of if their father holds their mother's purse for a moment. Once this basic gender identity as boy or girl is cemented, the process of gender role formation begins.

Identification and Modeling

According to Nathan Kagan (1958, 1964), children are "identifying" when they believe that some of the attributes of a model (parents, siblings, relatives, peers) belong to the self. If a girl identifies with her mother, she takes it for granted that she thinks like her mother, feels as she feels, or acts as she acts. She shares in her mother's joys and sorrows, successes and failures. The same is true of the boy who identifies with his father.

Parents as Models.   Three factors determine whether or not children identify "optimally" with their parents: (1) Early in life, do the children feel that they are similar to their parents in the way they look, think, feel, or act? In Hawaii, for example, where Japanese, Chinese, Caucasians, Hawaiians, and other ethnic groups mix freely, more than 50 percent of marriages involve men and women of different ethnic groups. Some children report that the fact that they *look like* their mother or their father is critically important in which ethnic group they identify with. (2) Are the parents nurturant? (3) Are the parents powerful people who seem capable of getting the things they want from the world? Presumably, children identify with their parents in part because they assume that if they become like the parents, they, too, will be able to secure the things they want. Since parents are usually the most nurturant and most powerful people in the child's world, it is not surprising that most children identify so profoundly with their parents.

Parents and others with whom children identify serve as important models of what it means to be a boy or girl, man or woman. Children are great mimics, either because the tendency to imitate is inherent in all of us, or because we are rewarded early in life for imitating others. Observation and imitation of male and female models contribute in important ways to children's formation of gender roles.

Other Models.   Parents are children's most important models, but almost anyone can serve as "an example." Psychologist Albert Bandura (1977) and his colleagues

Children frequently learn gender roles by modeling the behavior of parents or other adults.

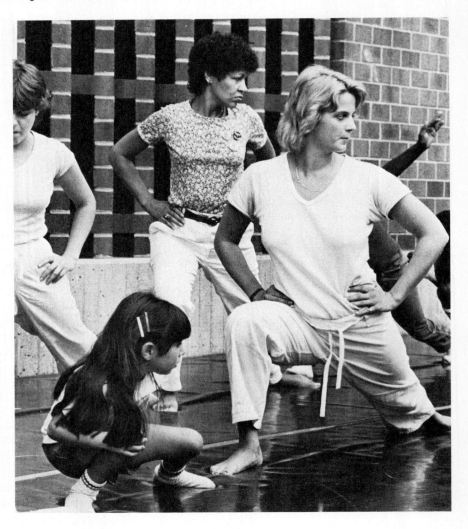

have systematically studied the modeling process. Bandura, Ross, and Ross (1963) conducted a typical study. One group of nursery school children watched an adult model play with a BoBo doll in an unusually violent way. The adult sat on the doll, punched it in the nose, pummeled it on the head with a mallet, and kicked it around the room. Other children saw a film of this violent activity. Still others saw the cartoon character *Herman the Cat* engaging in these rowdy activities. Children in a control condition saw none of all this. The next day, all the children were mildly frustrated. The scientists found that the children exposed to the aggressive models *were* far more aggressive than their peers in their response to the frustration experienced. Boys and girls had learned to be aggressive by simply observing the actions of models.

Friends and parents provide clear role models for how boys and girls and men and women *ought* to behave—and so, too, do the media. A number of critics have observed that books, magazines, television, movies, songs, newspapers, and professional journals consistently depict boys' and girls' and men's and women's roles in stereotyped ways (Weitzman, Eifler, Hokada, & Ross, 1972; U'Ren, 1971; Sternglanz & Serbin, 1974). In many children's books, boys are the central characters. Boys do things, they are smart, calm in emergencies, adventurous, brave, and successful. Girls are often peripheral characters. They sit quietly and watch, and ask other people to solve their problems for them. Indeed, Women on Words and Images (1972), a New Jersey group that studies sexual stereotypes, surveyed 2750 stories in 134 children's books and found that in those stories men's lives were depicted as broad and women's as narrow. For example, men were shown in 147 different professions while women were limited to 26 jobs including acrobat, circus fat lady, and witch.

McArthur and Resko (1975) analyzed 200 television commercials. Again, men were featured prominently but women were not. Men and women were depicted in stereotyped roles in the commercials; men were experts while women were appreciative consumers. Moreover, the advertisers used very different "bait" to tempt men and women to use their products. Men were promised career and social advancement. Women were promised that, if they used Brand X, their families, husbands, or male friends would approve of them.

What do children learn from all these different models? To some extent, children do learn to behave "appropriately" by observing and mimicking models. If a boy often plays football with his father, he is naturally going to imitate the mannerisms with respect to that sport that he sees in his father. A girl who has never seen her father in action on the football field obviously has no chance to learn to imitate the way he hitches up his pants as he walks to the sidelines. Similarly, a boy who has never helped his mother bake brownies cannot imitate the way she purses her lips as she concentrates on the recipe. On a number of specific, sex-typed tasks, then, boys *are* more likely to resemble their fathers, and girls their mothers (Tavris & Offir, 1977; Pleck & Brannon, 1978).

Yet most actions are not performed in isolation. Children have ample opportunity to observe both their parents in operation. And, by observation, children learn how *both* men and women behave. As Walter Mischel (1970) has noted, "Both men and women know how to curse or fight or use cosmetics or primp in front of mirrors." Children pick up *both* their parents' ways of thinking, speech habits, emotional expressions, and behaviors. Researchers who have compared personality traits common to parents and children worldwide have discovered that boys and girls are likely to possess traits of *both* their parents (Maccoby & Jacklin, 1974).

Reinforcement

The basic principle of *reinforcement* is a simple one—we learn to do those things that are rewarding and to avoid doing those things that are not. In a typical animal experiment, for example, a hungry pigeon that gets a pellet of food (a reinforcement) when it taps a certain spot will quickly learn to peck at that spot again and again. A pigeon that gets a painful electric shock (a punishment), or gets nothing (a nonreinforcement), each time it taps at a spot, will quickly learn to quit pecking. Of course, the same is true of people.

There are a variety of ways parents can reinforce children for acting properly. Sometimes, parents send subtle messages. For example, they may become acutely embarrassed when their child asks about sex. The child realizes she has done *something* she is not supposed to do, but she is not sure exactly what. Sometimes, she learns it is smarter to avoid the whole issue. Sometimes parents are more direct. They simply tell their children what they want: "Big boys don't cry—don't be such a sissy!" "Act like a lady—take your feet off that coffee table!" They praise their children when they act properly and criticize them when they do not. Sometimes parents provide even more concrete rewards and punishments for proper behavior. They give their daughter an allowance if she helps with the dishes and baby-sits. They pay their son when he rakes leaves. Both children are punished when they fail to perform their assigned chores.

In all societies, parents use reinforcement techniques to mold their children into the people they want them to be. Anthropologists give us some idea as to the traits most cultures encourage boys and girls and men and women to possess. In one study, Barry, Bacon, and Child (1957) tabulated anthropologists' descriptions of the socialization practices of 110 societies. They analyzed these descriptions with respect to whether or not boys and girls received similar or different training in five areas: (1) responsibility and dutifulness training, (2) nurturance training—training the child to be nurturant or helpful toward younger siblings and other dependent people, (3) obedience training, (4) self-reliance training, and (5) achievement training—training the child to achieve as excellent a performance as possible. The authors found that in most societies girls are taught to be nurturant, responsible, and obedient, while boys are encouraged to be achieving and self-reliant.

What about gender role training in our own society? It has been suggested that in our society, too, boys and girls are socialized in very distinct ways. Girls are encouraged to be warm and expressive specialists in love and intimacy. Boys are encouraged to be rational, controlled, specialists in achievement (Firestone, 1970). But is it this clear-cut? More systematic observation suggests that boys and girls are not reared as differently as might be expected.

In a monumental work, Eleanor Maccoby and Carol Jacklin (1974) reviewed more than 1600 studies that have been conducted to find out how boys and girls are reared and to determine how their differential rearing affects their personalities. Their conclusions follow:

Our review of the socialization pressures directed at the two sexes revealed a surprising degree of similarity in the rearing of boys and girls. The two sexes appear to be treated with equal affection, at least in the first five years of life (the period for which most information is available); they are equally allowed and encouraged to be independent, equally discouraged from dependent behavior; as noted above, there is even, surprisingly, no evidence of distinctive parental reaction to aggressive behavior in the two sexes. There are differences, however. Boys are handled and played with somewhat more roughly. They also receive more physical punishment. In several studies boys were found to receive both more praise and more criticism from their caretakers—socialization pressure, in other words, was somewhat more intense for boys—but the evidence on this point is inconsistent. The area of greatest

The process of socialization may contribute to the formation of sex-typed behaviors and attitudes, such as the belief that males should be strong and muscular.

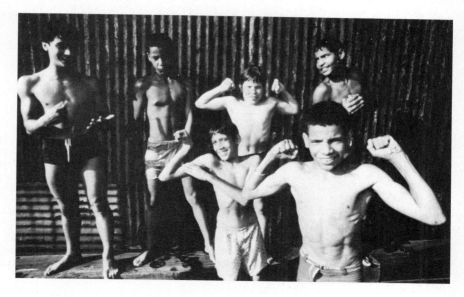

differentiation is in very specifically sex-typed behavior. Parents show considerably more concern over a boy's being a "sissy" than over a girl's being a tomboy. This is especially true of fathers, who seem to take the lead in actively discouraging any interest a son might have in feminine toys, activities, or attire. (Maccoby & Jacklin, 1974, p. 362)

GENDER ROLE PATTERNS

By providing models for and reinforcing certain patterns of behavior, society attempts to shape children into particular types of boys and girls, men and women. What are the outcomes of this gender role training? Do males and females in our society actually differ in their behavior and characteristics?

There has been a tremendous amount of research devoted to examining differences between boys and girls or men and women in behavior and characteristics. Maccoby and Jacklin (1974) reviewed about 1600 scientific studies that have been conducted to determine how males and females differ. They attempted to determine whether, for whatever reason (nature or nurture), men and women differ in intellect, achievement, temperament, sociability, desire for power, and other variables. Their conclusions regarding gender differences that are fairly well established, areas where the evidence is ambiguous, and unfounded beliefs about sex differences are summarized in Table 7–1.

Maccoby and Jacklin's findings indicate that there are relatively few characteristics that have been found to differ substantially in males and females. (Girls have greater verbal ability; boys have greater visual-spatial ability, greater mathematical ability, and are more aggressive.) This suggests that what appear to be quite different patterns of gender role training for males and females result in relatively

Table 7–1.

Summary of research evidence concerning gender role differences in the United States.

Gender Differences That Are Fairly Well Established

1. Girls have greater verbal ability.
2. Boys have greater visual-spatial ability.
3. Boys have greater mathematical ability.
4. Boys are more aggressive: Until 2 to 2½ years of age boys and girls are equally aggressive. Boys are more aggressive, both verbally and physically, from 2½ years on.

Areas Where the Evidence Is Ambiguous

1. Tactile sensitivity: Probably no differences between males and females.
2. Fear, timidity, and anxiety: According to self-ratings and teacher ratings, girls are more timid and anxious. Observational studies, however, fail to find such differences.
3. Activity level: In infancy boys and girls are equally active. By the preschool years boys *may* be more active—especially in social settings.
4. Competitiveness: A few studies indicate that boys are more competitive, but many studies have failed to secure such differences.
5. Dominance: In childhood, since the sexes are segregated, one sex rarely has a chance to try to dominate the other. By adulthood, in most groups, males are initially ceded formal leadership. With the passage of time, however, the most competent person—male or female—emerges as the leader.
6. Compliance: In childhood, girls are more compliant with the directions of adults than are boys. Both sexes are equally willing to comply with one another's wishes, however.
7. Nurturance and maternal behavior: Research indicates that sometimes men are more willing to help younger children, animals, or those in distress. Sometimes women are more willing to help.

Unfounded Beliefs About Gender Differences

1. Girls are more "social" than boys: Actually, in early childhood girls and boys are both quite dependent on their parents; they remain very close to them. Later, both spend equal time with playmates; both are equally empathetic in understanding emotional reactions of others; both work equally hard for social approval.
2. Girls are more suggestible than boys: In fact, the two are equally susceptible to persuasive communications and in face-to-face social influence situations.
3. Girls have lower self-esteem: In fact, the sexes are similar in their *overall* self-satisfaction and self-confidence. There are some differences in the *areas* in which the two have the greatest self-confidence. Girls rate themselves higher in social competence; boys rate themselves as stronger, more powerful, dominant, and "potent."
4. Girls are better at simple, repetitive tasks: The sexes do not, in reality, differ in ability in such tasks.
5. Boys excel at tasks requiring more complex cognitive processing and the inhibition of previously learned responses: The sexes do not actually differ in ability in such tasks.
6. Girls are more affected by heredity and boys by environment: No evidence supports this presumed difference.
7. Girls are less motivated toward achievement: Observational studies of achievement strivings either find no sex differences or find girls to be superior to boys.
8. Girls are more auditorially oriented while boys are more visually oriented: In fact, the sexes do not differ in sensory orientations.

SOURCE: Adapted from Maccoby & Jacklin, 1974.

---

minor differences in the actual characteristics of males and females. Thus, men and women do not seem to differ as much as might be expected. But how well do our perceptions and beliefs concerning men and women match the "reality" of the research evidence? Let us now examine gender role perceptions and stereotypes and how they influence our behavior.

GENDER ROLE PERCEPTIONS AND STEREOTYPES

A stereotype is a relatively rigid, biased perception of people or social groups (see English & English, 1958). There is a substantial amount of evidence that the ways in which we view people are influenced by our stereotypes.

Stereotypes

Gender role standards specify that the ideal man and the ideal woman *should* be different. Not surprisingly, nearly everyone *perceives* men and women as the stereotypes they are supposed to be. Investigators have found that the majority of people believe that men and women should be very different and that they are very different (Brannon, 1976; de Beauvoir, 1952; Fasteau, 1974; Goldberg, 1979; Tavris & Offir, 1977). Some gender stereotypes are discussed in the Research Highlight. Nevertheless, research findings indicate that most of the male-female differences that are taken for granted exist more in fantasy than in fact (Maccoby & Jacklin, 1974; Unger & Siiter, 1974).

How can one explain the fact that most Americans are so convinced that there *are* enormous psychological differences between boys and girls and men and women when the evidence suggests that surprisingly few differences exist? Maccoby and Jacklin propose one possible explanation:

However, a more likely explanation for the perpetuation of "myths," we believe, is the fact that stereotypes are such powerful things. An ancient truth is worth restating here: if a generalization about a group of people is believed, whenever a member of that group behaves in the expected way the observer notes it and his belief is confirmed and strengthened; when a member of the group behaves in a way that is not consistent with the observer's expectations, the instance is likely to pass unnoticed. (1974, p. 355)

There is evidence for Maccoby and Jacklin's contention that people *do* tend to see gender differences when they do not exist at all. Let us review this evidence.

Perceptions

Our perceptions of people are sometimes heavily influenced by prevailing stereotypes. This is particularly true when we have little or no direct experience with them or information about them as individuals. Even with such direct experience and information, however, our perceptions of ourselves and of others are often biased by other factors.

Self-Perceptions.   In recent years the processes by which people form impressions of themselves and of their behavior have been studied extensively. Males and females appear to use very different standards in judging their own performance. One of the more pervasive findings in the social psychological literature is that women *expect* to perform more poorly than do men on most tasks (Crandall, 1969; Deaux & Farris, in press; Montanelli & Hill, 1969). Men and women evidently accept popular stereotypes about their ability.

RESEARCH HIGHLIGHT

Gender Role Stereotypes

Broverman, Vogel, Broverman, Clarkson, and Rosenkrantz (1972) found that gender role stereotypes are pervasive. They asked mental health professionals (psychiatrists, clinical psychologists, and psychiatric social workers) and men and women of widely varying ages, religions, and education to indicate what they thought the typical man and typical woman were like. They found that most people uncritically accept gender role stereotypes. They believe that the typical man and the typical woman are very different.

Men are perceived to be rational, competent, independent, and assertive. Unfortunately, they are also branded as insensitive and rough. Women are perceived to be warm and expressive. Unfortunately they are also seen as illogical, emotional, noncompetitive, and submissive. Those characteristics that Broverman and associates found are identified by most people as typically masculine or typically feminine are listed here in tabular form.

These perceived gender role differences contrast sharply with more objective evidence showing few actual gender differences in behavior and characteristics. An important feature of the stereotypes summarized here in the table should be noted. Both men and women agree that men have many more admirable characteristics than do women.

A number of other investigators have confirmed this finding (Ellis & Bentler, 1973; Frieze, 1974). This suggests that, in our society, the value placed on males is greater than that placed on females. Evidence discussed later in this chapter supports this view.

Competency Cluster

Masculine Pole Is More Desirable

Feminine	Masculine
Not at all aggressive	Very aggressive
Not at all independent	Very independent
Very emotional	Not at all emotional
Does not hide emotions at all	Almost always hides emotions
Very subjective	Very objective
Very easily influenced	Not at all easily influenced
Very submissive	Very dominant
Dislikes math and science very much	Likes math and science very much
Very excitable in a minor crisis	Not at all excitable in a minor crisis
Very passive	Very active
Not at all competitive	Very competitive
Very illogical	Very logical
Very home oriented	Very worldly
Not at all skilled in business	Very skilled in business
Very sneaky	Very direct
Does not know the way of the world	Knows the way of the world
Feelings easily hurt	Feelings not easily hurt
Not at all adventurous	Very adventurous
Has difficulty making decisions	Can make decisions easily
Cries very easily	Never cries
Almost never acts as a leader	Almost always acts as a leader
Not at all self-confident	Very self-confident
Very uncomfortable about being aggressive	Not at all uncomfortable about being aggressive
Not at all ambitious	Very ambitious
Unable to separate feelings from ideas	Easily able to separate feelings from ideas
Very dependent	Not at all dependent
Very conceited about appearance	Never conceited about appearance
Thinks women are always superior to men	Thinks men are always superior to women
Does not talk freely about sex with men	Talks freely about sex with men

Warmth-Expressiveness Cluster

Feminine Pole Is More Desirable

Feminine	Masculine
Doesn't use harsh language at all	Uses very harsh language
Very talkative	Not at all talkative
Very tactful	Very blunt
Very gentle	Very rough
Very aware of feelings of others	Not at all aware of feelings of others
Very religious	Not at all religious
Very interested in own appearance	Not at all interested in own appearance
Very neat in habits	Very sloppy in habits
Very quiet	Very loud
Very strong need for security	Very little need for security
Enjoys art and literature	Does not enjoy art and literature at all
Easily expresses tender feelings	Does not express tender feelings at all easily

Stereotypes of characteristics of men and women.
SOURCE: Summarized from Broverman et al., 1972.

But what happens when people's perceptions of their own competence (or lack of it) are challenged by reality? The data suggest that men and women tend to maintain their stereotyped beliefs in spite of compelling evidence to the contrary. Bernard Weiner and his colleagues (1971) studied college men and women's attributions of their own academic successes and failures. When students succeed or fail they can explain their performances in a variety of ways: They can attribute their success or failure to *personal factors* such as their own ability or lack of it ("I am smart," or ". . . not so smart") or their own effort or lack of it ("I tried hard," or ". . . not so hard"). Alternatively, they can attribute it to *external factors* such as the exam's difficulty ("That exam was such a snap, anyone could have passed it," or "That test was so hard no one could have passed it") or to luck ("I was lucky," or "I was unlucky").

Weiner and his colleagues have found that men and women seem to explain their successes or failures in very different ways. In one study, for example, these researchers asked college students to take a series of tests. They scored the tests and gave the students their "results." In fact, the tests were rigged. Half the time students were told they had done unusually well on the tests and half the time they were told they had failed. The scientists found that men and women came to quite different conclusions as to what caused their successes and failures. When men were told they had succeeded on a task, they generally attributed their success to their ability and motivation. When they were told they had failed, they attributed their failure to external causes—the test was too hard or their luck was bad. Women reacted in just the opposite way. When women were told they had succeeded on a test, they tended to explain away their successes by attributing them to environmental factors, saying "The test was easy" or "I was lucky." It was when they "failed" that they took full responsibility for their performance. Similar results have been secured by Deaux and Emswiller (1974) and Nicholls (1975). Some commentators have observed that men's and women's biased attributions mean that men end up thinking of themselves as successes and women end up thinking of themselves as failures, regardless of actual performance (Crandall, 1969; Deaux, 1976; Feather, 1969).

Perceptions of Others.   Men and women may be biased when assessing their own behavior and characteristics but they are at least equally biased by stereotypes when judging the behavior and characteristics of others. For example, tendencies to see infants acting "just like a boy" or "just like a girl" regardless of the infant's actual behavior are widespread. Psychologists studied parents' reactions to their firstborn infants. According to the objective hospital data, the boys and girls were identical at birth. They were the same height and weight and received an identical Apgar score. (The Apgar score measures an infant's color, muscle tone, reflex irritability, and heart and respiratory rates.) Yet their parents saw the boys and girls as markedly different. They insisted their sons were larger-featured, bigger, firmer, better coordinated, more alert, stronger, and heartier. Their daughters were viewed as weaker, more delicate, cuter, more awkward, and more inattentive (Rubin, Provenzano, & Luria, 1974).

Although *both* fathers and mothers saw what they expected to see, it was fathers who saw their children in the most stereotyped ways. Why? Psychologists offer one explanation:

As we know from our experience, hospitals are reluctant to allow fathers "handling" privileges, thus excluding fathers from the early interaction and nurturance of infants. If fathers were more involved in infant care would they perceive more similarities between their infant sons and daughters? Perhaps including fathers directly in child rearing would change their perceptions and would lead to less stereotyped expectations. Future parents, then, might be more responsive to the existence of sex similarities—androgyny—than the differences dictated by cultural sex roles. (Kaplan & Bean, 1976, p. 173)

A number of studies indicate that even when people are trying their hardest to be objective, they are still influenced by prevailing stereotypes (Goldberg, 1968). People simply react very differently to ideas, emotions, and behavior if they think they came from a man than if they think they came from a woman (Deaux & Emswiller, 1974; Feldman-Summers & Kiesler, 1974; Etaugh & Brown, 1975).

A trio of social psychologists (Pheterson, Kiesler, & Goldberg, 1971) have proposed that unless a woman is a person of unusual ability or an acknowledged success, she will be discriminated against. Further, they suggest that when a woman is merely *trying* to accomplish something, her performance will be judged harshly. Once she overcomes the barriers of discrimination and "makes it," however, discrimination should disappear. The researchers tested this idea in a simple experiment: They asked Connecticut college women to take a look at several paintings. Sometimes, they claimed a woman artist had created the painting, sometimes a man. The alleged status of the painters whose paintings they were shown was also systematically varied. Half of the time, the women were told that the painting was an *entry* in an art show. (This was a clear indication that the artist was *trying* to become established.) The rest of the time they were told that the painting had won a prestigious prize. (This was to indicate that the artist had obviously become established.) How did the woman like the painting? When the painting was merely an entry, women liked it better if they thought a man had done it than if a woman had. Once the experts had put their stamp of approval on a painting and it had won a prize, however, discrimination disappeared. It did not matter who had done it—they liked it.

Considerable research exists, then, to document that even today people believe that men and women *should* be different and that they *are*. Women are believed to be warmer and more expressive than men. Men are seen as more competent than women. Social scientists, such as Maccoby and Jacklin, find that men and women *do* differ in some ways, but not in such major ways as people think. Many of the differences that people think they see exist more in fantasy than in fact.

THE FUTURE OF GENDER DIFFERENCES

American men and women are in a period of difficult transition concerning gender roles. Traditionally, most Americans have believed that a "real man" should be emotionally controlled, independent, rational, primarily concerned with achievement, and not very concerned with emotional intimacy. A "real woman" should be emotionally expressive, tender, an expert at intimate relationships, unconcerned with her own achievement, and content to live through the achievements of her husband and sons (Fasteau, 1974; Firestone, 1970; Friedan, 1963; Goldberg, 1979).

Gender roles are, however, in a period of transition. Both men and women now cite desires for intimacy and companionship as the major reasons for marriage. Both husbands and wives now feel responsible for child rearing. The majority of women now are employed (Unger, 1979). Thus, it is not surprising that traditional men and women who were trained to feel uncomfortable when behaving "inappropriately" feel uncomfortable when today's world requires them to do just that. Many traditional men experience discomfort at the prospect of establishing intimate relations with others. An important concern for many traditional women arises from the emphasis that is now being placed on women's achievement and success. Let us briefly consider each of these issues.

Intimacy: A Problem for Men?

According to Kaplan (1978), all people spend much of their lives resolving the dilemma between their need for independence and their need for closeness: "All . . . human love and dialogue is a striving to reconcile our longings to restore the lost bliss of oneness with our equally intense need for separateness and individual self-hood" (p. 27). For everyone, working out an appropriate balance between independence and intimacy is difficult. For some men, the task is even more difficult, if not impossible.

Some traditional men try to be fully independent and to avoid intimacy. This is virtually impossible. Intimacy is generally considered to be a basic human need (Boszormenyi-Nagy & Spark, 1973; Erikson, 1964). There is accumulating evidence that intimate relations are critically important in protecting people against the stresses of life. Scientists have found that the quality of one's intimate life is related to one's satisfaction with marriage and physical health (Bernard, 1973; George, 1978; Traupmann & Hatfield, 1979). Today, the traditional man's inability to express emotions and establish intimate relationships may be lethal.

Achievement and Success: Problems for Women?

Matina Horner (1972) observed that some women are caught in a dilemma—they want to be successful, but not too successful. Horner tested her notion that women are more ambivalent than men concerning success. She provided college students with the opening sentence of a story and asked them to complete it. The women were given this sentence: "After first-term finals, Anne finds herself at the top of her medical school class." The men were given the same sentence, except that it was "John" who found himself at the head of *his* class. Horner argued that men and women should be labeled as "fearing success" if the manner in which they completed the story indicated they assumed that to be successful is a mixed blessing—that Anne or John would suffer as a consequence of their high grades in medical school.

Horner found that women displayed much more fear of success than did men. Fewer than 10 percent of the men wrote stories containing fear-of-success imagery, while over 65 percent of the women did so.

Here is a typical woman's story (pp. 162–163):

Anne has a boyfriend Carl in the same class and they are quite serious. Anne met Carl at college and they started dating around their sophomore year in undergraduate school. Anne is rather upset and so is Carl. She wants him to be higher scholastically than she is. Anne will deliberately lower her academic standing the next term, while she does all she subtly can to help Carl. . . . His grades come up and Anne soon drops out of med school. They marry and he goes on in school while she raises their family.

Here is a typical man's story (p. 162):

John is a conscientious young man who worked hard. He is pleased with himself. John has always wanted to go into medicine and is very dedicated. His hard work has paid off. He is thinking that he must not let up now, but must work even harder than he did before. His good marks have encouraged him. (He may even consider going into research now.) While others with good first term marks sluff off, John continues working hard and eventually graduates at the top of the class. (Specializing in neurology.)

Today, then, many women face a dilemma—they are afraid to succeed and afraid not to. Recently, Horner's research has been criticized by other investigators (Tresemer, 1974; Unger, 1979; Zuckerman & Wheeler, 1975). They argue that things have changed since Horner's day; that both men and women face such dilemmas. Only subsequent research can determine whether male-female differences in fear of success *and* desire for success still exist.

The Promise of Androgyny

In traditional societies, men and women are gently nudged, firmly pushed, or roughly forced to conform to tightly constrained gender roles. These gender role socialization pressures and much of the research on gender roles have been based on the notion that people are *either* masculine or feminine. In other words, from this point of view, most males are masculine but not in any way feminine and most females are feminine but not in any way masculine. Masculinity and femininity thus are considered mutually exclusive characteristics; people cannot be both masculine and feminine.

Recently, however, it has become evident that many people do not conform to

Traditionally, women were supposed to be specialists in love and intimacy; men in achievement.

CATHY

by Cathy Guisewite

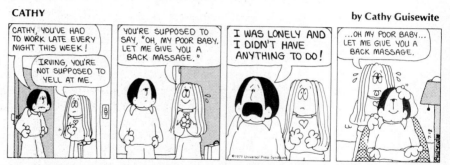

traditional stereotypes of masculinity and femininity. Many women have numerous characteristics that are traditionally viewed as feminine but also many characteristics viewed as masculine. Similarly, many men exhibit a mixture of both masculine and feminine characteristics. These people are referred to as **androgynous** (Bem, 1976; Spence & Helmreich, 1978). The term *androgyny* is derived from the Greek words *andro*, meaning "man," and *gyne*, meaning "woman."

Among others, Sandra Bem (1976) has forcefully argued that it is restrictive for people to adhere rigidly to traditional stereotypes of masculinity and femininity. She suggests, "For a fully effective and healthy human functioning, both masculinity and femininity must be tempered by the other, and the two must be integrated into a more balanced, a more fully human, a truly androgynous personality" (p. 51). She further observes that traditional gender roles limit the range of behaviors and characteristics available to men and women:

Both historically and cross-culturally, masculinity and femininity have represented complementary domains of positive traits and behaviors. Different theorists have different labels for these domains. According to Parsons . . . masculinity has been associated with an instrumental orientation, a cognitive focus on getting the job done or the problem solved, whereas femininity has been associated with an expressive orientation, an affective concern for the welfare of others and the harmony of the group. Similarly Bakan has suggested that masculinity is associated with an 'agentic' orientation, a concern for oneself as an individual, whereas femininity is associated with a 'communal' orientation, a concern for the relationship between oneself and others. Finally, Erikson's anatomical distinction between 'inner' (female) and 'outer' (male) space represents an analogue to a quite similar psychological distinction between a masculine 'fondness for what works and for what man can make, whether it helps to build or to destroy' and a more 'ethical' feminine commitment to 'resourcefulness in peacekeeping and devotion in healing.' (Bem, 1976, p. 49)

It appears, then, that the individual who strictly adheres to those gender role prescriptions defined as appropriate for his or her own sex (the sex-typed person) is handicapped in many ways. For example, the "real man" is at a disadvantage when he faces situations calling for nurturance and tenderness. The "real woman" is at a disadvantage when she faces a situation requiring leadership and problem-solving. In contrast, according to Bem (1976), androgynous people are capable of expressing a wide range of thoughts, emotions, and behaviors. They can be assertive and independent on some occasions and expressive and yielding on others. They can be instrumental when required, and expressive when expressiveness is required.

In order to investigate masculinity, femininity, and androgyny, Bem (1974) developed the Bem Sex-Role Inventory (BSRI), sample items from which are shown in Table 7–2, to measure gender roles. According to the scoring procedures for the test, if men and women agree with a large number of items on the masculinity scale and few items on the femininity scale, they are sex typed as masculine. If they agree with many of the items on the femininity scale and very few

Table 7–2.

Sample items from the Bem Sex-Role Inventory. Respondents indicate how well each characteristic describes them on a scale of 1 (never or almost never true) to 7 (always or almost always true). Femininity and masculinity scores are obtained by adding the ratings for the respective scale items.

Femininity Scale Items	Masculinity Scale Items
yielding	self-reliant
shy	independent
affectionate	assertive
flatterable	forceful
sympathetic	analytical
understanding	self-sufficient
compassionate	dominant

SOURCE: Bem, 1974.

on the masculinity scale, they are sex typed as feminine. If their scores on masculinity and femininity are relatively equal, they are androgynous.

By now, several thousand men and women have taken Bem's test. Bem (1976) found that approximately 50 percent of the Stanford University students tested are traditionally sex typed. About 15 percent are cross sex typed; that is, they score higher on traits associated with the opposite sex than on those associated with their own sex. About 35 percent are androgynous. They report approximately equal masculine and feminine qualities.

Two Texas psychologists, Janet Taylor Spence and Robert Helmreich (1978) have developed a newer, and possibly more sophisticated, measure of androgyny—The Personal Attributes Questionnaire. They point out that Bem labels men and women as "androgynous" if their scores on the masculinity and femininity scales are roughly equal. This, of course, includes those who possess many masculine and many feminine characteristics, those who possess a moderate number of both characteristics, and those who possess few of either type of characteristic. Spence and Helmreich sharply criticize this procedure. They argue that men and women should only be considered androgynous if they possess many typically masculine and many typically feminine traits. They label as "undifferentiated" those men and women who have neither masculine nor feminine traits. Recently, Bem (1977) responded to this criticism. She revised her scoring system to allow interviewers to distinguish between those who possess both male *and* female traits and those who possess neither. Nonetheless, Spence and Helmreich provide considerable evidence that theirs may be a superior measure of androgyny.

Bem (1976) cites an impressive array of evidence that traditional sex roles are unduly restricting and that it is the androgynous who will fare best in the world of the future. For example, in women, high femininity has consistently been correlated with low self-esteem, low social acceptance, and high anxiety (Cosentino & Heilbrun, 1964; Gall, 1969; Gray, 1957; Sears, 1970; Webb, 1963). In men, although high masculinity has been correlated with better psychological adjustment during adolescence, by adulthood it is connected with high anxiety, high neuroticism, and low self-acceptance (Mussen, 1962).

What are the behavioral correlates of masculinity, femininity, and androgyny? Bem (1978) summarizes a number of studies investigating independence and assertiveness, and nurturance and expressiveness. The initial evidence suggests that in situations requiring independence and assertiveness for effective functioning, highly masculine and androgynous people function more effectively than do highly feminine people. Situations calling for tenderness and nurturance pose difficulties for highly masculine men and women. Androgynous women function well in such situations. In response to direct requests for assistance, women sex typed as feminine are quite responsive and supportive. But, in situations where they must initiate nurturant assistance, women sex typed as feminine perform poorly. The apparent explanation for this seemingly paradoxical finding is that these women are low risk takers and hesitant to act unless social settings are well defined.

Spence and Helmreich (1978), too, have collected considerable data to support their contention that it is the androgynous person who is best adapted to life. They found that androgynous men and women—those who secured high scores on *both* their masculinity and femininity scales—had the highest self-esteem. Individuals traditionally sex typed either as masculine or feminine had self-esteem of a moderate level. Those who possessed few masculine or feminine traits had the lowest self-esteem. Spence and Helmreich also found that androgynous men and women date more, receive more honors and awards during their school years, and are mentally and physically healthier than are their more sex-typed peers.

The mid and late 1970s witnessed a flurry of research and speculation on the merits of psychological androgyny as an ideal model for gender roles. Most frequently androgyny was hailed as an optimal mode of adjustment to gender role standards. It was viewed as the very best that masculinity and femininity have to offer (Bem, 1976; Singer, 1977).

Recently, however, questions have been raised about the advantages of androgyny in gender roles and about the measurement of psychological androgyny as well. Some studies suggest that self-esteem, creativity, self-confidence, sexual maturity, and relative freedom from psychological problems are associated with

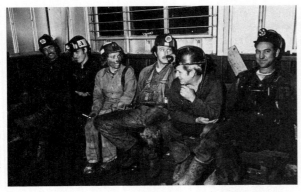
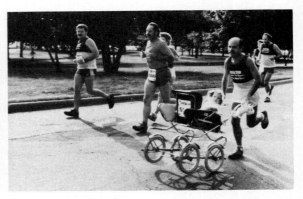

Research suggests that the people who fare best in society are those who are not restricted by traditional, stereotyped rules governing masculine and feminine behavior.

masculinity in both sexes rather than with androgyny (Antill & Cunningham, 1979; Jones, Chernovetz, & Hansson, 1978). Furthermore, some rather serious questions have been raised about procedures used to measure androgyny (Kelly, Furman, & Young, 1978) and the interpretation of scores on the most frequently used measures (Helmreich, Spence, & Holahan, 1979). Whether androgyny is destined to be the wave of the future in optimal gender role adjustment will be determined only by additional research.

SUMMARY

All societies possess gender role standards specifying the desired characteristics of ideal men and women, even though different societies have very different ideas as to what constitutes masculine or feminine behavior. Regardless of what gender role standards are, children must reach a certain level of cognitive development before they are capable of acquiring their own gender roles. Gender role standards and behaviors are transmitted from one generation to the next through the processes of identification, modeling, and reinforcement.

In a review of more than 1600 studies, Maccoby and Jacklin found that for the most part, in our own society, boys and girls are given surprisingly similar training. Boys and girls are given equal affection, at least in the first five years of life. Both are encouraged to be independent and discouraged from being dependent. Parents discourage both boys and girls from being aggressive with equal firmness. There are *some* differences however. Parents play more roughly with boys than with girls. They praise and criticize boys more than girls. When we consider those few behaviors that are considered specifically sex typed—for example, girls playing with dolls, boys playing with trucks—we note that parents are considerably more upset if their son is a "sissy" than if their daughter is a "tomboy."

How effective is society's training? Are most boys appropriately masculine and most girls appropriately feminine? It is clear that people *think* they are. When we look at the evidence, however, we find that, although men and women are different in some ways, many male-female differences exist more in fantasy than in fact. Society is effective in teaching men and women to perform specific sex role behaviors. Most women do carry purses and most men do carry wallets. In general, however, men and women are surprisingly similar. When Maccoby and Jacklin tried to determine whether the sexes differ in intellect, achievement, temperament, sociability, or other characteristics, they found that men and women are remarkably similar. Few consistent gender differences were found. Girls have greater verbal ability while boys have greater mathematical and visual-spatial ability and are more aggressive.

What does the future hold? Some have suggested that socialization efforts should be directed toward training people to be androgynous. This combination of masculine and feminine characteristics is seen by some as an optimal mode of gender role adjustment. Early research seemed to support this suggestion but more recent studies raise important questions concerning not only procedures for measuring psychological androgyny but also its value.

SUGGESTED READINGS

Bem, S. L. (1978). Beyond androgyny: Some presumptuous prescriptions for a liberated sexual identity. In J. Sherman & F. L. Denmark (Eds.), *Psychology of women: Future directions of research*. New York: Psychological Dimensions.

Maccoby, E. E., & Jacklin, C. N. (1974). *The psychology of sex differences*. Stanford: Stanford University Press.

Spence, J. T., & Helmreich, R. (1978). *Masculinity and femininity: Their psychological dimensions, correlates, and antecedents*. Austin: University of Texas Press.

Tavris, C., & Offir, C. (1977). *The longest war: Sex differences in perspective*. New York: Harcourt, Brace, Jovanovich.

PART 4

SEXUAL BEHAVIORS

CHAPTER OUTLINE

NOCTURNAL SEX DREAMS
Sex Dreams and Sex Dreamers
Origins and Characteristics of Sex Dreams and Orgasms
Significance of Sex Dreams and Orgasms

SEXUAL FANTASY
Origins and Incidence of Sexual Fantasies
Nature and Content of Sexual Fantasies
Significance and Consequences of Sexual Fantasies

MASTURBATION
Masturbation and Masturbators
Nature of Masturbation
Significance and Consequences of Masturbation

CHAPTER 8

AUTOSEXUAL BEHAVIORS

Once aroused, our sexual needs and desires may find expression in a variety of behaviors. These behaviors may be broadly categorized as *sociosexual* or *autosexual*. Sociosexual activities are those that involve interaction between two or more people. If those people are of the opposite sex, we call the activities *heterosexual*. If they are of the same sex, we call the activities *homosexual*.

Autosexual activities are those we do alone. The most common are *nocturnal sex dreams, sexual fantasies*, and *masturbation*. In this chapter we will consider these solitary types of sexual expression, examining their prevalence, their origin, and their significance. We will also consider the personal and social characteristics of people who engage in them. Let us begin our discussion with nocturnal sex dreams.

NOCTURNAL SEX DREAMS

About one third of our lives is spent in sleep. Yet, despite centuries of attention from philosophers, physicians, religious thinkers, and more recently, physiologists, psychologists, and pharmaceutical companies, we know very little about the mechanisms underlying sleep. Even more puzzling are the dreams that occur at least four or five times during an ordinary night's sleep and account for nearly one fourth of our total sleeping time (Dement, 1964; Kleitman, 1963). Dreams usually coincide with recurrent periods of sleep characterized by rapid eye movements (REM) and electroencephalogram (EEG) tracings of brain wave activity resembling the fast rhythms during waking states. The most vivid dreams occur during REM sleep periods, as evidenced by reports from people who are awakened in the midst of such periods. In addition, over 80 percent of the instances of REM sleep are accompanied by partial or full erections in males, even though such erections are not always associated with sex dreams (Karacan, Williams, Guerrero, Salis, Thornby, & Hursch, 1974). In women REM sleep is associated with increases in vaginal congestion (Abel, Murphy, Becker, & Bitar, 1979). The consistency and apparent universality of recurrent REM periods during sleep suggest that everyone dreams several times every night, even though the dreams may not be remembered upon awakening in the morning.

An unknown proportion of dreams are sexual in content and potentially important sources of sexual arousal. Like nonsexual dreams, sexual dreams consist of rather fragmentary and fleeting images, thoughts, and perceptions that rarely "fit together" to form coherent or logical plots. Sometimes, even though the sexual nature of dreams is not immediately obvious, the dreams are still accompanied by the subjective and physiological manifestations of sexual arousal and, perhaps, orgasm. On other occasions the content of dreams may include blatantly sexual activities but produce few, if any, sexual sensations at all. More often, however, the erotic elements of sexual dreams are clearly evident and correspond in some degree to sexual activities the dreaming person has actually experienced in reality or in fantasy while awake. Most of what is known about sex dreams concerns those of the latter type. Following a brief consideration of available data on their incidence, frequency, and correlates, we will return to a more detailed examination of the characteristics, causes, and significance of sex dreams.

Sex Dreams and Sex Dreamers

Although they have been studied, analyzed and written about for several centuries (Ellis, 1942), most of our current (though limited) understanding of sex dreams must be credited to the extensive and systematic investigations of the Indiana University Institute of Sex Research (Kinsey, Pomeroy, & Martin, 1948; Kinsey, Pomeroy, Martin, & Gebhard, 1953). The discussion that follows, unless otherwise indicated, is based mostly upon data obtained in these studies.

Sex Dreams: Incidence and Frequency.   As is generally true of most other types of sexual activities, more males than females report having sex dreams. The data reveal that virtually all males and nearly 70 percent of females dream about sex at some time in their lives. Dreams leading to orgasm are less common but, nevertheless, experienced by over 80 percent of males and nearly 40 percent of females by the time they have reached the age of forty-five.

The percentages of males and females who experience nocturnal orgasm by various age levels are shown in Figure 8–1. Shortly after the onset of adolescence, the average male who will ever dream to orgasm has his first nocturnal orgasm. Virtually all males who dream to orgasm do so within five years after the onset of adolescence. The average female who experiences nocturnal orgasm does not do so until about fifteen years after the beginning of adolescence. Thus, not only do fewer females than males dream to orgasm, but those who do generally do not begin until much later in their lives than the average male.

The peak incidence of dreaming to orgasm among males occurs during the late teens and early twenties. During this time 70 percent of all males who ever do so are having nocturnal orgasms at an average frequency of once every month. Beyond the age of thirty, the percentage of men having orgasmic dreams drops

Figure 8–1.

Accumulative (total) percentage of males and females who have experienced nocturnal orgasm relative to age.

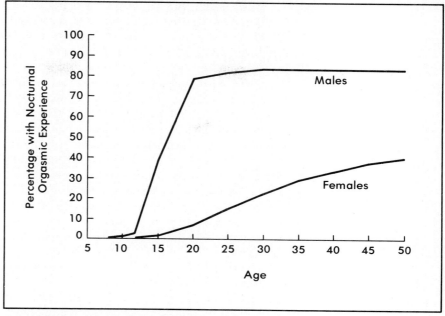

SOURCE: Data from Kinsey et al., 1948.

rather sharply. After fifty years of age, less than one third ever dream to orgasm and among those the average frequency is no more than once or twice a year. The peak of involvement for females does not occur until the late thirties and early forties when between 20 and 40 percent are dreaming to orgasm at an average rate of once every three or four months. Beyond the forties the percent of women having nocturnal orgasms gradually decreases but the average frequency remains at once every three or four months. Though important for a number of other reasons, sex dreams are never an important source of sexual outlet for either males or females. Depending on age, marital status, and other factors, sex dreams account for only 2 to 15 percent of the male and 1 to 14 percent of the female total orgasmic outlet.

Sex Dreamers: Personal and Social Characteristics.   In the preceding section rather substantial sex differences in dreaming to orgasm were noted. More males than females experience nocturnal orgasms and, at virtually all ages, male frequency of orgasmic dreaming exceeds that of females. In more recent studies, such sex differences continue to be evident (Gravitz, 1970; Wilson, 1975). In addition to differences between males and females, however, there are wide variations within the sexes in the incidence and frequency of dreaming to orgasm. For example, although the overall incidence of nocturnal orgasm in males is 83 percent, there are subgroups in which the incidence ranges between 99 and 75 percent. Similarly, some males average as many as twelve dreams to orgasm per week while others may have only a few such dreams in their lives. There are some females who average nearly two orgasmic dreams per week and others who may experience only one such dream in their lives.

Among males, high incidences and frequencies of orgasmic dreaming are found in those who are highly educated, unmarried, and relatively young. Almost all (99 percent) of those males who go to college dream to orgasm sometime in their lives, while 85 percent of those who complete high school only and 75 percent of those who never go beyond grade school ever do so. At all age levels, those who have gone or ultimately do go to college have substantially higher frequencies of nocturnal orgasms than those with only high school or grade school educations. Utilizing fantasy as a source of arousal and orgasm, whether during sleep or while awake, requires at least a minimal degree of imaginative capacity. It is possible that college-educated males have more experience or training with creative and imaginative endeavors. A second possibility is that the incidence and frequency of sexual activities that stop short of orgasm are higher among college-level males and the accumulated tensions from an evening of prolonged petting are more frequently released during sleep. At any rate, similar educational level differences continue to be reported in more recent studies (Wilson, 1975).

Marriage seems to reduce the occurrence of nocturnal orgasm in males. Although over 70 percent of single men dream to orgasm between the ages of twenty-one and twenty-five, less than 60 percent of married men at the same ages do so and their orgasmic dreams occur at a lower frequency. Thus, nocturnal orgasms constitute a lower portion of the sexual outlet for married than for single males. These data support (but do not confirm) the theories of some (for example, Ellis, 1942) that as other sources of sexual outlet become available, dreaming to orgasm becomes less probable. Conversely, in this view, as the availability of other outlets decreases, the probability of nocturnal orgasms increases, suggesting that sex dreams serve some sort of compensatory function. We will return to this issue in later sections of this chapter.

Regardless of age, marital status, educational level, religious affiliation, or religious devoutness, females who dream to orgasm do so at a relatively constant frequency of three to four times per year. The percentage of women who ever experience orgasm from dreams is, however, related to their degree of religious devoutness and marital status. Whether Protestant, Catholic, or Jew, fewer of those women who are religiously active and devoted dream to orgasm than those who are only nominally religious. In contrast to the findings for males, more married and previously married than single females dream to orgasm. This suggests that female capacities for fantasy-produced arousal and orgasm are enhanced by sexual experience. That is, the relatively higher degree of sexual experience associated with marriage and with religious inactivity increases the pool of overt experiences about which one can dream as well as one's erotic responsiveness to fantasy images (Griffitt, 1975; Kinsey et al., 1953).

Origins and Characteristics of Sex Dreams and Orgasms

A variety of explanations ranging from the supernatural to the glandular have been offered from time to time to account for erotic dreams and orgasms. For example, the ancient Babylonians and medieval Christians believed in succubi ("maids of the night") and incubi ("little men of the night") who aroused nocturnal passions in men and women (Ellis, 1942). More recently Davenport (1965) reported beliefs among East Bay inhabitants of the Melanesian Islands in "Crooked Men" spirits who have intercourse with sleeping women and in the female spirit Inelwa who seduces young men during sleep.

Glandular explanations of nocturnal orgasm are based on two erroneous assumptions concerning the physiological functioning of the male and female sexual apparatus. First, it was once thought that nocturnal orgasms (emissions) in males results from the pressure created by accumulated semen in the testes or other reproductive glands and structures. Of course, seminal fluid does not accumulate in the testes, and there is no evidence showing that pressure buildups in the prostate, seminal vesicles, vasa deferentia, or other structures stimulate any sexual responses. A second mistaken assumption, quite prevalent in early literature (Ellis, 1942), is that orgasm in females is always accompanied by an emission parallel to ejaculation in males and that, as in males, glandular pressures are responsible for both nocturnal dreams and orgasms.

Though physical stimulation from tight-fitting night clothing, bed covers, one's bed partner, certain sleeping positions, or an overly warm bed have also been suggested as causal factors, it now seems clear that nocturnal orgasms are triggered primarily by psychosocial rather than biological processes. The psychosocial processes of primary importance are needs, thoughts, memories, wishes, and impulses that supply the fuel for sleeping fantasies. Virtually all experiences of arousal and orgasm during sleep are connected to dreams; the rare instances when dreams are not reported probably represent failures of recall.

Dream content in both males and females usually parallels the actual experiences of the individual dreamer. In some cases strongly desired experiences that have not actually occurred may appear in dreams. When other persons are involved, they are often obscure and unidentifiable and may actually represent combinations of several different people or epitomize some general type of person. In some cases, the dreamer does not participate in the dream activities but merely observes. On other occasions, the dreamer may act as both participant and observer. One of the most striking aspects of sex dreams is the speed with which the dreamer may be brought to high levels of arousal and orgasm by the fantasized activities. The specific activities themselves may seem to be only minimally erotic. An event as seemingly innocuous as a look, a touch, holding hands, a kiss, a word, or a conversation may trigger an orgasm. That such activities (fantasized or real) rarely produce orgasm during the waking state suggests that, whether due to weakened inhibitions or other factors, the threshold for sexual responses is remarkably low during sleep (Money, 1974).

We have noted that the content of sexual dreams is usually a reflection of the actual experiences of the dreamer. When the waking activities or desires of the person are heterosexual, the dreams are most often heterosexual. Homosexual dreams are most frequent in those whose overt experiences are limited to the homosexual. The dreams of the individual with mixed heterosexual and homosexual experiences are sometimes heterosexual, sometimes homosexual, and sometimes even heterosexual and homosexual in the same dream. Interestingly, very few males or females ever dream of masturbation. Thus, the dreams of most males and females are heterosexual, those of 5 to 10 percent are homosexual, and those of an even smaller percentage are of animal contacts, sadomasochistic activities, and so forth, depending on the overt experiences of the dreamer (Kinsey et al., 1948, 1953).

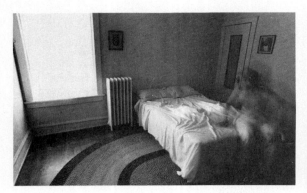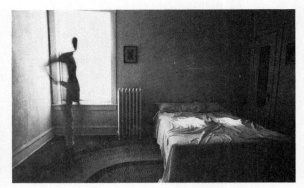

Activities or images that would not normally be considered erotic may seem highly arousing to a person in a dream

The content of some dreams, however, extends beyond the actual experiences of the individual. It *may* represent experiences that the dreamer may desire to have but, because of lack of opportunity or rejection of the activity in actual life, has not experienced. The psychoanalytic position on dreams generally asserts that most dream content represents repressed and unconscious, often forbidden, desires of which the person may be unaware during the waking state, but which find expression during sleep when ego defenses against awareness of such desires are relaxed (Freud, 1900). In light of the frequency with which dream contents are incoherent, contradictory, absurd, or even outrageous, aversive, and morally reprehensible to the dreamer, there may be some merit in this view. Caution should be exercised in the wholesale interpretation of one's dreams as indicative of deep-seated desires, however, since scientific support for the psychoanalytic view is far from conclusive (Klinger, 1971). Thus, while dream content may sometimes provide cues to a person's sexual orientation or preferences, it is by no means inevitable that homosexual dreams in heterosexual men or women, heterosexual dreams in homosexual men or women, or dreams of rape in women reveal hidden homosexual or heterosexual tendencies or secret desires to be raped.

Significance of Sex Dreams and Orgasms

Despite their infrequency, nocturnal sex dreams are of interest and significance for a number of reasons. Historically, orgasmic dreams have received tacit approval, if not wholehearted endorsement, from both the Jewish and Catholic codes of sexual conduct as the only acceptable form of sexual outlet other than vaginal coitus with one's marital partner. Due to the long-standing assumption that abstinence from sexual activity leads to a buildup of some sort of "sexual energy," nocturnal orgasms have been viewed as relatively "natural" safety valves that preserve chastity and prevent participation in morally unacceptable or nonprocreative sexual acts such as nonmarital coitus, masturbation, and homosexual behaviors (Bullough & Bullough, 1977; Ellis, 1942; Kinsey et al., 1948, 1953). Their acceptability stems from the fact that they are viewed as involuntary and "naturally compensatory" for abstinence.

The notion that nocturnal orgasms compensate for the lack of other sexual outlets implies that those people who are sexually active should have fewer nocturnal orgasms than those who, by choice or circumstances, are sexually inactive. The data concerning this issue are mixed and inconclusive. Among the females of the Kinsey sample who had ever dreamed to orgasm, a *compensatory* relationship between such dreams and other outlets was found in about 14 percent of the dreamers. When other outlets were drastically reduced through imprisonment or the loss or absence of a spouse, nocturnal orgasms became somewhat more frequent. But, the "increase in the frequencies of nocturnal orgasms is usually not more than a few per year, although the outlets for which they were supposed to be compensating may have averaged several times per week" (Kinsey et al., 1953, p. 209). Thus, sex dreams are certainly inadequate substitutes for high levels of sexual activity. In some women (about 7 percent of the sample) increases in sexual activity were associated with increased frequency of dreaming to orgasm. In the vast majority (79 percent) there was simply no relationship between dream frequency and frequency of other sexual outlets. The data for males are equally inconclusive and the question of whether nocturnal orgasms are compensatory or not remains unanswered.

Perhaps the greatest significance of nocturnal orgasms is in their meaning to the individual. Although feelings of guilt or shame often accompany other forms of sexual activity, most males and females react to sexual dreams without any disturbance or concern over their moral significance. In those few (less than 10 percent) cases in which sex dreams provide the first orgasmic experience of a person's life, however, some degree of bewilderment, confusion, and even anxiety may follow. This is particularly true for males who, prior to such an experience, may be totally unaware of the process of ejaculation. They may interpret their emission as indicative of injury or disease.

For the most part, however, orgasmic dreams are accepted and even welcomed as pleasurable experiences. Some people even deliberately attempt to induce sex dreams by thinking sexy thoughts or perusing erotic materials prior to sleep. Exposure to erotic stimuli sometimes increases the frequency of sex dreams (Amoroso, Brown, Pruesse, Ware, & Pilkey, 1971; Mosher, 1971) but the feat of actually programming oneself or others to dream of sex (or anything else) has yet to be accomplished. An efficient method of doing so would surely be welcomed by those who wish to make the most of their twenty years of sleeping.

SEXUAL FANTASY

Because of our intellectual endowment, we have access to a whole world of activity that is confined to our minds and generally regarded as unavailable to lower animals because of their inferior neocortical development (Beach, 1969). In this world of fantasy we are able to mentally experience the impossible, relive and reshape the past, plan and rehearse for the future, and enrich or add spice to what otherwise might be a dull, humdrum, or unpleasant present. Through the creation, addition, subtraction, and modification of images and thoughts, that which is forbidden, unattainable, or aversive in reality becomes acceptable, reachable, and desirable in the secret world of fantasy.

It is probably safe to say that virtually everyone engages in fantasy at one time or another. Singer (1966) has indicated that 96 percent of adult Americans report having fantasies or daydreams several times a day. The contents or themes of fantasies typically revolve around experiences that the daydreamer has had, would like to have, or are otherwise of importance to him or her. They may be concerned with goal attainment, personal appearance, social interactions, material possessions, heroic acts, or personal acclaim, as well as a host of other topics. Fantasies may range from the realistically logical and possible to the totally fantastic and illogical. Some portion of these fantasies may also be concerned with sexual activities and themes and may contribute significantly to a person's sexual life. The discussion that follows concentrates on the incidence, nature, and significance of sexual fantasies. For a more thorough discussion of fantasy and daydreaming in general, the interested reader should see Klinger (1971) or Singer (1966).

Origins and Incidence of Sexual Fantasies

Data concerning the origins and incidence of sexual fantasies are relatively scarce and sometimes contradictory. Kinsey and his associates (1953) reported that a majority of both males (84 percent) and females (69 percent) experience fantasies that are at least sometimes sexually arousing. Of twenty-four categories of daytime fantasies originating from unspecified sources, Wagman (1967) reported that nearly 16 percent of those of male and 13 percent of those of female college students concerned sexual matters. Others (for example, Gravitz, 1970) have reported relatively high incidences of sexual thoughts, images, and fantasies among normal adult males and females.

Such thoughts are often triggered by everyday encounters with erotic stimuli such as attractive men or women, odors, sounds, or commercially produced visual or literary erotica. For example, Nancy Friday (1974) collected reports of sexual fantasies from a nonrandom sample of over four hundred women in the United States and Europe. Among the events reported by these women as activating sexual fantasies were the sight of attractive male strangers, former lovers, male movie stars or athletes, and male models in magazines such as *Cosmopolitan* or *Playgirl*. Other cues such as overhearing or seeing others engaged in sexual activity or scenes reminiscent of earlier sexual experiences were also mentioned by many women as potent fantasy stimuli. It is well known that comparable stimuli are effective stimulants to sexual fantasies in most males (Kinsey et al., 1953). Thus, it is clear that a multitude of cues to which we are exposed on a regular basis are potentially capable of triggering fleeting thoughts or images of sex, or in some cases, fairly elaborate and intricate sexual dramas that unfold in the private theaters of our minds (Friday, 1980).

It was suggested earlier that commercial erotica in the form of photographs, stories, tape recordings or records, and so-called stag movies derive their power to sexually arouse by activating sexual fantasies, images, or thoughts in observers (see Chapter 4). For example, Hunt (1974) and Kinsey and colleagues (1953) have found that both males and females recall engaging in fantasies following exposure to erotic photos, movies, and literary works. In experimental work conducted in recent years, several investigators (Mosher, 1971; Schmidt & Sigusch, 1971, 1973; Schmidt, Sigusch, & Schäfer, 1973) have reported increased frequencies of sexual fantasy in up to 40 percent of both males and females following exposure to a variety of erotic stimuli. Furthermore, when such fantasies occur during masturbation or intercourse, the content of the erotic stimuli (actors, settings, and activities) is often incorporated into them or used as a basis for them (Schmidt & Sigusch, 1973). Thus, the fantasies or images produced by others in the form of erotica are capable of activating and influencing our own fantasy productions (Sachs & Duffy, 1976).

That masturbation is frequently accompanied by fantasy has long been recognized. For example, Kinsey and his colleagues (1948, 1953) reported that 89 percent of males engage in fantasy at least part of the time while masturbating. Almost three fourths (72 percent) always fantasize during masturbation, and 17 percent do so at least part of the time. According to these investigators (1953), 64 percent of females have fantasies at least sometimes when they masturbate. Smaller, but still substantial, proportions of men and women who are married fantasize while masturbating (Hesselund, 1976). Studies that are more limited but more recent than the Kinsey investigations suggest that the majority of men and women who masturbate fantasize while doing so (Hite, 1976, 1981; Hunt, 1974; McCauley & Swann, 1978; Sorensen, 1973).

The somewhat romantic notion that heterosexual intercourse should constitute a mystical, divine, all-consuming union and blending of two otherwise separate individuals for spiritual, existential, or procreative purposes has tended to obscure the fact that many males and females alike are deeply engrossed in fantasy during coitus. Recent data suggest that up to 65 percent of married women engage in sexual fantasies during intercourse with their husbands (Hariton & Singer, 1974; Hesselund, 1976). Over one third (37 percent) of the women studied by Hariton and Singer (1974), for example, stated that coitus with their husbands was always or very often accompanied by fantasy. Though few precise figures are available, it has also been noted that "many" males (Auerback, 1975) have fantasies during intercourse with their wives. Fantasies during intercourse are also common among unmarried men and women (McCauley & Swann, 1978, 1980). The nature and significance of such fantasies will be considered in more detail in following sections.

In Chapter 4 we noted the existence of rather widespread beliefs and survey data supporting these beliefs that males substantially exceed females in terms of sexual responsiveness to psychogenic sex stimuli such as erotica. Similar beliefs (Comfort, 1972; Ellis, 1942) and data (Kinsey et al., 1953) are found in analyses of male and female differences concerning the incidence of sexual fantasy. Traditionally, it has been assumed that, because of their relative disinterest in sex and their dependency on physical stimulation as a source of sex arousal, most women have little use for erotic fantasies (Kinsey et al., 1953). Dallying with sexual fantasy was thus viewed primarily as a male activity. Indeed, those women who admitted to engaging in such fantasies were frequently regarded as "loose," "sinful," or psychosexually disturbed (Ellis, 1942; Friday, 1974).

While sometimes contradictory, most recent studies reveal relatively few male-female differences in the incidence of sexual fantasy. In fact, some studies even report a slightly higher incidence among females than among males of fantasy during masturbation (Hunt, 1974; Sorensen, 1973) and during coitus (Hesselund, 1976). It seems clear that, although previously reported sex differences may have been quite accurate for their time (Kinsey et al., 1953), converging standards of male and female sexual expression are drawing the sexes closer and closer together in the use and importance of erotic fantasies in their sexual lives (McCauley & Swann, 1980; Crépault & Couture, 1980).

Among males and females, who are those most likely to have sexual fantasies? The few data available concerning this question suggest that the highly educated are more likely to fantasize about sex than are those with more limited education (Kinsey et al., 1948; Wilson, 1975). Those who are most sexually responsive and have a wide range of sexual experience have more extensive and varied sexual fantasies than do the less responsive and experienced (Clopper, Adelson, & Money, 1976; Hariton & Singer, 1974; Kinsey et al., 1953). Finally, it has been found that those who are relatively guilt-free concerning sexual matters and those who actively seek new and stimulating experiences frequently experience sexual images and fantasies (Galbraith & Mosher, 1968; Hariton & Singer, 1974; Moreault & Follingstad, 1978). Although it is sometimes suggested that sexual fantasies are more frequent in the sexually frustrated and disturbed (Ellis, 1942; Friday, 1974), no systematic data support these assumptions.

Nature and Content of Sexual Fantasies

The sexual fantasies we have while awake share many characteristics with those that occur during sleep. They often include rather vague and fleeting images of obscure people and places representing fictional and sometimes changing combinations of familiar figures and settings. They may vary in detail and coherence from momentary and quickly passing scenes to highly detailed and intricate plots involving multiple characters, actions, and settings. In some cases the actors are known and in others they may be total strangers. The fantasized activities may violate all known laws of physics and anatomy or simply be reruns of conventional activities actually experienced by the daydreamer.

In a few important ways, however, waking fantasies differ from dreams that occur during sleep. First, in waking fantasies the individual having the fantasy is more often the central figure rather than merely an observer as in many nocturnal dreams. Second, considerably more "conscious" control is exerted over the waking fantasy. In much the same way as a movie director might, the daydreamer selects and maneuvers the cast of characters, the setting, and the action with more authority than in nocturnal sex dreams. As a result of this increased conscious control, the daydreamer is able to rerun sexual fantasies at will whenever and wherever desired. Finally, the degree of sexual arousal accompanying waking fantasies is frequently much less than that which occurs during dreams. Even though we may attempt to "let our imaginations run wild," our inhibitions and ego defenses while awake are rarely as relaxed as during sleep.

The contents of sexual fantasies are as varied as the individual daydreamers themselves. Relatively few systematic studies of sexual fantasy content have been conducted and, because of procedural and sampling differences, the comparability of results from such studies is unclear. Most often, fantasy content has been studied in connection with masturbation or intercourse; little is actually known about those fantasies that arise under other circumstances. Furthermore, most of this research has focused on female fantasies (Friday, 1974; Hariton & Singer, 1974) and until

The content of a sexual fantasy is limited only to the individual's imagination.

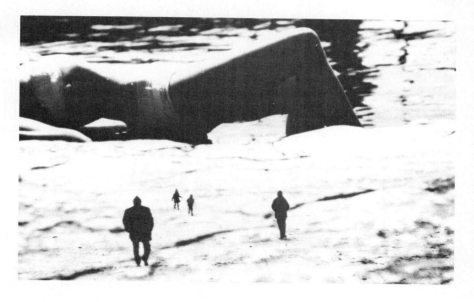

recently (Friday, 1980), little detailed information concerning male fantasies has been available. With these difficulties in mind, let us examine some of the more common aspects of fantasy content in men and women.

The erotic fantasies of both men and women often reflect sexual experiences that they have actually had. For example, the masturbatory fantasies of heterosexual men and women are most often heterosexual, those of homosexuals most often homosexual, and those of people with both heterosexual and homosexual experience in their histories are frequently mixed in terms of heterosexual and homosexual content. However, it is also true that heterosexuals have fantasies of homosexual acts and homosexuals have fantasies of heterosexual acts (Masters & Johnson, 1979). Those few individuals who have sexual contacts with animals do sometimes include such content in their fantasies, and sadomasochistic themes are reported by those with such experiences (Kinsey et al., 1948, 1953). Sometimes, however, fantasy content may go well beyond the actual experiences of the individual and reflect anticipated, desired, or otherwise significant activities (Crépault & Couture, 1980; McCauley & Swann, 1978, 1980).

There are some differences in the types of fantasy content utilized by males and females. For example, Kinsey and associates (1953) reported that fantasies that transcend actual sexual experiences are more frequent in males than in females. That is, males studied were more likely to have fantasies concerning unconventional or forbidden sexual acts than were females studied, who seemed closely tied to their personal experiences. John Gagnon and William Simon (1973) have proposed that the socialization experiences of males and females in our society might account for such differences. They suggest that men and women have distinctly different culturally shaped "scripts" or images and language for sexuality. For men, the usual script is a genitally oriented one in which physical unions of penis, vagina, mouth, hand, and other body orifices or parts are of primary importance. For females, on the other hand, the usual script is one involving interpersonal unions providing romantic, affectionate, and secure relationships, which may, in part, be cemented by sexual favors or submission.

Are these different emphases apparent in the sexual fantasies of men and women? In at least one study the answer was clearly yes. Andrew Barclay (1973) asked undergraduate males and females at Michigan State University to record their own sexual fantasies in writing. The male fantasies bore a striking resemblance to so-called hard-core pornography in which uncaring and highly sexed individuals engaged in vividly described sexual marathons. The most salient characteristic of female fantasies, however, was that they more frequently involved elements of romantic and affectionate ties between the participants in heterosexual activities in which females were either sexually submissive or taken by force.

Other findings suggest that, though there may be some sex differences, the sexual fantasies of men do not always involve frantically paced orgies nor are the fantasies of women always limited to sexual intercourse with the one they love. The masturbation fantasies of men and women reported by Hunt (1974) are shown in Table 8–1. The most common fantasy for both men and women was of heterosexual intercourse with a loved person. Men, however, were more likely than women to imagine intercourse with strangers, group sex with multiple opposite-sex partners, and forcing someone to have sex. Women were more likely than men to have fantasies of performing sexual activities that they would never really engage in, of being forced to have sex, and of homosexual activities. It is clear that fantasies of daring and unconventional sexual acts are not limited to males. Females' fantasies during masturbation sometimes go well beyond their actual experiences (Hite, 1974). As with other forms of sexual expression, convergence of male and female norms since the Kinsey studies is evident in fantasy content (Hunt, 1974). Other evidence suggests that contemporary women have (or are willing to admit) considerably more fantasies involving daring, unconventional, or forbidden themes than those of the previous two or three decades. For example, Hariton and Singer (1974) studied the coital fantasies of 141 married females residing in the New York City suburbs. The incidences of several types of their fantasy themes are shown in Table 8–2. As noted earlier, it was found that 65 percent of these women reported fantasizing during intercourse with their husbands at least some of the

Table 8–1.

Self-reported masturbation fantasies of males and females.

Reported Fantasy Themes	Percentage Reporting Each Type of Fantasy	
	Males	Females
Equally Frequent in Males and Females		
Intercourse with a loved person	75	80
More Frequent in Males than Females		
Intercourse with strangers	47	21
Group sex—multiple partners of the opposite sex	33	18
Forcing someone to have sex	13	3
More Frequent in Females than Males		
Doing sexual things you would never do in reality	19	28
Being forced to have sex	10	19
Homosexual activities	7	11

SOURCE: Data from Hunt, 1974.

Table 8–2.

Married females' sexual fantasies during intercourse.

Reported Fantasy Theme	Percentage Reporting Each Type of Fantasy
Having an imaginary romantic lover	56.0
Reliving a previous sexual experience	52.0
Pretending to do something wicked or forbidden	49.6
Being overpowered or forced to surrender	48.9
Sex in different place (car, motel, beach, woods, etc.)	46.8
Delighting many men	43.2
Resisting sex, becoming aroused, then surrendering	39.7
Observing self or others having sex	38.3
Pretending to be another irresistibly sexy female	37.6
Sex with multiple males simultaneously	35.5
Feeling weak or helpless	33.3
Imagining self as harem girl or striptease dancer	28.4
Imagining self as a whore or prostitute	24.9
Being forced to expose body to seducer	19.1
Fantasies concerning urination or defecation	2.1

SOURCE: Data from Hariton & Singer, 1974.

time. It is clear that the minds as well as the bodies of many of these women are occupied during coitus. They are, in fact, imagining one or more of a whole array of sexual acts in addition to, or instead of, the ones that are actually occurring.

There is, of course, limitless variety in the details of fantasies that both men and women have. As in the Hariton and Singer (1974) study, however, most investigators have used prepared lists containing a limited array of themes and asked respondents to indicate whether or not they have ever experienced each fantasy. When Friday (1974) simply asked women to report on their fantasies without limiting the categories, the potential range of fantasy themes was more apparent. For example, in addition to those previously reported, fantasies concerning exhibition of genitals, physical pain and suffering, humiliation, fertility, incest, sex with animals, pedophilia, homosexuality, and many other sexual activities were relatively common. Though Friday (1974) reported no statistics concerning the incidence of various fantasies, it seems clear that the previously recognized range of sexual fantasies in males (Kinsey et al., 1948) is at least matched in contemporary females (Crépault & Couture, 1980; Masters & Johnson, 1979; McCauley & Swann, 1978, 1980).

Significance and Consequences of Sexual Fantasies

There are several dimensions to the significance of sexual fantasies. First, they are readily accessible and demonstrably effective sources of sexual arousal and pleasure. Even though only 2 percent of females and even fewer males are able to reach orgasm through fantasy alone (Kinsey et al., 1953), several studies have demonstrated the effectiveness of the imagination as a source of moderately intense levels of sexual arousal (for example, Byrne & Lamberth, 1971; Laws & Rubin, 1969). By merely thinking the appropriate thoughts or visualizing the appropriate scenes, we may become sexually aroused at any time at any place. On the other hand, we may voluntarily inhibit and control sexual arousal with fantasies that focus on asexual stimuli (Geer & Fuhr, 1976; Henson & Rubin, 1971). Thus, it is in fantasy that human sexual expression most clearly manifests its independence from the control of hormonal and other biological processes (Beach, 1969).

Second, due to sociocultural constraints, lack of opportunity, and physiological and anatomical limitations, a wide variety of potentially pleasant and desirable sexual activities are available to most people only in fantasy. But, in fantasy, socially condemned acts such as incest, bestiality, exhibitionism, voyeurism, sadomasochism, homosexual activities, and rape may be engaged in with absolute secrecy and impunity from external censure. Missed or absent sexual opportunities may be realized in fantasies in which we have sex with the man or woman next door, an attractive grocery store clerk, motion picture stars, a casual acquaintance, a favorite teacher, or the entire defensive line of the Pittsburgh Steelers. Physiologically or anatomically impossible sexual acts such as rapid-fire ejaculations and intercourse in fantastic positions or with dozens of people simultaneously may readily be imagined without the restrictions imposed by biological realities.

At a less sensational level, sexual fantasies may simplify some of the more common, but nevertheless bothersome, details of sexual activities. One need not worry about asphyxiation in the cramped seats of an auto with exhaust leaks, the unexpected arrival of a roommate, birth control precautions, wrinkled clothing, or balky zippers. Sex becomes simple, spontaneous, and uninhibited as in Erica Jong's fantasy of the "zipless fuck." To Jong this fantasy sexual experience was "more than a fuck. It was a platonic ideal. Zipless because when you come together zippers fell away like rose petals, underwear blew off in one breath like dandelion fluff. Tongues intertwined and turned liquid" (1973, p. 11). In short, acts that are impossible or unattainable in reality may become commonplace in fantasy and substantially enrich our sexual lives.

Fantasies may also provide a convenient and safe means of planning and rehearsing future courses of action (Gagnon & Simon, 1973). In anticipation of a date or other sociosexual interaction, one may "try out" various sexual techniques or approaches in fantasy, comfortable with the knowledge that any of these trial gestures that seem foolish, clumsy, ill timed, or that backfire and lead to rejection are only fantasies. By this trial-and-error approach, one's strategy for dealing with the sexual interaction may be repeatedly altered and reshaped to allow for various contingencies. Thus, at least some of the anxiety and fear associated with looking foolish or being rejected in reality is reduced. Though some of the "best-laid plans" often go wrong, it is comforting to know that one has at least considered some of the "what if" ("if he or she says or does this, I will do this") aspects of sexual interactions.

We have seen that masturbatory, heterosexual, homosexual, and other forms of sexual activity are often accompanied by fantasy. It seems clear that such fantasies may significantly enrich or enhance the pleasure and arousal associated with these sexual acts. In fantasy, masturbation may be transformed into a wild, uninhibited, and passionate affair with Robert Redford or Farrah Fawcett. One's coital partner may be transformed from a slightly overweight, unattractive, disinterested, and dull bedmate into a fantastic combination of beauty and excitement. What do such coital fantasies reveal? Studies of coital fantasies have identified several possibilities (Hariton & Singer, 1974; McCauley & Swann, 1978, 1980). First, some who engage in fantasy during intercourse do so simply as part of their general tendency to be creative and imaginative in all of their social interactions. Others use fantasies of different partners or other acts to compensate for their general dissatisfaction with their own partners or their negative feelings about sex (Moreault & Follingstad, 1978). Still others are quite satisfied with their sexual relationship and simply use fantasy as "icing on the cake" or embellishment.

Generally, however, women seem more likely than men to use fantasy to increase their degree of arousal during intercourse, to enhance an ongoing sexual experience, or to compensate for less than ideal experiences. Men, on the other hand, are more likely than women to use fantasies to control their own arousal or the direction of the sexual interaction (McCauley & Swann, 1978, 1980). In any case, the presence or absence of coital fantasies does not automatically reveal satisfaction or dissatisfaction with one's partner or sexual activity. Thus, equating the presence of fantasy with dissatisfaction (Freud, 1908) is, in many cases, unjustified (McCauley & Swann, 1980).

What are the consequences of sexual fantasy for the individual? Beyond the immediate personal satisfaction that may be gained from fantasy, little is actually known concerning the answer to this difficult question. Most people take a generally positive or at least benign view of their own fantasies and accept them as pleasantly enriching experiences. In some people, however, sexual fantasies may lead to feelings of shame, guilt, or embarrassment. These negative feelings may have little to do with the specific acts imagined but concern the experience of sexual pleasure itself (Moreault & Follingstad, 1978). For example, as one woman reported:

I imagine it is a man making love to me, that he kisses me passionately all over my body, concentrating most of his ardor on my cunt, teasing the outer lips, loving me totally and expertly. I simply lie there in ecstasy, which makes me feel a little guilty later at having such a selfish fantasy. (Friday, 1974, p. 251)

Sometimes guilt is associated with imagining and desiring experiences that one's partner will not or does not provide:

We've been married seven years, and our sexual life is no different now than it was when we were first married, except that there's less of it. . . . But it's only when I imagine that someone is performing cunnilingus on me, which my husband will not do, that sex becomes exciting, and I've always felt too guilty to discuss this with anyone. (Friday, 1974, p. 254)

Fantasies of socially forbidden acts may leave an individual with lingering feelings of guilt, shame, or disgust:

Most of the time I imagine someone very slowly approaching me and moving closer to kiss my genitals. . . . Sometimes this imaginary person is female—which makes me feel guilty. These lesbian feelings do worry me. . . . All my lesbian feelings are imaginary; I would probably be disgusted if I were approached by a lesbian in reality. (Friday, 1974, p. 253)

Taken together, these excerpts from the fantasies of a sample of women reveal an undercurrent of guilt associated with sex itself as well as with these women's concerns about the meaning of their fantasies. Similar reactions have also been reported in men (Crépault & Couture, 1980). Do such imaginary activities reveal underlying desires for cunnilingus or homosexual activity that might find expression in actual behavior? Might someone be overwhelmed by his or her fantasies and driven to acting them out in reality? The answer to this question depends on the nature of the fantasy itself. Some fantasies may be of relatively innocuous and acceptable acts, which, if carried out in reality would pose no particular threats to the actor. In such cases sexual fantasies may well become realities. Other acts, such as rape, being raped, or sadomasochistic behaviors may be exciting in fantasy; actual rape and sadomasochism, in contrast, involve very real pain, fear, and humiliation and few people are likely to actively seek such experiences. In other words most people are capable of clearly distinguishing that which is real and dangerous from that which is imaginary and safe:

But act my fantasies out? Make them come true? No, absolutely not. My real life's not what they're about. I don't want those things to really happen to me, I simply want to imagine what it would be like. (Friday, 1974, p. 288)

MASTURBATION

Strictly speaking, the term **masturbation** should be reserved for reference to those behaviors that involve *deliberate self-stimulation that is intended to produce sexual arousal* (Kinsey et al., 1948, 1953). Since wider definitions of this term have been implied in other contexts (Freud, 1905), it is important to note some of the implications of the present usage. First, by including the word "deliberate" we are excluding accidental acts that may sometimes lead to sexual arousal. Second, the term refers exclusively to self-stimulation, and not to stimulation applied by another person. One masturbates oneself and is neither masturbated by nor masturbates someone else. Third, the definition insists that the goal or intention of the behavior is that of producing sexual arousal. Deliberately scratching oneself to relieve a nagging itch and self-massage to reduce pain do not constitute masturbatory acts. Although each of these points may appear to be self-evident, they are emphasized here because of the frequency with which both the nature and significance of masturbation are misunderstood. This will become especially clear when we discuss the "meaning" of masturbatory acts later in the chapter.

Masturbation and Masturbators

Of all the possible activities a person might engage in that lead to orgasm, masturbation is surpassed only by heterosexual petting and intercourse in the number of people involved both before and after marriage. Thus, masturbation constitutes a significant mode of sexual expression and outlet for both males and females. In this section we will first discuss the incidence and frequency of masturbation and then turn to a consideration of the personal and social correlates of masturbatory activity.

Masturbation: Incidence and Frequency. Although a multitude of studies have been conducted in attempts to establish the prevalence of masturbation, we must, once again, turn to the Kinsey investigations (1948, 1953) as the most comprehensive sources of information concerning this topic. These studies, as well as more recent ones (Hunt, 1974), reveal that by the time they reach the age of forty-five, over 90 percent of males and at least 60 percent of females in America will have masturbated to orgasm at least once. Figure 8–2 shows the incidence curves for masturbation to orgasm as a function of age for both males and females. Beyond the age of ten the discrepancy in the curves for males and females is obvious. By the age of thirteen half of all those males who will ever masturbate to orgasm have done so, but only about a third of the females who will ultimately masturbate to orgasm have had the experience. It is not until the age of twenty that the average female who will ever masturbate begins doing so.

More recent figures (Hunt, 1974) indicate that both males and females who ever masturbate are beginning at earlier ages. In comparison with the median ages of first experience for males (thirteen) and females (twenty) reported by Kinsey and colleagues, Hunt reported drops to around age twelve for males and age thirteen for females. Thus, even though the percentages of males (94 percent) and females (63 percent) who ever masturbate remain about the same, both sexes are beginning to masturbate at younger ages.

The peak period of involvement in masturbation for males occurs during the late teens when 88 percent of those single males who will ever masturbate are actively doing so (the active incidence). Hunt's more recent data indicate that the peak period of male involvement in masturbation still occurs during the late teens

Figure 8–2.

Accumulative (total) percentage of males and females who have masturbated to orgasm relative to age.

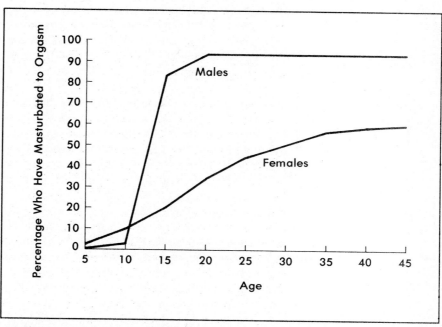

SOURCE: Data from Kinsey et al., 1948.

and early twenties. The active incidence declines steadily with age, and beyond age fifty less than half of single males masturbate (Kinsey et al., 1948). While more males are involved with masturbation between the ages of sixteen and twenty than at any other age, the peak *frequency* in single males occurs between the onset of adolescence and fifteen years of age when the average active male masturbates about once every four days. This rate steadily declines with age until the average male who masturbates after age fifty does so less often than twice a month. Recent findings (Hunt, 1974) suggest that the frequency of masturbation in contemporary older men may be somewhat higher than the Kinsey figures.

Masturbation is both less pervasive and less frequent in married men although the Kinsey data revealed that between 40 and 50 percent of husbands between the ages of twenty-one and thirty-five masturbate at a frequency of once every six to eight weeks. Hunt's data show a striking increase in masturbation among contemporary married men, with 72 percent of husbands of comparable age masturbating at a frequency of twice a month.

The peak of female involvement in masturbation (50 to 60 percent) occurs between the ages of thirty-six and forty, some twenty years later than the male peak, although recent findings (Hunt, 1974) suggest that the peak for contemporary women may have shifted to the late twenties and early thirties. In any case, it is still true that widespread masturbation occurs substantially earlier in males than in females. More older than younger females masturbate while just the opposite is true of males. The frequency of masturbation among females shows no clear peak during any age period. Across all ages the females who masturbate do so at a rate of once every two to three weeks. Slightly higher rates are apparent in contemporary females than in those studied by Kinsey.

In the Kinsey sample approximately one third of married females between the ages of twenty-one and thirty-five were masturbating about once a month. Although the rates among contemporary married women are about the same, far more of today's wives (approximately two thirds) in the same age range masturbate at least occasionally (Hunt, 1974). Thus, it is clear that masturbation during marriage is relatively common in women as well as in men.

Masturbators: Personal and Social Characteristics.   Despite the fact that nearly all males and a substantial majority of females masturbate at some time in their lives, there are wide variations among people and groups of people in the incidence and frequency of this form of autosexual behavior. The "average" male exceeds the "average" female in both the incidence and frequency of masturbation but the degree of variation among females is much greater than that among males. For example, though data show that 58 percent of all women do sometime masturbate, among some groups the incidence is as low as 34 percent and among others as high as 67 percent—a twofold difference. Among males, the range of variation is considerably smaller (89 to 99 percent). Variations among individuals in frequency of masturbation are even more striking for both sexes. Some males and females may masturbate to orgasm only once in their lives while others may do so several thousand times (Kinsey et al., 1948, 1953). What factors might account for such remarkable differences among people in their masturbatory practices? Although data concerning this question are relatively scarce, there are a few personal and social characteristics that have been identified as correlates of masturbation incidence and frequency. Let us briefly consider some of these findings.

Masturbation is both more widespread and more frequent in males who attend college than in those who obtain only an eighth grade or high school education. Those women who attend college and graduate school are much more likely than those who attend only high school or grade school to ever masturbate (Hunt, 1974; Kinsey et al., 1948, 1953; Miller & Lief, 1976). These findings, as well as those indicating that the highly educated begin masturbating at an earlier age than those with little education, are well established in both the United States and Europe (Schmidt & Sigusch, 1971; Wilson, 1975). There are several potential explanations for the educational differences and at least three should be mentioned. The first concerns differing attitudes toward masturbation across educational groups. Males and females with only grade school or high school educations tend to regard masturbation an an "unnatural" and inadequate substitute for sexual intercourse done only by those who are incapable of attracting a sexual partner. In contrast, those with college educations tend more to accept masturbation as a "natural" sexual outlet that may be used to supplement or complement heterosexual activities (Kinsey et al., 1948, 1953; Miller & Lief, 1976; Wilson, 1975). Second, the highly educated are more knowledgeable concerning the actual effects of masturbation on the individual. They are less likely to believe that masturbation causes insanity, pimples, or some physical harm than are the less educated (Miller & Lief, 1976). A third possibility is, of course, that the more educated are simply more willing to admit to masturbation.

Religious practices are also important determinants of differences in masturbatory behavior. Regardless of denominational affiliation (Jewish, Catholic, Protestant), those individuals who most closely adhere to and are active in their faith are less likely to masturbate than the inactive or less devout (Kinsey et al., 1948, 1953; Hunt, 1974). Although contemporary religious views of masturbation are less restrictive than they once were (Bullough & Bullough, 1977), deep and powerful religious commitments seem to inhibit masturbatory behavior.

The inhibitory factor involved would appear to be an emotional one in which masturbation becomes an aversive act producing guilt in those who violate or contemplate violating strong religious or cultural taboos against the practice. Support for this interpretation is provided in studies demonstrating the inhibitory influence of sex guilt (Abramson & Mosher, 1975) and negative attitudes on masturbatory practices (Miller & Lief, 1976). Not surprisingly, those individuals who endorse statements that "masturbation is a sin against myself" and "I feel guilty about masturbating" (Abramson & Mosher, 1975, p. 487) are less likely to masturbate than those who do not subscribe to such attitudes. Furthermore, strong dispositions toward guilt concerning sexual matters in general tend to inhibit sexual arousal and promote negative emotional responses to depictions of masturbation by others (Mosher & Abramson, 1977; Ray & Walker, 1973). The guilt-ridden person not only condemns himself or herself for masturbation but also tends to attribute a variety of pernicious effects to masturbation itself, as the following letter to Ann Landers clearly indicates:

Dear Ann Landers:

Masturbation is sinful. I tried it and the consequences were extremely damaging. It made me suspicious, jumpy, fearful, unkind, and highly critical of everyone I came in contact with.

Because of this terrible habit my judgment became warped and I lost out on many good opportunities that will never come again. By praying a great deal and engaging in strenuous physical exercise I have regained my mental and spiritual balance. I am once again serene, kind, ready to smile and can now enjoy the friendship of people. (Ann Landers Advises, Mercury, *Manhattan, Kansas, December 16, 1976, p. 8)*

That many contemporary theologians no longer view such behavior as sinful suggests that future generations may suffer less conflict and guilt concerning their masturbatory practices.

In Chapter 4 we saw that people differ a great deal in sexual responsiveness or readiness to become aroused by erotic stimuli. A high degree of sexual responsiveness is associated with frequent masturbation. For example, Abramson (1973) obtained measures of masturbation frequency and "sex drive" from a sample of male and female college students. Those with high monthly frequencies of masturbation scored significantly higher on the measure of sex drive and interest than did infrequent masturbators. In a different type of study Griffitt (1975) found that men and women who are most sexually responsive to erotic stimuli masturbate more often than do less responsive individuals.

It is generally agreed (Griffitt, 1975; Kinsey et al., 1953) that sexual responsiveness tends to increase with sexual experience. For example, many women begin masturbating only after they have had extensive heterosexual or homosexual experience (Kinsey et al., 1953). Similarly, Miller and Lief (1976) found that virginal males and females are less likely to masturbate than are nonvirgins of either sex. An additional set of findings (Money & Ehrhardt, 1972) indicates that sexual apathy, whether the result of biological or social influences, is associated with low-frequency masturbation.

Though it seems safe to conclude that highly sexually responsive individuals are more likely to masturbate than less responsive ones, the direction of causality in this relationship is unclear. It could be that highly responsive people are more prone to masturbate because of their responsiveness to and interest in all aspects of sexual expression. On the other hand, it could be that masturbation experience increases sexual responsiveness (LoPiccolo & Lobitz, 1972). Still another possibility is that some third variable exerts an influence on both sexual responsiveness and masturbatory practices (Griffitt, 1975).

In the latter case, various attitudinal and personality characteristics might act to promote or inhibit both responsiveness and masturbation. Several studies, for example, have shown that introverted individuals are more likely to masturbate than extraverts (Giese & Schmidt, 1968; Husted & Edwards, 1976). Introversion is associated both with a high degree of sensitivity to bodily sensations and a tendency to engage in solitary activities (Eysenck, 1971). This combination may dispose introverts to be highly reactive to sexual urges and to seek satisfaction through self-stimulation (Abramson, 1973). Indeed, any personality characteristic that increases our sensitivity or reactiveness to our feelings or sensations but draws us away from interpersonal contacts may increase the likelihood of masturbation (Eysenck, 1971; Hart, 1975). As a final example, generally positive and liberal attitudes toward sexuality in general might facilitate both sexual responsiveness and masturbation (Griffitt, 1975).

Finally, a few points should be made concerning the psychoanalytic viewpoint of masturbation. The traditional position taken by analysts (Freud, 1905) has been that masturbation is a normal and widespread activity during childhood and adolescence. But, in the usual course of events, it is replaced by heterosexual involvement during adulthood. Continued and frequent masturbation during adulthood is seen as reflecting psychosexual immaturity and maladjustment. Unless one is willing to accept the notion that a majority of male and female adults are psychosexually maladjusted, the data we have reviewed stand in contradiction to this view. *It is the well-educated, the well-informed, the sexually responsive, and the liberal segment of the American and European populations that is most likely to masturbate.* There is little, if any, evidence linking masturbation in itself to immaturity or maladjustment. The guilt and conflict that sometimes accompany masturbation may, however, be very real sources of personal and social difficulty for some people.

Nature of Masturbation

Despite some arguments to the contrary (see Ellis, 1942, for a review), it is erroneous to view masturbation as a uniquely human perversion resulting from twisted and misdirected sexual drives or desires. Masturbation, is, in fact, not limited to humans but widespread across several mammalian species. Masturbation has been recorded in male and female monkeys, chimpanzees, apes, baboons, porcupines, and several other animals (Ford & Beach, 1951). In the case of some male primates it is usually obvious that the self-stimulative activities are engaged in specifically for the purpose of producing orgasm since ejaculation often occurs. Female primates masturbate less frequently than do males and, though orgasm from masturbation does sometimes occur in a few species (Gebhard, 1975), it is relatively rare (Ford & Beach, 1951).

Masturbation techniques in animals are quite varied but, of course, limited by the anatomical characteristics of a particular species. Male chimps and apes usually rely on manual or oral stimulation of the penis while spider monkeys frequently take advantage of their long prehensile tails for genital stimulation. Male elephants manipulate and rub their penis with the trunk and other animals may rub their penis against the ground or some other object. Females of many species are sometimes observed stimulating their own genitals with their paws, fingers, tongues, lips, or various objects in their environment. In some cases the techniques used may show considerable ingenuity and creativity. Female porcupines in heat, for example, have been observed walking about holding, in one forepaw, a stick that extends between the hind legs. As the stick bumps against the ground its vibrations are transmitted to the animal's genital area (Ford & Beach, 1951).

Masturbation occurs in virtually all human cultures that have been studied. In their extensive review of anthropological literature, Ford and Beach (1951) reported masturbation in about forty primitive cultures and the practice is well documented for several ancient civilizations including the Babylonian, Greek, Roman, Egyptian, and Hebrew (Ellis, 1942). Contemporary studies record the occurrence of masturbation in Japan (Asayama, 1975), China (Edwards, 1976), West Germany (Sigusch & Schmidt, 1973), France (Athanasiou, 1972), Ireland (Messenger, 1971), and, of course, the United States. It is, in fact, doubtful that masturbation is absent in any modern society.

Although it is true that most societies condemn masturbation (particularly in adults) as sinful, perverted, immature, or silly, it is clear that self-stimulation for erotic purposes is widespread. But how do such activities originate? Even though no complete answer may be given to this question, it is generally agreed that neither masturbatory urges nor masturbatory techniques spring full-blown from instinctual or other biologically based predispositions. Masturbatory behavior is, in short, learned.

Learning to Masturbate.   In the normal course of exploring their own bodies, most infants and children eventually become aware of the satisfaction that may be derived from tactile stimulation of their genitals. Such a discovery probably provides the foundation for future masturbatory practices. Though we have previously noted the sexual response capacity of very young children and infants (see Chapter 5), there is some question as to whether the preadolescent genital stimulation practiced by virtually all males and females is, in the strictest sense, masturbation. That is, there is good reason to question whether such practices in most children meet all the criteria for masturbation demanded by our earlier definition.

To be sure, genital stimulation often becomes quite deliberate in children following their early incidental and seemingly accidental experiences. Furthermore, it seems clear that children continue to engage in self-stimulation with the apparent intention of producing some sort of pleasurable sensation. The critical issue is whether or not such sensations are in any way appreciated by the child as sexual or erotic. This is a controversial issue on which at least two opposing stances have been assumed.

The biological position represented by Freud (1905) asserts that many of the behaviors and gratifications of infancy and childhood are at their core sexual. A biologically based sexual drive is assumed to be the underlying origin of the pleasures derived from oral, anal, phallic, and genital stimulation. (In Freud's view both the penis and clitoris are phallic structures. He considered only the primary copulatory organs, the penis and vagina, as true genitals. In males the penis is both a phallus and genital; in females only the vagina is a genital organ.) Thus, the child engages in genital self-stimulation for the specific purpose of experiencing erotic gratification.

In contrast, others (Gagnon & Simon, 1973; Martinson, 1976) argue that in order to have a specifically sexual experience one must have learned a system of "scripts" or labels that distinguish the sexual from the nonsexual. A person's experiences become sexually scripted (Gagnon & Simon, 1973), "eroticized" (Martinson, 1976), or sexual only when he or she consciously recognizes or labels them as such. The scripts or labels follow cultural conventions that are largely established by the adult world and, according to this view, unavailable to the very young child or infant.

The proponents of this position explain it further thus. When children engage in inherently pleasurable acts of genital stimulation, parental or other adult reactions are often those of disgust or embarrassment. Pleasurable self-stimulation of the genitals is therefore scripted or labeled for the child as dirty, disgusting, forbidden, or otherwise undesirable. Relying on their own adult scripts, parents, in reality, view the child's behavior as sexual. For most adults, however, sexual scripts contain cognitive ("this is sexual behavior") as well as emotional ("this is bad, dirty") elements. The emotional rather than the cognitive elements are most often transmitted to the child. It is only when the child is exposed to sexual interpretations of his or her behavior through movies, literature, peer-supplied information, or other means that genital pleasures and acts become fully eroticized. Recognition of the sexual nature of such experiences is usually delayed until late preadolescence, early adolescence, or even longer in some cases. From this point of view, then, it is not a specific set of acts but those acts plus a specific set of associated meanings that determine whether or not behaviors are truly masturbatory (Gagnon & Simon, 1973).

Although the fact that coordinated and concentrated masturbatory activities rarely appear prior to adolescence (Kinsey et al., 1948, 1953) appears to support the latter position, it must be emphasized that it is difficult, if not impossible, to "prove" or "disprove" either the biological or learning viewpoint. There are no currently acceptable methods for identifying biological drives or instincts or for detecting scripts or meanings in preverbal or minimally verbal children. In any case, it is clear that specific masturbatory techniques are not biologically programmed but emerge as acquired or learned behaviors.

As Figure 8–3 indicates, males and females differ somewhat in how they acquire their information concerning masturbation and masturbation methods (Kinsey et al., 1953). Most boys learn about masturbation by hearing about it or reading about it before they try it themselves. Sex is a frequent conversational topic among adolescent males and many learn from their more informed peers or older boys that erections and pleasurable sensations may be self-induced through masturbation. Others may learn about the possibility by reading sexual wall inscriptions, erotic publications, or sex education literature specifically intended to discourage masturbation. The second most important source of information about masturbation for males in the Kinsey sample was found to be watching other boys masturbate. Once they discover that they can voluntarily produce erections and ejaculations through self-stimulation, many boys are proud and boastful of their new accomplishment and some seek to demonstrate their prowess to others or actually engage in masturbatory competition. In these group efforts, or "circle jerks," the boy who can ejaculate the fastest, the farthest, or the most times in rapid succession is declared winner. Newcomers to these events may learn of masturbation for the first time. Other boys may receive specific instructions from the older and more experienced:

An older cousin of mine took two of us out to the garage and did it in front of us. I remember thinking that it seemed a very strange thing to do, . . . but it left a powerful impression on me. . . . I wanted to do it, . . . I worried and held back, and fought it, but finally I gave in. (Hunt, 1974, p. 79)

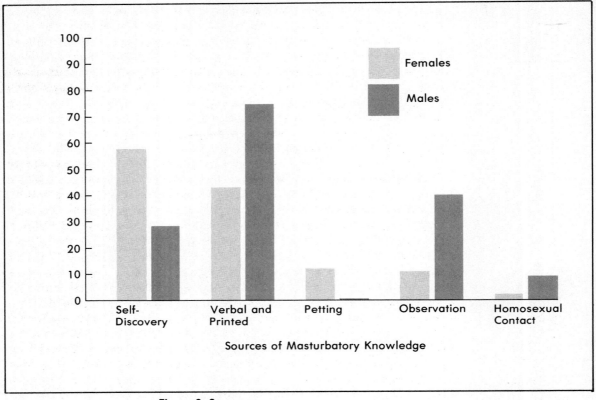

Figure 8–3.

Percentage of females (F) and males (M) reporting various sources of information concerning masturbatory practices.
SOURCE: Data from Kinsey et al., 1953.

Few boys discover masturbation as a result of homosexual experiences and virtually none do in the course of heterosexual petting activities. Somewhat surprisingly, less than a third report that they discover how to masturbate on their own.

Most of the Kinsey sample of women reported self-discovery as their primary source of information about masturbation. This was particularly true of those few females who began masturbating before adolescence. Self-discovery may also, however, be an important source for older girls:

It was sort of an accident. I first discovered how when I was about eighteen, as the result of reading a book. Not a book on sex.... I was reading in bed and in a state of excitement over one of the chapters I started rubbing my genitals. When I achieved an orgasm, it came as a great surprise. (Kronhausen & Kronhausen, 1964, p. 124)

Only in recent years has a substantial body of scientific and popular literature concerning female sexuality appeared. It is, perhaps, because of this that less than half of the Kinsey women reported discovering the possibility of masturbation from printed or verbal sources. Well into their graduate school years, over a fourth of these women made their first discovery of masturbation entirely on their own. Sex and moral education literature or lectures were, however, important sources of information for those who began masturbating after the age of twenty. While some women are, even today, ignorant of the fact that women can and do masturbate, the popularity of books such as *The Sensuous Woman* ("J," 1969) and *My Secret Garden* (Friday, 1974), articles in leading women's magazines, and explicit courses in human sexuality may be expected to increase the importance of literature and verbal information as sources of masturbatory knowledge as well as impetus (Zuckerman, Tushup, & Finner, 1976).

Few women ever have the opportunity to observe other women masturbating and such observation was important as an inspiration to masturbation for only 11 percent of the Kinsey sample. Some females learned that masturbation was possible following petting or precoital experiences with male partners who manually or orally stimulated their genitals and brought them to orgasm. Only about 3 percent learned of masturbation as a result of homosexual experiences.

Techniques of Masturbation. While it may seem unnecessary to enter into detailed descriptions of an activity that 90 percent of the average male and half or more of the average female readers of this book have already practiced, there are important reasons for doing so. Among the most important is the existence of widespread ignorance on the part of both males and females concerning the sexual lives of people of the opposite sex. This is particularly true where masturbation is concerned. Very few people are eager or even willing to engage in revealing conversations about their masturbatory habits even though they may admit to violations of speeding laws, cheating on exams, and readily discuss the intimate details of their sociosexual relationships. Most masturbators never really "come out of the closet" and, because of such secrecy, most of us know very little about the masturbation of others of our own sex, let alone the practices of the opposite sex.

How do people masturbate? It would be impossible to compile an exhaustive list of methods of masturbation. There are some common elements to the masturbatory techniques of both men and women but the details vary enormously from person to person. Some people are quite ingenious and creative but, of course, limited in their efforts by anatomical and physiological realities.

For the most part, masturbation in both men and women has a genital focus even though the specifics differ due to differing anatomy. In males the techniques are usually manual and less varied than those of females. Most males simply grasp the penis and stroke it back and forth from base to glans in what has been described as a "milking" motion (Katchadourian & Lunde, 1975). Stroking is slow and gentle at first until full erection is achieved, at which time a stronger grip may be applied and hand movements become more rapid. Light stimulation of the glans and coronal ridge may occur at low levels of arousal but, as tension increases, is usually abandoned due to the extreme sensitivity of these areas. At high levels of arousal (late plateau) most men stroke the shaft with a firm grip as rapidly as possible being careful not to pass their hand over the swollen and sensitive coronal ridge. Immediately prior to orgasm the strokes may become extremely short and rapid.

During ejaculation most men suddenly cease or slow their stroking movements and many grip and squeeze the shaft just below the coronal ridge as ejaculation takes place. (Similarly, in intercourse, most men will penetrate deeply and "hold" rather than continue thrusting during orgasm.) A minority of men (estimated at no more than 10 percent by Masters and Johnson, 1966) continue slow and light stroking of the penile shaft during ejaculation. During coitus these men also continue slow vaginal thrusting as they ejaculate. Following ejaculation the glans is extremely sensitive and painful to touch or pressure and most men avoid continued contact with this area for some time.

What we have described is, of course, the usual pattern of male masturbation and some men vary markedly from this pattern. Some prefer to stroke lightly only the ventral (under) surface of the penis and others gently manipulate and pull on the glans with their fingers. Some prefer to lubricate the penis using Vaseline, soap, body lotions, oils, or other materials while others rarely do so. During the early stages of masturbation some men may rub the scrotum or use their fingers or other objects for anal stimulation. As arousal increases, however, most abandon scrotal or anal stimulation and devote full attention to stimulation of the penis (Masters & Johnson, 1966, 1979).

Fully 95 percent of men studied by Kinsey and his associates (1948) practiced masturbation by manual manipulation, as described above. Most males have, in fact, never used any technique other than manual stimulation. Autofellatio (oral stimulation of one's own penis) is attempted by many but it is a rare man who is able to accomplish the task. Some, believing that manual masturbation is somehow sinful or degrading, use other objects such as pillows, bed coverings, or mattresses to supply penile stimulation. This may enable them to maintain their conviction that they really do not masturbate:

After a while I got to the point where I'd be half awake, and deriving great pleasure from moving my penis back and forth against the sheets until I'd have an orgasm without ever touching it with my hand, even though I wanted to and had to fight myself not to. . . . I told myself I wasn't masturbating, the way I did it . . . I never did use my hand on it until I was eighteen or nineteen—and that made me feel even worse, at first. (Hunt, 1974, p. 79)

More esoteric methods sometimes include the use of various objects to simulate the female vagina. These may range from the commonplace, such as the uncooked liver used by Roth's (1967) hero Portnoy, to speciality items such as commercially available inflatable plastic dolls equipped with vibrator-powered artificial vagina, anus, or mouth, or electrically powered pneumatic suction devices. The possibilities are limited only by anatomy, technology, and individual creativity.

Females use a greater variety of methods in their masturbation than do males. Kinsey and associates (1953) reported the regular or occasional use of about a half-dozen techniques by their sample of women. More recently, Hite (1976) described more than twenty different female masturbation techniques. Most women settle on and use only one method in all of their masturbation but some regularly masturbate in two or more ways (Hite, 1976; Kinsey et al., 1953). Like males, however, most (84 percent) females rely on direct stimulation of their external genitals. Most frequently involved are the clitoris, labia minora, and mons.

When the stimulation is manual one or more fingers are used to gently stroke and manipulate the clitoral shaft. Right-handed women usually manipulate the right side of the shaft and left-handed women the left side. Direct glans stimulation is usually avoided because of the extreme sensitivity of this structure. Masters and Johnson (1966) have reported that most women actually stimulate the entire mons area with rhythmic strokes, circular motions, or pressures rather than directly concentrating on the clitoris. In their view most women do so because they prefer the slow buildup of tensions associated with mons stimulation over the sometimes overwhelming and rapidly developing sensations produced by direct clitoral contact.

Mons and clitoral stimulation is sometimes combined with manipulation of the minor labia; in a to-and-fro motion the woman moves her fingers forward over the mons and clitoris and rubs or pulls the inner lips. The erotic sensitivity of the minor labia is well documented (Kinsey et al., 1953), and with this technique women are simultaneously able to stimulate all three of these highly erotic structures. The outer lips (labia majora) are less erotically sensitive and less frequently stimulated. When they are stimulated, it is usually during the course of masturbatory techniques which apply pressure to the entire genital area (Masters & Johnson, 1966, 1979).

Like males, most females begin masturbating with light and gentle manual stroking but increase both the pace and intensity of stimulation as arousal increases. As orgasm is approached, manipulation becomes more and more rapid, and during orgasm most women continue to actively apply stimulation to the mons, clitoris, and labia until the orgasmic contractions subside. Continued stimulation may be effective in producing a second, third, or even more orgasms in some women. In some women, however, the genital area becomes painfully sensitive to touch or pressure following orgasm and these women may avoid attempts at multiple orgasm.

Females are more likely than males to masturbate by stimulating their genitals in ways that do not involve using the hands. For example, the use of electric vibrators is becoming fairly widespread among sexually liberal women. A variety of such devices are available but the most popular appear to be those that are shaped rather like a penis and are battery powered. Some are equipped with interchangeable attachments, each of which provides somewhat different sensations. The effectiveness of the vibrator as a masturbatory aid has been widely acclaimed ("J", 1969; Masters & Johnson, 1966). Still other methods of nonmanual stimulation involve directing a stream of water over the vulval area from a bathtub faucet, shower, or whirlpool bath device ("J," 1969; Kronhausen & Kronhausen, 1964) and rubbing the genitals against pillows, blankets, or other objects (Kinsey et al., 1953).

Some women may masturbate by crossing their legs tightly and rhythmically contracting their thigh muscles or rocking their top leg so that pressure is exerted on the entire genital area. Stimulation of the mons, clitoris, and labia in this way leads to arousal and sometimes orgasm. The Kinsey studies (1953) revealed as many as 10 percent of the women sampled used this method. This technique is rarely used by men.

A small proportion (5 percent) of women are able to reach orgasm by the creation of extremely high levels of muscular tension. A woman may lie face down with her knees drawn up against her abdomen and rhythmically thrust back and

RESEARCH HIGHLIGHT

Becoming Orgasmic Through Masturbation

In recent years the failure of a substantial proportion of women to regularly experience orgasm during coitus has attracted the attention of an increasing number of sex educators and therapists. It has been reported (Kinsey et al., 1953), for example, that during the first year of their marriages fully one fourth of all women never have orgasms during coitus and even after thirty years of marriage there are still

some 10 percent who have never experienced coital orgasm. Within the last decade a variety of therapeutic procedures have evolved for the treatment of such orgasmic dysfunctions (Heiman, LoPiccolo, & LoPiccolo, 1976; Kaplan, 1974; Masters & Johnson, 1970). Some of these procedures are described in Chapter 13. The central assumption in such therapies is that orgasmically dysfunctional women have failed

to learn to respond sexually and that treatment should center around training procedures designed to correct the faulty learning (Barbach, 1976).

As an adjunct to such regimes, LoPiccolo and Lobitz (1972) developed a technique called "directed masturbation" for use in the treatment of women who have never experienced orgasm from any source of physical sexual stimulation (primary

orgasmic dysfunction). The primary inorgasmic woman is particularly difficult to successfully treat by the more traditional sex therapies (Masters & Johnson, 1970) since she has no experience whatsoever with orgasm and may have never become intensely aroused by any of her sexual activities. Since masturbation is the most effective means by which women may reach orgasm, it forms the core

Primary inorgasmic females' self ratings of sexual arousal during marital sexual interactions for four weeks before and seven weeks after beginning treatment through directed masturbation.

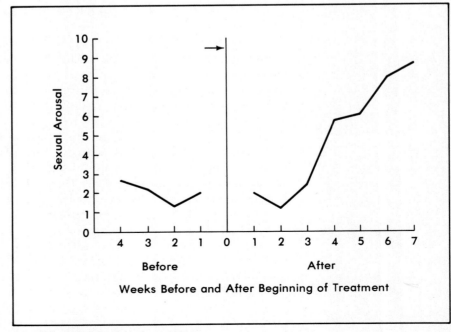

SOURCE: Data from Kohlenberg, 1974.

of the LoPiccolo and Lobitz procedure.

Robert Kohlenberg (1974) has described the use of directed masturbation in the treatment of three primary inorgasmic women who had failed to respond to the basic treatment procedures developed by Masters and Johnson (1970). Several steps are involved in the masturbation procedure: (1) the patient is first given basic information concerning masturbation and desensitized to her negative feelings about it; (2) the patient is instructed to familiarize herself with her genital anatomy by examining herself in the nude using a mirror and to touch and stroke her genitals to learn which parts are most sensitive; (3) she is then encouraged to experiment with various stroking methods to obtain the maximum amount of pleasure and to gradually increase the time devoted to auto-stimulation; (4) with her husband present, the patient is directed to show him how she obtains the maximum pleasure; and (5) the couple is encouraged to engage in sexual encounters involving mutual genital stimulation and coitus if pleasurable for both. To assess the effectiveness of the procedure the women were asked both before and after treatment began to rate how sexually aroused they became during sexual interactions with their husbands and to report on the occurrence of orgasm in their interactions.

The average sexual arousal ratings of the sexual encounters of these women for the four weeks before and seven weeks after the beginning of treatment are shown in the graph on page 242.

The effectiveness of the procedure is readily apparent in these data and from the fact that each woman became orgasmic for the first time in her life within seven weeks of the beginning of the directed masturbation technique. By learning to masturbate effectively the women became more aroused by and capable of responding orgasmically in their marital sexual encounters.

forth with her pelvis while tightening and squeezing her buttocks together. Simulating coital thrusting motions, these actions must be performed with considerable force if they are to be effective (Kinsey et al., 1953).

Only about 20 percent of women ever insert anything into their vaginas while masturbating (Kinsey et al., 1953). When such insertions are used it is most often one or more fingers, which shallowly penetrate the opening of the vagina in order to provide a firm hold while the women stimulates the outer genitals with the rest of her hand. Some females, however, derive erotic pleasure from penetration. Others use vaginal insertions in order to simulate coitus because it was recommended by either a male friend or a specialist urging them to acquire "vaginal orgasmic" capacity (see Chapter 5 for a discussion of this topic). Others do so simply to entertain male partners who are sexually aroused by observing such insertions (Kinsey et al., 1953). Even though a variety of artificial penislike devices **(dildos)** are widely available, their use is much less frequent than is often assumed.

Only a small percentage of women are able to reach orgasm through breast stimulation alone. The breasts and nipples of many women, however, are erotically sensitive and at least 11 percent of the Kinsey females manipulated their breasts while simultaneously stimulating their genitals. Some women are able to suck on their own nipples and may occasionally do so for erotic pleasure. It is apparent that women have a much richer repertoire of masturbatory techniques than do men.

Significance and Consequences of Masturbation

Virtually no aspect of human sexual expression has escaped the condemnation of one or more religious, medical, or scientific "authorities." This is particularly true of masturbation, which has variously been called "self-abuse," "pollution," the "ultimate sin against nature," and a host of other pejorative names (Kinsey et al., 1948, 1953). The origins of the taboos against masturbation are to be found in the complex and often interacting forces of theology, medicine, and science (Bullough, 1975). Contemporary attitudes toward masturbation, however, seem to be founded on at least two influential beliefs concerning this form of sexual behavior.

First, the theological view has been that masturbation is sinful or wrong because it represents the height of hedonism in which the masturbator pursues pleasure for its own sake through an act that is nonprocreative and inconsistent with the ultimate purpose of sex—to multiply and expand the human population. From this standpoint nonprocreative sex is viewed, at best, as a diversion for both males and females from fruitful reproduction and, at worst, as a wasteful loss of limited supplies of precious semen by males. Semen wastage through masturbation is condemned as sinful because it results in reduced fertility and ultimately restricts population growth.

Second, the moral objections to masturbation were bolstered by eighteenth-century medical beliefs that, if not sinful, masturbation and loss of semen actually endangered the health of the masturbator. Most noteworthy in this respect was a monograph published in 1758 by the Swiss physician Samuel Tissot entitled *Onania, or a Treatise upon the Disorders Produced by Masturbation*. This influential work carried the message that masturbation was a dangerous habit capable of producing every "illness" known, including pimples, blisters, constipation, con-

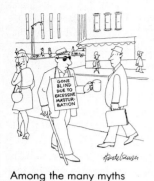

Among the many myths about masturbation was that, in excess, it would lead to blindness.

sumption, blindness, insomnia, headaches, genital cancer, feeblemindedness, weakness, jaundice, nose pain, intestinal disorders, confusion, insanity, and a host of additional rather grotesque maladies (Bullough, 1975; Kinsey et al., 1948, 1953).

Taken together, theology and medical "science" acted in concert to convince people that masturbation was not only sinful and immoral but also dangerous to one's health. When we add the influential view of late nineteenth- and early twentieth-century psychological theorists (Freud, 1905) that masturbation is infantile and immature, it becomes clear why this form of sexual behavior is so widely condemned. It is equally clear, however, that such views have been relatively ineffective in eliminating masturbation. Almost all males and most females do masturbate at some time in their lives and it is important to briefly examine the moral, biological, and psychosocial significance of this form of sexual behavior.

Let us first consider the biological issue. There is no evidence that the biological effects of masturbation differ in any fundamental way from the biological effects of any other form of sexual behavior. In short, beliefs that masturbation causes pimples, jaundice, feeblemindedness, and other maladies have been fully discredited as erroneous by contemporary biological scientists. Some, however, reach the conclusion that "excess" masturbation may be harmful and should be carefully avoided. At what point masturbation becomes excessive is rarely defined, although it appears that people are likely to consider any masturbatory frequency that exceeds their own as excessive (Masters & Johnson, 1966). Once again, however, there is no evidence that high rates of masturbation are physically harmful. In any case, when individuals reach the point of sexual satiation, additional sexual activity becomes aversive or impossible because they no longer respond erotically (Kinsey et al, 1948; Masters & Johnson, 1966). When this happens people will simply quit masturbating for a time. Despite the rather widespread dissemination of information concerning the lack of harm associated with masturbation, as many as 15 percent of surveyed males and females (including medical students and resident physicians) continue to believe that the act leads to mental instability or insanity (Arafat & Cotton, 1974; Miller & Lief, 1976). Such beliefs are, of course, most prevalent in those who never or rarely masturbate (Miller & Lief, 1976).

On a more positive side is evidence suggesting that masturbation may even be physiologically beneficial. As we noted in Chapter 5, high levels of sexual arousal are associated with severe internal and external genital vasocongestion which, if unrelieved by orgasm, sometimes produces feelings of discomfort or pain. When other orgasmic outlets are unavailable or ineffective, masturbation may provide convenient and effective relief to accumulated sexual tensions and discomfort (Masters & Johnson, 1966). Indeed, high levels of sexual tension (Hunt, 1974), or "feeling horny" (Arafat & Cotton, 1974), are the most frequently cited reasons for masturbating.

Whether masturbation is moral or immoral is a theological or philosophical question that is scientifically unanswerable. Transgressions or anticipated transgressions of moral codes, however, often produce psychosocial disturbances reflected by feelings of guilt which may be investigated scientifically. There is little question that masturbatory desires and practices are potent sources of guilt and moral conflict for many males and females. Even in this era of sexual enlightenment and liberation, between 30 and 80 percent of those surveyed feel that masturbation is morally wrong and should be discouraged (Greenberg & Archambault, 1973; Hunt, 1974; Miller & Lief, 1976; Wilson, 1975). While some people refrain from masturbating because of such feelings (Arafat & Cotton, 1974; Kinsey et al., 1953), many more masturbate in spite of their moral objections and suffer the consequences of guilt. Depending on the populations sampled, various studies have placed the incidence of feelings of guilt and depression following masturbation at between 25 percent (Arafat & Cotton, 1974) and 81 percent (Sorensen, 1973). Such feelings are generally most prevalent among the less educated (Wilson, 1975), older (Hunt, 1974), and most religiously devout (Kinsey et al., 1948, 1953) segments of the population. The effects of masturbatory guilt on various individuals range from mild twinges of conscience to severe emotional conflict and depression sometimes resulting in attempted suicide (Gordon, 1972; Kinsey et al., 1948). That masturbation is becoming more and more acceptable (Hunt, 1974) suggests that the clouds of guilt surrounding this practice are beginning to dissipate.

Those individuals who do not suffer guilt, shame, or anxiety from their masturbatory practices may expect to derive some psychosocial benefits from the practice. For both men and women masturbation provides a safe, convenient, and highly effective outlet for sexual tensions. It is the most effective means by which females may reach orgasm. Although women may achieve orgasm in less than half of their coital experiences, they do so in 95 percent or more of their masturbation activities (Kinsey et al., 1953) and the orgasms resulting from masturbation are frequently more *physiologically* intense and satisfying (Masters & Johnson, 1966).

There is also evidence that orgasmic experience in masturbation may facilitate a woman's orgasmic responsiveness in marital coitus. Among the married females in the Kinsey sample who had never masturbated to orgasm before marriage, almost a third failed to reach orgasm from coitus during the first few years of their marriage. In contrast, less than a fifth of those who had masturbated to orgasm before marriage were coitally nonorgasmic during their early marital years. One possible explanation for this finding is that through masturbation a woman is able to learn what stimulative techniques are most effective in "turning her on" and this knowledge and experience transfers positively to her responses and actions during intercourse. At any rate, it is clear that learning to masturbate effectively is sometimes a significant aid to the development of orgasmic responsiveness in females (Kohlenberg, 1974).

SUMMARY

The most significant forms of autosexual behavior are nocturnal sex dreams, sexual fantasy, and masturbation. Almost all males and nearly three fourths of females dream about sex at some time in their lives. Smaller percentages of each sex sometimes reach orgasm during such dreams. Sex dream content most frequently, but not always, is a reflection of the actual sexual experiences of the dreamer such that heterosexuals have heterosexual dreams, homosexuals have homosexual dreams, and so forth.

Most males and females indulge in waking sexual fantasies at least occasionally. Masturbation and coitus are particularly potent activators of sexual fantasies in both men and women. Research during the 1930s and 1940s indicated that sexual fantasies are more common in males than in females but more recent investigations reveal a genuine convergence between the sexes in terms of fantasy use. The most highly educated, most sexually responsive, and least sexually guilty of both sexes are most likely to engage in sexual fantasies. Waking sexual fantasy content most often parallels people's sexual experiences and preferences even though it sometimes includes forbidden, physically impossible, or risky sexual activities which transcend their actual experiences.

Masturbation is deliberate self-stimulation that is intended to produce sexual arousal. Over 90 percent of all males masturbate at some time in their lives and the average boy begins masturbating between the ages of twelve and thirteen. Between 60 and 70 percent of all females masturbate but the average girl begins later than the average boy. The peak incidence of masturbation in males occurs during the late teens and early twenties while peak female involvement does not occur until the late twenties and early thirties. Contrary to some views, it is the well-educated, the well-informed, and the sexually responsive segment of the population which is most likely to masturbate. Masturbation is widespread among nonhuman mammals and primitive cultures. Humans learn to masturbate; American males are most likely to acquire their knowledge by hearing or reading about it and American females are most likely to discover masturbation on their own. The popularity of contemporary sex-oriented literature should increase the probability that women will learn to masturbate from such sources. Male and female masturbatory techniques are mostly manual but females use a greater variety of genital stimulation methods than do men. While the morality or immorality of masturbation is an issue that cannot be addressed by science, it is clear that masturbation produces none of the harmful physiological effects that have frequently been credited to it. Many people may feel guilty about their masturbation habits but the practice is becoming more and more acceptable and presumably less troublesome to those who engage in it.

SUGGESTED READINGS

Barclay, A. M. (1973). Sexual fantasies in men and women. *Medical Aspects of Human Sexuality, 7,* 205–216.

Ellis, H. (1942). *Studies in the psychology of sex* (2 vols.). New York: Random House. (See especially Volume 1, Part 1, pp. 161–325.)

Friday, N. (1974). *My secret garden: Women's sexual fantasies.* New York: Pocket Books.

Kinsey, A., Pomeroy, W., & Martin, C. (1948). *Sexual behavior in the human male.* Philadelphia: Saunders. (See especially Chapters 14 and 15.)

Kinsey, A., Pomeroy, W., Martin, C., & Gebhard, P. (1953). *Sexual behavior in the human female.* Philadelphia: Saunders. (See especially Chapters 5 and 6.)

CHAPTER OUTLINE

CHAPTER 9

HETEROSEXUAL BEHAVIORS: SEX PLAY AND PETTING

During this period I was exposed to many members of the opposite sex who were approximately my age. The one who held the strongest attraction for me was my cousin. . . . It was my brother's idea to play doctor. The three of us covered as much of ourselves as we could with a blanket. When my cousin's pants were off, he examined her while I watched. After a short time of feeling her between the legs, my brother and I opened up our pants so she could feel us as well. Finally, I had my turn with her. (Ribal, 1973, pp. 67–68)

Although most adults tend to think of sexual intercourse or coitus as the essence of heterosexual expression, many Americans live out nearly two decades of their lives before experiencing coitus. Yet there are few whose existence prior to coitus is totally devoid of sexual activity. Heterosexual intercourse is not, of course, the only avenue of sexual expression. Furthermore, there is more to heterosexual behavior than coitus. In this chapter we consider those patterns of heterosexual interaction that do not involve intercourse. More specifically, we shall examine those forms of behavior referred to as *heterosexual play* and *heterosexual petting*.

PREADOLESCENT HETEROSEXUAL PLAY

Most of us tend to think of our sexual feelings, desires, and behaviors as truly emerging during that period of life extending from the onset of puberty to adulthood known as adolescence. Even though we may recall instances of behavior during preadolescence that we now think of as sexual, there is a tendency to regard that time as one of limited sexual involvement. Indeed, prior to the twentieth century, the traditional view was that our sexual impulses remain dormant until awakened by the physiological changes of puberty and then mature into fully adult patterns of sexuality after a few years of adolescent cultivation.

There is no longer any doubt, however, that at least some people are physiologically capable of sexual responses long before puberty (Kinsey et al., 1948, 1953). With the exception of ejaculation in the male, all of the outward physical manifestations of orgasm have been documented in both males and females under one year of age. Kinsey et al. (1948) estimated that at least half of all boys are physiologically capable of orgasm by the time they are three or four years old and virtually all boys *could* reach orgasm by the age of ten. The available data suggest that less than one third of males have actually experienced orgasm before puberty although two thirds report becoming sexually aroused prior to puberty (Kinsey et al., 1948). In contrast, less than one fifth of adult females recall orgasm and only one third report becoming sexually aroused prior to puberty (Kinsey et al., 1953).

The earliest childhood activities that bear any resemblance to sexual behavior are, of course, autosexual. Around age three or four, however, children begin to interact more frequently and intimately with other children, and their sexual explorations may extend to these relationships. Most of these interactions take the form of play, and it is in this context that sociosexual behaviors first occur. At least half of all adults recall engaging in some form of sociosexual play prior to adolescence. Around 40 percent of males and 30 percent of females report heterosexual play and 44 percent and 33 percent of males and females, respectively, recall homosexual play activities. In actuality, the percentage of both males and females who ever engage in preadolescent sex play is probably higher but many adults may intentionally or unintentionally fail to recall such experiences (Kinsey et al., 1948, 1953). In this chapter our primary concern is with heterosexual activities, and it is to this topic that we now turn.

Heterosexual Play and Heterosexual Players

Up to now our use of the term "sexual" in connection with the activities of preadolescents has been somewhat casual. Investigators, however, have yet to arrive at a consensus as to just what is meant by the term when it is applied to childhood behaviors (Broderick, 1966). Because of the nature of the available data concerning this topic, we will judge as heterosexual *the play activities of opposite-sex peers that involve deliberate genital-genital contacts, or genital exhibition, viewing, or stimulation.*

Heterosexual Play: Incidence, Frequency, and Techniques.   The most comprehensive investigations of preadolescent heterosexual play are those conducted by the Kinsey team in which adults were asked to retrospectively report on their childhood sexual experiences. Although Kinsey et al. (1948, 1953) suggested that the use of retrospective reports from adults might result in substantial underestimates of the incidence of preadolescent sex play, subsequent analyses of actual interviews with preadolescents (Elias & Gebhard, 1969) provide results that are remarkably similar to the adult reports. In Figure 9–1 the percentages of males and

Figure 9–1.

Accumulative (total) percentage of males and females reporting preadolescent heterosexual play experience relative to age.

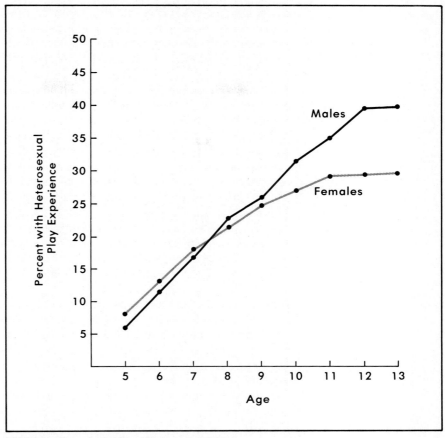

SOURCE: Data adapted from Kinsey et al., 1948.

females who report engaging in heterosexual play at various preadolescent ages are shown.

Before puberty, 40 percent of males and 30 percent of females are involved in some form of heterosexual play, although most do not have their first experience until they are seven to nine years old. Even following their initial experiences, very few children establish regular and consistent patterns of sex play. For over one third of males and two thirds of females, heterosexual play is confined to only a single year. Around 15 percent of both sexes engage in such play over a time span of two years. For many there is only a single experience prior to puberty. Others have multiple experiences which occur sporadically. A few individuals of each sex have their first experiences at an early age and continue heterosexual play on a regular basis for five or more years before reaching adolescence (Kinsey et al., 1948, 1953). The usual pattern for both males and females, however, is one of infrequent and irregular episodes spanning no more than one or two years of their preadolescent lives.

Most of these experiences occur in games such as "you show me yours and I'll show you mine," "doctor and patient," and "mama and daddy." The most prevalent form of heterosexual play involves nothing more than the exhibition of genitals. In some 20 percent of males and 40 percent of females, genital exhibition is all that is ever involved. Curiosity is probably the primary motivator for most mutual genital displays.

Genital manipulation is less common than exhibition, but nearly one third of boys and one fifth of girls manually touch and manipulate the genitals of their play partners. The touching may be motivated by curiosity concerning how penises and vulvas feel or, in some children, by specific desires to produce erotic pleasure. A substantial percentage of boys attempt to insert objects (usually their fingers) into the vaginas of their playmates but very few girls ever actually have their vaginas penetrated by boys prior to adolescence. In a small percentage of cases during the late preadolescent years, oral-genital contacts may occur. Many more boys than girls report attempts at coitus during their preadolescent years. In most cases the success of the effort is restricted by the small size of the penis. Male-female genital contact may occur but the depth of vaginal penetration is limited to such an extent that complete genital union rarely occurs. Incidence figures for various heterosexual play techniques are summarized in Table 9–1.

Heterosexual Players: Personal and Social Characteristics. Who are the children most likely to engage in preadolescent heterosexual play? It is clear that not all do, and among those with such experiences there are wide variations in the frequency and extensiveness of the activities involved. Little, in fact, is known concerning either the situational or psychosocial factors that promote or inhibit heterosexual play.

Among the higher primates there is a widespread tendency for both prepubertal males and females to engage in mutual genital stimulation as well as attempts at coitus:

Like human children, little male and female chimpanzees play sexual games involving erotic advances by either or both partners and including attempts to effect actual copulation. Several different copulatory positions are experimented with and partial intromission is sometimes achieved. Some young males practice manual and oral stimulation of the feminine genitalia and females may handle the erect penis of their immature partners. (Ford & Beach, 1951, p. 199)

Prepubertal sexual experimentation among primates is strongly influenced by observation of the sexual activities of others. For example, the sex play of young monkeys and chimpanzees usually resembles acts that they have observed in sexually mature adults (Ford & Beach, 1951). When deprived of such observational opportunities, male and female monkeys are totally inept sexually upon reaching adulthood (Harlow, 1975). Under natural rearing conditions, however, there are ample opportunities for the young to observe the sexual practices of adults as well as other prepubescents. No cultural restrictions are imposed, and sex play emerges in the normal course of growing up.

Similar forces seem to be involved when we consider heterosexual play among human children. Children reared in societies characterized by sexual restrictiveness and secrecy rarely engage in any form of prepubertal sex play. They are carefully "protected" from observing adult sexual interaction and rather severely punished

Table 9–1.

Percentage of preadolescent males and females experiencing various heterosexual play techniques.

Heterosexual Play Technique	Percentage Reporting Each Type of Experience	
	Males	Females
Genital exhibition	39.4	29.7
Manual genital stimulation	32.2	15.6
Vaginal insertions	19.4	1.0
Oral-genital stimulation	3.5	1.0
Attempts at coitus	21.9	5.1

SOURCE: Data adapted from Kinsey et al., 1948, 1953.

if detected in sex play. In contrast, sex play is fairly widespread in more permissive societies in which children are allowed to observe adult sexual activities or are provided with specific sexual training during childhood (Ford & Beach, 1951).

Our own society is characterized by moderately restrictive attitudes toward childhood sexual expression which tend to inhibit sex play among preadolescents. There are, of course, wide variations among cultural subgroups, families, and individuals even within Western societies, and such differences presumably influence the incidence of sex play. For example, childhood sexual expression is more frequently regarded as "natural" and expected by those from the higher than those from the lower social and educational strata. Perhaps as a consequence, preadolescent heterosexual play is most widespread among those from the higher socio-economic brackets who will ultimately attend college and graduate school (Kinsey et al., 1948, 1953).

In the United States the degree of sexual restrictiveness imposed on children varies both with sex and with age. The taboos against sexual expression are more severe for girls than for boys and, as Figure 9–1 indicates, fewer preadolescent girls than boys ever become involved in heterosexual play. Furthermore, the restrictions become more and more strict for girls but tend to relax for boys as they approach puberty. This results in distinctly different age patterns of involvement in heterosexual play, as shown in Figure 9–2. The percent of girls actively involved declines just prior to puberty while in boys it increases steadily up until puberty.

Significance of Heterosexual Play

Despite what appears to be a genuine liberalization of views regarding sexuality (Griffitt, 1977), Western attitudes toward childhood sexual expression are characterized by ambivalence and conflict. Many adults are now aware that some sort of sexual experimentation is relatively common among preadolescents and try to suppress their own overt manifestations of shock, dismay, anger, or embarrassment when they discover children involved in such activities. Yet, no matter how sexually "liberated" they may be, many adults are also plagued by nagging doubts concerning whether children are "ready" for or should engage in what appear to be miniature rehearsals of adult sexual behaviors. Our sexual heritage is one based on the views of several preceding generations that sexual activity is a prerogative and privilege reserved for adults. It is earned only by long years of abstinence and psychosocial and physical maturation. Viewed from this perspective, childhood sexuality assumes great significance in the eyes of adults. What are the effects of early sexual experience on adolescent and adult sexual patterns? What do such experiences "mean" to the child? Are preadolescents old enough to "handle" sex? Even though complete answers to these questions have yet to be formulated, let us examine what is known concerning the significance of heterosexual play.

Sex Education.   For many individuals the sex play of childhood provides the first, if not the only, preadolescent information about the genital anatomy of those of the opposite sex. Most children are provided few parentally sanctioned opportunities to closely examine or touch the genitals of others. Clandestine sexual play episodes often provide their first detailed educational experiences concerning sexuality (Elias & Gebhard, 1969).

Sex knowledge may, of course, be acquired in a number of ways. The current tendency is to urge parents to actively participate in, if not initiate, the sex education of their children. This is a troublesome prospect for most parents, who are uncertain as to both their knowledge about and attitudes toward sexuality. For many parents "sex education" consists of a collection of "thou shalts" and "thou shalt nots." Unemotional adult reactions to childhood sexual explorations or inquiries are rare. Usually children are not taught "this is a penis," "that is a vagina," and "that is sexual behavior," but told "don't touch that, it's dirty," "that's not nice," and "good boys and girls don't do that." In short, many parents are ill-equipped to deal unemotionally with the sexuality of their children. They frequently convey emotional but content-free "information" when responding to the sexually curious child. One result is that parents often teach the attitudinal and

Societies that are relatively permissive view sexual expression in young children as natural and acceptable.

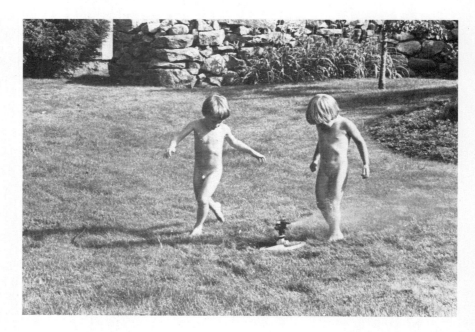

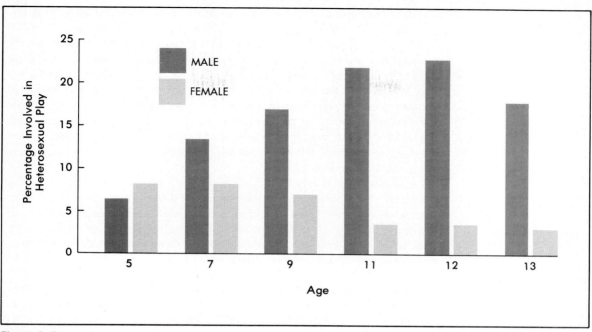

Figure 9–2.

Percentage of males and females who ever experience heterosexual play who actively engage in such play at various preadolescent ages.
SOURCE: Data from Kinsey et al., 1948.

emotional (and frequently negative) but not the intellectual content of sex knowledge (Gagnon & Simon, 1973).

Most children do, however, acquire at least a limited amount of information about sexuality prior to puberty. For example, almost all boys and girls have a minimal understanding of coitus by the time they are thirteen. As might be expected, more preadolescent girls than boys know that babies result from pregnancy. But very few of either sex have learned at these stages that pregnancy results from fertilization or the fusion of a sperm and an ovum. Many may associate coitus with the possibility of pregnancy, but detailed technical knowledge concerning how they are linked is relatively rare (Elias & Gebhard, 1969).

How is this limited, and in many cases inaccurate, information acquired? Until recently, at least, most boys and many girls obtained most of their sex knowledge from their peer group. This has been particularly true among those children reared in homes where the level of education is relatively low and parental communication concerning sexual matters rarely occurs (Elias & Gebhard, 1969).

An obvious difficulty involved in relying on peers for sex information is that the "teachers" are frequently as poorly informed as the students. Although parents are reluctant to speak frankly and openly with their children about the details of petting, coitus, pregnancy, and especially contraception, playmates and classmates are often eager to do so. Most children acquire a slang vocabulary for sexual anatomy and functions during the course of their peer interactions. Frequently, however, the words are learned independently of their specific sexual connotations. Thus, many children may count "prick," "prod," "dick," "peter," "fuck," "screw," "ball," "cocksucker," "pussy," "cunt," "twat," and other terms in their arsenal of words that impress other children and shock most adults. The casual use of such terms in peer interactions, though, does not necessarily imply that children know the sexual meaning of the words. They have learned from the emotional reactions of others to such words that these words are, indeed, important. Until the child learns the connection between them and certain of the forbidden sexual play activities that parents react to so emotionally, however, neither the activities nor the words are "eroticized" and imbedded into a specifically sexual script (Gagnon & Simon, 1973; Martinson, 1976).

Thus, from their parents many children learn first that many of their sex play activities are "bad" and then from their peers that these activities are "sexual." The dilemma of this form of "sex education" is that powerful emotions and inadequate knowledge become associated with sex and sexual behavior. It is when accurate labels and explanations are unemotionally provided that childhood play best serves as a medium for early sex education.

Sexual and Emotional Reactions.   Most adults and adolescents have fairly clear-cut ideas of what is sexual and when they are engaging in sexual behavior. Genitals are sexual, and the deliberate touching, fondling, manipulating, mouthing, or uniting of genitals is sexual behavior, as are those behaviors such as nongenital kissing and caressing that precede genital activities. The adult sexual experience is also one that is associated with salient physiological reactions and powerful emotions.

What about the sex play activities of children? Are they really sexual in the eyes of the children themselves? Do children experience genuine erotic arousal and satisfactions when they do what adults view as sexual? At least two competing viewpoints exist with regard to these questions. The psychoanalytic position postulates the existence of an instinctually based sexual (libidinal) energy that manifests itself from birth onwards (Freud, 1905). The specific modes of sexual expression and gratification are seen as sequentially changing and unfolding in various stages. The erotic sensations and activities of infancy are largely autosexual. During the first year of life sexual pleasure is *oral* in nature, and the mouth is the primary erogenous (erotically pleasurable) zone. During the second year of life autosexual interests continue to predominate, but the erotic focus becomes *anal* and important gratifications are associated with fecal elimination.

It is during the *phallic* stage, between the ages of two and five, that the erotic interests of children first become sociosexual. The penis and clitoris emerge as the primary erotic structures, and children become aware of the opposite-sex parent as a potential sex object. Because of sexual attraction to the opposite-sex parent, phallic-stage children enter a period—the so-called Oedipal period—of sexual competition with the same-sex parent. Because of the futility and potentially negative consequences of such competition, the children abandon their sexual desire for the opposite-sex parent as well as their newly emergent heterosexual orientation. This is followed by a period of *latency*, or asexuality, in which sexual urges are placed on the back burner until reawakened by the biological changes

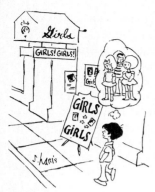

What adults consider to have a sexual meaning may have no such significance for children.
SOURCE: Sydney Harris.

associated with puberty. The *genital* stage begins at puberty, when the theoretically "normal" course of psychosexual development results in the reemergence of heterosexual interests.

Thus, psychoanalytic theory assumes the existence of very real erotic responses and sexual experiences from birth onward. These are progressively channeled through *autosexual, heterosexual, asexual,* and, once again, *heterosexual* phases (Freud, 1905). The implication is, of course, that the sex play experiences of even young children are truly sexual as the meaning of sexual is understood by adults. Modes of expression may vary, but sex is sex whether it occurs during preadolescence, adolescence, or adulthood.

A contrasting view (Gagnon, 1977; Gagnon & Simon, 1973; Martinson, 1976) argues that what is sexual for an individual is determined not by instinctual urges or templates but by culturally supplied meanings or scripts:

Most people assume that children give the same or similar meanings to activities that adults interpret as sexual. Nearly all theories of psycho-sexual development ignore the fundamental problem of how the organism learns to label, experience, and desire what it is doing as sexual. . . . Imputing an adult version of a sexual experience to a child is an error. It is equally an error to assume that the meanings given to the activity early in life have any simple or direct connection with what the activity will mean in the future. . . . The meanings are not fixed; if they were, we would feel like children all our lives. (Gagnon, 1977, p. 81)

This increasingly popular conception implies that sex play will be sexual in the eyes of children only when such meaning is supplied by parents, peers, or others of significance. Since most adults find it difficult to define young children as sexual, such meanings are withheld until late preadolescence or longer. Thus, for the majority of children sex play is more play than sex until puberty. A major social redefinition of both males and females begins at puberty and sex play becomes eroticized, elaborated, and fully sexual during adolescence (Gagnon & Simon, 1973).

Ideally, such contrasting viewpoints could be resolved by reference to relevant empirical data. For a number of reasons, however, data that zero in on this issue are not currently available nor will they be in the near future. No methodologies exist by which the "meanings" of activities to preverbal children may be assessed. With older children, ethical considerations make specific investigations problematic. If, in fact, adult inputs are responsible for creating sexuality, investigative techniques may well shape preadolescent sexual activities in molds that are unacceptable to the current social order. For example, interviewing children about their understanding of coitus *may* have the effect of inducing them to engage in this form of behavior—an outcome that many parents would view as unacceptable.

Given these difficulties, retrospective reports from adults, though perhaps distorted by redefinitions of or failures to recall childhood sex play experiences, are our primary source of information. We have already noted that at least some adults recall experiencing what they consider to be sexual arousal prior to puberty. Among the Kinsey (1948, 1953) informants, 12 percent of the females reported becoming erotically aroused during the course of their heterosexual play experiences. Preadolescent heterosexual arousal was reported to be "much more common" in boys than in girls, although no specific percentage figures were reported. Thus, for at least some boys and girls, heterosexual play is of sexual significance, but mostly during the late preadolescent years.

As puberty nears, some children do become involved in extensive sex play activities. These may be relatively continuous and may carry over into and provide an early foundation for adolescent petting and coitus. This is more frequent among boys than girls, but for many of each sex there are clear breaks between the sex play of childhood and the petting of adolescence (Kinsey et al., 1948, 1953). There is no evidence that childhood sex play exerts any notable influence on later patterns of sexuality. Those with sex play experience are no more sexually "driven" or active than those without such experience.

HETEROSEXUAL PETTING

For most individuals, sexual activities prior to puberty are truly playful in character and sporadic in occurrence. Few children develop patterns of behavior in which sexual play is actively and regularly pursued. In short, preadolescent sex is not really "serious business" for many children. Even those who experience erotic arousal and orgasm at early ages rarely become seriously committed to seeking sexual expression. In this way sexual behaviors differ little from many other activities which, from time to time, occupy the interests of young children. Indeed, sometimes to the distress of parents and teachers, few children prior to the ages of ten or eleven seem capable of enduring involvement in any endeavor. The six- or seven-year-old who plays baseball all day on Tuesday may abandon the game on Wednesday to play with dolls. Learning to read, tell time, or play the piano may be fun for a few minutes but soon become tedious.

Even though mildly frustrating at times, the apparent fickleness of interest among children is not too disturbing to most adults. After all, they are children rather than "real people," and what they do need not be taken too seriously. As Gagnon (1977) suggests, it is as if there is a "childhood exemption" in which what children do or fail to do is protected by the status of childhood. By social definition, children are irresponsible and innocent and thus not accountable for their activities. As part of this exemption, sex play activities are not viewed as evidence of any "real" sexual potential.

All of this begins to change, however, around the age of eleven or twelve, when most children are approaching and some are experiencing the biological changes associated with puberty. The visible changes of puberty such as the appearance of underarm hair, a "growth spurt," and, in girls, breast development provide signals to parents as well as the larger society that the asexuality of childhood is rapidly fading and will soon be replaced by reproductive capacity and a true sexual potential. For the first time, the individual is viewed, defined, and reacted to as a "real" sexual being.

This newly acquired status marks the end of the young person's social existence as a child and the beginning of the transitional period of adolescence. He or she is now expected to "mature" sexually, intellectually, socially, and emotionally until the status of adulthood is achieved. The "childhood exemption" is lost forever and adolescents are expected to develop lasting and serious commitments to interests and activities that foster the childhood-adulthood transition. Sexual activities are no longer viewed as playful, but rather as serious business. Young people are expected to evidence a serious but gradually developing commitment to heterosexuality. This can be a confusing and frustrating time for adolescents. They are expected or at least permitted to become sexually active but only in a limited way. Although most adolescents are aware of coitus by age thirteen (Elias & Gebhard, 1969), the act does not become fully socially legitimized for them until they marry. On the average this will be from four to twelve years later, depending on social class, religion, educational attainments, and other factors (Kinsey et al., 1953).

That many adults (particularly parents) regard coitus as undesirable prior to marriage is clearly understood by most adolescents. Indeed, most girls and some boys are told that they shouldn't "do it" or "go all the way" until they are married. Less clearly communicated, however, is just what form of sexual activity is permissible for young people. The many sexual behaviors that are permissible are generally learned through experience or from peers, and most parents have little, if any, knowledge of the details of the sexual experiences of their children.

As a result of these exploratory experiences and information exchanges, the compromise between complete heterosexual abstinence and coitus reached by most adolescents takes the form of heterosexual petting. *Heterosexual petting is any heterosexual physical contact that involves deliberate attempts to produce erotic arousal but does not involve coitus* (Kinsey et al., 1948, 1953). The key element of this definition is the phrase "deliberate attempts to produce erotic arousal." It is the level of commitment to erotic gratification involved that distinguishes petting from sex play. For most preadolescents the commitment is more often to the play rather than to the sexual aspects of behaviors. The behaviors then

With adolescence comes an increased interest in establishing mature, satisfying heterosexual relationships.

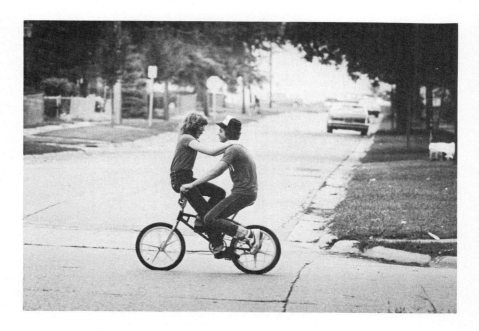

become eroticized during adolescence as a result of the individual's emerging definition of himself or herself as a sexual being.

Heterosexual Petting and Heterosexual Petters

In a society such as ours, which values heterosexuality but condemns coitus prior to marriage, the adolescent with newly emerging sexual interests and expectations is in a position of conflict. Socially created and reinforced desires to be heterosexual and do heterosexual things stand in opposition to societal insistence that coitus be postponed until marriage. For many, heterosexual petting provides a partial and sometimes temporary compromise solution to this dilemma. Petting allows people opportunities to engage in all of the highly stimulating and gratifying physical contacts that precede or are associated with coitus without violating what appears to be the most important norm—that coitus should be confined to marriage. Petting encompasses a wide array of sexual activities, some of which we shall consider in detail after first examining the incidence and frequency of heterosexual petting and the characteristics of people who engage in it.

Heterosexual Petting: Incidence and Frequency.   It has long been recognized that some sort of petting activity is an integral part of the adolescent sexual experience. Referred to by various generations as "spooning," "mooning," "sparking," "smooching," or other terms that now seem archaic, what we refer to here as petting has been recognized as a common if not totally acceptable element in the courtship behaviors of American youth. Prior to the appearance of the Kinsey Reports in 1948 and 1953, the prevalence of premarital coitus was not widely recognized. Considerable attention was devoted to petting activities, which, along with masturbation, were viewed as issues of major moral and social significance. With the appearance of the Kinsey revelations that rather substantial proportions of both males and females actually engage in coitus prior to marriage, public and scientific attention was diverted from petting to premarital coitus. Since then a seemingly endless list of investigations designed to keep track of the percentage of males and females with premarital coital experience has developed and continues to do so. We discuss some of these studies in Chapter 10.

One of the unfortunate side effects of this preoccupation with premarital coitus has been that petting, which continues to be a substantial and significant element in the sexual lives of adolescents, has been somewhat neglected in research since the Kinsey projects. Data from the Kinsey investigations in some ways still offer the most comprehensive view of the petting practices of American males and females. That petting is a widespread form of sexual expression is evident from Figure 9–3, which shows the accumulative incidence of petting at various age levels for males and females.

These data, based on interviews with married and unmarried individuals during the 1940s and early 1950s, reveal that by the time they reach the age of thirty, about 90 percent of both males and females will have had at least one premarital petting experience with or without orgasm. For the average male the first petting experience occurs between the ages of fourteen and fifteen, while the average female has her first experience between her fifteenth and sixteenth birthdays. At all

Figure 9–3.

Accumulated (total) percentage of males and females with premarital petting and petting to orgasm experience relative to age.

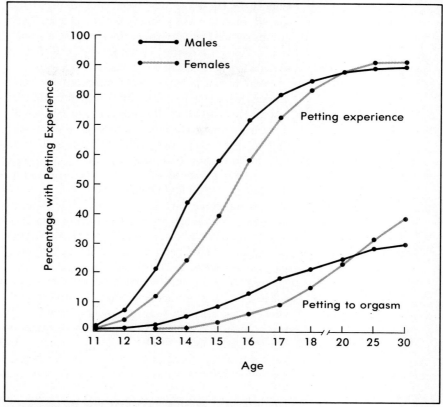

SOURCE: Data from Kinsey et al., 1948.

age levels until age twenty the percentage of males with petting experience exceeds that of females.

Recent findings suggest that both males and females are beginning to pet at earlier ages. For example, a large study involving nearly two thousand boys and girls in junior and senior high schools revealed that half of both sexes reported engaging in "prolonged hugging and kissing" between the ages of thirteen and fourteen (Vener & Stewart, 1974). Similar drops in median age at first petting experience among American adolescents are reported by Kantner and Zelnik (1972), Sorenson (1973), and Wagner, Fujita, and Pion (1973).

American youth are beginning to pet at earlier ages and other data make it clear that higher percentages of contemporary males and females are ultimately involved in petting than ever before (DeLamater & MacCorquodale, 1979). A similar trend was evident even in the Kinsey studies in which steady increases in petting incidence from the oldest to youngest generations were reported for both males and females (Kinsey et al., 1948, 1953). Recent studies of premarital petting practices suggest that by the age of twenty-one, between 95 and 100 percent of both males and females have engaged in some sort of petting (Istvan & Griffitt, 1980;

Hunt, 1974; Luckey & Nass, 1969). Most of these studies, however, rely on college student or otherwise sexually liberal samples. Even in the Kinsey studies these groups showed higher incidences of petting than did those with lower educational levels. Thus, it is unclear whether the incidence of petting has increased at all societal levels or just at those studied.

More unmarried males and females are involved in petting between the ages of sixteen and twenty-five than during any other age period. It is during this peak time that nearly one half of all males and one third of all females who will ever pet to orgasm are doing so at median rates of seven to fifteen times per year for males and four to seven times per year for females. The average male who is petting to orgasm during this time receives about 10 percent of his total orgasms from this source. Petting leads to 18 percent of the orgasms for active female petters between the ages of sixteen and twenty-five.

It is apparent from Figure 9–3 that only about one third of those with petting experience ever reach orgasm as a result of petting. While there are data suggesting that this percentage has increased substantially (Hunt, 1974), it is clear that much petting never culminates in orgasm. Among unmarried males and females between the ages of sixteen and thirty only the roughest of estimates are available concerning frequency of petting which does not lead to orgasm. These estimates, however, suggest that the average unmarried person is involved in nonorgasmic petting between two and five times per month. There are, of course, wide variations with some males and females petting without orgasm every day or night and others doing so only once or twice a year (Kinsey et al., 1948, 1953). The significance of petting is in the opportunities it provides for heterosexual education and experimentation, rather than in its role as an orgasmic outlet.

Heterosexual Petters: Personal and Social Characteristics.   The near universality of some sort of premarital heterosexual petting experience in the lives of American (see Figure 9–3), Canadian (Hobart, 1972; Herold, 1984), and European (Luckey & Nass, 1969; Schmidt & Sigusch, 1971) males and females should not obscure the existence of wide variations among particular individuals and groups of individuals in the incidence, frequency, and extent of petting practices. There are some people of each sex who never engage in any form of petting prior to marriage, others who may have only a single experience with a future marital partner, and still others who begin petting at early ages and ultimately pet extensively with a hundred or more partners. Are there identifiable personal and social characteristics which might act to promote or inhibit petting behavior and thus be associated with such wide variations? Let us now turn to what is presently known concerning correlates of individual differences in petting.

Despite the obvious fact that every heterosexual petting episode requires the involvement of at least one male and one female, there are some differences between the sexes in the details of their petting experiences. As evident in Figure 9–3, among the generations of people studied by Kinsey et al. (1948, 1953), there was a clear tendency for males to begin petting at younger ages than did females. The youngest of these people are now in their forties and fifties, and in younger generations there is evidence suggesting that some of these age-related sex differences are beginning to disappear. More recent data (Vener & Stewart, 1974) indicate that for both males and females the median age for first "prolonged hugging and kissing" is between thirteen and fourteen years, and the average girl actually experiences her first "lower level" heterosexual contacts such as holding hands and simple kissing at a younger age than does the average boy.

Males, however, do become involved in the more intimate forms of petting such as breast and genital contact at earlier ages than do females. By the age of fourteen more than half of all boys but only 40 percent of all girls studied by Vener and Stewart (1974) had engaged in "above the waist feeling." Over 40 percent of boys but less than 30 percent of girls had petted "below the waist." These differences between the sexes do not begin to fade until the late teens and early twenties. But, even at these ages, slightly more males than females have engaged in the more intimate forms of contact such as nude breast petting, nude female genital petting, mutual petting of nude genitals, petting with both partners nude, fellatio, cunnilingus, and mutual oral-genital contacts (Griffitt, 1975; Istvan & Griffitt, 1980; Luckey & Nass, 1969). In short, while as many females as males ultimately have some sort of petting experience, young males are more likely than young females to participate in the "advanced" techniques mentioned above. Similar sex differences have been observed in virtually all countries studied in recent years including Canada (Hobart, 1972; Herold, 1984), England, Norway, Germany (Luckey & Nass, 1969), Japan (Asayama, 1975, 1976), and China (Edwards, 1976).

Male premarital petting experiences are not only more extensive in terms of techniques but also in terms of number of partners (Hunt, 1974; Zuckerman, Tuschup, & Finner, 1976). In the Kinsey (1953) sample of married women who had petting experience prior to marriage, 10 percent of them had petted with only one person—usually their future marital partner. Nearly one third had petted with two to five males and one fourth had between six and ten petting partners prior to marriage. A small proportion (5 percent) had been involved in petting with fifty or more males. While the average number of partners for all married women was around eight, the numbers varied considerably depending on the age at which the women married. Those who married between the ages of sixteen and twenty averaged fewer than seven petting partners, but those who did not marry until between the ages of twenty-six and thirty had petted with an average of more than 9 men. For the majority (65 percent), petting was first begun in high school and involved between 4 and 5 males. Those who went on to college had an additional 5 to 6 partners before marrying.

Kinsey et al. (1948) reported no specific figures concerning the number of petting partners for males but clearly implied that the average numbers exceeded those for females. More recent data are consistent with this view. For example, married males over 35 studied by Hunt (1974) reported a median of 15 petting partners prior to marriage. These men were just entering adolescence at the completion of the Kinsey (1948) project and the data suggest that males at that time had substantially more petting partners than did females. Curiously, Hunt (1974) found that contemporary young people report fewer petting partners than did the previous generation. Females continue to report fewer (an average of 3) than males (an average of 12) but both sexes show decreases from those of the Kinsey generations.

It has been suggested that heterosexual partnerships in which petting is the highest or terminal degree of sexual intimacy achieved are both fewer in number and shorter in duration than formerly (Luckey & Nass, 1969). That is, rather than accepting petting as a long-term compromise activity that is more intimate than abstinence or simple kissing but less intimate and more morally acceptable than coitus, contemporary young people of both sexes are "moving on" to regular patterns of coitus at younger ages than previously (Hunt, 1974).

Overall, then, the available data suggest that males begin petting earlier, engage in "advanced" petting techniques earlier, and have more petting partners than do females. The origins of these differences appear to be found in those psychosocial processes that instill in males and females differing attitudes and meanings associated with sexual activities (Staples, 1973). The general tendency within our culture to oppose premarital sexual involvement has been unevenly applied. At least limited sexual experimentation is tolerated or even tacitly encouraged for males but strongly discouraged for females. At relatively early ages, adolescent boys learn that among the central elements of what is socially defined as "manliness" or "masculinity" are sexual experience and sophistication. Encouraged and reinforced by same-sex peer approval and popularized media images of the masculine male, boys learn to value extensive sexual experience positively. By the same token, however, many also learn to place little, if any, value on the establishment and maintenance of emotional ties with their sexual partners.

In contrast, the socially created and reinforced model of "femininity" emphasizes the values of affection, romance, and love as prerequisites to sexual involvement. Adolescent girls first learn a commitment to romantic love relationships in which sexual intimacy becomes partially legitimized. "Good girls" are those who limit their sexual experimentation and involvement to males to whom they are emotionally tied. "Bad girls" are those for whom emotional bonds are not necessary for sexual intimacy. For the majority of young females, however, extensive sexual involvement (advanced petting and coitus) is positively valued only in strongly bonded relationships.

With such differing orientations toward sexual activities more or less firmly established during adolescence, it is not surprising that virtually all surveys of sexual standards and attitudes show males to be more positive toward and accepting of premarital petting activities than females (e.g., Bauman & Wilson, 1976; Eysenck, 1974; Hunt, 1974). On the other hand, there is substantial evidence that female attitudes and standards of acceptance regarding premarital petting are becoming more liberal (Bauman & Wilson, 1976; Croake & James, 1973). As a consequence, male and female patterns of premarital petting are beginning to converge (Curran, 1977). That is, at least college-age females are approaching and in some instances equaling or surpassing males in terms of experience with a variety of petting behaviors.

There is, then, little doubt that males and females as groups are becoming increasingly similar in terms of their petting practices. This does not mean, however, that the experiences of all males and females are identical. The "average" male and "average" female are, of course, mythical creatures. Within the sexes there are substantial variations among people and groups of people in the details of their petting histories. As we noted previously, there are those of both sexes who pet frequently and extensively with a large number of partners and others whose petting activities are infrequent and limited in both scope and number of partners.

A major influence on both sexual attitudes and practices is religion. A number of studies (Reiss, 1967; Zuckerman et al., 1976) have shown that those people who are deeply religious and attend religious services regularly are less permissive in their attitudes toward premarital petting than are the less devout. Furthermore, the most devout are those who are least likely to engage in intimate forms of sexual contact (Curran, Neff, & Lippold, 1973; Kinsey et al., 1953; Spanier, 1977). Generally, however, the inhibiting effect of religion on petting is stronger for females than for males (Kinsey et al., 1953; Reiss, 1967) and for white than for black Americans (Reiss, 1967).

To some extent, degree of religious devoutness is an indicator of an individual's style of life. The least religious generally maintain more liberal and nontraditional views, while the most religious are more traditional and conservative in their social and political outlooks. Several studies have investigated the relationships between liberalism-conservatism and sexual attitudes and practices. Generally, it has been found that conservatives tend to be less permissive and to engage in less premarital petting than do liberals (Curran et al., 1973; D'Augelli & Cross, 1975; Eysenck, 1976). For example, Joe and Kostyla (1975) administered a scale of conservatism and Zuckerman's (1973) sex experience scales to male and female college students. Overall, conservatives reported less premarital sex experience than did liberals. More specifically, liberal males and females were more likely than conservatives to have engaged in the petting techniques listed in Table 9–2.

These and other findings suggest that it is those who are generally most reserved and traditional in their life-style who are least likely to engage in extensive premarital petting. Taken together, the results of a number of studies that are summarized in Table 9–3 support this view. It may be seen that those personal and social characteristics that reflect adherence to rather conventional values and codes of conduct are associated with low levels of petting. More unconventional and somewhat "rebellious" values and actions promote, or at least are associated with, extensive petting experience.

Several studies indicate that premarital petting attitudes and practices are associated with individual differences in personality. The characteristics of those with low and high petting experience listed in Table 9–3 suggest that those with

Table 9–2.

Premarital petting experiences more common among liberals than conservatives.
A comparison of the premarital petting experiences of social and political liberals with those of conservatives indicates that liberal males and females are more likely than conservatives to experience each of the listed petting acts prior to marriage.

Males	Females
Feeling covered breasts of female	Covered breast felt by male
Feeling nude breasts of female	Nude breast felt by male
Lying prone on female without penetration	Male prone on female without penetration
Mouth contact with breast of female	Mouth contact with breast by male
Penis manipulated by female	Vagina manipulated by male
Manual manipulation of vagina	
Mouth contact with vagina	

SOURCE: Adapted from Joe & Kostyla, 1975.

extensive petting experience tend to be people who rather actively seek stimulating experiences in a variety of ways. That is, the fact that they engage in exciting, daring, and perhaps delinquent acts, consume alcohol and drugs, approve the use of pornography as an erotic stimulant, and so forth implies a desire for new and varied experiences. From this perspective, engaging in frequent and varied petting with a number of partners may be viewed as one expression of a general need for physical and social stimulation.

Eysenck (1976) has described the *extravert* as a person who, because of rather low characteristic levels of cortical and physiological arousal, tends to seek out a variety of stimulating social and physical experiences. In contrast, the *introvert* is viewed as a person whose physiological arousal level is chronically high and who tends to withdraw from or avoid situations which may lead to excess stimulation from external sources. Extraverts are more likely than introverts to have permissive attitudes toward premarital petting, to be highly excited and stimulated by sexual activities, to derive physical satisfaction from sex, to pet to orgasm, to engage in lengthy petting, to engage in intimate petting such as fellatio and cunnilingus, and to pet with a large number of partners (Eysenck, 1974, 1976; Giese & Schmidt, 1968).

Similar findings were obtained in another study (Zuckerman et al., 1976), using a variety of personality instruments with male and female college students as subjects. Among the tests were measures tapping several components of a general need for variety in sensory and emotional experiences. It was found that those people most prone to seeking thrills and adventures through sports, entertainment, and other activities were also those who were permissive in their petting attitudes. In addition, they were the most frequently orgasmic in their petting activities, had the largest number of petting partners, and had experienced the greatest variety in their petting behavior. Other findings revealed that, for males, strong *hedonistic needs* (for change, exhibitionism, impulsivity, play) were associated with high petting experience. For females, strong and extraverted *social needs* (for dominance, affiliation, social recognition) were predictive of extensive petting experience.

Table 9–3.

Characteristics of people with limited and extensive petting experience.
The results of several studies suggest that traditional life-styles are associated with low levels of petting, and nontraditional life-styles with high levels of petting.

Limited Petting Experience	Extensive Petting Experience
Positive attitudes toward religion, police, school, teachers	Negative attitudes toward religion, police, school, teachers
No use of alcohol and drugs	Use of alcohol and drugs
No cigarette smoking	Cigarette smoking
Nondelinquency	Delinquency
Friends who do not smoke	Friends who smoke
Opposition to pornography	Approval of pornography
Opposition to nudity in the home	Approval of nudity in the home
Conservative political attitudes	Liberal political attitudes

SOURCE: Summarized from Curran et al., 1973; D'Augelli & Cross, 1975; Eysenck, 1976; Vener & Stewart, 1974; Zuckerman et al., 1976.

Nature and Significance of Heterosexual Petting

As our earlier definition suggests, heterosexual petting is a goal-directed activity. While a number of additional motives may exist, most petting occurs because of its potential for producing erotic arousal. Our previous discussions (particularly Chapters 4 and 8) have indicated that sexual arousal may be produced by a variety of stimuli and chaneled through all sensory modalities. In petting, however, it is the tactile (touch) stimulation of various parts of the body which is the most salient mode of erotic stimulation.

The Petting Sequence.   Sometime between the ages of thirteen and sixteen, most American males and females begin the pattern of heterosocial and heterosexual interaction known as dating. For the first time they are thrust into situations in which they are alone with a person of the opposite sex and which are defined by parents, peers, and the larger society as potentially sexual. Early dating experiences frequently involve little, if any, sexual activity. The dances, parties, and other social activities of the young are often chaperoned and monitored by parents or teachers and transportation to and from them is provided by adults. As a result, there are few opportunities for couple privacy until dating practices become more independent.

The sexual potential of such relationships begins to be realized, however, as the dating activities of young people become more and more independent of parental control and supervision. Even though most adolescents are not specifically trained concerning "what to do," they are vaguely aware that some sexual experimentation is now permissible and, to some extent, expected. In most modern societies males are expected to and do take the lead in initiating sexual experimentation. More so than for females, the dating "scripts" (Gagnon & Simon, 1973) of males are dominated by sexual themes and to be masculine is to be sexually knowledgeable and aggressive. In contrast, females are socialized to view dating relationships more in terms of their potential for the development of affection and attachment. The initiation of or even active participation in sexual expression by young females is frequently viewed by both sexes as unseemly or indicative of moral defect.

Most young males are, however, ill-prepared for their "leading role" in sexual expression (Masters & Johnson, 1979). Neither they nor females are biologically equipped with "natural tendencies" to engage in specific sexual acts. Furthermore, specific sexual instruction is rarely provided by reliable and knowledgeable sources. The information that is acquired usually originates with equally uninformed peers or incomplete and perhaps misleading media representations. Thus, when it comes to learning what to do sexually both sexes are, for the most part, on their own.

In spite of all of this, however, there is a surprising degree of commonality both within and between the sexes in the order in which particular petting practices emerge. The most frequent petting pattern in both sexes is one that begins with very general body contacts such as holding hands and hugging. This is followed by kissing—at first light and then deeper—the male touching the female breasts and then her genitals, the male orally stimulating the female breasts, the female touching the male genitals, the pair rubbing their genitals together without penile-vaginal penetration, and finally, perhaps, oral contact with the genitals.

Though neither this nor any other sequence can be said to apply to all individuals, the findings of a number of studies in which the premarital petting practices of males and females up to the age of twenty-one have been examined reveal a fairly common developmental pattern for both sexes. These findings are summarized in Table 9–4, which shows the usual order in which American male and female college students experience specific petting practices.

Variations in these general patterns, of course, occur in many ways. Those with permissive sexual attitudes, a nontraditional life-style, a liberal orientation, and an extraverted nature are more likely to experience the full range of petting practices listed in Table 9–4 than are the nonpermissive, traditional, conservative, and introverted. Some may participate in all of these acts but in a different order than indicated. In many cases, for example, oral-genital contacts may not occur until after intercourse has been experienced. Furthermore, the intimacy of the petting acts performed often depends on the nature of the relationship between petting partners. The more intimate techniques (those with higher numbers) are often limited to relationships defined as affectionate or loving. A number of other factors including age and number of previous sexual partners are important determinants of petting practices.

Clearly, as people accumulate petting experience by progressing through the sequences shown in Table 9–4, the degree of sexual intimacy and involvement in the acts steadily increases. Similarly, the erotic potential of the acts steadily grows with increasing experience; the more intimate and "advanced" techniques such as mutual oral-genital contacts are more sexually stimulating than "elementary" techniques such as simple kissing. This is because the more intimate techniques involve direct and concentrated stimulation of the most sensitive erogenous zones of the body. Still, in any given petting episode the most intimate acts are almost always accompanied or preceded by each of the less intimate but, nevertheless, erotically arousing stimulation techniques.

That it is possible to plot what appear to be rather orderly progressions of petting experiences for both sexes does not mean that the actual transitions from one experience to the next and on through the sequence are smooth and trouble-free. In fact, the very act of entering the petting sequence is a difficult task for many people. The first petting efforts are often hesitant, clumsy, embarrassing, and even guilt producing for both participants. Consider, for example, the ageless and multifaceted dilemma of the "first kiss," which can be a terrifying experience for both males and females. In his sometimes unwelcome leading role the young male is expected to assume the initiative. In doing so he faces a number of troublesome questions. They include but are not limited to the following: "Is kissing right or wrong?" "Will she let me kiss her?" "What is the 'correct' way to kiss?" "Will she enjoy it?" "Will I enjoy it?" "What next?"

It is only when these and other similar questions are at least partially answered that the male will summon sufficient "nerve" to attempt the kiss. Females are, of course, faced with a similar dilemma but the specific questions are somewhat different. In her socially prescribed role as "gatekeeper" (Gagnon, 1977), the female is expected to set limits on "how far to go," and the limits are in part determined by her answers to questions such as "Is kissing right or wrong?" "Will he try to kiss me?" "Should I let him kiss me?" "What is the correct way to kiss?"

Table 9–4.

Studies of the premarital petting experiences of college males and females up to the approximate age of 21 reveal a great deal of commonality in the order in which both sexes experience particular petting acts.

College Males		College Females	
Petting Acts, in Order of Experience	Percentage with Experience by Age 21[1]	Petting Acts, in Order of Experience	Percentage with Experience by Age 21[1]
1. Light embracing and hugging	99	1. Light embracing and hugging	98
2. "Simple kissing"	97	2. "Simple kissing"	97
3. "Deep kissing" (tongue contact)	93	3. "Deep kissing" (tongue contact)	93
4. Prone embrace (clothed)	90	4. Prone embrace (clothed)	83
5. Manual contact with clothed female breasts	88	5. Male manual contact with clothed breasts	78
6. Manual contact with nude female breasts	81	6. Genital apposition (clothed)	77
7. Manual contact with clothed female genitals	78	7. Male manual contact with nude breasts	70
8. Genital apposition (clothed)	77	8. Male manual contact with clothed female genitals	64
9. Oral contact with female breasts	73	9. Male oral contact with breasts	63
10. Manual contact with nude female genitals	72	10. Male manual contact with nude female genitals	60
11. Female manual contact with clothed male genitals	65	11. Female manual contact with clothed male genitals	54
12. Female manual contact with nude male genitals	63	12. Female manual contact with nude male genitals	52
13. Female oral contact with male genitals	46	13. Male oral contact with female genitals	40
14. Oral contact with female genitals	43	14. Female oral contact with male genitals	36
15. Female oral contact with male genitals (male orgasm)	27	15. Mutual oral-genital contact with male	24
16. Mutual oral-genital contact with female	25	16. Female oral contact with male genitals (male orgasm)	21
17. Mutual oral-genital contact with female (mutual orgasm)	14	17. Mutual oral-genital contact with male (mutual orgasm)	10

[1]These percentage figures were obtained by averaging the findings of the studies on which this table is based.

SOURCE: Findings compiled and summarized from Bentler, 1968a, b; Curran, 1977; Curran et al., 1973; Griffitt, 1975; Istvan & Griffitt, 1980; Hunt, 1974; Kinsey et al., 1948, 1953; Luckey & Nass, 1969; Zuckerman, 1973.

"Will he enjoy it?" "Will I enjoy it?" "What will he do next and should I let him?" As with males, the list of questions confronting females could be expanded substantially, but it is only when at least some satisfactory answers are forthcoming that female participation in the venture will occur. Similar questions, of course, arise for each of the activities involved in the petting sequence.

What we have described for both sexes is what is known as an *approach-avoidance conflict* where the desire to engage in kissing is in conflict with pressures not to kiss. The erotic and emotional satisfaction anticipated—the approach forces—create the desire to kiss. The opposing pressures, real or imagined—the avoidance forces—are those stemming from acquired moral sanctions against sexual experimentation, from fears concerning possible rejection, from fears that one's technique will be clumsy or ineffective, and from a number of additional sources. The vast majority of people, of course, ultimately resolve the conflict in favor of kissing and perhaps experience some degree of guilt and embarrassment along with the erotic pleasures associated with the act. If, however, the positive aspects of the experience outweigh the negative, kissing will continue, with both people becoming more and more adept until relatively high levels of sexual arousal result from increasingly passionate kissing.

This pattern of conflict intervenes between each and every sequential petting act. Generally, the intensity of conflict increases as the intimacy of the acts increases. The lower percentages of people experiencing the more intimate acts (those with higher numbers) suggest that the avoidance forces strengthen at a faster pace than do the approach forces for many people. Thus, relatively few college males and females under age twenty-one (14 and 10 percent, respectively) report experience in the most intimate petting act listed in Table 9–4, mutual oral-genital contact with orgasm for both sexes.

What has been described here is the most usual pattern of petting experience for a hypothetical couple. Most people, of course, have more than one petting partner and each new relationship progresses through similar stages. With increasing experience, however, people find that the importance of the specific questions they must deal with changes. Those concerning morality and technique become less troublesome while those involving negotiation of the interpersonal aspects of the situation acquire renewed importance with each new relationship. They must essentially start over with each new partner and ask the same questions about the relationship: "Will she let me?" "Will he try?" "Should I let him?" Those who have a substantial amount of previous experience with other partners progress through the various steps of the petting sequence at a faster and perhaps smoother pace than do a pair of novices.

Consequences of Petting. The most immediate outcome of petting is at least some degree of *sexual arousal*. The degree of arousal reached depends on many factors, including the duration of time and the intimacy of the techniques involved. Nearly all of the males and females interviewed in the Kinsey (1948, 1953) projects indicated that their petting experiences had resulted in erotic arousal although less than half reported reaching orgasm through petting and then only infrequently. Given the trend toward greater permissiveness regarding some of the more intimate petting techniques (Croake & James, 1973), it is not surprising that orgasm resulting from petting is becoming more and more common. At least one study (Hunt, 1974) suggests that over half of unmarried females and two thirds of unmarried males experience orgasm in at least some of their petting. Regardless of whether orgasm is achieved or not, it is clear that most young men and women regard petting as a pleasurable and sexually satisfying experience and look forward to it (Sigusch & Schmidt, 1973).

While petting can be and is a pleasurable and erotic experience for both sexes, it is often accompanied by mild to severe *feelings of guilt* for some. By the time we reach early adolescence, most of us have internalized some rather vague moral proscriptions against premarital sexual experimentation. When we violate or anticipate violating these proscriptions, the result is some degree of guilt.

The many approach pressures or incentives for petting, however, are sufficiently powerful for most people to overcome their inhibitions and enter the petting sequence. The erotic and interpersonal rewards associated with the earliest, least intimate, and least taboo acts eventually overshadow or neutralize guilt feelings. We are then motivated to "move on" to more intimate (and more taboo) techniques which are once again inhibited by guilt (as well as the other factors discussed previously). How far one progresses through the sequence depends, of course, on the relative strengths of the inhibitory guilt feelings and the actual or imagined rewards of petting, as well as other factors (Mosher & Cross, 1971).

Perhaps the most significant consequence of petting is the education or training it provides in the management of the complexities of sexual expression in an interpersonal context. Regardless of what they have read, fantasized, or been told, both sexes gain their first real understanding of a heterosexual experience in petting. Most males bring with them to this context an established history of sexual response and expression through masturbation. Often their masturbation has been accompanied by fantasies concerning what heterosexual relationships might be like and what their own roles in such interactions should be. They anticipate sexual gratification from petting and expect to take an active, perhaps conquering, role in initiating petting behaviors. In contrast, because of their limited masturbatory histories at this age, most females have less experience in sexual arousal and expect little erotic reward from petting. Most tend to view their role as one of establishing limits in which they attempt to maintain control of the action, anticipate the moves of the male, and limit access to their bodies (Gagnon & Simon, 1973).

In the early stages of petting, the active, initiating role of the male and the passive but controlling role of the female are clearly evident. He attempts to do something to her (kiss her, touch her breasts, touch her genitals) and she may or may not allow him to do something to her (kiss her, touch her breasts, touch her genitals). While much of this early petting may not be very arousing to the female, as the male's techniques become more and more insistent and intimate, her own erotic sensations gradually begin to emerge. Perhaps hesitantly at first, she begins to take a more active role in the petting by touching and manipulating his genitals (see Table 9–4).

Throughout all of this both sexes learn something of the realities involved in heterosexual interactions. The male's preexisting fantasies and peer- or media-supplied "knowledge" are all put to the test. Many of his fantasies and much of his

RESEARCH HIGHLIGHT

The Erotic Effectiveness of Petting Techniques

It has frequently been observed (Kaplan, 1974; Masters & Johnson, 1970) that one of the major obstacles to mutually satisfying heterosexual interactions is the failure of one or both participants to understand precisely which sexual techniques are sexually stimulating and enjoyable to the other. There are several factors which contribute to such misunderstanding. The most obvious one is our inability to "get inside the skin" of others and actually experience sensations as they do. Another is the fact that much of what we "know" about the sexual preferences and reactions of the opposite sex is first acquired in the context of peer interactions. Young males share secret sexual techniques which are guaranteed to "drive girls wild" and young females learn what acts to avoid so as to prevent boys from becoming too excited. Perhaps most important, however, is the almost total lack of verbal communication between the sexes during sexual interactions. Rarely do we directly tell each other which techniques we find

highly arousing and enjoyable. Instead, we tend to rely on ambiguous body movements which are intended to increase or decrease the chance of certain types of stimulation. Or, we emit vague and incoherent gutteral sounds such as moans and groans which we hope our partners will understand. But does a moan indicate erotic ecstasy or excruciating pain? It may, of course, mean either.

There is little in the way of systematic research which has been directed at discovery of how erotically stimulating particular sexual techniques are to most males and females. A recent study, however, (Griffitt, 1978) sought to determine on the basis of self-reports how sexually arousing and enjoyable particular petting techniques are to average male and female college students. The students were asked to rate on scales of 0 (low) to 5 (high) how arousing they found several petting practices. The average ratings obtained from males and females are

shown in the bar graph here. It may be seen that both sexes reported considerable sex arousal from and enjoyment of hand and oral stimulation of the female breasts. This finding is of particular interest since it is often reported that few females are highly responsive to breast stimulation (Kinsey et al., 1953; Masters & Johnson, 1966). The remaining techniques rated involve hand and oral stimulation of the genitals of each sex. Rather consistently men reported being more aroused by these techniques than females, regardless of whose genitals were being stimulated. Not too surprising, however, is the finding that both men and women are more aroused by the "recipient," or passive, roles when their own genitals are being stimulated than by the "donor," or active, roles of stimulating the genitals of their partners. For example, men are considerably more aroused by fellatio (oral stimulation of the penis) than by cunnilingus (oral stimulation of the female genitals) but the opposite is

true for females. It is of interest to note that the least arousing and enjoyable act for females is fellatio resulting in ejaculation.

It should be emphasized that these data profile the "average" male and female college student and that marked variations among individuals exist. Nevertheless, such findings provide useful preliminary guidelines for understanding the petting technique preferences and reactions of males and females in general.

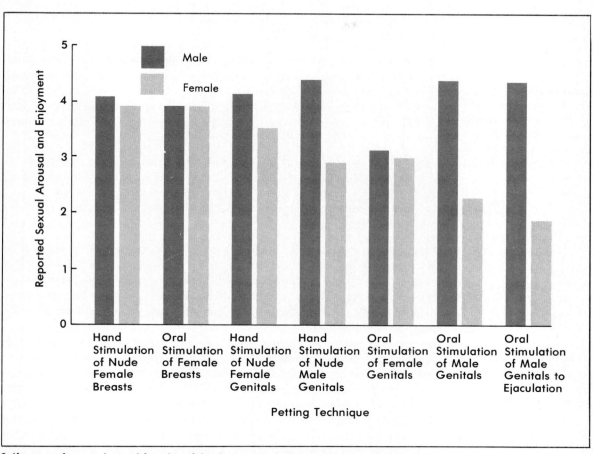

Self-reports from males and females of the degree to which they are sexually aroused by and enjoy various petting techniques.

SOURCE: Data from Griffitt, 1978.

knowledge may have to be modified. And, as many have discovered, the female body holds many surprises (Ribal, 1973):

For the last date we had, I was determined to give her the finger if I could, but when I finally made it to the objective with my hand, I got turned off. Her panties were all wet. I thought she had urinated. . . . I couldn't wait to get to the John to wash my hand. I was even worried that I might get a disease. (p. 157)

Betty taught me that wetness between a girl's legs was normal when she got excited. Away went the myth I had been harboring since feeling Boobie in the movie. Cunts are not just hot, they're juicy. (p. 159)

The usual female experience with petting is, of course, a similar one. She may find males more or less demanding and forward in their sexual advances than expected. As her experience widens, she learns to adapt to various male partners who differ widely in their aggressiveness, preferences, and emotional reactions in petting. In addition, the anatomical lessons to be learned are no less significant for females than for males:

Hank pulled off my pants and in a mad whirl of arms and legs had dropped his own pants to the car floor and suddenly showed me the thing I had only gingerly felt through the insulation of wash-and-wear slacks. Let's just say that I was something less than thrilled. It was a lot bigger than I thought one of those could be. (Ribal, 1973, p. 99)

Thus, petting experiences may be seen, in part, as providing training grounds on which both sexes learn the topography of the genitals and erogenous zones of those of the opposite sex and learn to negotiate the give-and-take relationships inherent in heterosexual interaction. At the same time, however, the significance attached to heterosexual expression undergoes some basic transformations for both males and females.

The early sexual socialization experiences of males are characterized by an emphasis on "scoring" in which females are viewed primarily as sexual targets. In early adolescence the average male is most fully committed to the sexual aspects of heterosexual relationships to which his sexual role is closely tied. To be "masculine" is to be sexually successful with as many females as possible and females are valued primarily to the extent that they afford opportunities for the young male to repeatedly affirm his masculinity. In contrast, to feel affection, attachment, or love for females is often regarded as a rather unmanly trap into which the unwary might fall. Such attitudes toward heterosexuality originate in and are reinforced by same-sex peers as well as popularized media images of the "man's man" whose sexual credo is guided by the "Four F" philosophy: "Find 'em, Feel 'em, Fuck 'em, Forget 'em."

Young females, however, are trained (socialized) to value dating and courtship for the opportunities they provide for the establishment of stable relationships characterized by affection, love, and possible future marriage. There is little early commitment to or interest in sexuality itself. To be "feminine" is to love and be loved but to remain sexually pure until such time that sexual involvement is legitimized by marriage.

Men are often trained to focus on the physical aspects of a relationship, whereas women tend to be more concerned with the emotional aspects.

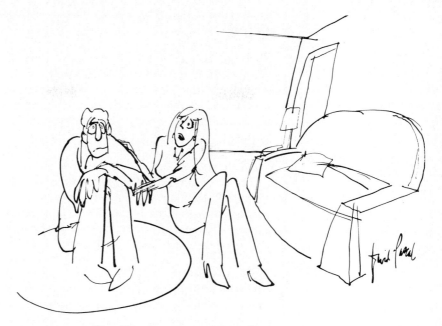

"Is there a yearning with the churning, or is it mostly just churning?"

Drawing by David Pascal; © 1984 The New Yorker Magazine, Inc.

Thus, males and females are socialized in essentially opposite ways and enter the dating and petting arena with what frequently are conflicting goals. With males committed to sex rather than romance and females to romance rather than sex, a marketplace atmosphere develops in which testimonials of affection are bartered for sexual involvement and vice versa. What rather commonly happens during this exchange, of course, is that males find themselves becoming emotionally involved with their partners and females find themselves enjoying and becoming sexually aroused by the petting activities (Ehrmann, 1959; Gagnon & Simon, 1973).

For males, then, sexual involvement leads to affectionate involvement, and the "Four F" philosophy somehow no longer seems as appropriate. In fact, because of the prevalence of the "good girl–bad girl" distinction at this age, some males are reluctant to press for increasing sexual intimacy once they become attached to their partners. Sex becomes less a game and is embedded in a matrix of emotional commitment in which the girl's feelings are important. She is not only a sex object but also a love object.

In contrast, females find that growing affectionate involvement more fully legitimizes sexual involvement, and they often become more interested in sexual activity as they perceive their partners' protestations of affection as more genuine. Sexual "advances" are no longer so vigorously defended against but are, rather, participated in or even initiated by the female, who now begins to learn to fully appreciate the erotic pleasures of petting. In essence she learns to respond sexually. Around one third of all females experience their first erotic response as a result of petting (Kinsey et al., 1953).

SUMMARY

Nearly half of both sexes report engaging in sexual play with those of the opposite sex prior to adolescence. Preadolescent heterosexual activities first occur in the context of games and most frequently involve genital exhibition or genital manipulation. Attempts at coitus are rare. More males than females recall preadolescent heterosexual play. It is through sex play that most boys and girls are first exposed to information concerning the anatomy of the opposite sex. For most children sex play is more play than sex even though some recall becoming sexually aroused during such play. The effects of early sex play on adolescent and adult sexual expression are poorly understood but there is no evidence to suggest that sex play interferes with later adjustment.

Between the ages of twelve and fifteen most males and females begin to engage in rather deliberate sexual interactions in the form of petting. Prior to marriage, at least 90 percent of both sexes have petted at least once. Males generally begin petting earlier, have more petting partners, and progress to intimate forms of petting sooner than do females. Recent studies suggest that the petting attitudes and practices of males and females are beginning to converge.

Those most likely to begin petting early, to pet with many partners, and to utilize highly intimate petting techniques are those who are most attitudinally permissive regarding sexual expression, least religiously devout, most likely to go to college, politically and socially liberal, and perhaps somewhat rebellious in their life-styles. They are active seekers of physical and social stimulation, extraverted, and relatively low in guilt concerning sexual matters.

Petting experience gradually unfolds in a sequential pattern in which acts characterized by a relatively low degree of intimacy (hugging, kissing) serve as prerequisites to more intimate behaviors involving manual and oral stimulation of the genitals. For both sexes even the least intimate of petting activities such as kissing involve approach-avoidance conflicts. In other words, the actual or imagined rewards of petting are in conflict with avoidance pressures associated with moral and social inhibitions as well as uncertainties regarding effective techniques. As a temporary compromise between sexual abstinence and coitus, petting is a highly sexually arousing activity which may be erotically rewarding to both sexes.

Petting provides an arena in which both males and females first come to understand what is involved in heterosexual interaction. In addition to learning something of the anatomy of the opposite sex, they also gain valuable experience in negotiating the very real complexities involved in managing the physical, social, and emotional aspects of heterosexual expression.

SUGGESTED READINGS

DeLameter, J., & MacCorquodale, P. (1979). *Premarital sexuality: Ideology, interaction, and behavior.* Madison: University of Wisconsin Press.

Gagnon, J. H., & Simon, W. (1973). *Sexual conduct.* Chicago: Aldine. (See especially Chapters 1, 2, and 4.)

Kinsey, A., Pomeroy, W., & Martin, C. (1948). *Sexual behavior in the human male.* Philadelphia: Saunders. (See especially Chapters 5 and 16.)

Kinsey, A., Pomeroy, W., Martin, C., & Gebhard, P. (1953). *Sexual behavior in the human female.* Philadelphia: Saunders. (See especially Chapters 4 and 7.)

Ribal, J. E. (1973). *Learning sex roles.* San Francisco: Canfield Press.

CHAPTER OUTLINE

CHAPTER 10

HETEROSEXUAL BEHAVIORS: COITUS

Although there are many forms of sexual expression, for most heterosexually oriented adults "sex" means coitus or sexual intercourse involving the union of a penis and a vagina. In contemporary societies virtually all males and females are socialized to believe and feel that coitus is the only "normal" and "natural" form of sexual activity. Even so, our attitudes concerning this most acceptable of sexual acts are a mixture of positive and negative elements as revealed by the dual meanings attached to terms such as "fuck," "screw," and "ball" often used to refer to coitus. In this chapter we will consider patterns of coitus first by an examination of techniques and functions of *precoital stimulation and arousal (foreplay)*. Next we will turn our attention to the nature and techniques of *coitus* itself and to the issue of *orgasm in coitus*. Finally, we will examine the *social context* in which coitus occurs through considerations of premarital, marital, extramarital, and postmarital coital partnerships.

PRECOITAL STIMULATION AND AROUSAL

Like other forms of sexual activity, intercourse does not simply happen. Instead it is embedded in a complex array of physical and psychosocial erotic as well as nonerotic elements. Initially, sexual interests and desires may be aroused by a variety of internal or external cues. Events as diverse as the sight, smell, or sound of one's sexual partner, the erotic thoughts and images generated by soft music and candlelight or the driving beats of disco music, conversations about sex, exposure to erotic reading or visual material, massage parlor signs, and a host of other stimuli are all capable of activating sexual longings.

Atmosphere

Whether or not the relatively mild levels of sexual excitement produced by such events lead to overt sexual acts depends on a variety of factors. For example, sexual expression is a relatively private matter for most people and will be delayed or avoided unless the circumstances allow for at least some degree of isolation from possible onlookers. Similarly, what is often rather vaguely described as atmosphere has an important bearing on whether or not sexual desires are translated into behavior. As it is most frequently used with reference to sexual interaction the term *"atmosphere"* refers to the physical as well as the psychosocial context within which sexual behavior might occur. There are wide variations among people in terms of what type of atmosphere is most conducive to sexual expression.

In spite of such variations, media representations of sex found in movies, magazines, and novels have effectively created an almost stereotyped image of the "ideal" sexual (always heterosexual) atmosphere. With some variations this atmosphere is one which nearly always includes soft music, a warm fireplace in an expensively furnished room, wine or other alcoholic beverage, and an incredibly attractive man and woman both dressed in sexually appealing, if not revealing, clothing. Common variations include an isolated beach, mountain, or meadow as other physical backdrops. Such settings almost "ooze" sexuality and because of media popularity are frequently aspired to in fantasy or reality but rarely attained by most people. For most of us the realities are that we lack the money, the time, the uninterrupted privacy, or the physical attractiveness to duplicate such settings.

Even in the rather less glamorous world outside the movie theater and the pages of *Playboy, Esquire,* and *Cosmopolitan*, however, atmosphere is important. Even though sexually aroused, some people, for example, may find it difficult to initiate sexual activity outside of marriage or out of the confines of a locked bedroom, with an unloved or unloving partner, when they or their partners have not recently bathed, with a physically unattractive partner, without a preparatory alcoholic drink, with the lights on, when the children are home, or in the homes of strangers or parents. All of these factors and more are important components of the atmosphere for sex for many people. What is important for people is determined by their individual learned sexual preferences, responses, and expectations and cannot be prescribed with any precision for all men or women. In short, what is sexual atmosphere for one person or couple may well be an asexual or even antisexual one for another person or couple.

Given a sexually conducive atmosphere and the availability of a willing partner, even relatively low levels of sexual excitement will motivate an individual or couple to begin overt sexual contact. At first such contact may involve only moving closer together physically or perhaps psychosocially through eye contact (Griffitt, May, & Veitch, 1974) or other nonverbal or verbal means. There may be a period of uncertainty during which each person attempts to discern the willingness and desires of the other without specifically asking or verbally revealing his or her own. Some people, on the other hand, may be quite forthright and open in stating their wishes to engage in sexual contact. As a general rule, the most sexually experienced and most positively oriented toward sex are most comfortable in conversing openly about their sexual intentions and desires (Fisher, Miller, Byrne, & White,

Although couples seek out the most romantic setting possible, they usually must settle for something less than the ideal.

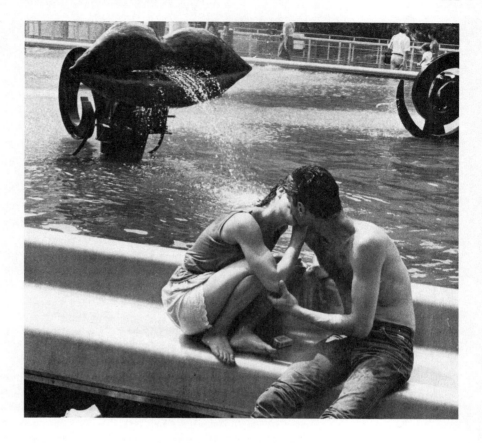

1978). At any rate, the physical contact that results serves to further heighten the subjective as well as the physiological sexual excitement in both partners. The sexual activities involved in this contact are identical to those discussed as petting in Chapter 9, but when they precede coitus they are popularly and most frequently referred to as *foreplay*.

Techniques of Arousal and Foreplay

Some form of foreplay prior to coitus is almost universal among nonhuman as well as human mammals (Ford & Beach, 1951) and is found among many species of insects and birds as well (Bermant & Davidson, 1974). In a functional sense the purpose of foreplay is clear—at least a minimal degree of sexual excitement is necessary for coitus to occur. Males must erect sufficiently to accomplish vaginal penetration which, in humans at least, is easier and more pleasant for both sexes if the female has reached a level of arousal which results in vaginal lubrication and separation of the labia. The petting activities of foreplay serve to dramatically increase the degree of sexual excitement and thus facilitate actual coital activity. There are, of course, a multitude of physical stimulation methods by which sexual arousal may be enhanced and it would be impossible to describe or even enumer-

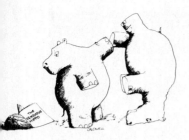

Religiously following the instructions in a sex manual does not necessarily result in a better sex life.
SOURCE: John Caldwell.

ate all of them. There are, however, a few which are fairly common, perhaps because they have stood the test of time across several millenia of human sexual interaction. It is these on which we will concentrate in the present section.

Before proceeding, a few words are necessary concerning the purposes and contents of this section. The proliferation of sex and marriage manuals such as *The Sensuous Woman* ("J," 1969), *The Sensuous Man* ("M," 1971), and Comfort's *The Joy of Sex* (1972) and *More Joy* (1974) is due, in part, to the assumption that most people are really quite uninformed when it comes to sexual technique and that without proper instruction they will be unable to manage more than a clumsy kiss followed by a joyless act of coitus. If this were true, we would not be facing a world population crisis of frightening proportions. Clearly, many people learn enough to perform the act of coitus and often to enjoy it or they would not keep repeating it.

What, then, is the value of discussions of sexual technique? Such discussions are important for at least two reasons. First, there are some people for whom sex is difficult and even distasteful because of their ignorance of pleasant and arousing sexual techniques. Technical information concerning erogenous zones, sexual anatomy, and sexual response cycles can help those individuals overcome their negative responses to sex. Second, even if people's knowledge of technique is adequate, they may still have inhibitions that detract from their enjoyment of sex. The fact that most sex manuals and texts with how-to-do-it descriptions are written from a positive, approving, and accepting stance helps such individuals allay anxiety, fear, and guilt they may feel concerning the "normality" or appropriateness of most specific sexual acts.

One potential disadvantage of instructions in technique, however, is that some are written much like a recipe for a cake. The implication, then, is that if *all* ingredients are not present or properly mixed, sex, like a cake, will fail. In recent years many of the required ingredients have included such sexual techniques as oral-genital contact and anal stimulation, which traditionally have been rather taboo. If, because the book says so, a couple feels compelled to perform sexual acts that they find distasteful, painful, guilt-producing, or otherwise aversive, their experience of sex will be bad even though they have followed the recipe. In short, there is no single or magical set of sexual techniques that will be pleasurable to all people. Perhaps the best advice a couple can take to enhance their sexual pleasure is to be open to experimentation with a variety of techniques but not feel compelled to perform any particular ones simply because "the book" says they should or could. It follows, then, that the primary purpose of the present discussion is not to prescribe, recommend, or promote but rather to describe some of the fairly common foreplay techniques along with research findings relevant to their incidence, correlates, and demonstrated or presumed effects.

Kissing.   The role of kissing in American and most Western cultures is an interesting one. On the one hand it is frequently used as an expression of affection between parents and children or as a greeting or expression of affection and friendship between opposite-sex and sometimes between same-sex (mostly female) adults. By social convention such kisses are supposed to and usually do mean little erotically. At the same time, however, kissing for erotic purposes is an important part of petting and foreplay in most, but not all, cultures (Ford & Beach, 1951; Marshall & Suggs, 1971). Indeed, beyond light embracing, lip kissing with the mouth closed ("simple" kissing) is the initial intimate heterosexual experience for most American (Vener & Stewart, 1974) as well as European (Luckey & Nass, 1969) youth and first occurs around the age of twelve for the average male and female. By the time they reach the age of twenty-one virtually all American males and females have engaged in such kissing.

Simple lip kissing can be quite erotically arousing particularly for those just beginning their sexual careers and as part of a person's first sexual experience with a new partner. As their kissing and other sexual experience accumulates, however, most people move on to the more erotic deep, or "French," kiss in which their lips are parted and used to gently stroke or nibble those of their partners. This is frequently followed or accompanied by light and tentative, then firm and bold, tongue exploration of the partner's lips, tongue, and inner mouth as well as sucking on the partner's lips and tongue. For those who practice it, this type of kissing is highly erotic and sometimes may result in orgasm. Frequently the deep kiss not only serves as arousing foreplay but continues throughout intercourse.

While almost all men and women engage in some sort of kissing prior to coitus, there are wide variations in the extent to which it is elaborated during foreplay. For example, the Kinsey (1948) survey of males indicated that deep kissing prior to intercourse was more widely practiced by those with some college education (77 percent) than those with only a grade school education (41 percent). Kissing, when it did precede coitus, tended to be rather perfunctory in males with lower levels of education; intercourse often followed a single kiss. More recent data (Hunt, 1974) suggest that extended kissing and foreplay is becoming somewhat more common at the lower educational and social levels.

Kissing is often extended beyond the lips and mouth of one's sexual partner to the neck, ears, back, abdomen, breasts, thighs, and virtually all other body areas including, for some, the genitals, buttocks, and anus. For some, the phrase "showering with kisses" is an appropriate one, for the escalation in sexual excitement produced by prolonged deep kissing often leads to a passionate frenzy of rapidly shifting mouth-body contact.

Breast Stimulation.   Foreplay usually begins in earnest with kissing and even among those who are not "total body kissers" leads to and blends with exploration and stimulation of other body parts. As noted in Chapter 9, both males and females report a great deal of pleasure and excitement associated with stimulation of the female breasts. Furthermore, some males experience erotic pleasure when their own breasts are stimulated (Masters & Johnson, 1966). The special significance of the female breasts for both the young adolescent male and female is, of course, well known. Breasts are the primary visible distinction between males and females and so acquire a high degree of sexual symbolism. For many males and females, young and old, access to the female breasts represents an important "breakthrough" in petting and suggests the promise (or threat) of advancing intimacy. Thus, for both sexes stimulation of the female breasts has psychosocial as well as physiological erotic significance.

It is not surprising, then, that recent surveys (cited in Chapter 9) indicate that some sort of stimulation of the female breasts is a common and important element of the premarital petting experiences of both sexes. When such petting is a prelude or accompaniment to coitus, stimulation of the female breasts is almost universal among Americans, with over 90 percent of both sexes reporting manual as well as oral breast stimulation in marital coital foreplay (Hunt, 1974; Kinsey et al., 1948; Kinsey et al., 1953). Premaritally, when coitus is involved mouth-breast stimulation is somewhat less common (approximately 80 percent of both sexes) but hand stimulation of the female breasts is found in over 90 percent of those with premarital coital experience (Kinsey et al., 1948, 1953).

Breast stimulation often begins with manual fondling, massage, and perhaps squeezing of the entire breast mass followed by gentle brushing, rubbing, and squeezing of the nipples with the fingers. In the early stages of arousal, at least, most women prefer a gentle approach in which the caresses are light and intermittent rather than rough and potentially painful. The nipples are, of course, highly sensitive to painful as well as erotic stimulation and must be manipulated with care. Some women, in fact, avoid direct nipple stimulation, preferring instead that the man's fingers gently circle their nipples in a brushing fashion to stimulate the areolae. Similarly, the breast mass must be carefully stimulated since strong squeezing and rough handling can be painful and even injurious.

Mouth-breast contact in which the man kisses, nibbles, licks, or sucks the nipples or entire breast is a highly erotic and sensuous experience for most men and women. This is frequently interspersed with manual breast contact or takes place as part of more widespread manual and oral body stimulation. As with manual breast stimulation, for most women gentleness is important in stimulating the breasts orally at low levels of arousal. Biting or otherwise rough stimulation can be painful as well as harmful. As arousal escalates, however, some women do enjoy tender biting of the nipples and breast and many men experience pleasure from sucking powerfully on the entire breast. Breast stimulation may continue throughout a coital episode, and one advantage of some coital positions is that they allow continual manual or oral breast contact.

Generally speaking, those who are well-educated, extraverted, eager for a wide range of experiences, and without guilt concerning sexual matters are most likely to practice and enjoy breast stimulation during petting and foreplay (see Chapter 9). Some women who are dissatisfied with the size or appearance of their breasts (Berscheid, Walster, & Bohrnstedt, 1973) may seek to avoid breast stimulation not because small and large breasts differ in erotic sensitivity but because they are embarrassed by their breasts. Finally, it should be noted that even though most women find breast stimulation enjoyable and erotically satisfying (Griffitt, 1978), relatively few are able to reach orgasm through breast stimulation alone (Masters & Johnson, 1966).

Genital Stimulation.   Direct genital stimulation is perhaps the most effective means of producing erotic arousal through petting and foreplay and, not surprisingly, is a common part of the sexual repertoire of both men and women. For example, the Kinsey research (1948) revealed that nearly 90 percent of all males with at least a high school education reported manually stimulating their partner's genitals as a prelude to premarital intercourse. As a part of premarital intercourse 80 percent of females reported hand stimulation of the male genitals. In marital intercourse the percentages are higher with 95 percent of males and 91 percent of females reporting manual stimulation of their partner's genitals. More recent research (Hunt, 1974) indicates that these already high percentages have not increased substantially in recent years.

In the most common and traditional course of events in foreplay, manual genital stimulation is initiated by the male following a period of kissing and breast stimulation. His hands may freely roam over his partner's body, gradually moving closer and closer to her genitals. The contact becomes more genitally focused as he first rubs and caresses her entire vulval area and simultaneously separates the labia and inserts one or more fingers into her vagina. The most effective form of manual stimulation is that which focuses on the clitoris and labia minora, usually the most sensitive erogenous zones in women (Fisher, 1973; Kinsey et al., 1953) and those most frequently involved in female masturbation (Hite, 1976). There are, of course, wide variations among women in the particular techniques of genital stimulation they prefer. For example, reported preferences include "gentle but firm with a rhythm," "shaking my clitoral area with the palm," "firm, quick, constant movements," "a light, teasing, tentative touch, not too regular," "indirect clitoral stimulation," "direct clitoral stimulation with a regular rhythm," and "a rhythm with syncopation" (Hite, 1976, pp. 347, 348, 349). Such a list could, of course, be extended seemingly indefinitely. As a general rule, however, the manual stimulation techniques preferred by most women parallel those they utilize in their autosexual activities. Communication about such matters, while difficult for some, can be a great aid to their partner's understanding of their individual sexual preferences.

Most men enjoy having their genitals stimulated by their female partner and, like females, prefer to be stimulated in a manner that resembles their own masturbatory practices. Thus, the most preferred and effective technique is one in which the woman grasps and gently strokes in a to-and-fro motion the shaft and glans of the penis. At low levels of arousal the glans is highly sensitive to pain and gentle stimulation is preferred. The penis has no natural lubricant and the application of lotions, saliva, or other lubricating substances can be of value in reducing irritation and pain. Some men enjoy light stimulation of the scrotum but the testes are so sensitive to pressure-induced pain that they should be caressed with great care.

For those who are comfortable with it, oral genital stimulation is an extremely effective means of heightening sexual arousal and producing orgasm. Incidence figures from the Kinsey studies regarding premarital oral stimulation of the male genitals **(fellatio)** and of the female genitals **(cunnilingus)** are difficult to interpret because of inconsistencies in the manner in which male and female data were reported. Rough estimates based on recomputations of the reported figures, however, suggest that nearly 30 percent of both sexes experienced fellatio and cunnilingus as part of their premarital coital foreplay. As with many other forms of stimulation, fellatio and cunnilingus were more common among those at the upper than at the lower educational levels. There is little doubt that attitudes regarding the acceptability of fellatio and cunnilingus are becoming more and more permissive (Croake & James, 1973). Recent surveys suggest that the actual premarital practice of these foreplay techniques is now more widespread than at the time of the Kinsey surveys. For example, in the *Playboy*-sponsored survey (Hunt, 1974), 60 percent of both sexes reported engaging in cunnilingus as part of their premarital coital foreplay while 70 percent and 60 percent of the unmarried males and females, respectively, reported fellatio experience. These are rather remarkable increases and probably exaggerate the actual changes due to the likely overrepresentation of sexually active and liberal men and women in the *Playboy* sample (Gagnon, 1977).

Data from the Kinsey sample indicated that approximately half of all couples at least occasionally used cunnilingus and fellatio in their marital foreplay, with more of those at the upper than the lower educational levels reporting such practices. The most comparable figures from Hunt (1974) are those based on his entire sample, which included married couples age eighteen and older. Among those with high school but no college education both cunnilingus and fellatio were practiced by between 50 and 60 percent of both males and females. As in the Kinsey data, both forms of oral-genital stimulation were more common in those with at least some college education and occurred in from 60 to 75 percent of the marriages in this group. Both cunnilingus and fellatio were more widespread among those under the age of twenty-five; over 90 percent of the married couples in this group reported both activities.

Other large-scale studies which are overrepresented by the young, highly educated, and sexually and politically liberal such as the *Psychology Today* (Athanasiou, Shaver, & Tavris, 1970) and *Redbook* (Tavris & Sadd, 1977) surveys also report the incidence of cunnilingus and fellatio ranging between 77 and 93 percent. Given the fact that these surveys include high proportions of well-educated, liberal, nonreligious, and nontraditional men and women who voluntarily and actively reveal the intimate details of their sex lives, it is most appropriate to consider the reported figures as estimates of the upper limits of the incidence of oral-genital foreplay (Gagnon, 1977). Inclusion of their less well-educated, conservative, deeply religious, and traditional counterparts would undoubtedly lower the figures (see Chapter 9).

Generally speaking, the range of foreplay techniques used in marital sex is greater than that in either premarital or extramarital sex. In comparison with both premarital and extramarital partnerships, married couples are usually more familiar with the sexual preferences of their partners, and their relative freedom from guilt and anxiety concerning possible discovery allows for more extensive experimentation with various sexual techniques. Thus, it is not surprising that both cunnilingus and fellatio are less widespread and frequent in extramarital than in marital foreplay. For example, Tavris and Sadd (1977) reported that less than half of their sample with extramarital intercourse experience "occasionally" or "often" engaged in oral-genital contacts in such relationships and an additional 15 percent reported doing so only once. For many, the intimacy involved in oral-genital stimulation is so great that it is possible only in well-established, familiar, and secure relationships.

Though there are no standardized rules for oral-genital stimulation, there are enough commonalities in technique to summarize the most usual forms of cunnilingus and fellatio. In cunnilingus, the man usually kisses, licks, or sucks the clitoris and labia and occasionally endeavors to penetrate the vagina with his tongue. Both the saliva and vaginal fluids produced by such stimulation aid in lubrication and the prevention of irritation. As with other forms of stimulation, the progression is usually from light and gentle caresses to more bold, rapid, and deliberate stimulation. Many women find it relatively easy to reach one or more orgasms through cunnilingus and it is most readily produced by constant and steady tongue or lip stimulation of the clitoral area (Hite, 1976; Masters & Johnson, 1966).

In fellatio, it is the glans of the penis which is the primary focus of stimulation. The woman usually kisses, licks, and sucks on the glans while stroking or grasping the penile shaft and perhaps gently stimulating the scrotum. Many men find it particularly exciting to have their partners take the entire penis into their mouths in the manner popularized and sensationalized by Linda Lovelace in the movie *Deep Throat* and described step-by-titillating-step in her book *Inside Linda Lovelace* (Lovelace, 1973). Some women, of course, find complete mouth-penile penetration impossible, uncomfortable, or degrading and prefer not to attempt it even though they may freely participate in and enjoy other forms of fellatio. As indicated in Chapter 9, a major dilemma for many women is the possibility of male orgasm during fellatio and the consequent ejaculation into the mouth. Though this is a concern that must be dealt with by the individual couple, it should be pointed out that there are no harmful substances in semen which on hygienic or health grounds would dictate against swallowing it. Similarly, of course, there are no harmful ingredients in vaginal fluids. Our reservations about such substances are a product of ambivalent feelings about our own and our partner's genitals, including their smells and secretions.

Elaborations. The preceding brief discussion has concentrated on those foreplay techniques that, according to numerous investigations (Hunt, 1974; Kinsey et al., 1948, 1953; Pietropinto & Simenauer, 1977; Tavris & Sadd, 1977), are most common among American and European men and women. The available evidence suggests that these acts are also the central elements of foreplay in some of the major Asian countries, including Japan (Asayama, 1975) and China (Edwards, 1976).

There are, of course, endless variations and elaborations of these basic techniques which are practiced by some people some of the time. For example, it has been estimated (Tavris & Sadd, 1977) that up to 50 percent of married couples use erotic books, movies, or pictures as an added source of stimulation during foreplay. These materials not only *enhance sexual arousal* but also suggest unusual or untried foreplay techniques and intercourse positions.

Some couples find the use of various oils, lotions, jellies, and other lubricants particularly exciting. When applied to the genitals, these substances reduce the chance of painful irritation, and many are aroused by spreading them over their entire bodies. For related reasons some people enjoy taking baths or showers together in which they cover their bodies with soap or bath oils. Some recent sex manuals ("J," 1969; "M," 1971) recommend that couples combine dining and foreplay by covering each other's bodies with whipped cream, jellies, jams, butter, or other tasty delights and then licking or sucking them off. While the use of lotions, soaps, or other substances in foreplay and intercourse sometimes adds novelty and excitement to sexual encounters, some degree of caution in the selection of what is used is necessary. Genital tissues are very susceptible to irritation, and foreign substances that are highly acidic or alkaline may be quite painful or injurious when applied to these areas.

Some men and women are aroused by inserting various objects in the vagina. Most often, these are objects that in some way resemble a penis, such as hot dogs, carrots, bananas, small round tubes, and commercially available artificial phalluses, or dildos. Even though potentially exciting, such insertions should be attempted with great care for the walls of the vagina are very thin and may be easily ruptured (Masters & Johnson, 1966).

The electric vibrator is becoming more and more popular as an aid to enhancing female sexual arousal and orgasm (Hite, 1976; "J," 1969), and an increasing number of couples are including such devices in their repertoire of sexual techniques. Some men, however, are a bit threatened by women's use of vibrators, fearing that their own sexual techniques might seem less exciting or somewhat humdrum to the woman who has become experienced in the delights of electric sex. For the most part such fears are unfounded since, in spite of highly publicized testimonials (Hite, 1976), most women prefer the living and loving hands, fingers, tongue, lips, and penis of their partners as sexual stimulants (Tavris & Sadd, 1977).

Those who use oils, lotions, vibrators, and other aids in their lovemaking are fairly uniform in praising their effectiveness ("J," 1969; "M," 1971; Tavris & Sadd, 1977). The available evidence, however, suggests that their use is not widespread. For example, Tavris and Sadd (1977) found that only 21 percent of their sample of women reported that they or their partners ever employed "sex aids" in their foreplay or intercourse and their use was rather infrequent. Even though rated as enjoyable by over 90 percent of these women, the irregular use of such devices is understandable. Oils, lotions, whipped cream, and strawberry preserves are messy. Few people are eager to change and launder bedding following each episode of lovemaking. Many vibrators are rather noisy and their use is often limited to those occasions that guarantee substantial privacy and freedom from being overheard by children or others.

Throughout recorded history the sexually adventurous have sought and devised innumerable aids to sexual pleasure. Those we have described here constitute only a small portion of the items used by some people some of the time. To this list could be added a variety of penile attachments with rubber or plastic protrusions ("French ticklers") designed to increase intravaginal stimulation, rubber-pronged attachments for the base of the penis which facilitate clitoral stimulation, penis extenders, *ben-wa* eggs (small stainless-steel balls for vaginal insertion), penis rings designed to produce and prolong erections, and anesthetics for application to the glans of the penis to prevent premature ejaculation. Most of these aids are intended to enhance female excitement by prolonging, concentrating, or intensifying genital stimulation. Some undoubtedly accomplish their goal but many people view their use as patently absurd. In a *Playboy* informal test of some of these devices ("The Great Playboy," 1978), the conclusion of one respondent reflected the feelings of many:

With most of these products my interest lasted as long as the first set of batteries. I doubt if I will incorporate many of them into my sex life. Maybe the Prelude 3 [a vibrator]. Maybe the oils. But the rest are disposable. Great for one date, but you wouldn't want to live with them. (p. 208)

Recent data suggest that anal stimulation as a part of coital sex play may not be as rare as most might have suspected. For example, Hunt (1974) found that over half of his married sample under the age of thirty-five occasionally engaged in manual stimulation of the anus and nearly 25 percent practiced oral-anal stimulation **(anilingus)** but only infrequently. Even though it is one of the most taboo of sexual acts, **anal intercourse,** in which the penis is inserted into the anus and rectum, is sometimes practiced by a minority of men and women. Because it is such a controversial and sensitive topic, however, reliable data concerning its incidence are difficult to obtain and the available figures must be interpreted with some caution. A *Playboy* poll of college students conducted in 1976 indicated that between 20 and 25 percent of those surveyed had engaged in heterosexual anal intercourse at least once ("What's Really Happening," 1976). Hunt (1974) found that 17 percent of his unmarried sample of males and females under twenty-five with coital experience had tried anal intercourse while 25 percent of his married couples under the age of twenty-five practiced anal intercourse on rare occasions. An anomaly among recent large-scale surveys is a finding in the *Redbook* (Tavris & Sadd, 1977) study that 43 percent of the married female respondents had engaged in anal intercourse at least once. Considering the relative similarity of the Hunt (1974) and *Redbook* samples, the reasons for this discrepancy are not immediately apparent. It is probably most accurate to conclude that the "truth" lies somewhere between the two figures. That is, perhaps a third of young, well-educated, and sexually liberal married couples engage in anal intercourse on rare occasions.

Among those who have experienced it, males are two to three times more likely than females to report that they enjoy anal intercourse. Similarly, even if they have not tried it, nearly twice as many males as females indicate an interest in doing so ("What's Really Happening," 1976). Less than 5 percent of males, however, indicate strong desires for such activity in their heterosexual practices (Pietropinto & Simenauer, 1977).

Anal stimulation is rarely a central component of sex play activities. It generally occurs sporadically or perhaps only once in the lives of people who report they have experienced it. Like other forms of sexual activity it is neither inherently "natural" nor "unnatural" but one among many possible avenues of sexual expression. The only potential physical hazards of anal and rectal stimulation are the possibilities of infection and pain. Masters and Johnson (1970) suggest that the bacterial content of the rectum might be transferred to the vagina by the fingers or penis in the course of anal stimulation resulting in vaginal infections. Recent clinical evidence suggests that such infections are not as likely as once believed (Tavris & Sadd, 1977).

Significance of Arousal and Foreplay

As with other forms of sexual expression, there are many dimensions to the significance of coital foreplay. Most frequently, however, it is described and discussed in the context of its importance for producing or enhancing female sexual arousal, orgasm, and pleasure from intercourse. The basis for this focus on females is reasonably clear and we have alluded to it often. It generally has been assumed and affirmed by "experts" that, in contrast to males, most females are difficult to arouse sexually, become aroused slowly, do not really enjoy sex, and reach orgasm in intercourse only as a result of heroic, sophisticated, and patient efforts on the part of their partners (Gordon & Shankweiler, 1971). From this standpoint, in order to become competent lovers males must learn to employ varied and exotic techniques of stimulation. They must control or pace their own rapidly accelerating arousal levels (Comfort, 1972) so that they are capable of the lengthy periods of foreplay required for female orgasm during intercourse. This view, of course, places the major burden of responsibility for female orgasm on males. More recent analyses of sexual partnerships, however, fully recognize the necessity of females taking active roles in reaching orgasm (Hite, 1976).

But what, if any, effects do foreplay technique and duration actually have on the probability of female orgasm during intercourse? This is a complex question that is difficult to answer with any certainty on the basis of available research findings. The "typical" married couple devotes ten to fifteen minutes to foreplay although many may spend fewer than three minutes or more than an hour prior to coitus (Fisher, 1973; Hunt, 1974; Kinsey et al., 1953). Perhaps because intercourse is somewhat less acceptable and more reluctantly performed outside of marriage, foreplay lasts an average of five to ten minutes longer when single individuals are involved (Hunt, 1974; Kinsey et al., 1953).

Kinsey et al. (1953) found little, if any, consistent relationship between the amount of time devoted to foreplay and the occurrence of female orgasm in intercourse. Although no detailed data were presented, it was suggested that lengthy foreplay might even interfere with female sexual response and pleasure, an opinion which has also been voiced by Eichenlaub (1961). In a more recent investigation with a smaller sample, Fisher (1973) was also unable to detect any relationship between foreplay duration and female coital orgasm. In a reexamination of some of the Kinsey data, however, Gebhard (1966) found a weak positive correlation between the length of time spent in foreplay and the probability of female orgasm during intercourse. As foreplay duration increased from ten minutes or less to over twenty minutes, the percent of women who almost always reached orgasm in the intercourse that followed increased steadily from 40 to 60 percent. (In this case, "almost always" was defined as 90 to 100 percent of the time. Still others, however, find no relationship between foreplay duration and coital orgasm in women (Huey, Kline-Graber, & Graber, 1981).

What these rather mixed findings seem to suggest is that extended foreplay may be of some benefit if female orgasm during intercourse is desired. At the same time, however, it is clear that lengthy foreplay prior to intercourse offers no guarantee of female orgasm and may possibly even reduce its probability if fatigue and boredom set in (Blood, 1969).

There is, of course, more to sexual interaction than coitus and coital orgasm. Indeed, the sex play that precedes intercourse is of great importance to most people. Even if coital orgasm for each partner is a primary goal, foreplay can still offer both partners at least as much enjoyment as orgasm. The buildup of sexual arousal, after all, is in many ways as pleasurable as its release in orgasm. That is, both receiving and giving sexual stimulation through varied, extended, and effective erotic techniques are pleasurable and may, as in petting, be pursued for their own sake. Furthermore, many women find it easier to reach orgasm through the uninterrupted clitoral stimulation involved in genitally oriented sex play techniques than through the less intense and intermittent stimulation most coital positions offer (Masters & Johnson, 1966). In fact, sex play frequently serves as a means to orgasm for females and males either before, after, or rather than intercourse (Fisher, 1973; Hite, 1976; Pietropinto & Simenauer, 1977; Tavris & Sadd, 1977).

Beyond its purely physiological effects, however, foreplay is of substantial psychosocial significance for most men and women. Sexual interaction is among the most intimate of all interpersonal interactions. When relating sexually we bare ourselves psychologically as well as physically to our partners. We are highly vulnerable to their acceptance or rejection of us as people, as lovers, and as desirable or undesirable sexual partners. For most couples, reaching this level of intimacy requires a transitional period during which the nature of their relationship is transformed from a somewhat impersonal preoccupation with aspects of everyday life such as job, household, finances, education, and auto repairs to a concern for highly personal and intimate forms of human exhange. Sudden transformations of this magnitude are usually difficult, if not impossible, to achieve and foreplay, therefore, has an important role in providing the opportunity for a graduated entry into intimacy.

As sexual arousal grows, so may feelings of intimacy, affection, tenderness, trust, and the desire to please and be pleased by one's sexual partner. Gradually, rather than abruptly, during foreplay sexual partners may shed some of their vulnerabilities, abandon some of their concerns with the mundane or troublesome aspects of everyday life, and become increasingly absorbed in the mutual sensual and emotional pleasures they derive from sexual relations.

Clearly, then, the time spent in sex play prior to coitus is important for both men and women. In spite of widespread media reports of an increasing incidence of casual and noncaring sexual encounters, the most desirable and satisfying sexual interactions for most people are those characterized by mutual feelings of affection, tenderness, trust and acceptance. Regardless of popular stereotypes (Gordon & Shankweiler, 1971; Hite, 1976), this is true for the majority of men (Hunt, 1974; Pietropinto & Simenauer, 1977; Tavris, 1978) as well as women (Tavris & Sadd, 1977; Schaefer, 1973). Indeed, much of the gratification that both sexes derive from sexual interaction results from feelings of warmth and closeness and perceptions that their partners genuinely care for them personally, desire and want to please them sexually, and are sexually and emotionally involved in and pleased by the interaction.

Such feelings and perceptions, as well as others, are created and communicated in many ways during foreplay. While little is actually known about communication patterns during sexual interaction, it is often asserted that the ability and willingness of sexual partners to verbalize their feelings for one another and their preferences and aversions concerning sexual techniques are important keys to sexual and interpersonal satisfaction (Comfort, 1972; McCary, 1978; Shope, 1975). Yet verbal communication concerning such matters is difficult for most people. Recent estimates indicate that, even within marriage, only about half of all couples regularly vocalize their sexual and emotional feelings before, during, or after sexual interaction (Pietropinto & Simenauer, 1977; Tavris & Sadd, 1977). Among contemporary couples, those who are most likely to do so are relatively young, well educated (Pietropinto & Simenauer, 1977), and relatively free of negative feelings concerning sexual matters in general (Fisher et al., 1978).

Much of the communication that takes place during foreplay as well as coitus is nonverbal. A great deal is actually "said," intentionally or unintentionally, by what one does and how one does it. Correctly or incorrectly, most people interpret active involvement, responsiveness, and apparent eagerness to engage in exciting sexual acts as indicators that their partners desire, value, and want to please them sexually and are experiencing pleasure from sexual interaction. In contrast, passivity, unresponsiveness, and reluctance to experiment with potentially pleasurable techniques often imply lack of concern and care as well as sexual or general disinterest in the partner.

That the nature of feelings communicated (mostly nonverbally) during foreplay and coitus is a crucial element involved in sexual satisfaction is demonstrated forcefully by the results of several recent large-scale surveys of men (Pietropinto & Simenauer, 1977; Tavris, 1978a, b) and women (Tavris & Sadd, 1977). These surveys find that sexual satisfaction in men, as well as in women, is clearly tied to feelings that one's partner is sexually satisfied, actively involved, responsive to one's sexual techniques, and truly desires and enjoys all elements of the sexual interaction.

The importance of such feelings and related ones to men are evident in personal testimonials:

I want the woman to be more passionate. I would like her to be more active and do whatever she felt like rather than being inhibited by convention. Having my partner happy would give me the most pleasure. (Pietropinto & Simenauer, 1977, p. 50)

I enjoy the feeling that I get when I make my partner very excited and I enjoy making her have an orgasm or more than one if possible. It is very important that my partner be satisfied. (Pietropinto & Simenauer, 1977, p. 43)

I would get the title deed to the moon for my wife if she would just once make me feel that I was sexually desirable. (Tavris, 1978a, p. 179)

Similar sentiments are revealed in comments from women:

Having a man love me and want to have sex with me is necessary to my happiness. It gives me a feeling of being worthwhile if I can turn a man on. (Hite, 1976, p. 426)

I love to hear him panting, groaning, moving, getting crazy. I like the feeling of closeness it produces, and I am excited by my partner's excitation. (Hite, 1976, p. 426)

If I feel that he has tried to communicate with me and give something to me emotionally, that he's enjoying me and I'm enjoying him, then I don't care whether I have a climax or not. (Schaefer, 1973, p. 147)

COITUS

Coitus is the union of male and female genitals in which the penis is inserted into the vagina. The relative positions of the male and female genitals in the most common (face-to-face) coital position are shown in Figure 10–1. Considered objectively it is a remarkably simple act well within the physical and cognitive capabilities of most normally functioning and sexually mature men and women. In spite of this basic simplicity, for the majority of heterosexually oriented men and women, coitus is regarded as the essence of sexual expression. The significance of coitus beyond its potential reproductive function rests on considerations concerning how, how often, why, and with whom it does (or should) occur and what the biological and psychosocial consequences of it are (or should be). The remaining sections of this chapter are devoted to considerations of some of the "is and are" rather than the "should be" aspects of coitus since the latter are largely matters of individual values, attitudes, and judgments. First, we will examine some of the many variations in how coitus takes place. Then we will turn to a brief consideration of orgasm during coitus. Finally, our attention will shift to the social context in which coitus occurs.

The Ways of Coitus

The basic act of penile-vaginal union can be accomplished in a variety of ways. Indeed, ancient (Vatsyayana, 1964), classic (Van de Velde, 1965), and contemporary (Comfort, 1972, 1974) marriage and sex manuals list and describe dozens of

Figure 10–1.

Relative positions of male and female genital structures in face-to-face coitus shown in longitudinal cross section.

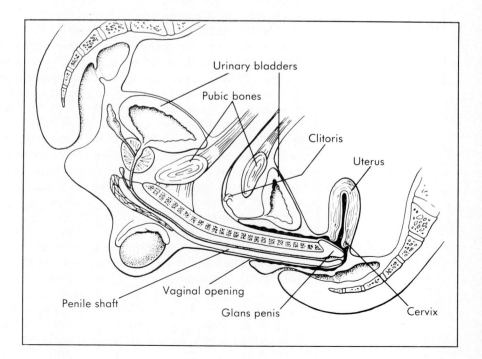

possible positions, variations on such positions, and variations on the variations of body arrangements in which human coitus can occur. This degree of variation contrasts sharply with the relatively invariant use of the rear-entry approach found among most nonhuman mammals (Ford & Beach, 1951).

The tremendous amount of attention devoted to human coital positions and approaches by marital and sex manuals is based on biological as well as psychosocial considerations. Biologically, the primary element involved in triggering orgasm in females is the stimulation received by the clitoris (Kinsey et al., 1953; Masters & Johnson, 1966), and certain coital positions offer a greater chance of clitoral stimulation than do others.

The extent to which coital positioning influences the probability of female orgasm is, however, a matter of some debate (e.g., Hite, 1976; Kinsey et al., 1953; Masters & Johnson, 1966) and will be considered in more detail later in this chapter. A second biological consideration is related to the likelihood of conception in various coital positions. For example, those positions in which the male is above the female are more conducive to conception than are female above or standing or sitting positions although neither the latter nor any other positions offer more than chance levels of contraceptive protection (Langmyhr, 1976). Yet another consideration from a biological point of view is the physical and medical condition of sexual partners. For example, during the late stages of pregnancy, some forms of the rear entry or face-to-face side positions which limit depth of vaginal penetration are often recommended (McCary, 1978).

Even though biological factors sometimes play a role in the choice and variation of coital positions, for most people psychosocial considerations are of equal or greater importance. For instance, coital positions are often varied for the sake of variety itself. As astonishing as it may seem to those who have just become sexually active, sex—like any other form of human activity—can grow somewhat monotonous, boring, and unexciting when it is routinized and ritualized in form. Under such circumstances, the novelty provided by variations in coital technique sometimes serves to renew, revitalize, and maintain enjoyment of sexual interaction (Comfort, 1972, 1974). Choice of coital techniques is also influenced in important ways by beliefs and attitudes concerning the "meanings" of various positions. For example, those whose attitudes and beliefs favor male dominance in heterosexual relationships tend to prefer coital positions in which the male is above the female. Beliefs in sexual equality are associated with frequent variation from the male superior approach (Beigel, 1953). Recent evidence, however, suggests that while such generalizations may hold at the cultural level, differences in sex roles at the individual level have negligible effects on coital position preferences. That is, individual differences in measured masculinity and femininity are unrelated to position preferences (Allgeier & Fogel, 1978).

Personality and social characteristics also play some role in determining the extent to which couples vary their positions in intercourse. Research has indicated that those who are relatively young and well educated (Hunt, 1974; Kinsey et al., 1948, 1953), sexually responsive (Griffitt, 1975), sexually liberal (Joe & Kostyla, 1975), extraverted (Eysenck, 1976), free from sex guilt (Mosher & Cross, 1971), adventuresome, nonreligious (Zuckerman, Tushup, & Finner, 1976), and nontraditional in their views of male-female relationships (Fisher, 1973) are most likely to seek and practice variety in their use of coital positions.

Although numerous possibilities exist, only a few basic positions in coitus are actually practiced with any great frequency by most people and it is these few on which the following sections concentrate. Before proceeding, however, it is appropriate to reiterate our intention to describe and discuss rather than to prescribe, recommend, or promote the use of certain coital techniques.

Face-to-Face, Male Above Positions.   Some variant of the face-to-face, male above ("missionary position") configurations shown in Figure 10–2 is the most widely used coital position at all age, educational, and socioeconomic levels in the United States and other modern societies. This was also true in the majority of primitive societies surveyed by Ford and Beach (1951). Virtually all people with any intercourse experience utilize this position at least once in a while. Kinsey and his associates (1953) reported that it was the only position assumed by 10 percent of married and 20 percent of unmarried individuals surveyed in the 1940s. The

Figure 10–2.

Some face-to-face, male-above coital positions.

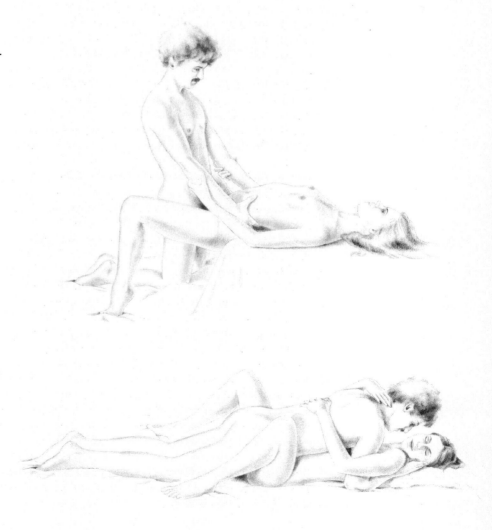

exclusive use of this position is, however, less widespread among contemporary couples (Hunt, 1974).

There are several potential advantages to the male above positions. Penetration is relatively simple and for those couples who enjoy it, male pelvic thrusting can be quite powerful, rapid, deep, and active. There is a great deal of freedom of movement possible for the man and the woman's position is a relaxing one. Furthermore, face-to-face positions (male or female above) enhance the possibility of communication through eye contact and facial gestures, which are sometimes valuable cues for a couple concerning each other's reactions and feelings. Finally, for those couples who desire pregnancy, these positions may be conducive to conception if, following ejaculation, penetration is maintained for some time and the woman remains lying on her back with her legs slightly elevated for a few minutes. This allows the sperm an extended opportunity to pass through the cervix and enter the uterus (see Figure 10–1).

Of course, the advantages for one couple or under one set of circumstances may be disadvantages for another couple or under a different set of circumstances. In male above positions the man's weight is either directly on the usually smaller woman or he must support his body with his arms. In either case, his opportunity to engage in manual caresses or stimulation of his partner's breasts, arms, face, buttocks, or clitoris is restricted. Furthermore, the woman's movement is some-what limited in these positions and, because of the possible pressure exerted on the fetus, penetration may be too deep during the later stages of pregnancy. Finally, some males find it difficult to control or delay ejaculation in this position due to the rapid buildup of relatively high levels of muscular tension, which enhance arousal and tend to hasten orgasm (Kinsey et al., 1953; Masters & Johnson, 1966).

Face-to-Face, Female Above Positions.   When other than the male above position is used, it is most frequently some variation of the face-to-face, female above positions depicted in Figure 10–3. This is true for modern (Hunt, 1974; Kinsey et al., 1953) as well as primitive societies, where the female above position is sometimes the most preferred (Ford & Beach, 1951). Kinsey and his associates (1953) reported the use of this position by nearly half of all married couples and in premarital coitus by nearly one third of all those with premarital coital experience. Continuing a trend noted in the Kinsey investigations (1953), the female above position was found by Hunt (1975) to be more widespread in the marital (75 percent) and premarital (70 percent) coitus of recent generations.

In female above positions the woman has considerably more freedom of movement than in male above positions and is able to regulate the depth of penetration (which can be maximal in this position) to suit her own comfort and desires. She can also participate in coitus more vigorously. Furthermore, when she assumes a sitting posture (see Figure 10–3) the man's hands are free to caress and stimulate her breasts, face, clitoris, buttocks, thighs, and most other parts of her body. Similarly, her own hands are free to caress the man (chest, scrotum, abdomen) as well as herself (breasts, clitoris) to heighten her own arousal and, in some cases, enhance the possibility of her reaching orgasm during penetration (Hite, 1976; Kaplan, 1974; Masters & Johnson, 1970). In addition, since less muscular tension is required of the man to maintain this position, he may find he is more able to control ejaculation.

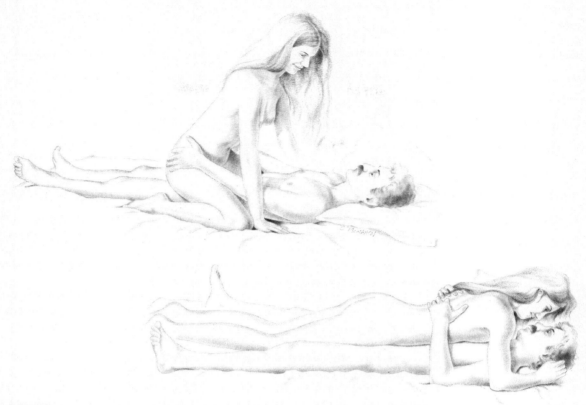

Figure 10–3.

Some face-to-face, female-above coital positions.

Among the potential disadvantages of female above positions are the restrictions they impose on male movement and ability to control pelvic thrusting and penetration. The penis may, thus, repeatedly slip from the vagina, interrupting the rhythm and pace of intercourse. While it is sometimes tempting to hastily reinsert the penis, some care should be exercised to avoid potential injury to the genitals of either or both partners (Kaplan, 1974; Masters & Johnson, 1970). Coitus in these positions is not recommended for the later stages of pregnancy since it could exert harmful pressure on the fetus. Finally, the chances of conception are lowered when female above positions are used due to the possibility of the semen and sperm seeping from the depths of the vagina (Langmyhr, 1976). This, of course, will be a disadvantage only to those wishing for conception to occur.

Face-to-Face, Side Positions. Over half of all married couples and nearly 40 percent of those who engage in premarital coitus (Hunt, 1974) at least occasionally engage in intercourse in one of the positions in which both partners are lying on their sides facing one another (Figure 10–4). Again, these percentages represent increases over those reported from the Kinsey survey (1953), when less than one

Figure 10–4.

Face-to-face, side coital positions.

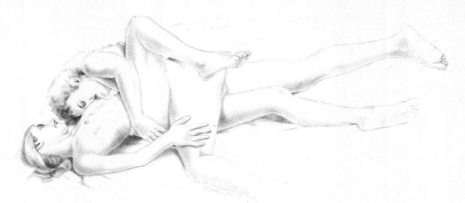

third of married couples and 20 percent of coitally experienced single couples used such positions. Even today, however, facing, side positions are more often used by relatively young (eighteen to twenty-four) than by older (fifty-five and over) couples (Hunt, 1974). While not unusual, side positions are the preferred ones in only a few societies (Ford & Beach, 1951).

In comparison with others, these are relatively comfortable and relaxing positions for both partners. Neither partner supports either his or her own weight or that of the partner, and the hands of both are free for use in caressing and stimulating (partner or self).

The pace of thrusting and depth of penetration may be controlled easily by either partner. It is often easier for a man to delay ejaculation and prolong coitus in these positions than in others because of his relative freedom from muscular tension and ability to regulate the pace of thrusting. Because of these advantages, one variant of the side positions, called the *lateral coital position*, is recommended by Masters and Johnson (1970) as an aid in overcoming ejaculatory control difficulties in males and coital orgasmic difficulties in females (see Chapter 13).

Despite the apparent advantages of face-to-face side positions, people do, on occasion, experience problems with them. Unless they first assume one of the other face-to-face orientations and then roll into side positions, some people find it difficult to effect penile-vaginal entry in these postures. Once entry is achieved, penetration depth is somewhat limited and, since both partners are in control of thrusting, it is rather easy for the penis to slip out of the vagina. In addition, neither partner is able to obtain much in the way of foot or leg leverage and when vigorous and deep thrusting is desired these positions will be somewhat unsatisfying.

Rear Vaginal Entry Positions.   Because of the posterior placement of the female genitals, the most usual coital position assumed by virtually all nonhuman mammals is one in which vaginal entry is achieved from the rear of the female (Ford & Beach, 1951). Perhaps because of the more frontal location of the human female genitals, rear vaginal entry positions are not the preferred postures in any human societies studied in any depth (Ford & Beach, 1951). Indeed, Kinsey and his colleagues (1953) reported the occasional use of such positions by only 15 percent of surveyed married couples and premaritally by only 6 percent of those with premarital coital experience. Hunt (1974), however, found that 40 percent of married couples and 37 percent of coitally experienced unmarried people surveyed in the early 1970s assumed rear entry positions for coitus (see Figure 10–5) at least occasionally, with more younger than older people doing so. This marked increase reflects the growing trend for people to seek variety in sexual expression.

In spite of their rather infrequent use, rear entry positions offer a number of benefits. The man may find the pressure of the woman's buttocks against his abdomen and thighs particularly exciting and he is able to thrust rapidly and powerfully in these positions. In addition, the man's hands are free to caress and stimulate his partner's buttocks, thighs, back, breasts, and especially clitoris thus enhancing her degree of sexual arousal and facilitating orgasm. Direct manual stimulation of the clitoris is rather difficult in most other positions due to obstacles posed by the man's body. Because of this, rear entry positions are frequently used in the treatment of female coital orgasmic difficulty where manual-clitoral stimulation by either the man or the woman is desirable (Kaplan, 1974; Masters & Johnson, 1970). Rear vaginal entry with both partners lying on their sides is a particularly relaxing position in which coitus can proceed at the leisurely pace that is often preferable during pregnancy or ill health. Finally, the "knee-chest position," which is shown at the top of Figure 10–5, is particularly conducive to conception when the woman remains in this posture for some time following ejaculation (Langmyhr, 1976).

The primary disadvantage of rear entry positions is in the attitudes of some people who regard them as demeaning and "animalistic" because of their resemblance to the usual form of coitus in animals or to positions that might be assumed

Figure 10–5.

Some rear vaginal-entry coital positions.

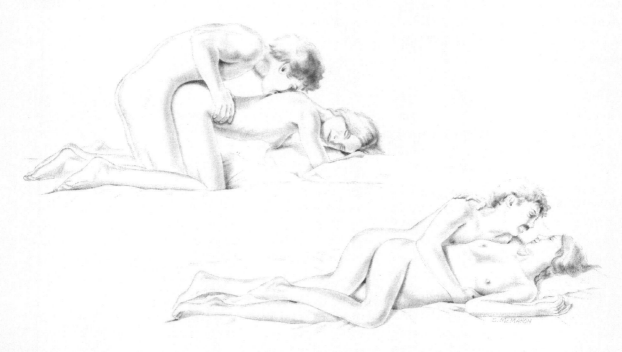

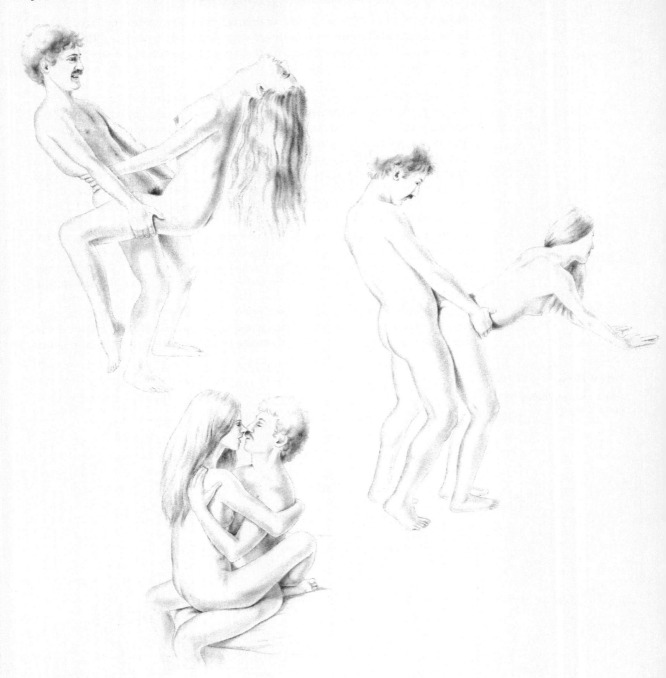

Figure 10–6.

Sitting and standing coital positions.

for anal intercourse. Generally, rear entry positions are not very suitable for obese couples, for a man with a very short penis, or when erection is not complete. Under these circumstances achieving and maintaining penetration is difficult, if not impossible.

Sitting, Standing, and Other Positions. The basic coital postures we have described are, of course, subject to endless variations. While many of them are rather minor in that they involve only slight differences in leg or arm positions, sitting and standing variations are noteworthy since they involve rather deliberate attempts at variety and cannot simply be "rolled into" (Katchadourian & Lunde, 1980). As illustrated in Figure 10–6, both face-to-face and rear vaginal entry positions are possible while sitting and standing as well as while lying prone as discussed previously. The best available estimates suggest that sitting and standing positions are sometimes used by between 10 and 25 percent of married and coitally experienced unmarried couples (Hunt, 1974; Kinsey et al., 1948, 1953).

There is little to be gained by more detailed discussion of the many possible variations in coital positions. A couple truly interested in positional variety will experience little difficulty in discovering or creating a vast repertoire of interesting and pleasurable postures and movements for intercourse. Furthermore, a number of sources exist to which people might turn for additional suggestions concerning coital techniques (e.g., Comfort, 1972, 1974; Kaplan, 1974; Masters & Johnson, 1970). As with foreplay techniques, however, it should be emphasized that there are no magical coital postures that guarantee sexual ecstasy or even pleasure and satisfaction for all people or for a given person or couple on all occasions. Indeed, as we suggested earlier, a sexual recipe that includes coital techniques that one or both partners find disgusting, immoral, painful, guilt producing, absurd, or aversive in other ways will, if followed, result in unpleasant sex.

Similarly, it must be recognized that even though many men and women enjoy and often wish for more variety in coital positions, locations, and times (Hite, 1976; Hunt, 1974; Pietropinto & Simenauer, 1977; Tavris & Sadd, 1977), variety itself offers no foolproof promise of sexual pleasure. Ritualistically varied coitus in which couples assume and switch positions "by the numbers" (1 to ?) can easily become as tedious, boring, and unexciting as that which is rigidly limited to a single position. In fact, most couples do most of their experimenting with variations in coital postures early in their relationship and then settle into a pattern in which no more than two or three positions are regularly used (Fisher, 1973; Kinsey et al., 1953). Most such people are well satisfied with their sex lives (Pietropinto & Simenauer, 1977; Tavris, 1978a; Tavris & Sadd, 1977).

For the majority of men and women alike, the origins of such satisfaction are to be found not in obsessive concerns with the mechanics of foreplay and coitus but in the shared physical and emotional pleasures that are derived from whatever sexual techniques that are employed. Whether intercourse takes place standing up in a canoe or in the missionary position in the privacy of a locked bedroom, the crucial factors involved in sexual pleasure for most people are feelings of being desired and valued as a person as well as an effective sexual partner (Pietropinto & Simenauer, 1977; Tavris & Sadd, 1977).

Coitus and Orgasm

We have characterized "complete" sexual activity episodes as consisting of at least three phases: (1) the stimulation and arousal of sexual desires, (2) performance of behaviors motivated by sexual arousal and (3) the culmination of sexual activity in orgasm. The available evidence indicates that men and women differ very little in their physiological capacities to carry sexual activity episodes through to completion in orgasm. It has long been recognized, however, that the likelihood of reaching orgasm in coitus is much lower for women than for men. Kinsey and his associates (1948, 1953) estimated that men reach orgasm in virtually all their coital contacts although more recent data indicate that at every age level small percentages of men do not reach orgasm in every coital experience (Hunt, 1974). Indeed, it is likely that almost all men at some time will not reach orgasm as a result of intercourse. Most, however, will do so most of the time (Hunt, 1974).

In contrast, several decades of research have revealed that only around half of all women reach orgasm in all or almost all of their coital experiences. Table 10–1 summarizes the findings of several studies conducted since the 1920s concerning the percentages of coital encounters in which women reach orgasm. Since various methodologies, data reporting methods, and sampling techniques are represented in these studies, they are not strictly comparable. Even so, it is clear that about one fourth of all women experience orgasms in less than half of their coital experiences with about 10 percent never reaching orgasm as a result of intercourse.

At various times in history, and as recently as the beginning of this century, it has been assumed that, in comparison with males, most females are relatively insensitive to sexual stimuli, experience little pleasure from sexual activities, and are inherently inferior in orgasmic capacities (Williams, 1977). From this perspective, low coital orgasmic rates in females are neither surprising nor a source of concern. Growing recognition that the inherent sexual capacities of women actually equal or exceed those of men (Kinsey et al., 1953; Masters & Johnson, 1966; Sherfey, 1973), and contemporary views that women have a definite "right" to and "need" for orgasm equaling that of men (Hite, 1976) have, however, produced a very real concern for the large percentage of women who experience orgasm in coitus infrequently.

As a result, in recent years a substantial amount of speculation and research has been devoted to discovering those factors associated with variations in coital orgasmic regularity among women. Such research and speculation has taken two major directions. The first has involved a search for *personal and social characteristics of women* that might act to facilitate or interfere with the occurrence of coital orgasm. We have already reviewed much of this research in Chapter 5. To summarize briefly, it is generally those women who are relatively well educated, happy, self-confident, independent, interpersonally secure, not guilty or inhibited sexually from religious or other sources, and highly sexually experienced who are most likely to experience orgasm from coitus (Fisher, 1973; Shope, 1975).

A second major line of speculation and research has focused on the *nature and circumstances of coitus itself*. As noted in Chapter 5, it is now well established (Kinsey et al., 1953; Masters & Johnson, 1966) that high levels of sexual arousal and orgasm in most females are created primarily, if not wholly, by constant direct or indirect stimulation of the clitoris and adjacent areas. As may be seen in Figure

10–1, penile-vaginal penetration offers a somewhat inefficient means by which to achieve such stimulation. Indeed, direct stimulation of the clitoral area is possible only when the male and female pubic bones and tissues are firmly pressed together. With the most usual methods of coitus involving rhythmic thrusting of the penis in and out of the vagina, direct clitoral stimulation is, at best, irregular and occurs only during full penetration.

We might expect, then, that intercourse techniques that provide the most direct and constant stimulation to the clitoral area would be most likely to produce female coital orgasm. Some support for this theory is provided by the reports of consistently orgasmic women studied by Hite (1976). For many, the most effective techniques were those in which penile-vaginal thrusting was minimized and clitoral-pubic area contact was emphasized (Hite, 1976):

How I orgasm involves being on top and moving back and forth so my clitoris rubs against the base of the penis without the penis moving in and out of the vagina. (pp. 276–277)

I have an orgasm during intercourse when I assume the 'dominant' position and rub my clitoris against his belly and pubic area. (p. 277)

Very close body contact. I enjoy it when the penis is completely inserted and when we sort of rub together more than making bouncing motions. (p. 278)

I lie on the bottom with my legs around him, then grind my pelvis and pubic areas against his. (p. 279)

In some coital positions, of course, direct contact is impossible. Masters and Johnson (1966) have shown, however, that the clitoral glans and shaft are always *indirectly* stimulated in coital thrusting by the rhythmic movements of the labia and clitoral hood, which are alternately tugged and released by the in-and-out motions of the penis. Since such stimulation is indirect, the likelihood of female orgasm might be expected to increase as the duration of penetration increases. Recent studies provide some support for this expectation. Gebhard (1966), for example, found that only around a quarter of married women were consistently able to reach orgasm when penetration lasted one minute or less. In contrast, some 50 percent of the women were consistently orgasmic in coitus lasting from one to eleven minutes and two thirds of all women reached orgasm when penetration was extended for sixteen minutes or longer. More recently, Tavris and Sadd (1977) reported that a majority of women require between five and ten minutes of penetration to reach orgasm and that, when it is extended to at least fifteen minutes, fully 85 percent of women who ever have orgasms from coitus do so. Similar findings have been reported by Fisher (1973). The importance of extended penetration and thrusting to some women is apparent in the statements of one of Hite's (1976) respondents:

My most recent steady boyfriend is the best lover I've ever had (i.e., I respond best), and I think it is because he fucks me rhythmically and continuously for long periods (e.g., half an hour to an hour). This steady rhythmical uninterrupted thrusting by him is over-all very soothing, and enables that degree of relaxation necessary for the delicate quivering response of the vaginal walls to begin. (p. 282)

Table 10–1.

Estimates of percentages of marital, premarital, extramarital, and postmarital coital encounters resulting in female orgasm.

Reported percentages of coitus resulting in orgasm have been classified as ranging from "very low" to "very high." Phrases in parentheses are terms used by various investigators to describe the percentages of coital encounters resulting in female orgasm. The numbers above those in parentheses are the percentages of women in each category.

	Coital Orgasm Rates of Women				
	Percentage with Very Low Rate	Percentage with Low Rate	Percentage with Medium Rate	Percentage with High Rate	Percentage with Very High Rate
Marital					
Hamilton (1929)[1]		21 (Sometimes)		38 (Usually or always)	
Dickinson & Beam (1931)[1]				61 (Usually)	
Kopp (1933)[1]	20 (Never)		46 (Occasionally)	34 (Usually)	
Terman (1938)[1]	8 (Never)	25 (Sometimes)		45 (Usually)	22 (Always)
Terman (1951)[1]		30 (Never or sometimes)		70 (Usually or always)	
Stone & Stone (1952)[1]	16 (Never)	43 (Rarely or occasionally)		41 (Regularly)	
Kinsey et al. (1953)	16 (None)	13 (1–29% of encounters)	13 (30–59% of encounters)	15 (60–89% of encounters)	43 (90–100% of encounters)
Gebhard (1966)	11 (None)	17 (1–39% of encounters)	11 (40–59% of encounters)	15 (60–89% of encounters)	46 (90–100% of encounters)
Athanasiou, Shaver, & Tavris (1970)[2]	20 (Never or almost never)	10 (About ¼ of encounters)	10 (About ½ of encounters)	15 (About ¾ of encounters)	45 (Almost every time)
Fisher (1973)	5 (Never)		56 (Rarely, occasionally, frequently)		39 (Always or nearly always)
Hunt (1974)	7 (None or almost none)	8 (About ¼ of encounters)	11 (About ½ of encounters)	21 (About ¾ of encounters)	53 (All or almost all)
Hite (1976)	29 (None)	22 (Rarely)			30 (Regularly; 49% *with* manual-clitoral stimulation)

	Coital Orgasm Rates of Women				
	Percentage with Very Low Rate	Percentage with Low Rate	Percentage with Medium Rate	Percentage with High Rate	Percentage with Very High Rate
Tavris & Sadd (1977)	7 (Never)	11 (Once in a while)	19 (Sometimes)		63 (Most or all encounters)
Pietropinto & Simenauer (1977) Estimated by husbands	9 (0–19% of encounters)	9 (20–39% of encounters)	23 (40–69% of encounters)	10 (70–79% of encounters)	48 (80–100% of encounters)
Tavris (1978b) Estimated by husbands	8 (Never)	23 (Sometimes)		48 (Most times)	21 (All encounters)
Premarital Kinsey et al. (1953)			50 (At least some of the time)		
Hunt (1974)			75 (More than 50% of encounters)		
Tavris & Sadd (1977)	34 (Never)	37 (Sometimes)		23 (Most of the time)	7 (Always)
Extramarital Kinsey et al. (1953)			85 (At least some of the time)		
Hunt (1974)	35 (None or almost none)	7 (About ¼ of encounters)	7 (About ½ of encounters)	12 (About ¾ of encounters)	39 (All or almost all)
Postmarital Gebhard (1971) Divorced	17 (Never)	13 (1–39% of encounters)		16 (40–89% of encounters)	55 (90–100% of encounters)
Widowed	16 (Never)	7 (1–39% of encounters)		17 (40–89% of encounters)	60 (90–100% of encounters)
Hunt (1974) Divorced/ Widowed		15 (0–75% of encounters)		85 (75%–all of encounters)	

[1]Figures cited in Kinsey et al., 1953, p. 375.   [2]Marital and nonmarital.

Without some deliberate attempts at control, however, most men will reach orgasm during coitus within two to seven minutes (Fisher, 1973; Gebhard, 1966; Kinsey et al., 1948). Recent estimates that the median duration of penetration prior to ejaculation now approaches ten minutes (Hunt, 1974) suggest that many men attempt to delay ejaculation to increase the likelihood of their partners reaching orgasm. Most men, in fact, do not consider intercourse to be fully complete unless their partners reach orgasm (Pietropinto & Simenauer, 1977) and the data of Table 10–1 suggest that female coital orgasm has become more likely in recent years as intercourse duration has increased (Hunt, 1974). As is true of foreplay, however, coital duration (or endurance) is not necessarily *the secret* to orgasm for all women (Hite, 1976, p. 297):

If intercourse lasts more than ten-fifteen minutes, it begins to irritate me and the next time I urinate I get a burning feeling.

After too long my lubrication decreases.

If the man is grinding away in a boring fashion, then I get bored.

To be sure, the importance of coital duration is a complex issue, and other data suggest that duration may not be closely related to female orgasm (Huey, Kline-Graber, & Graber, 1981).

For many women orgasm during coitus is unlikely or impossible unless the stimulation provided by penetration and thrusting is supplemented by direct manual manipulation of the clitoral area. For example, both Fisher (1973) and Hite (1976) reported higher coital orgasm rates among women whose intercourse was accompanied by simultaneous manual-clitoral stimulation supplied either by their partners or by the women themselves. Indeed, in both of these studies, a majority of women, at least sometimes, could not reach coital orgasm without such added stimulation.

In summary, all of these findings point to the conclusion that orgasm from coitus is far from automatic for most women. Related findings also suggest, however, that the probability of any given woman reaching coital orgasm may potentially be enhanced by the learning that is possible through experience. For example, among the unmarried, those women with the greatest amount of coital experience are more likely to reach orgasm in their intercourse than are those with only limited experience (Kinsey et al., 1953; Shope, 1975). Similarly, as marriage duration increases (and coital experience accumulates), there is a small but steady increase in the percentage of women who regularly reach orgasm during intercourse (Fisher, 1973; Hunt, 1974; Kinsey et al., 1953) and this increase continues through the postmarital coitus of those women whose marriages terminate due to divorce or death of the husband (Gebhard, 1971; Hunt, 1974; Table 10–1).

In addition, prior experience with orgasm itself, regardless of its origins, seems to enhance the probability of female coital orgasm. Kinsey and his fellow researchers (1953) reported that women with premarital orgasmic experience through masturbation, petting, or coitus were substantially more likely to experience coital orgasm during the first few years of their marriage than were women with no such orgasmic experience. These and similar findings (Shope, 1975) indicate that experiences that allow a woman (and her sexual partners) to learn precisely which types of stimulation are most arousing for her will tend to increase her chances of reaching orgasm during intercourse.

Because of the sometimes obsessive attention the issue of female orgasm during coitus has received in recent years, it is necessary to maintain some degree of perspective. Many women and men view lack of female coital orgasm as "failure," with the almost inevitable result that blame for the perceived failure is attributed to one or both partners. When the woman is blamed for failure (by herself or her partner), the term "frigid" is often used, even though its "definition" has changed somewhat over the years:

In the old days a "frigid" woman was a woman who hated sex and wouldn't have anything of it, she was probably truly "not sexy." Now a woman who doesn't have orgasms regularly, but who may love sex, still often fears she is "frigid": not sexy. (Cobrun, 1978, p. 229)

An alternate view holds the man responsible for failure. This is, perhaps, best epitomized by a frequently used statement of advice columnist Ann Landers that "there are no frigid women, only clumsy men."

Little is to be gained by such extreme views. Orgasm cannot be taken as the sole criterion of either female or male satisfaction from coitus (Waterman & Chiauzzi, 1982). In spite of the seemingly low rates of female coital orgasm discussed above, it is clear that the vast majority of both women and men derive a great deal of pleasure and satisfaction from intercourse (Hite, 1976; Hunt, 1974; Tavris & Sadd, 1977). To be sure, satisfaction may be heightened when both partners reach orgasm, but it must be recognized that, for most women, coitus is simply not the most effective way to do so. The intensely pleasurable satisfaction possible through orgasm is, however, "needed" by women as much as by men and may as legitimately be achieved through noncoital as through coital stimulation.

The Social Context of Coitus

The traditional moral, religious, ethical, and legal codes of most contemporary societies impose limitations on the social contexts within which coitus is permissible. According to these codes, whose origins are somewhat obscure, it is only within marriage that coitus is fully acceptable. Yet in reality, intercourse does occur and presumably always has occurred outside of marriage (Kinsey et al., 1948, 1953). Thus, with whom one has coitus has been, is, and promises to remain an issue of some psychosocial and moral significance at the individual as well as at the societal level. This, of course, does not mean that the quality of coitus should be evaluated in terms of whether or not the partners are married. As previously noted, coitus is just one among many avenues to sexual expression and pleasure. In the remaining sections of this chapter we will briefly consider some of the research relevant to coitus as it occurs in various types of partnerships.

Premarital Coitus.   The formal standard regarding premarital coitus in our society has traditionally been one that demands abstinence. At the same time, however, it is clear that adherence to such a strict code has never been and probably never will be complete (Reiss, 1967). Indeed, the majority of available evidence reveals a steadily increasing degree of both attitudinal and behavioral permissiveness concerning premarital coitus since at least the 1920s (Hunt, 1974; Kinsey et al., 1953; Reiss, 1967). In national samples of adults surveyed in the late '30s and again in the late '50s only 22 percent approved of premarital coitus for both males and females, with an additional 8 percent offering approval for males only (Hunt, 1974). This low approval rate held through the early sixties (Reiss, 1967), increased somewhat to 32 percent in 1968, but rose dramatically in 1973 when over half of a sample of American adults approved of premarital intercourse (Hunt, 1974).

In 1967 Reiss noted the predominance of two major premarital coital standards. According to the *double standard* coitus (or other sexual behavior) is acceptable for one sex (usually male) but unacceptable for the other. A second, the *permissiveness with affection standard*, defines premarital intercourse as more acceptable when an affectionate or loving relationship exists than when sexual partners do not feel particularly affectionate toward one another. The degree to which each of these standards operated during the early '60s, late '60s, and early to mid '70s is illustrated by the data summarized in Table 10–2. At least three features of these data are of interest. First, fairly dramatic changes in the rates of approval of premarital intercourse occurred between the early and late 1960s with less dramatic but still steady increases into the 1970s. Second, the standards during all three time periods were more permissive for males than for females. At the same time, however, it is clear that the double standard is weakening with time and standards for females are approaching those for males (Bauman & Wilson, 1976; Curran, 1977; Hunt, 1974; Singh, 1980). Third, the predominant standard for both sexes is still one of permissiveness within an affectionate relationship even though being engaged and in love are now viewed as equally acceptable contexts for premarital coitus.

These figures are, of course, only averages and there are wide differences among people in their premarital coital permissiveness. Most permissive are those

Table 10–2.

Percentage approval by college students of premarital coitus for males and females at various levels of affection in the early 1960s, late 1960s, and early to mid-1970s.

	Percentage Approving Premarital Coitus		
Level of Affection	Early 1960s (1)	Late 1960s (2)	Early and Mid-1970s (3)
For males			
No strong affection for partner	21	51	50
Strong affection for partner	37	65	73
In love with partner	48	76	84
Engaged to partner	52	76	85
For females			
No strong affection	11	28	38
Strong affection	27	50	70
In love	39	70	75
Engaged	44	70	75

SOURCE: Data in Column 1 from Reiss, 1967; in Column 2 combined from Bauman & Wilson, 1976, and Kaats & Davis, 1970; in Column 3 combined from Bauman & Wilson, 1976, and Hunt, 1974.

Table 10–3.

Percentages of young people with premarital coital experience.
Surveys since the Kinsey studies reveal that intercourse prior to marriage has become more prevalent among contemporary American youth.

		Age												Ever Before Marriage
	Sex	15	16	17	18	19	20	21	22	23	24	25	30	
Kinsey et al. (1948)[1]	M	19	28	35	42	48	53	57	61	64	66	71	78	82
Kinsey et al. (1953)[2]	F	3	5	9	14	17	20	25	29	30	32	33	44	50
Wagner et al. (1973)	M		15											
	F		11											
Udry et al. (1974)	M						—							
	F						45							
College students[3]	M				Ages 18–21 = 62									
	F				Ages 18–21 = 37									
Athanasiou et al. (1970)	M													80
	F													78
Simon et al. (1972)	M		—		—									
	F	10		27	38									
Vener & Stewart (1974)	M	38	38	34										
	F	24	31	35										
Hunt (1974)	M			50–75										84–95
	F			20–33								50–75		31–81
College students[4]	M				Ages 18–21 = 67									
	F				Ages 18–21 = 55									
Zelnik & Kantner (1977)	M	—	—	—	—	—								
	F	14	23	36	44	49								
Tavris & Sadd (1977)	M													—
	F													80
Tavris (1978b)	M													90
	F													—

[1]Based on uncorrected data calculated from Kinsey et al. (1948).
[2]Data from Kinsey et al. (1953).
[3]Average figures calculated from data reported in Bauman & Wilson (1974); Christensen & Gregg (1970); D'Augelli & Cross (1975); Diamant (1970); Finger (1975); Kaats & Davis (1970); Lewis (1973); Lewis & Burr (1975); Luckey & Nass (1969); Robinson, King, & Balswick (1972); Simon, Berger, & Gagnon (1972); Touhey (1971); and Zuckerman (1973). Data collected between 1965 and 1969.
[4]Average figures calculated from data reported in Abramson (1973); Arafat & Yorburg (1973); Bauman & Wilson (1974); Curran (1977); Curran, Neff, & Lippold (1973); Finger (1975); Griffitt (1975); Istvan & Griffitt (1980); Jackson & Potkay (1973); Jessor & Jessor (1975); King & Sobel (1975); and Zuckerman, Tushup, & Finner (1976). Data collected from 1970 on.

who are male, relatively young, well educated, nonreligious, extraverted, and politically and socially liberal, and those who have sexually permissive parents (Alston & Tucker, 1973; Bauman & Wilson, 1976; Hunt, 1974; Levitt & Klassen, 1973; Zuckerman et al., 1976).

Prior to the appearance of the Kinsey surveys in the late 1940s and early 1950s it was generally assumed that the vast majority of Americans (particularly females) remained virgins until the time of marriage (Griffitt, 1977). The Kinsey data for males (1948) and for females (1953), however, revealed a startlingly different picture. As shown in Table 10–3 one fifth of all surveyed white females and over one half of all white males who were unmarried at the age of twenty had experienced intercourse at least once. These percentages steadily increased with age for both sexes so that, as Table 10–3 indicates, of those who remained unmarried the longest, 50 percent of females and over 80 percent of males ultimately had premarital intercourse. It is apparent, however, that substantially larger percentages of females and slightly larger percentages of males now report premarital intercourse than at the time of the Kinsey surveys.

A number of personal and social characteristics seem to predict not only people's attitudes toward premarital coitus but also how likely they are to have premarital coital experiences. For both males and females, the likelihood of premarital coitus is generally higher among those who are least religious (Hunt, 1974; Kinsey et al., 1948, 1953; Simon et al., 1972; Tavris & Sadd, 1977), those who are most unconventional and somewhat alienated from parents and traditional institutions (Arafat & Yorburg, 1973; Joe & Kostyla, 1975; Simon et al., 1972; Vener & Stewart, 1974), and those who live in large urban centers (Kinsey et al., 1948, 1953). Furthermore, those who date frequently and report having been "in love" (Kaats & Davis, 1970; Simon et al., 1972), are extraverted (Zuckerman et al., 1976), and are relatively low in sex-related guilt (Mosher & Cross, 1971) are also likely to engage in premarital intercourse.

Although the prevalence of premarital coitus has clearly undergone rather dramatic changes in the last several years, the nature of the partnerships in which it occurs has changed very little. For example, the number of premarital coital partners for females shown in Table 10–4 has remained remarkably stable over more than a quarter of a century. Most married women with premarital intercourse experience have only one coital partner prior to marriage and that one partner is most often a man they subsequently marry. Kinsey et al. (1953) found that 46 percent of all married women with premarital coital experience had had intercourse only with their future husband, 41 percent with their future husband as well as other men, and 13 percent with other men but not with their future husband. Comparable figures of 51 percent, 43 percent, and 6 percent, respectively, were obtained in the more recent study by Hunt (1974).

Even though detailed data concerning males are relatively scarce, it is, nevertheless, clear that those with premarital coital experience have more partners than do females. Recent estimates, for example, suggest that the median number of partners for men is somewhere between three and six (Athanasiou et al., 1970; Hunt, 1974; Tavris, 1978b). For the most part, however, men's as well as women's partners in premarital intercourse are those who are loved or toward whom some degree of affection is felt (Hunt, 1974; Lewis & Burr, 1975; Reiss, 1968).

In spite of increased liberalization in premarital coital attitudes and behaviors, the first intercourse experience for many is not an ecstatically joyous occasion

Table 10–4.

Married and unmarried females with any premarital coital experience.

Number of Premarital Intercourse Partners	Kinsey et al. (1953)	Tavris & Sadd (1977)	Zelnik & Kantner (1977)
1	53%	51%	50%
2–5	34	34	40
6 or more	13	15	10

(Eastman, 1972; Hunt, 1974; Schaefer, 1973). Hunt (1974), for example, reported that 20 percent of all men regarded their first coitus in indifferent or unpleasant terms while over half of all females felt that it was neutral or unpleasant. Over a third of the males and nearly two thirds of the females reported at least some regret following their initial experience. Similar figures are reported by Eastman (1972), who, like Hunt (1974), found that the primary sources of concern and regret were fears of pregnancy, guilt and uneasiness concerning the morality of the experience, and fears of discovery by parents and peers. As with other forms of sexual intimacy, however, repeated experience seems to dull the sting of guilt, replacing it with enjoyment and more confident and enthusiastic participation (Kinsey et al., 1953; Reiss, 1967). Those who are most likely to continue feeling guilty or regretful are, not surprisingly, those who are highly religious (Hunt, 1974) or whose attitudes concerning the acceptability of premarital intercourse are strongly at odds with their actual behavior (Christensen & Gregg, 1970). The majority of men and women, however, experience no long-lasting regret concerning their premarital experiences (Kinsey et al., 1953).

What are the effects of premarital coital experience on marital adjustment? This question and the answer(s) to it are among the more hotly debated but inadequately researched issues concerning premarital intercourse. In spite of the paucity of relevant evidence, many "experts" have shown no lack of willingness to offer answers based on little more than speculation and common sense argument (see Lief, 1975, pp. 242–248, and Scoresby, 1972, for a variety of opinions). Realistically, however, it is an extremely difficult question to answer because marital adjustment is not easily defined and because, if there are any relationships between premarital coital experience and marital adjustment, they are undoubtedly complex.

Some relevant data do exist, though, and we will briefly summarize them here. As noted, the 1953 Kinsey study found that women with premarital coital experience *with orgasm* were more likely to reach orgasm in their marital coitus than were women without such experience. Among other things, this finding suggests that premarital coitus which leads to orgasm provides a learning opportunity for the enhancement of coital orgasm in marriage. Even though orgasm in coitus is far from a perfect indicant of sexual satisfaction, it thus seems possible that premarital intercourse experiences might be of benefit for some women. Yet the same study (Kinsey et al., 1953) revealed a potentially negative consequence of premarital coitus. Those women who engaged in premarital intercourse *without orgasm*, it was found, were less likely to reach orgasm in marital coitus than women who remained virginal until marriage. Thus, premarital coitus itself seems to have little effect on marital coital orgasm. The crucial factor is whether or not that premarital intercourse leads to orgasm.

At least three studies suggest the possibility of a very weak negative effect of premarital coital experience on subsequent marital happiness. These studies suggest that those with many premarital coital partners and whose first experience occurs quite early (before age fifteen) and is with someone other than their future spouse describe their marital lives as somewhat unhappy (Athanasiou & Sarkin, 1974; Shope & Broderick, 1969; Tavris & Sadd, 1977). Other studies (Ard, 1974), however, report no connection between premarital coitus and marital satisfaction. It seems very much an individual matter whether premarital intercourse has positive, negative, mixed, or no effects on marital satisfaction.

Singles and Coitus.   The term premarital coitus is a bit imprecise and value laden. It implies that partners who engage in coitus ultimately will (or should) marry each other or someone else. Even though between 85 and 90 percent of Americans marry (usually for the first time between the ages of twenty-one and twenty-five), the appropriateness of the term for those who do not marry or marry at later ages is questionable and perhaps misleading.

Little is known about the sexual lives of those people who remain unmarried in their late twenties and later. On the one hand, there is the traditional stereotype of singles as lonely seekers of marital partners. On the other is the media-popularized image of the swinging singles who have access to an endless supply of sexual partners through singles bars and apartment complexes. Undoubtedly, the "truth" for the majority of single men and women lies between these extremes. Though many singles actively seek relatively permanent intimate relationships, many also value the opportunity for varied sexual experience, independence, and alternative relationships provided by single living (Stein, 1975). Ultimately, however, most people do marry and much of what is studied about coitus is that which occurs in marriage.

Marital Coitus.   Because marriage is the only fully acceptable context for intercourse in most contemporary societies, virtually all marital partners at least occasionally have or have had coitus with one another. Consequently, research questions concerning marital coitus focus not on the percentages of married individuals who *ever* have intercourse but primarily on the percentages of people in different age brackets who do so and how often they do so.

A popular adage concerning marital sex suggests rather dramatic changes in the incidence and frequency of coitus as marriages progress:

Starting on your wedding night and continuing through the first year of marriage, put one bean in a jar every time you have intercourse. Starting with the beginning of your second year of marriage, take one bean out of the jar every time you have intercourse. When you die there will still be some beans left in the jar.

While it is unlikely that many have ever actually tested this prediction, there is evidence that, as marriages increase in duration, both the percentages of men and women who remain coitally active and the frequencies with which they have intercourse decline. For example, Kinsey and his associates (1948, 1953) found that up to the age of forty virtually all married men (99 percent) and women (98 percent) continued to have intercourse at least occasionally with their spouses. Beyond forty, however, there was a tendency for the percentages of men and women who remained coitally active to decline so that by the age of sixty some 6 percent of men and nearly 20 percent of women had discontinued marital intercourse. Other data suggest that by age sixty-five, 20 percent of all men and 40 percent of all women are coitally inactive in their marriages, with the percentages increasing to 24 percent of men and nearly 50 percent of women by the age of seventy (Pfeiffer, Verwoerdt, & Davis, 1972). The primary reason that fewer married women than married men at these ages are coitally active is that in most marriages the husband is older than the wife. For example, a woman of sixty may be married to a man of sixty-five.

Figure 10–7.

Average frequencies of marital coitus per week between the ages of 16 and 60.

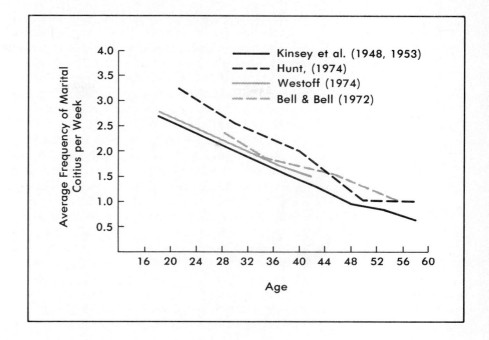

Even among those married people who remain coitally active in their later years, most early studies found declines in the frequency with which they have intercourse. As shown in Figure 10–7, average rates of marital intercourse prior to the age of thirty have been reported as twice the rates for coitally active couples who are in their late fifties. A more recent study, however, suggests that the declines may not be as great as those earlier studies have indicated (Weiler, 1981).

There are at least two possible explanations for the steeper declines reported in earlier studies. First is that early studies used what is called a cross-sectional methodology in which the couples studied at any given age are different couples from those studied at another age. The differences in coital frequencies at different ages could thus be due to actual declines with age or to the fact that different generations of people reared in different sexual climates engage in different frequencies of marital coitus. That is, sixty-year-old couples studied in 1970 were born in 1910 while twenty-year-old couples were born in 1950. Sexual attitudes, beliefs, and practices differed substantially in the eras in which these two age groups grew up. In contrast, the more recent study (Weiler, 1981) used a longitudinal method in which the same couples were studied at various ages and the reported declines were less. Thus, people born in 1910 were compared with themselves as they grew older and they reported relatively little decline in coital frequency with age. In short, the different findings could be due to the use of different study methods. The second possible explanation is that there actually is a trend for contemporary married couples to remain more coitally active than was true in the past. Both explanations are probably true to some extent.

It should be emphasized that these figures represent average frequencies and that there are wide variations among people in terms of coital frequency. For example, average rates ranging from zero to over twenty-nine coital contacts per week were reported by the Kinsey (1953) respondents. Such variations in marital coital frequency as well as the declines with age illustrated in Figure 10–7 are, of course, determined by a number of factors. Among the factors identified as associated with low frequencies of marital coitus are marital unhappiness and conflict (Edwards & Booth, 1974; Tavris & Sadd, 1977), large numbers of children (James, 1974), and the use of relatively ineffective or no contraceptive practices among those wishing to avoid pregnancy (Westoff, 1974).

But, by and large, the most important determinants of marital coital rates are related to the desires and capacities of husbands rather than wives. Several studies, for instance, have suggested that age-related declines in intercourse frequencies are due more to declining interest and sexual responsivity in men than in women (James, 1974; Kinsey et al., 1953; Masters & Johnson, 1966; Pfeiffer et al., 1972) and both husbands and wives tend to attribute cessation of marital intercourse more to the husband than to the wife (Pfeiffer et al., 1972). This is, in part, due to differences in the rates of decline in sexual response capacities among men and women. That is, erectile and ejaculatory capacities in men begin a rather steady decline beyond the age of thirty-five (Solnick & Birren, 1977) until at seventy-five nearly half of all men are at least occasionally unable to achieve erection (Kinsey et al., 1948). In contrast, female erotic responsiveness shows no such sharp decline with age but gradually diminishes with advancing years (Kinsey et al., 1953; Masters & Johnson, 1966). One result of these differences is that in the early years of marriage many men wish for higher frequencies of intercourse and in the later years of marriage many women prefer to have more intercourse than they actually have (Rubin, 1965).

Intercourse need not, however, disappear in marriage simply due to the advancing age of the married couple. Physiologically, most men and women remain capable of sexual responses in their later years although such responses may be slower in coming and less intense than when they were younger. Declines in sexual activity with age most often result from boredom, preoccupation with nonsexual matters, and culturally supported attitudes that sex is somehow unseemly in older persons (Griffitt, 1981). Those who establish regular and vigorous patterns of sexual activity in their early years and maintain such patterns during middle age are likely to continue to enjoy active sexual lives well into their seventies or even nineties (Kinsey et al., 1948, 1953; Masters & Johnson, 1966). In addition, such people are more likely than the sexually inactive to regard their marital relationships as happy and satisfying (Tavris, 1978a, b; Tavris & Sadd, 1977).

Extramarital Coitus.   Among the most restrictive sexual codes in contemporary societies are those condemning intercourse between a married man or woman and someone other than his or her spouse. Traditionally, however, sanctions against extramarital coitus have been more stringently applied to females than to males, presumably due to the historic practice of granting husbands property rights to their wives at the time of marriage (Kinsey et al., 1948).

In spite of more than a decade of public testimonials proclaiming the impending demise of norms of sexual exclusivity in marriage, the available evidence

Older couples who enjoy an active physical relationship are more likely to consider their marriage a happy and fulfilling one.

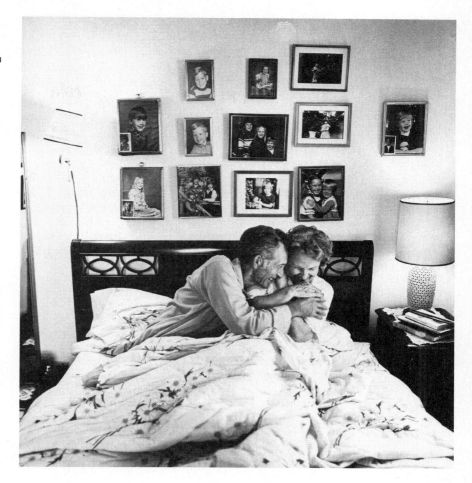

indicates that the attitudes of most contemporary Americans are firmly against extramarital intercourse (Hunt, 1974). For example, large-scale national surveys conducted in the 1970s show that upwards of 80 percent of all males and females view extramarital intercourse as wrong (Levitt & Klassen, 1973; Snyder & Spreitzer, 1976). Nearly half of all respondents in one survey (Levitt & Klassen, 1973) favor legal punishment (including the possibility of imprisonment) for those who engage in extramarital coitus. Predictably, those who are relatively young, male, well educated, nonreligious, and otherwise liberal are least opposed to extramarital intercourse (Levitt & Klassen, 1973; Snyder & Spreitzer, 1976).

Thus, despite the persuasive publicity, it seems clear that attitudinal norms of sexual fidelity have not been abandoned in recent years. Similarly, the available evidence indicates that there has been little in the way of change in extramarital coital behavior since the publication of the Kinsey (1948, 1953) findings. Kinsey and his associates (1948) estimated that under the age of twenty-five about a fourth (26 percent) of married males had at least one extramarital coital experience and that about 50 percent eventually have intercourse with someone other than their

RESEARCH HIGHLIGHT

Equity and Extramarital Coitus

One of the most stable and predictable findings in research concerning extramarital coitus is that it is most widespread and frequent among those who are unhappy or dissatisfied with their marriages. There are, of course, many sources of possible distress in marriage and many possible ways of dealing with distress when it occurs.

In recent years, social psychologists have formalized what is referred to as equity theory (Walster, Walster, & Berscheid, 1978) as a general framework for understanding sources of distress and reactions to distress in interpersonal relationships. While there are several formal propositions to equity theory, one basic assumption is that in all relationships each person contributes something of value (incurs a "cost") and receives something of value ("reward"). The relative balance of costs incurred and rewards received determines his or her perception of how equitable the relationship is. When an individual's costs (inputs) are roughly equal to his or her rewards (outcomes) the relationship is perceived as equitable. When one

person's inputs far exceed his or her outcomes, the relationship is referred to as inequitable, with one person deprived (having inputs that exceed outcomes) and the other person overbenefited (having outcomes that exceed inputs). According to the theory, inequitable relationships are distressing to the overbenefited as well as to the deprived partner. For the overbenefited, distress results from mild guilt that arises from the feeling of not contributing his or her share as well as from fear that the favored position will be lost. The deprived partner feels greater distress due to anger or resentment that he or she is not getting all that is deserved from the relationship. When people perceive that their relationships are inequitable, they attempt to eliminate the resultant distress by restoring equity.

Elaine Walster, Jane Traupmann, and William Walster (1978) suggested that, in inequitable marriage relationships, one way a person who perceives himself or herself as deprived might attempt to restore equity is through engaging in extramarital intercourse. They suggested that the

deprived partner, resenting the fact that he or she is already contributing more than his or her share to the relationship, would feel that his or her partner should be tolerant of the deprived partner's extramarital affairs but refrain from creating further inequity by having any of his or her own. Extramarital intercourse would thus be a vehicle by which equity could be restored to the marriage and should be more likely in deprived than in either overbenefited partners or those who perceive their marriages as equitable.

In order to test these ideas, the authors analyzed data from a large-scale *Psychology Today* study (Berscheid et al., 1973) in which couples were asked to indicate, on a global rating measure, how desirable their partner was in comparison with themselves. Those who rated their partners as less desirable as a mate than themselves were classified as deprived; those who saw their partners as more desirable were considered overbenefited; those who saw themselves and their mates as equal in desirability were classified as

being in equitable relationships. The respondents were then asked two questions: how long in their relationship they had waited before engaging in extramarital intercourse and how many extramarital intercourse partners they had had. Answers to these questions were considered indicants of their eagerness to engage in extramarital intercourse.

The researchers found that, in fact, those who perceived themselves as deprived in their relationships were substantially more prone to extramarital affairs than were the overbenefited and those in equitable marriages. That is, the deprived were more likely to have extramarital affairs, to begin these affairs sooner in their marriages, and to have more extramarital partners than were the overbenefited or the equitably treated. These findings strongly suggest that marital and sexual dissatisfaction may lead to extramarital intercourse because such intercourse is perceived as "deserved" by the most dissatisfied and deprived mate in the marriage.

wives while they are married. Strikingly similar figures are reported by Hunt (1974), who found that 32 percent of married males had extramarital experience by age twenty-four and estimated that ultimately 50 percent of males would have some experience during their marriages. Comparable figures for males were reported by other researchers (Athanasiou et al., 1970; Pietropinto & Simenauer, 1977). Thus, it seems clear that there has been no dramatic increase in the prevalence of extramarital coitus among males within the past two decades.

The changes that have occurred in extramarital coital rates since the Kinsey surveys are, for the most part, confined to women. Kinsey and his associates (1953) found that by the age of twenty-five less than 10 percent of married women had had extramarital intercourse and that only between 20 and 26 percent ever did so. In contrast, Hunt (1974) reported a 24 percent rate for women up to twenty-four years of age with little increase beyond that age. Similarly, other studies in the 1970s have reported female extramarital coital incidences of between 25 and 30 percent (Bell, Turner, & Rosen, 1974; Tavris & Sadd, 1977). In short, among younger females (up to age twenty-five) extramarital coital rates have increased dramatically and now approach those for males at this age. Currently, taking all age groups into account, however, nearly twice as many men as women have extramarital intercourse.

Who are those people most likely to engage in extramarital intercourse? Among males and females alike, those who are relatively nonreligious are more probable than their devout counterparts to have extramarital affairs (Athanasiou et al., 1970; Hunt, 1974; Kinsey et al., 1948, 1953; Tavris & Sadd, 1977). This is, of course, not too surprising since all major religions severely condemn adultery. Further, as we might expect, extramarital coitus is most likely among those with sexually liberal attitudes and extensive premarital coital experience (Athanasiou & Sarkin, 1974; Athanasiou et al., 1970; Kinsey et al., 1953; Reiss, Anderson, & Sponaugle, 1980).

One of the more obvious, but nevertheless important, reasons men and women venture into extramarital coital relationships is dissatisfaction with the sexual, emotional, or other elements of their marriages. These are individuals who are generally bored and unhappy with many aspects of their marriages (Bell et al., 1975; Hunt, 1969) and are particularly dissatisfied with the frequency or quality of their marital sex (Bell et al., 1975; Hunt, 1974; Tavris, 1978b; Tavris & Sadd, 1977). In general, those who feel that they are putting more into a marriage than they are getting out of it (see Research Highlight) are more likely to seek extramarital relationships than those whose rewards and costs are more evenly balanced (Edwards, 1973; Edwards & Booth, 1974; Walster, Traupmann, & Walster, 1978).

But not all people who have extramarital intercourse are unhappy in their marriages. Indeed, some are quite satisfied (Hunt, 1974; Tavris & Sadd, 1977) but seek an extra degree of variety and excitement through coitus with others. Whether happily married and seeking variety or reacting to an unhappy marriage, most people avoid extramarital promiscuity and publicly flaunting their extramarital coital experiences. Most women's experiences are confined to one partner and around a third have between two and five partners (Hunt, 1974; Kinsey et al., 1953; Tavris & Sadd, 1977) while men who engage in extramarital coitus typically have two to three partners (Athanasiou et al., 1970; Pietropinto & Simenauer, 1977). Very small minorities of either sex have more than ten extramarital partners (Kinsey et al., 1953; Tavris, 1978b; Tavris & Sadd, 1977).

Even though most extramarital coitus is carried out with the intent to maintain secrecy, discovery occurs in from 20 to 40 percent of the cases (Hunt, 1974; Kinsey et al., 1953). Discovery is often a precipitating factor in divorce, particularly when a man discovers his wife involved with other men (Hunt, 1974; Kinsey et al., 1953). Because there are the added elements of fear of discovery and excitement associated with engaging in forbidden behavior, it is widely thought that extramarital intercourse provides ecstatic pleasures and joys that far surpass those available in marital sex. For some people this seems to be true, but most men and women with extramarital coital experience regard these experiences as somewhat less pleasurable than their marital coitus. For many, the fears, the dangers, and unfamiliarity with the extramarital partners detract from the sensuous pleasures they anticipate from extramarital intercourse.

This brief discussion has been limited to the most common form of extramarital coitus in our society—that which is clandestine or kept secret from others, particularly the uninvolved spouse. There are, however, other arrangements in which extramarital coitus occurs with the partial or full consent and knowledge of both marital partners. Among such arrangements are those referred to as "swinging" (mate swapping), open marriages in which each spouse is permitted an occasional "affair," and extended, or group, marriages in which several men and women live together as a single marital unit with shared sexual privileges. Despite the widespread public fascination with such activities, most data indicate that less than 5 percent of all men and women ever participate in such exchanges (Bartell, 1971; Hunt, 1974; Spanier & Cole, 1975). Because of the relative rarity of such activities, interested readers are referred to Bartell (1971) for a detailed discussion of "swinging," to O'Neill and O'Neill (1972) for information concerning "open marriages," and to Constantine and Constantine (1973) for a consideration of "group marriage."

Postmarital Coitus. At any given time in the United States approximately 5 percent of the population over the age of eighteen are divorced or separated and another 5 percent are single by virtue of being widowed. Of the widowed, roughly 90 percent are female. Very little is known, however, about the sex lives of the previously married people who compose this 10 percent of our adult population. Most of the available evidence concerns the coital activities of those who are divorced.

The divorce rate in the United States more than doubled between 1966 and 1981 so that in 1981 there was one divorce granted for every two marriages performed (*"Births, Marriages, Divorces,"* March 30, 1982). In more familiar terms, there were 2,438,000 marriages and 1,219,000 divorces during 1981. Stereotypes of the sex-starved divorced woman who is easy sexual prey and of the wildly libidinous and promiscuous divorced man are well known. But what are the postmarital coital lives of such people actually like? There is little doubt that divorced people of both sexes do lead reasonably active sex lives. Hunt (1974), for example, found that 100 percent of all divorced men had had coitus at least once during the year preceding the survey. On the average these men had intercourse twice a week and eight different partners during the year. Most men (85 percent) had begun postmarital coital activity within the first year after their divorce and 90 percent of them reported that they found such intercourse very pleasurable.

Among divorced women, 90 percent had been coitally active within the year preceding the survey at a median frequency of twice a week and the average woman had had intercourse with four different men during the year. Most of the divorced women (85 percent, as in the case of divorced men) had begun post-marital coitus within the first year following their divorce and the vast majority reported enjoying their intercourse very much, with 80 percent reaching orgasm in 75 percent of their coital contacts (Hunt, 1974). As with married women, both the percentage of divorced women who remain coitally active and the frequency with which they have intercourse steadily declines as they grow older (Gebhard, 1971; Kinsey et al., 1953). The same is, of course, true for divorced men (Kinsey et al., 1948). While these data seem to reinforce the image of divorced persons as happy, carefree, hedonists, it should be emphasized that most eventually tire of their single lives and nearly 80 percent choose to remarry (Katchadourian & Lunde, 1980).

Those who become single due to the death of a spouse find themselves in a different social and emotional situation than do the divorced. Their single status usually has not been preceded by the period of relative sexual deprivation and marital conflict which characterizes the waning months or years of marriages which terminate in divorce. They often retain strong emotional ties to the memory of the deceased spouse, are pressured from relatives and children to remain "faithful" to this memory, and observe a "respectable" period of mourning during which new emotional and sexual relationships are postponed temporarily or permanently. Thus, it is not surprising that in comparison with divorced women, fewer widowed women engage in coitus following the end of their marriages (Gebhard, 1971). Those who do resume coital activity before or without remarrying wait longer than the divorced and do so less frequently. Ultimately, however, nearly half of all widowed women do have intercourse, enjoy it, and reach orgasm in it as often or more often than they did with their husbands (Gebhard, 1971).

No comparable data are available concerning the postmarital intercourse of widowed men. In line with other sex differences, however, we would expect that in comparison with women a higher percentage of widowed men would engage in intercourse, would begin sooner following the spouse's death, and would do so more frequently. It should be clear that substantially more needs to be known about the sexual lives and problems of the divorced and widowed.

SUMMARY

Coitus is a form of heterosexual expression in which male and female genitals are united through the insertion of a penis into a vagina. Before coitus, most people engage in a period of "foreplay" involving various petting activities that intensify both subjective and physiological levels of erotic arousal as well as help create an atmosphere which is conducive to intimate sexual interaction. The average duration of foreplay is between ten and fifteen minutes, although some couples may devote as little as one minute or up to several hours to petting prior to intercourse.

The most common sequence of foreplay activities begins with general bodily contacts, leading to kissing, manual and oral contact with the female breasts, manual and perhaps oral fondling of the genitals, followed by coitus. Most couples utilize kissing, manual breast contact, and manual-genital stimulation as part of their foreplay repertoire, although oral contact with the breasts and oral-genital stimulation are somewhat less common.

Coitus is a relatively simple act but one that may be accomplished in a variety of ways and that is of tremendous significance to most people. The most common position for intercourse for Americans is one in which the couple lies face to face with the man above the woman. Increasing numbers of couples are now using positions in which the female is above the male. Facing side-by-side positions are used by nearly half of all single couples and over half of all married couples at least once in a while. Rear vaginal entry positions are used by less than half of married and unmarried coital partners. More and more people are now engaging in intercourse while standing and sitting in various positions.

Although most men reach orgasm in almost all their coitus, various estimates suggest that nearly one fourth of all women do so less than half the time and about one tenth never reach orgasm during intercourse. It appears that the degree of clitoral area stimulation that occurs in coitus is the most important determinant of whether or not most women reach orgasm. For many women direct manual-clitoral stimulation is necessary for orgasm to occur during intercourse.

Although coitus is fully approved only within marriage, it often occurs in premarital, extramarital, and postmarital social contexts as well. Attitudes toward premarital coitus have become increasingly permissive during the last two decades, particularly among the young, well educated, and liberal. In addition, the available evidence suggests that in the late 1960s the percentage of never married young people having intercourse began a dramatic rise such that now by the middle of the college years nearly two thirds of all males and around half of all college females will have experienced premarital coitus. Ultimately, nearly 80 percent of both sexes have intercourse sometime before they marry.

During the early years of marriage virtually all men and women at least occasionally have intercourse with their mates but the percentages of married men and women who remain coitally active steadily decrease until around the age of seventy nearly one fourth of all men and one half of all women have ceased marital intercourse. During their early twenties coitally active married couples have intercourse an average of two to three times per week, a frequency which steadily declines with age to an average of around once a week for coitally active couples in their fifties.

Extramarital intercourse is more prevalent among men than among women although recent studies indicate that as many young (under age twenty-five) married women have extramarital "affairs" as do husbands in the same age range. Ultimately, however, more men (nearly half) than women (one fourth) engage in extramarital coitus at some time during their marriages.

Virtually all men and women whose marriages terminate in divorce continue to be coitally active postmaritally. As with premarital and extramarital coitus, men are more active postmaritally and have more coital partners than do women. Nearly 80 percent of all divorced men and women, however, eventually remarry. Postmarital coitus is less common in widowed than in divorced women and the widowed resume coital activity more slowly than do the divorced.

SUGGESTED READINGS

Hite, S. (1976). *The Hite report*. New York: Dell. (See especially pp. 225–384.)

Hunt, M. (1974). *Sexual behavior in the 1970s*. Chicago: Playboy Press. (See especially Chapters 3, 4, and 5.)

Kinsey, A., Pomeroy, W., & Martin, C. (1948). *Sexual behavior in the human male*. Philadelphia: Saunders. (See especially Chapters 17, 18, and 19.)

Kinsey, A., Pomeroy, W., Martin, C., & Gebhard, P. (1953). *Sexual behavior in the human female*. Philadelphia: Saunders. (See especially Chapters 8, 9, and 10.)

Pietropinto, A., & Simenauer, J. (1977). *Beyond the male myth*. New York: Times Books. (See especially Chapters 1–7.)

Tavris, C., & Sadd, S. (1977). *The Redbook report on female sexuality*. New York: Delacorte Press. (See especially Chapters 2, 3, and 4.)

CHAPTER OUTLINE

CHAPTER 11

HOMOSEXUAL BEHAVIORS AND HOMOSEXUALITY

Most human societies expect that men will choose women and women will choose men as sex partners. In most human societies rather large numbers of people violate this norm by engaging in sexual behavior with others of their own sex. Although there have been and continue to be some societies that approve of homosexual behavior under some circumstances (Ford & Beach, 1951), it is widely thought of in most societies (including our own) as unnatural, abnormal, perverted, and sinful.

This chapter is devoted to a consideration of homosexual behaviors and homosexuality. It is important to distinguish between "homosexual behaviors" and "homosexuality." **Homosexual behaviors** are sexual responses or behaviors that are directed toward people of one's own sex. **Homosexuality** refers to the sexual orientation in which an individual forms an *identity* (a definition of self) as a person who is sexually attracted to same-sex people and prefers them as sexual partners. The importance of the distinction will become apparent later in this chapter as we see that homosexual behaviors are rather common but relatively few people form homosexual identities and label themselves as homosexuals. In this chapter we will first examine the nature and incidence of homosexual behavior and then turn to considerations of male and female homosexuality.

HOMOSEXUAL BEHAVIORS

Homosexual behaviors are sexual responses to or overt sexual contacts between people of the same sex. In this section we will examine the incidence of homosexual behavior in the general population of males and females and briefly describe the specific types of sexual acts that take place in homosexual relationships.

Incidence of Homosexual Behaviors

Because of the controversy and stigma associated with it, there has been great interest, and sometimes great dismay, generated by estimates of the prevalence of homosexual behavior. How widespread is homosexual behavior? This innocent and seemingly simple question is actually a very complex one with many different answers depending, among other things, on the age of the people being studied and the nature of the figures cited. In spite of the fact that they may be and have been criticized on many grounds, the Kinsey studies (1948, 1953) still provide the most comprehensive view of the incidence of homosexual behaviors among white Americans. Because of serious limitations in sample size and characteristics, the Kinsey data provide no information concerning the incidence of homosexual behavior among blacks. Other more recent data (Bell & Weinberg, 1978) suggest the existence of a substantial degree of similarity between blacks and whites in terms of homosexual behavior. Let us first examine homosexual behaviors among preadolescents and then turn our attention to adult homosexual experiences.

Preadolescent Homosexual Behaviors.   As we have seen in Chapters 8 and 9, childhood is not a period of total asexuality. It is a time during which many children discover and experiment with their emerging erotic potential through autosexual behaviors and heterosexual play. It is also a time during which many engage in sexual acts and experimentation with others of their own sex.

Between 50 and 60 percent of males recall engaging in homosexual activities during their preadolescent years. Most boys who ever have such experiences first do so around the age of nine and less than half continue their homosexual contacts into adolescence or adulthood. The most common form of homosexual play involves deliberate exhibition of the genitals. One third of all boys with childhood homosexual experiences go no further than this. About two thirds, however, extend their contacts to manual-genital manipulation. Oral-genital contacts or attempts at anal intercourse occur in less than 20 percent of homosexually experienced boys and less than 10 percent of involved boys attempt the potentially dangerous practice of inserting objects into the penile urethra. Thus, while over half of all males recall some sort of preadolescent homosexual behavior, such experiences are usually casual, sporadic, and involve little in the way of a commitment to homosexuality (Gagnon & Simon, 1973; Kinsey et al., 1948).

Although less prevalent than among males, preadolescent homosexual experiences are reported by a third of all women (Kinsey et al., 1953). As in males, the most common form of behavior is exhibition and examination of genitalia ("You show me yours and I'll show you mine") and for one third nothing more than exhibition is involved. Nearly two thirds progress to manual-genital manipulations but less than 20 percent report vaginal insertions (usually with fingers). Oral-genital contacts are extremely rare, occurring in less than 5 percent of all girls with any childhood homosexual experience. For most girls these experiences are infrequent, sporadic, of short duration, and involve little or no erotic arousal. As puberty nears, most girls temporarily abandon sexual activities of any sort and only 5 percent of homosexually experienced girls continue their homosexual practices into adolescence and adulthood (Kinsey et al., 1953).

Adult Homosexual Behaviors. Among the most controversial figures reported by Kinsey and his colleagues (1948, 1953) were those dealing with the prevalence of homosexual behavior among adults. Between the onset of adolescence and the age of forty-five, the Kinsey study researchers (1948) found that 37 percent of all men (single, married, divorced, widowed) interviewed had at least one homosexual experience involving physical contact to the point of orgasm. Among those men who remained unmarried until the age of thirty-five, about 50 percent had homosexual contacts to orgasm by that age and about 10 percent of all married men reported such experiences sometime during their marriages. To many, of course, these figures are shockingly high and even Kinsey and his fellow researchers (1948) expressed surprise at their findings.

In fact, it now appears that the original and widely quoted figure of 37 percent was somewhat of an overestimate of the incidence of homosexual experience to orgasm among adult males. Men from groups that were almost entirely homosexual in "membership," poorly educated men, and men with experience in prison (where the incidence of homosexual behavior is particularly high) were over-represented in the Kinsey sample. In recent years it has been estimated that the more accurate figure is between 25 percent and 30 percent (Gagnon & Simon, 1973; Pomeroy, 1972). The 25 to 30 percent estimate has been supported by Hunt's (1974) more recent large-scale survey.

For nearly five out of every six adult men with homosexual experience, such experience is confined largely to those years between the onset of puberty and the age of twenty (Gagnon & Simon, 1973). Of the remaining men, between 2 and 3 percent have exclusively homosexual histories throughout their lives and the rest (3 percent) have predominantly homosexual behavioral histories mixed with some heterosexual behavior (Athanasiou, Shaver, & Tavris, 1970; Gagnon & Simon, 1973; Hunt, 1974; Kinsey et al., 1948; Pietropinto & Simenauer, 1977).

All of the available evidence indicates that overt homosexual experiences are less common among females than among males. For example, Kinsey and his associates (1953) report that, by the age of forty-five, 13 percent of all women (single, married, divorced, widowed) have at least one homosexual experience to the point of orgasm. Subsequent studies (Athanasiou et al., 1970; Hunt, 1974) have reported similar figures and suggested that following adolescence between 10 and 15 percent of females have some overt homosexual experience. Not surprisingly, such experiences are more common among unmarried than married women. Around 20 percent of those women who remain unmarried until their thirties and 10 percent of those who marry before that age report homosexual contacts with or without orgasm (Hunt, 1974; Kinsey et al., 1953).

Most women who have homosexual contacts do so for relatively brief portions of their lives. Nearly a third of the homosexually experienced have 10 or fewer experiences in their lifetimes and half have such contacts for only one year or less. Another 25 percent confine their activities to a period of two to three years. Thus, as is true for men, the homosexual experiences of most women are sporadic, infrequent, and of short duration. They are not, however, concentrated in adolescence but, as is the case with most other forms of sexual expression, tend to emerge as women age. The available data suggest that between 1 and 2 percent of women are exclusively homosexual in their overt behavior for the whole of their adult lives. Another 2 to 3 percent may be predominantly homosexual with some heterosexual contacts as well (Athanasiou et al., 1970; Gagnon & Simon, 1973; Hunt, 1974; Kinsey et al., 1953).

Heterosexual-Homosexual Balance.   If we accept the figures discussed above as accurate, we may conclude that about 70 percent of all men in the United States have histories of exclusively heterosexual experience and 3 percent have exclusively homosexual histories. For women the comparable figures may be estimated at 85 percent with exclusively heterosexual experience and 2 percent with histories of exclusively homosexual experience. A bit of quick arithmetic reveals that these figures leave about a fourth (27 percent) of all men and a seventh (13 percent) of all women with mixed heterosexual and homosexual histories.

These data suggest that people vary substantially in their degree of commitment to or involvement in heterosexual and homosexual modes of sexual expression. Kinsey and his fellow researchers (1948, 1953) conceptualized these varying degrees of heterosexual and homosexual involvement as falling along a continuum ranging from exclusively heterosexual at one extreme to exclusively homosexual at the other, with mixed degrees of heterosexual and homosexual involvement between. A seven-point rating scale was devised to represent a person's position on the heterosexual-homosexual continuum. The *balance*, or *ratio*, between an individual's heterosexual and homosexual experience is used to determine placement on the scale. *It is important to note that in determining heterosexual-homosexual balance Kinsey and his associates (1948, 1953) defined "experience" as overt physical contacts and erotic responses with or without physical contacts.*

As shown in Table 11–1, the scale ranges from a rating of 0 to 6 (a total of seven categories). A rating of 0 is assigned to men and women whose erotic responses and physical contacts are exclusively directed to those of the other sex and a rating of 6 to those whose responses and contacts are exclusively directed toward those of their own sex. Between these extremes are those whose responses and contacts are mixed heterosexual and homosexual. The data provided in Table 11–1 are the percentages of men and women between the ages of twenty and thirty-five in the Kinsey studies (1948, 1953) with various heterosexual-homosexual ratings.

The notion of a heterosexual-homosexual balance is flexible and useful in that it adapts easily to changes that might take place throughout a person's life. For example, as we noted earlier, homosexual experimentation during early adolescence is fairly common among boys. Even though most boys of this age recognize societal expectations that their sexual needs, desires, and actions ultimately will be directed toward females, cooperative girls are not always readily available. Thus, circumstances may dictate heterosexual-homosexual balances of 4, 5, or 6 for some adolescent males. As they mature, however, their erotic responses and overt contacts usually become more and more heterosexual and ratings of 0, 1, or 2 are more appropriate. In short, to be meaningful, heterosexual-homosexual ratings must be specified within a particular time frame.

This scheme focuses on specific forms of *behavior* (heterosexual and homosexual) and avoids the pitfalls of imposing labels (as heterosexuals or homosexuals), which tend to stick for a lifetime, regardless of changes in actual behavior (Kinsey et al., 1948, 1953). Terms such as "heterosexual" and "homosexual" are more

Table 11–1.

Percentages of men and women receiving various heterosexual-homosexual balance ratings sometime between the ages of 20 and 35.

Ratings and balance descriptions are based on overt sexual contacts and erotic responses with or without overt contacts. Ranges of percentages are presented to represent variations associated with characteristics such as specific ages, marital status, and educational level.

Rating	Heterosexual-Homosexual Balance	Percentage Females	Males
0	Exclusively heterosexual Single Married Previously married	61–72 89–90 75–80	53–78 90–92
1	Predominantly heterosexual, only incidentally homosexual	11–20	18–42
2	Predominantly heterosexual, but more than incidentally homosexual	6–14	13–38
3	Equally heterosexual and homosexual	4–11	9–32
4	Predominantly homosexual, but more than incidentally heterosexual	3–8	7–26
5	Predominantly homosexual, but incidentally heterosexual	2–6	5–22
6	Exclusively homosexual	1–3	3–16

SOURCE: Adapted from Kinsey et al., 1948, 1953.

appropriately reserved for application by people to themselves in the process of defining themselves as sexual actors and establishing their identities as homosexuals or heterosexuals (Gagnon & Simon, 1973).

Bisexual Behavior and Bisexuality. As we noted above, about a fourth of men and a seventh of all women studied by Kinsey and his associates had sexual histories that included both heterosexual and homosexual involvement. Some of their sexual experience is with males and some is with females. The behavior of these individuals is best described as bisexual.

Bisexual biographies may follow many patterns. Philip Blumstein and Pepper Schwartz (1977) have documented the variety of erotic histories that are found in those with bisexual experiences. Some men and women live exclusively heterosexual lives for a period of time and later in life have homosexual experiences. Some follow a reverse pattern—their early lives are exclusively homosexual followed later in life by heterosexual experiences. Still others' lives are first heterosexual, then homosexual, and again heterosexual or homosexual, heterosexual, then homosexual. Yet another pattern is for a person to concurrently be involved in both heterosexual and homosexual relationships (Blumstein & Schwartz, 1977; Masters & Johnson, 1979).

That the objective facts of people's sexual behavior (heterosexual, homosexual, or bisexual) do not always coincide with their personal sexual identity is amply illustrated by the work of Blumstein and Schwartz (1977). Included in their research were men and women who, although sexually involved or experienced with both men and women, considered themselves to be heterosexual or homosexual. As one male reported,

Rock singer Elton John, shown at his wedding to Renata Blauel, has provided a well-known example of a person who is married, yet considers himself bisexual.

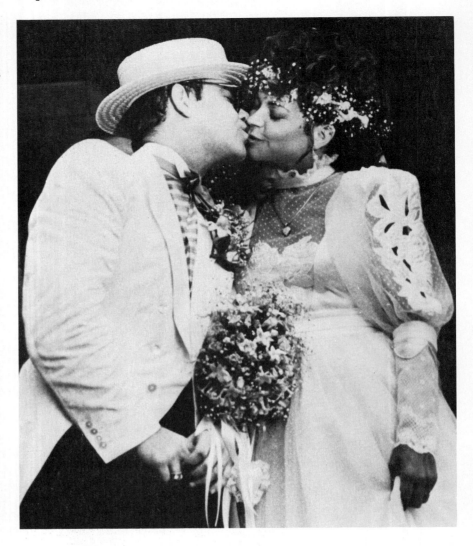

I had this affair with a gay guy for almost a year. We were good friends and we became identified as a couple after a while. I think he basically saw me as a straight person who was kind of stepping over the imaginary line for a while. I was also sleeping with a woman, and while I liked them both, I thought I was heterosexual as a person. (pp. 37–38)

Other examples of this type may be found in those who, while in prison, engage in substantial homosexual activity but continue to consider themselves heterosexual (Kassebaum, 1972). Similarly, some of those men who visit public restrooms or other locales for brief homosexual contacts are married and continue to consider themselves heterosexual (Humphreys, 1975).

Some people adopt bisexual identities, or at least bisexual philosophies as ideals, even though they have only heterosexual experiences. This pattern was sometimes noted in people who adhered to ideological positions in which sex is seen as a means of communication and "getting close to others" regardless of their sex. Similarly, some women, because of their feminist views regarding relationships with other women, adopt bisexual identities as an ideal even though their sexual activities are exclusively heterosexual (Blumstein & Schwartz, 1977).

Of course, some people evolve bisexual identities as a consequence of their actual sexual experiences. One male recounted how this happened to him:

"Well," I thought as this guy climbed in my bed, "What the hell? Why shouldn't I? There's no reason why I should cut off my nose to spite my face. It's going to be fun; it's been fun before, and why can't I have the best of both possible worlds?" Bisexuality seemed like me. (Blumstein & Schwartz, 1977, p. 38)

The findings on bisexual behaviors and bisexuality clearly illustrate the ways in which behavior and identity may or may not coincide. They also show how sexual behaviors and identities sometimes change rather dramatically across the lifespan.

Homosexual Behaviors and Roles

Many people are so accustomed to thinking of sexual expression in heterosexual terms that they find it difficult to picture what people of the same sex might do in a sexual encounter. Even though sexual relationships between men and women involve considerably more than coitus (Chapters 9 and 10), we are socialized to regard penile-vaginal penetration as the essence of sexual expression. Furthermore, our sexual heritage has been one that promotes stereotyped images of men as "active" and women as "passive" in their sexual roles. There is a rather pervasive tendency to generalize this stereotyped model of heterosexual expression to our thinking about homosexual behaviors and roles. Let us now turn to a brief examination of what is actually known about homosexual behaviors and roles in men and women.

Male Sexual Behaviors and Roles.   With two obvious exceptions (penile-vaginal penetration and cunnilingus), the behaviors involved in male homosexual contacts closely resemble those that occur between men and women. As Table 11–2 indicates, a number of sexual techniques are available to and widely used by homosexually active men. In addition to the preliminaries of kissing, hugging, and caressing, the most frequently practiced of the more "intimate" activities noted in Table 11–2 are, in decreasing order of frequency, fellatio, manual-genital stimulation, anal intercourse, and general body contacts involving genital stimulation (Bell & Weinberg, 1978).

The data summarized in Table 11–2 are based on studies of men who express more or less complete commitment to homosexual expression and who apply the label "homosexual" to themselves. Not surprisingly, their initial homosexual contacts frequently involve little more than manual-genital stimulation or **interfemoral intercourse**, in which one partner's penis is inserted and rubbed between the thighs of the other. Once they begin active homosexual involvement, however, young males quickly expand their sexual repertoires to include the full array of techniques listed in Table 11–2, only to eventually settle into patterns

Table 11–2.

Percentage of white men actively involved in homosexual contacts who, in the studies cited, reported use of various sexual techniques.
The Saghir & Robins data represent percentages of those ever actively engaging in the activities while the Hunt and Bell & Weinberg figures represent percentages of those with such experiences during the year prior to reporting.

Sexual Technique	Saghir & Robins (1973)	Hunt (1974)	Bell & Weinberg (1978)
Body contact and genital rubbing	51	—	41
Performing manual-genital stimulation	93	67	83
Receiving manual-genital stimulation	93	80	85
Performing fellatio	98	59	95
Receiving fellatio	96	67	94
Mutual fellatio	93	—	—
Performing anal intercourse	85	50	78
Receiving anal intercourse	93	50	67
Performing and receiving anal intercourse	—	50	—

involving less variety as they grow older or establish relatively long-lasting partnerships with another man (Bell & Weinberg, 1978).

It is widely believed that male homosexual activities involve clear-cut modes of sexual expression, with one man playing an "active" (doing it) role and the other assuming a "passive" (being done to) role. The similarity of such roles to stereotyped images of heterosexual coitus in which the man is seen as actively inserting his penis into the vagina of the passively receptive woman leads rather easily to views of the penis *insertor* in homosexual contacts as active and "masculine" and the penis *insertee* as passive and "feminine." Furthermore, it is often assumed that homosexual males have distinct preferences for and consistently adopt either the insertor (active, masculine) or insertee (passive, feminine) role in their homosexual activities.

To what extent do homosexually active men express preferences for and consistently play such roles? The available data indicate that exclusive role preferences or rigid role adoptions are relatively unusual among most American men who consider themselves homosexual. Well over half of the male homosexuals studied by Hooker (1965a) either expressed no preference for particular sex acts or roles or their preferences were so mild that they were disregarded as the situation required. The preferences that do exist appear to be for oral or for anal techniques rather than for roles that could be characterized as active-passive, masculine-feminine, or insertor-insertee (Harry, 1977). It should be noted, however, that distinct *sexual role preferences* are sometimes found among lower-class American males and males in cultures (Mexico, Brazil, Turkey) that maintain relatively rigid dichotomies between masculine and feminine *gender roles* (Carrier, 1971, 1977; Haist & Hewitt, 1974). The homosexual activities in prisons, moreover, often involve clear-cut distinctions in terms of sexual roles; some men ("wolves," "jocks," "daddies") virtually always act as insertors and others ("punks," "kids") as insertees. These roles are thought to be more reflective of dominance-submissiveness and power relations in the prison systems than of enduring role preferences. They also allow insertors to maintain images of themselves as "masculine" and "not really homosexual" (Gagnon & Simon, 1973; Kassebaum, 1972).

Female Sexual Behaviors and Roles.   Like those of males, the sexual practices of self-labeled female homosexuals (lesbians) and homosexually active women closely resemble the sexual activities of heterosexually involved women. Early in their homosexual histories most women limit their sexual practices to lip kissing and general body contacts, creating the widespread impression that female homosexual practices have a less genital and a less specifically erotic focus than do those of males (Kaye, 1971). But the data summarized in Table 11–3 indicate that women with more extensive commitments to and experience with homosexual activities commonly engage in highly intimate forms of sexual acts, including manual and oral breast and genital stimulation. Indeed, comparisons of Tables 11–2 and 11–3 suggest few differences in the degree to which the homosexual practices of men and women are genitally focused.

When questioned about the frequency of specific sexual acts and which acts are their "favorites," manual-genital stimulation and cunnilingus are most often mentioned by lesbians (Bell & Weinberg, 1978). The focus of these techniques is, of course, on the clitoris, labia, and mons, which are highly erotically sensitive. Contrary to what many might think, lesbian sexual activities rarely involve vaginal or anal penetrations with penis-like substitutes or dildos (Table 11–3). Furthermore, the fact that the practice of **tribadism**, in which one woman lies atop the other and the two then thrust their genitals together, is relatively rare reveals that lesbian activities are not mere imitations of heterosexual behavior. A related point worth noting is that women involved in homosexual activities more often reach orgasm in these contacts than do heterosexually married women in their coitus (Kinsey et al., 1953). This is not surprising considering the fact that one woman may be more likely to appreciate and understand the erotic preferences and erogenous zones of another woman than is a man (Masters & Johnson, 1979).

Like male homosexuals, the majority of lesbians do not adhere exclusively to one sexual role or another (Bell & Weinberg, 1978; Saghir & Robins, 1973). Lesbians, of course, are subjected to the same sexual socialization focus as are other women and early in their homosexual histories some tend to adopt sexual patterns that appear to mimic stereotypes of masculine and feminine roles in sexual expression (Gagnon & Simon, 1973). Those who adopt masculine roles are sometimes referred to as "dykes" or "butches" and tend to take the active approach to sex while those playing more passive roles are called "fem" (or "femme").

But such clearly defined sexual roles are not characteristic of most lesbian sexual relationships. Well over three fourths of lesbians alternate sexual practices, both performing and receiving manual-genital stimulation, cunnilingus, and breast stimulation (Saghir & Robins, 1973). Rigid role enactments and preferences, when they exist, are most likely to be found among lower-class women or others who adhere to distinctly traditional gender-role stereotypes (Gagnon & Simon, 1973; Saghir & Robins, 1973).

Before leaving this topic, we should note that, regardless of what specific sexual acts they perform, the physiological responses of homosexual men and women to

Table 11–3.

Percentage of white women actively involved in homosexual contacts who, in the studies
cited, reported use of various sexual techniques.
The Kinsey et al. and Saghir & Robins figures represent percentages reporting ever
experiencing the acts while the Hunt and Bell & Weinberg figures represent those
experiencing such acts during the year prior to reporting.

Sexual Technique	Kinsey et al. (1953)	Saghir & Robins (1973)	Hunt (1974)	Bell & Weinberg (1978)
Simple kissing	95	—	—	—
Deep kissing	77	—	—	—
Body contact and genital rubbing	56	33 (to orgasm)	80	40
Manual-breast stimulation	97	—	—	—
Oral-breast stimulation	85	—	"Majority"	—
Manual-genital stimulation	98			
Performing	—	100	—	79
Receiving	—	100	—	82
Mutual	—	100	—	—
Cunnilingus	78			
Performing	—	91	50	78
Receiving	—	96	50	75
Mutual	—	66	—	—
Use of dildo or other object for vaginal insertion	—	17	17	—

sexual stimulation are identical to those of heterosexual men and women. Furthermore, when observed under laboratory conditions, homosexuals and heterosexuals do not differ in orgasmic response capacity when masturbating or interacting
sexually with a partner. Interestingly, however, homosexual couples studied in the
laboratory tend to communicate their sexual preferences, aversions, and subjective
experiences verbally to their partners during sexual interaction more than do
heterosexual couples (Masters & Johnson, 1979).

MALE HOMOSEXUALITY

Contemporary estimates indicate that between 25 and 30 percent of males have at
least one overt homosexual experience during their postadolescent years. It is
clear, however, that not all men who have adult homosexual experiences have
homosexual identities. As we noted earlier, the adult homosexual behavior histories of most men are written while they are in their mid to late teens and consist
of little more than incidental or experimental contacts. The majority of men who
have such limited contacts consider themselves heterosexual.

What percentage of men, then, are homosexual in the sense that they have formed homosexual identities? It is virtually impossible to answer this question with more than rough estimates. One problem is that most studies have focused on overt homosexual experiences. Yet some men consider themselves homosexual even though they have never had any overt homosexual contact while others have extensive histories of predominantly homosexual contacts but consider themselves heterosexual (Humphreys, 1975; Lee, 1977; Warren, 1974). It is possible, however, to make what is probably a conservative estimate based on the 6 to 7 percent of men who received ratings of 5 or 6 on the Kinsey heterosexual-homosexual balance scale (Table 11–1). That is, it is likely that those men whose overt behavioral or erotic response histories are predominantly homosexual or exclusively homosexual are also homosexual in their identities. This, of course, suggests that between 3 million and 5 million American men consider themselves homosexual. Who are these men? In demographic terms, what are their social characteristics? What are their personal characteristics? What are their lives like? These questions are explored in the following sections.

Personal and Social Characteristics

In order to accurately describe the characteristics of any population it is necessary to draw a sample that is representative of that population in terms of all the characteristics of interest. In the study of homosexuals, or any other socially stigmatized group of people, it is probably impossible to obtain representative samples. Many potential respondents may feel that admitting their homosexuality (or other stigmatized characteristic) may involve extreme risk (Weinberg & Williams, 1975). Thus, much of what is known about male homosexuals comes from studies of men who cannot be described as representative of the total male homosexual population. These investigations include surveys of men associated with homosexual rights organizations, gay bars, and gay clubs (Weinberg & Williams, 1975), men identified as homosexual by other homosexuals (Bell & Weinberg, 1978; Bell, Weinberg, & Hammersmith, 1981), men in psychoanalysis (Bieber, Dain, Dince, Drellich, Grand, Gundlach, Kremer, Rifkin, Wilbur, & Bieber, 1962), men in prison (Gebhard, Gagnon, Pomeroy, & Christenson, 1965), and men willing to be observed in the laboratory (Masters & Johnson, 1979). These studies as well as the Kinsey (1948) study provide data concerning men whose homosexuality is known to at least one other person, but they suffer from an obvious bias in that nothing is revealed concerning the characteristics or lives of the unknown number of "secret" or "closet" homosexuals. There is also some question of bias introduced by the tendency of many investigators to compare homosexuals with heterosexuals (Morin, 1977).

Demographic Characteristics. The most general conclusion that can be reached from the available data is that homosexual men differ little from heterosexual men in terms of the usual demographic characteristics of education, occupation, social class, religion, age, and race (Bell & Weinberg, 1978; Kinsey et al., 1948). In the Kinsey (1948) survey of the male population in general, tendencies were noted for the *incidence of any homosexual experience* to be somewhat higher among men with moderate amounts of education (high school only), those who were least religiously devout, regardless of denominational preference, those living in large cities, and, of course, those who were unmarried.

It should be remembered that the Kinsey data refer to the male population in general (not just homosexuals). Although many of these tendencies continue to be evident in more recent studies (Athanasiou et al., 1970), investigations comparing homosexuals and heterosexuals reveal strikingly similar religious, educational, occupational, social, age, and racial patterns in the two groups. That is, in comparison with heterosexuals, homosexual men are neither overrepresented nor underrepresented in any particular religious, educational, occupational, social, age, or racial-ethnic group (Bell & Weinberg, 1978; Saghir & Robins, 1973; Weinberg, 1970).

Among the many stereotypes concerning homosexuality is the belief that some occupations or professions are heavily populated by homosexual men. These are occupations that are typically thought of as "feminine," such as hairdressing, clothing design, interior design, decorating, and professional dancing. Homosexuals are more likely to be tolerantly accepted in such occupations than in others. The available data (Bell & Weinberg, 1978), however, indicate that the percentage of homosexual men (8 percent) employed as hairdressers, nurses, designers, and decorators is quite similar to the percentage of heterosexual men (5 percent) in the same occupations. The existence of the stereotype can probably be traced to the fact that homosexual men who have such jobs are often those who are most open in revealing their homosexuality and who are more likely than homosexuals in other occupations to be highly effeminate in their behavior. In contrast, homosexual men in occupations less tolerant of homosexuality frequently remain covert and avoid "effeminate" clothing styles or behaviors (Leznoff & Westley, 1963). Thus, even though the percentage of homosexual men working in government or other "sensitive" positions is similar to the percentage of heterosexual men in similar jobs (Bell & Weinberg, 1978), the homosexuals in such occupations are less likely to be open concerning their homosexuality than are those in the stereotypically **"gay"** (homosexual) professions (Weinberg & Williams, 1975).

Homosexual men do differ from heterosexual men in some demographic characteristics. Not surprisingly, homosexual men are less likely than heterosexuals to ever marry a woman. Around 90 percent of all heterosexual men marry at some time during their lives but only between 10 and 20 percent of homosexual men ever do (Athanasiou et al., 1970; Bell & Weinberg, 1978; Saghir & Robins, 1973; Weinberg & Williams, 1975). These marriages are almost always to heterosexual women. "Marriages of convenience" between homosexual men and lesbians are very rare (Bell & Weinberg, 1978; Warren, 1976).

The marriages of homosexual men are relatively unhappy and dissolve relatively quickly, although over half of married homosexual men report their marriages were moderately to very happy relationships and nearly half of such marriages last five years or longer. More than half of the marriages of homosexuals that terminate do so because of the man's homosexuality. Marital dissolution may occur because of the man's sexual involvement with other men, his disinterest in sex with his wife, his inability to satisfy his wife sexually, or his wife's belated discovery of his homosexuality (Bell & Weinberg, 1978).

The relatively low degree of interest that many homosexual men have in sex with their wives is evident in Table 11–4. During the first year of their marriages nearly 10 percent have no coital contact with their wives at all. Although a substantial minority engage in coitus with their wives on almost a daily basis early in marriage, the overall frequency is not as great as it is for heterosexual men. Furthermore, over half of the married homosexual men studied by Bell and Weinberg (1978) report fantasizing about sex with men "sometimes" or "often" during coitus with their wives. Homosexual fantasies during heterosexual activity have also been reported by nearly 20 percent of heterosexual males in one study (Crépault & Couture, 1980) and as "common" by Masters and Johnson (1979).

Finally, we may conclude our consideration of demographic characteristics by noting that male homosexuals tend to be less religiously devout and more politically and socially liberal than are heterosexual men. They are also more likely to reside in large urban centers than in more rural areas. This, of course, does not suggest that low religiosity, liberalism, and living in cities leads to homosexuality. Indeed, quite the reverse "causal" connections seem to be involved. Homosexuals migrate from rural to urban areas where more anonymity and tolerance are possible, become less religious in the face of strong condemnation of homosexuality by traditional religions, and adopt liberal political and social views which are more consistent with a sexual orientation that is strongly at variance with traditional and conservative sexual ideology and morality (Bell & Weinberg, 1978; Gagnon & Simon, 1973).

Personal Characteristics.   Do homosexual men manifest identifiable personal characteristics which differentiate them from heterosexuals? This is a difficult and frustrating question to answer because the available research findings are extremely inconsistent and often derived from studies with serious methodological flaws. Since the question has most frequently been approached through attempts to discover the degree of "psychological adjustment" associated with homosexuality,

Table 11–4.

Frequency of coitus with spouse during first year of marriage for white homosexual and heterosexual married men and women.

Frequency of coitus	Married Homosexual Men	Married Heterosexual Men	Married Homosexual Women	Married Heterosexual Women
Never	9%	0%	10%	0%
Less than once a month	4	1	6	3
Less than once a week	8	3	10	5
1–2 times a week	10	10	19	9
2–4 times a week	31	30	30	36
4–6 times a week	19	32	14	27
6 or more times a week	18	24	11	19
Number of people studied	**116**	**208**	**80**	**74**

SOURCE: Data from Bell & Weinberg, 1978.

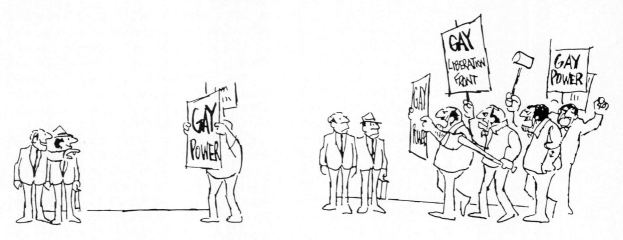

A common misconception among heterosexuals is that homosexual males are feminine in manner and appearance.

SOURCE: Sydney Harris.

the men studied have often been those involved in psychotherapy (Bieber et al., 1962) or imprisoned for sexual offenses (Gebhard et al., 1965). Almost "by definition" such men are likely to manifest a number of characteristics which are judged to reflect maladjustment or pathology. Studies of nonclinical and noninstitutionalized men are largely limited to samples consisting of those who are overtly involved in homosexual clubs, communities, or organizations, and those whose homosexuality is secret have not been studied. Given these limitations, the findings we will describe may or may not be representative of "homosexual men in general."

As noted earlier, many people tend to use a heterosexual model when thinking about sexual interactions. That is, men whose gender identities are male and gender roles are masculine have sex with women whose gender identities are female and gender roles are feminine. Thus, some think that if a man has or wishes to have sexual contact with another man he must think of himself as female and behave in a feminine manner or at least possess feminine characteristics.

A person's *gender identity* is his or her deep-seated conviction, knowledge, and awareness that he or she is either male or female (Chapter 6; Stoller, 1968). Are the gender identities of male homosexuals more "female" than those of heterosexual males? Although there is a considerable amount of disagreement concerning the answer to this question (Ross, Rogers, & McCulloch, 1978), most research has revealed that the gender identities of the majority of homosexual men are firmly male (Freund, Nagler, Langevin, Zajac, & Steiner, 1974; Hooker, 1965a; Townes, Ferguson, & Gillam, 1976). Even though they are erotically attracted to and prefer to have sex with males, they do not think of themselves as females nor do they desire to become females.

Gender role refers to a person's characteristics and overt behaviors that are regarded by the person and the larger society as *masculine* or *feminine*. One of the most prevalent stereotypes concerning homosexual men is that they are all effeminate in appearance, overt behavior, and underlying personality characteristics. Thus, it is widely thought that homosexuals may be recognized by their soft feminine features, limp wrists, swishy walks, dramatic gesturing, feminine clothing styles (or even female clothing itself), soft lisping speech patterns, and numerous other mannerisms that are usually thought of as feminine. To be sure, there are some homosexual men who manifest at least some of these characteristics but they constitute a small minority of homosexuals (Kinsey et al., 1948; Saghir &, Robins, 1973). Of course, some heterosexual males also display these same behaviors. If it does occur, effeminacy in homosexual men frequently appears during the period of "coming out" when a young man (age eighteen to twenty-five) first fully recognizes his homosexual identity and goes public in terms of overt sexual involvement with other men.

Gagnon and Simon (1973) have referred to this period of highly effeminate behavior as a "crisis of femininity" in which young male homosexuals "act out" the stereotyped view of homosexuality. They act the way they think homosexuals are supposed to act. Because such behavior is negatively sanctioned by the homosexual as well as the heterosexual community, most men soon abandon this "mask of femininity" in favor of a more comfortable personal style that is predominantly masculine.

Just as some homosexual men may adopt highly effeminate mannerisms, others sometimes enact "supermasculine" roles in dress, behavior, and even physical appearance. Of course, it is no more accurate to assume that muscular body-building enthusiasts, members of rough-looking motorcycle gangs, or those who dress in leather clothing are homosexuals than it is to assume that effeminate men are. Indeed, some homosexual men are hypermasculine in appearance or mannerisms but most are neither more nor less overtly masculine than are heterosexuals. In short, heterosexual-homosexual preferences and masculinity-feminity of overt behaviors are largely independent. It is erroneous to judge a man's sex preference by the masculinity or femininity of his appearance or mannerisms (Saghir & Robins, 1973).

Several investigators have used tests and questionnaires to assess masculine and feminine *personality characteristics* that are not necessarily apparent in a person's overt behavior. Some of these measures are designed to reveal people's conceptions of themselves as masculine or feminine (as socially defined). Others examine masculinity-femininity by comparing a person's self-reported interests, habits, traits, and desires with those of large samples of heterosexual men and women whose characteristics are considered as norms. With the latter type of test a person (male or female) whose characteristics closely resemble those of most males receives a high score for masculinity and a person who resembles females obtains a high score for femininity.

Studies using measures such as these have generally found that the average scores of samples of homosexual men are lower on indices of masculinity and higher on indices of femininity than are those of heterosexual men (Siegelman, 1972, 1978; Stringer & Grygier, 1976; Thompson, Schwartz, McCandless, & Edwards, 1973; Townes et al., 1976). It must be emphasized, however, that there is a great deal of overlap between the masculinity-femininity scores for homosexual and heterosexual samples of men. That is, the masculinity scores of some homosexuals are considerably higher than those of some heterosexuals. Furthermore, these measures tap the extent to which people match current conceptions of masculinity and femininity while societal views concerning masculinity and femininity are continually in flux. It should be evident, then, that measures of masculinity and femininity provide only weak clues to the hetersexuality or homosexuality of men (Storms, 1980).

Implicit or explicit in much of the psychological and psychiatric theorizing about the nature of homosexuality is an assumption that the personalities of homosexuals differ from those of heterosexuals. Putting aside the issue of personality adjustment for the time being, do the personality characteristics of samples of noninstitutionalized homosexuals who are not receiving counseling or psychotherapy differ from those of comparable samples of heterosexual men? Although a number of studies have addressed this question, it is difficult to draw any firm conclusions from the findings. One problem is that each investigation suffers in some way from its own unique sample bias. Another problem is that relatively few studies have been conducted in which either the same personality characteristic or the same measuring instruments have been used.

Because of these problems and because a detailed investigation of personality characteristics of homosexuals is beyond the scope of this book, we have simply summarized here in Table 11–5 some of the personality characteristics on which homosexual and heterosexual men have been found to differ. As before, it must be remembered that these differences are not absolute ones but rather differences between the average scores of samples of heterosexuals and homosexuals. None of the characteristics listed carry strong implications concerning personality adjustment or maladjustment. And again, we must emphasize that not all homosexual men fit these patterns.

Sexual and Social Lives

As we have noted several times in this chapter, most people see the world through "heterosexually colored glasses" that provide hazy and often distorted pictures of

Table 11–5.

Summary of some reported personality differences between samples of homosexual and heterosexual men.

Homosexuals Lower	Homosexuals Higher
Insistence on law and order	Liking for passivity, warmth, comfort, and mild sensual impressions
Drive for achievement	
Interest in exploration and adventure	Liking for seclusion and introspection
Interest in children	Impulsiveness and spontaneity
Initiative, self-reliance, and decisiveness	Unconventionality
Competitiveness	Narcissism
Interest in team sports	Creative and artistic interests
Tactile and handicraft interests	Tender-mindedness
	Submissiveness
	Dependency
	Nurturance
	Sensitivity
	Introversion
	Interest in individual sports

SOURCE: Findings summarized from Saghir & Robins, 1973; Siegelman, 1978; Stringer & Grygier, 1976.

what homosexuals do sexually and what they are like as individuals. Similarly, most people have only limited understanding of what the lives of homosexuals are like. Let us now examine some of the life patterns linked with male homosexuality.

Sexual Histories and "Coming Out."   When questioned as adults, most homosexual men report experiencing sexual or emotional attraction to other males prior to or near the onset of puberty. For example, during childhood, most are more interested in and receive more enjoyment from sex play (see Chapter 9) with other boys than with girls (Whitam, 1977a). Before the age of fourteen well over half have formed romantic attachments to other males (mostly schoolmates), have engaged in erotic fantasies concerning males, and have had at least one overt homosexual contact accompanied by sexual arousal (Saghir & Robins, 1973). By the age of seventeen, about 90 percent are aware of their attraction to males (Saghir & Robins, 1973; Whitam, 1977b) and nearly 80 percent have their first overt sexual contacts with other males (Whitam, 1977b). Less than 10 percent of homosexual men first become aware of their attraction to other men after they have reached the age of twenty. For many, there are no memories of heterosexual interest:

All my life I have felt emotionally attracted to boys. Even holding hands with them was pleasurable. . . . I remember forcing myself to go to school in order to see the boys, even if I was sick. (Saghir & Robins, 1973, p. 34)

These findings clearly indicate that homosexual interests in males emerge relatively early in life. Other data (Kinsey et al., 1948) suggest that the onset of puberty may be somewhat earlier in homosexual than in heterosexual men. This may, in part, account for findings that homosexual interests appear slightly earlier in homosexual men than do heterosexual interests in heterosexuals (Storms, 1981). Furthermore, homosexual men begin to masturbate at an earlier age and at a higher frequency than do heterosexuals (Saghir & Robins, 1973), a difference that is associated with early onset of puberty and that continues throughout the adult years (Kinsey et al., 1953; Saghir & Robins, 1973).

We should emphasize that the early sexual and emotional responses of adult homosexuals are not exclusively homosexual. Nor are the early response histories of adult heterosexuals exclusively heterosexual. Over half of adult homosexual men recall early emotional and sexual attraction to females accompanied by sexual contact or arousal. Similarly, nearly a third of adult heterosexual men report homosexual arousal before the age of twenty. The early heterosexual responses and interests of adult homosexuals and the homosexual responses of adult heterosexuals are, however, transient and short-lived (Saghir & Robins, 1973). These data make it clear that one cannot anticipate or judge an adult's sexual preference and identity solely on the basis of the nature of his early sexual contacts. Many adult heterosexuals have early homosexual experiences and many adult homosexuals have early heterosexual experiences. Furthermore, many adult homosexual men engage in heterosexual as well as homosexual activities (Bell & Weinberg, 1978).

How do people "become" homosexual? How do they make the transition from identifying themselves as people who experience homosexual feelings or perform homosexual acts to identifying themselves as homosexuals? Some, of course, never do, but several investigators (Dank, 1971; Gagnon & Simon, 1973; Hooker, 1965b; Lee, 1977) have described some of the more common stages involved among those who do.

Lee (1977) has presented a model of self-identification processes among male homosexuals that involves three stages. The first stage is referred to as *signification* and may include as many as four steps. Signification involves private recognition of one's sexual orientation toward others of the same sex. Private recognition may or may not be accompanied by overt homosexual contacts. The person may simply masturbate to homosexual fantasies or, if homosexual contact occurs, it is limited to anonymous sexual encounters in public rest rooms, parks, steam baths, or highway rest stops. The man may continue to live an ostensibly heterosexual or even married life, never coming into contact with the "gay world." Others may fully admit their sexual orientations to themselves but limit their homosexual contacts to only a small number of other homosexuals or to a single lover. These men are sometimes referred to as "closet queens" since their homosexual lives remain "in the closet" and unseen by the rest of the world as they "pass" as heterosexuals.

The second stage in Lee's (1977) analysis is referred to as *"coming out"* (of the closet). In this stage the individual reveals his identity as homosexual to others. Coming out usually occurs first within the gay community—among other homosexuals who have come out themselves. Some individuals make their "debut" (Hooker, 1965b) in the gay community by going to a gay bar or to parties or other functions held by members of the community (Dank, 1971; Lee, 1977). Many male homosexuals come out no further than this. Recent studies of men who are out in the gay community suggest that while only about 30 percent are out to family members and half to neighbors or employers, nearly three fourths reveal their homosexuality to at least a few heterosexual acquaintances and close friends (Bell & Weinberg, 1978; Weinberg & Williams, 1975). Relatively few join gay liberation organizations and openly work to promote the rights and welfare of homosexuals (Lee, 1977).

Finally, a third stage in homosexual identification that is reached by very few men is *going public*, or announcing one's homosexuality to the media. This may occur by allowing one's real name to be used in gay publications, permitting oneself to be identified as gay in the general press, appearing on television or radio as a representative of the gay community, or assuming the role of spokesperson for the gay movement (Lee, 1977).

It is probably safe to say that substantially more homosexual men have reached the stage of signification than have come out or gone public (Lee, 1977). It is often assumed that the degree to which a homosexual man reveals his homosexuality is related to the number of "problems" he encounters. Those who come out to heterosexual friends, family members, and employers are thought to encounter censure, rejection, loss of friends, and loss of jobs, all of which might contribute to adjustment problems. It may be, however, that secret or covert homosexuals encounter more problems due to the pressures and worries associated with the charade of passing as heterosexual. The available research findings are inconclusive on this issue, although they suggest that the more "overt" homosexual men are more self-accepting and less socially isolated and feel that they have more control over their lives than do closet or covert homosexuals (Myrick, 1974; Weinberg & Williams, 1975).

Though a relatively small percentage of homosexual men and women are involved in gay rights movements, thousands attended the first national gay rights demonstration in Washington, D.C., on October 14, 1979.

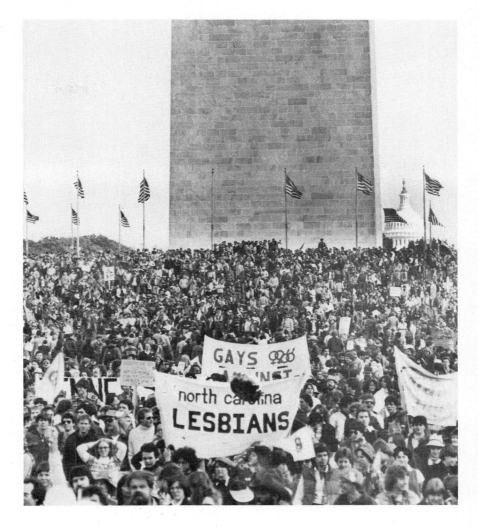

Sexual and Social Partnerships. A great deal has been written about the sexual and social activities of homosexual men but most of what is actually known is largely confined to those men who have come out in varying degrees. Covert, or closet, homosexuals are reluctant and unlikely to participate in research projects for the same reasons that they are in the closet. They anticipate that any sort of disclosure of their homosexuality will disrupt their lives or lead to public ridicule, loss of job, and rejection (Weinberg & Williams, 1975). Generally speaking, however, covert homosexuals often pass as heterosexuals most of their sexual and social lives, only making occasional journeys to public rest rooms, parks, or steam baths where anonymous homosexual contacts are available (Humphreys, 1975). A few men may establish long-term homosexual relationships with other men that are kept secret from all other acquaintances (Lee, 1977).

Coming out in the homosexual community involves a number of alterations in the personal, sexual, and social dimensions of a man's life. At the personal level, coming out almost always involves not only a redefinition of self, but also a redefinition of what it means to be homosexual (Dank, 1971; Lee, 1977). That is, many homosexuals share the stereotypes of homosexuals as unhappy, "perverted," "queer," "effeminate," and otherwise deviant people. Yet when they encounter other homosexuals who do not fit such stereotypes, they often abandon their definition of self as "homosexual" for a definition of self as "gay" or "homophile"—terms preferred by the gay community as tied to fewer negative stereotypes (Bell & Weinberg, 1978; Lee, 1977).

Participation in the gay community provides sexual and social possibilities that are generally unavailable to the covert homosexual. Gay communities are, for the most part, loose-knit networks of social relationships with no physical locations, although in larger cities such as New York, Chicago, San Francisco, and Los Angeles there may be entire neighborhoods, beaches, or sections that are mostly populated or frequented by gays (Bell & Weinberg, 1978; Weinberg & Williams, 1975). The gay community provides a number of social institutions ranging from gay bars to informal social groups that exert important influences on sexual and social partnerships.

It has been estimated that there are over two thousand bars and taverns in the United States that cater to and depend on gay communities for support. Most of these bars are located in large cities, although it is probable that any city of fifty thousand or more people has at least one gay bar (Harry, 1974). For some gay men, these *gay bars* serve as the focal points of their sexual and social lives. They provide convenient locales for recreation and socialization (dancing, drinking, making acquaintances) and for meeting sexual partners (Hooker, 1965b). Gay bars are sometimes described as "sexual marketplaces" (Bell & Weinberg, 1978) where men may go to find partners for brief sexual encounters involving no emotional commitments. In this way they are much like heterosexual "singles bars" where men and women go to "pick up" a sexual partner or be picked up. In gay bars sexual contacts are often initiated through nonverbal gestures such as lingering stares or smiles. When two men make contact, they generally go to one of the men's homes, engage in sex, and perhaps spend the night together, although many times the encounter lasts less than an hour (Bell & Weinberg, 1978). One or both men may then return to the bar (or another bar) and establish another contact (Hooker, 1965b). Nearly 70 percent of gay men at least occasionally "cruise" (seek sexual partners) in bars and about half of those who go to the bars do so at least once a week or more (Bell & Weinberg, 1978; Weinberg & Williams, 1975).

Gay baths are men's health clubs catering to gays that provide opportunities for quick and impersonal sex. They are most often found in large cities. Most contain a large room suitable for dancing and making sexual contacts as well as smaller more private rooms where sexual activities take place. Baths are not cruised as frequently as are bars in part because there are fewer of them. Nevertheless, they offer impersonal sexual contacts which may take place without an exchange of names or even words (Bell & Weinberg, 1978; Weinberg & Williams, 1975).

Though not establishments of the gay community like the gay bars and baths, *public toilets* (T-rooms or tearooms) are well known to gays as locations where brief, uncomplicated, and anonymous sexual contacts are available. Sexual interest may be conveyed by tapping on the stalls or by gesturing while urinating. Sexual acts are usually limited to manual stimulation or fellatio and the men part after sex without exchanging names or other personal information (Humphreys, 1975). The T-rooms are not very popular cruising locales for most adult members of the gay community but are often visited by young homosexuals or those who have not come out (Bell & Weinberg, 1978; Humphreys, 1975; Saghir & Robins, 1973).

Finally, we should mention that most gay communities possess a shared knowledge of certain streets, parks, beaches, or movie theaters where sexual contacts are available. Such places are, however, cruised for sexual partners by a relatively small percentage of gay community members (Bell & Weinberg, 1978).

The existence of all these sexually oriented "institutions" in association with gay communities suggests that gay males tend to engage in a great deal of sex and that much of it involves little or no emotional commitment. In fact, there is some accuracy in this common stereotype concerning gay males. For example, in two comprehensive studies it has been reported that between 60 percent and 70 percent of gay males engage in homosexual contacts at a rate of one or more per week and that about 20 percent have sex four or more times per week (Bell & Weinberg, 1978; Weinberg & Williams, 1975). Even more revealing are Bell and Weinberg's (1978) findings that nearly half of their sample of urban gay males in San Francisco, the "Gay Capital of the World," reported having sex with over five hundred men during their lives and 28 percent report having one thousand or more different sex partners. During the year prior to the survey, over one fourth of these men reported having more than fifty different partners. Other studies (Saghir & Robins, 1973; Schafer, 1977) have also reported high levels of sexual activity and numerous different partners for gay males.

Many of the sexual partners of gay males are strangers with whom sexual contact is made only once and who are not seen socially again even though personal information including telephone numbers and addresses might be exchanged (Bell & Weinberg, 1978). That these findings indicate that *some* gay males engage in a remarkable amount of sex with many different partners cannot be disputed. But do they mean, as some have implied (Bieber et al., 1962) that gay males neither want nor are capable of more enduring relationships? Such a conclusion seems unwarranted for at least two reasons. First, most recent studies (e.g., Bell & Weinberg, 1978; Saghir & Robins, 1973; Weinberg & Williams, 1975) indicate that the majority of gay males sometime in their lives do form relatively steady sexual and emotional relationships with one man lasting a year or more. Many of the relationships endure for four or more years and terminate due to problems that closely resemble those encountered by heterosexual couples, as the following accounts indicate (Bell & Weinberg, 1978, p. 87):

He became very jealous and antagonistic and bitchy and threw a violent tantrum one night. He thought I was cheating. His second tantrum was so violent, I moved out for my own safety.

We were too dissimilar. Different interests, different personalities. We just drifted apart.

I believe I was too possessive. I made unreasonable demands. Eventually he met someone else he was interested in and I wouldn't permit that, so I moved out.

RESEARCH HIGHLIGHT

Homosexual Attraction

What characteristics do gay men and women look for in a potential partner for sex or for deeper relationships? There are a number of stereotypes based in part on beliefs concerning gay life-styles and in part on misconceptions concerning the nature of homosexuality. For example, it is widely believed that gay men and women "really" want to have sex with opposite-sex people and that their same-sex choices resemble their "true" desire. Thus gay men are seen as desiring "feminine" men and gay women as desiring "masculine" women as sex partners. Another stereotype is that gays are so preoccupied with sex that any sexual partner will be acceptable.

Findings from a few studies shed some light upon the characteristics involved in homosexual attraction. In two studies (Laner & Kamel, 1977; Lee, 1976) advertisements for homosexual partners placed in issues of the *Advocate*, a widely circulated gay newspaper, were classified as to types of characteristics sought by gay men in their homosexual partners. Laner and Kamel (1977) compared the characteristics sought by gay men with those sought by het-

erosexual men and women in ads placed in the *Singles News Register*, a popular "singles" newspaper. As shown in the table here, the desired characteristics listed by gay and heterosexual men are remarkably similar but the heterosexual women placed less emphasis on the appearance and more on the occupation and financial status of their desired partners than did either group of men. It is also notable that the gay men were much more likely to specify the type of relationship sought (sex only or lasting, for example) than were the other groups.

In terms of physical characteristics, all groups express preferences for "attractive" partners and what is regarded as attractive coincides closely with our cultural norms for attractiveness (facial appearance, body build, weight, shape of buttocks, breast size, etc.). Gay men, however, more frequently express preferences as to genital appearance than do gay women (Bell & Weinberg, 1978).

In this and other studies (Bell & Weinberg, 1978; Lee, 1976) gay men express an overwhelming preference (over 90 percent) for "masculine" appearing and acting men

Second, Laner (1977) has reported that over 90 percent of gay males prefer permanent relationships to the multiple-partner sex that we have described above. This figure is virtually identical to that for heterosexual males, 92 percent of whom wish to establish a lasting relationship with one woman.

Why, then, are long-lasting relationships relatively less frequent among gay males than among heterosexual partners? At least three factors appear to be involved. First is the fact that gay relationships involve two men, both of whom—like other men—are generally socialized to seek diversity in their sexual lives (Hoffman, 1968, 1977). Heterosexual men are more likely than are women to engage in extramarital sex (see Chapter 10). When a sexual relationship involves two men, the potential problems associated with infidelity are compounded. Furthermore, the children and financial arrangements that often hold weak hetero-

and around two thirds of gay women seek "feminine" women as partners. Thus, it is clear that just like heterosexuals, gay men and women have distinct preferences for particular characteristics in their sex partners (not just anyone will do) and all prefer their partners to be appropriately "masculine" or "feminine." Other findings strongly reinforce these conclusions (Peplau, 1981).

Types of characteristics desired in partners as expressed in newspaper advertisements placed by homosexual men and heterosexual men and women.

Characteristics Desired in Partner	Percentage Listing Characteristics		
	Among Homosexual Men	Among Heterosexual Men	Among Heterosexual Women
Physical	50	75	67
Personality	32	60	72
Appearance	25	38	12
Recreation/interests	24	39	45
Occupation	4	3	24
Education	3	5	9
Financial status	1	4	16
Type of relationship desired	94	61	56

SOURCE: Findings from Athanasiou, Shaver, & Tavris, 1970; Greene, 1971; Ohlson & Wilson, 1974; Saghir & Robins, 1973; Thompson, McCandless, & Strickland, 1971.

sexual marriages together usually do not exist in gay relationships. Second, the **straight** (heterosexual) community exerts strong opposing forces against gay male relationships. Third, the same "institutions" within the gay community such as the bars and baths that make "promiscuous" sexual contacts possible tend to interfere with the maintenance of lasting relationships. Gay bars are notorious for "flirting" and sexual solicitation, which tends to evoke strong feelings of jealousy and rivalry among lovers who frequent the bars. Partly because of this, some gays carefully segregate their lovers from their social and friendship circles (Cotton, 1972). Long-term coupled gay male relationships do exist (Tuller, 1978) although not to the extent that long-term heterosexual relationships occur. Still, it is interesting to speculate concerning the proportion of heterosexual marriages that would endure for any length of time if they were not legally contracted but societally opposed, if they did not involve children or financial obligations, and if the couples regularly attended singles bars for entertainment. Clearly, "the social forces that bind married heterosexual partners together, sometimes even after love has dwindled, are weaker for coupled homosexuals" (Peplau, 1981, p. 37).

FEMALE HOMOSEXUALITY: LESBIANISM

As is true of males, more females have overt homosexual experiences at some time in their lives than form homosexual, or **lesbian**, identities. Based on data indicating that from 2 to 4 percent of adult women would receive ratings of 5 or 6 on the heterosexual-homosexual balance scale (Table 11–1), it may be roughly estimated that somewhere between 1 million and 3 million American women regard themselves as homosexuals. In the discussion that follows we will examine some of what is known about the personal and social characteristics of lesbians as well as what their sexual and social lives are like. As is true of research on male homosexuality, the findings we will describe have been obtained through studies of samples composed of lesbians who have come out in varying degrees and thus may not be representative of those whose lesbianism is fully secret.

Personal and Social Characteristics

Following the same format as was used in the preceding section on male homosexuals, let us first briefly examine some of the demographic and personal characteristics of lesbians.

Demographic Characteristics.   Like male homosexuals, lesbians are to be found in all educational, occupational, religious, social, age, and race categories (Bell & Weinberg, 1978; Saghir & Robins, 1973). In their survey of the general female population, Kinsey and his colleagues (1953) found that the percentages of women with *any adult homosexual contacts* were higher among those with greater amounts of education, those reared in urban environments, those who were least religiously devout, whether Protestant, Catholic, or Jewish, and, of course, those who were unmarried. Similar patterns continue to be apparent in more recent surveys (Athanasiou et al., 1970).

Recent studies reveal that lesbians and heterosexual women differ little with respect to membership in any particular educational, occupational, social, religious, age, or racial-ethnic group (Bell & Weinberg, 1978; Saghir & Robins, 1973). Relevant to an occupational stereotype are findings that lesbian women are only slightly more likely (13 percent compared to 6 percent) than heterosexual women to be engaged in traditionally "masculine" occupations such as engineering, skilled crafts, or other technical work (Bell & Weinberg, 1978). Approximately equal percentages of lesbians (23 percent) and heterosexual women (19 percent) are employed in positions of public trust—in fields such as medicine, law, teaching, counseling, or government jobs (Bell & Weinberg, 1978).

Lesbians are less likely than heterosexual women to marry a man, although recent studies (Bell & Weinberg, 1978; Saghir & Robins, 1973) suggest that between a fourth and a third of lesbians are married at least once and almost always to a heterosexual man (Warren, 1976). Perhaps because their homosexual identities tend to emerge later and they tend to come out later (Schafer, 1976, 1977), lesbians are more likely to enter heterosexual marriages than are homosexual men.

Over half of lesbians who marry rate their marriages as moderately or very unhappy and most such marriages last no longer than three years (Bell & Weinberg, 1978; Saghir & Robins, 1973). Over half of the marriages terminate as a result of the wife's lesbianism, either because she becomes sexually involved with other women or because she is completely uninterested in sex with her husband. Many married lesbians do occasionally or often reach orgasm through coitus with their husbands but still find it unsatisfactory (Saghir & Robins, 1973). Coital frequency in lesbian marriages to men is relatively low (see Table 11–4) and nearly half of married lesbians have fantasies of sex with other women during intercourse with their husband (Bell & Weinberg, 1978).

Like their male counterparts, homosexual women tend to be not very religiously devout, to be politically liberal, and to reside in large urban centers (Bell & Weinberg, 1978; Saghir & Robins, 1973). Each of these "affiliations" is, of course, associated with a rather more tolerant climate for homosexuality.

Personal Characteristics.   Like those of homosexual men, the *gender identities* of lesbians are clearly consistent with their biological gender. That is, most lesbians suffer from no doubts that they are, indeed, females even though they prefer other females as sexual partners (Wolff, 1971).

"Butch," "dyke," and "bull-dyke" are, among others, terms that reflect a popular stereotype that the *gender roles* of lesbians are more often masculine than feminine. That is, it is widely thought that lesbians may be distinguished from heterosexual women on the basis of lesbian tendencies to be highly aggressive and competitive, to be heavily and stockily built, to dress like men, and generally to act and look more like men than women in their walk, talk, gestures, and hairstyles. The data concerning this issue are quite limited but suggest that, on the basis of appearance and mannerisms alone, there are more "masculine" lesbians than "feminine" male homosexuals. In their study Saghir and Robins (1973) found that nearly a third of the lesbians appeared or acted masculine while only 16 percent of the homosexual men appeared feminine.

Just as male homosexuals may accept the common stereotypes of male homosexuality, lesbians may accept the common stereotypes of female homosexuality and act them out in exaggerated form soon after coming out. Thus, some lesbians engage in extremely "butchy" behavior early in their lesbian careers because they think that is how lesbians are supposed to act. Others, accepting the heterosexual model, adopt a highly feminine role to complement their partner's masculine role. Generally, however, unless such roles are compatible with the already established "personal styles" of the women involved, they are soon abandoned in favor of roles and relationships that "fit" more comfortably (Abbot & Love, 1972; Martin & Lyon, 1972).

Using tests and measures such as those described earlier for assessing the degree to which a person's self-image or personality characteristics reflect socially defined masculine and feminine components, it has been found that groups of lesbians score more in the masculine direction than do groups of heterosexual women. For example, 42 percent of the lesbians in the Saghir & Robins (1973) study considered themselves masculine and another 16 percent regarded themselves as "neuter" (neither masculine nor feminine) in gender role. All of the heterosexual women in the same study considered themselves "appropriately feminine." On the basis of indices derived from standardized personality inventories, lesbians emerged as more masculine than did heterosexual women in at least two other studies (Ohlson & Wilson, 1974; Thompson et al., 1973). Still, there is, of course, a substantial amount of overlap between the masculinity-femininity scores of lesbians and heterosexual women and it is, in any case, improper to consider such scores as indicants of lesbianism. Some lesbians are highly feminine in appearance, demeanor, self-image, and personality and some heterosexual women are highly masculine in the same dimensions.

In part because lesbians have been the focus of much less research than have homosexual men, less has been reported about the personality characteristics of lesbians than has been reported about homosexual men. Table 11–6 summarizes some of the reported differences between lesbian and heterosexual samples of women. These findings should be regarded as tentative and suggestive rather than conclusive and it must be emphasized that they characterize groups of people rather than individuals.

Sexual and Social Lives

The lives of lesbians have not been scrutinized as closely as have those of homosexual men. In part this is because lesbian sexual and social activities are not as "visible" as are those of gay men but also it is because lesbianism does not arouse the magnitude of social and moral passion that is stimulated by male homosexuality. Let us now examine some of what is known concerning the lives of lesbians.

Sexual Histories and "Coming Out." Like male homosexuals, most lesbians recall feeling emotionally attracted to others of their own sex around the age of puberty. Before the age of fourteen, four out of five have been romantically attracted to another girl, two thirds have fantasized relationships with other girls, and nearly half have become sexually aroused through physical contacts with girls. For about half, the first experience of homosexual arousal results from "casual" physical contacts such as holding hands or sleeping in the same bed. More deliberate contacts such as kissing and hugging are the first occasion for arousal for

Table 11–6.

Summary of some reported personality differences between samples of lesbians and samples of heterosexual women.

Lesbians Lower	Lesbians Higher
Tolerance of discord	Self confidence
Romanticism	Assertiveness
Conventionality	Recognition needs
Social extraversion	Positiveness of body image
Control of anger	Intellectual efficiency
	Competitiveness
	Interest in sports
	Artistic interests
	Intellectual interests

SOURCE: Data from Laner & Kamel, 1977.

a fourth and deliberate genital contacts for another fourth (Saghir & Robins, 1973). By the age of nineteen, about 90 percent of lesbians have formed emotional attraction to, have had erotic fantasies about, and have been sexually aroused by other females. That these feelings and responses are unmistakably erotic is evident for most girls:

I was 17 or 18 when I first had any homosexual attractions. I can remember then enjoying looking more at women's bodies in magazines than men's bodies. At 18 I would find myself looking at my 14-year old stepsister and enjoying seeing her naked in the bathtub but would try to avoid it. When I was 20 and in college, I became very close to a girl I had known. . . . My feelings were more than of friendship. I used to think about her a lot. She had a tendency to wander in the nude and it made me nervous. I would find myself enjoying looking at her body and would get sexually stimulated. I would wet myself without touching myself and I would feel like kissing and holding her. (Saghir & Robins, 1973, p. 206).

Emotional and sexual responses to other females appear earlier in the lives of lesbians than do comparable responses to males among heterosexual women. Early emergence of sexual interests among lesbians is also evident in data indicating higher frequencies of masturbation among lesbians than among heterosexuals prior to and during adolescence as well as in adulthood (Saghir & Robins, 1973). At the same time, however, it appears that homosexual responses and overt homosexual and masturbatory practices appear earlier in the lives of homosexual men than they do in those of lesbians (Saghir & Robins, 1973; Schafer, 1977).

Although many lesbians recall experiencing homosexual interests and activities when they were relatively young, their early sexual lives are usually not exclusively homosexual (McCauley & Ehrhardt, 1980). Over half experience heterosexual arousal or intercourse before their first overt homosexual contact. Because they "discover" their homosexuality at later ages than do males they are more likely to have relatively extensive heterosexual histories (dating, kissing, going steady, coitus) before their overt homosexual lives begin (Schafer, 1976, 1977). During adulthood, lesbians are more likely than male homosexuals to engage in heterosexual intercourse at least occasionally (Bell & Weinberg, 1978; Peplau, Cochran, Rook, & Padesky, 1978; Saghir & Robins, 1973; Schafer, 1977).

Less is known about the formation of homosexual identities in females than in males although it may be cautiously assumed that many of the processes and stages involved are similar (Lee, 1977). Generally, however, it is known that most homosexual men first think that they are homosexual at an earlier age (around fifteen) than do most lesbians (around eighteen). Furthermore, homosexual men tend to have their first overt homosexual experiences earlier than do lesbians; most homosexual men are certain of their homosexual identities by the time they reach nineteen while for lesbians such certainty does not emerge until they are about twenty-one (Saghir & Robins, 1973; Schafer, 1977).

Nearly half of all homosexual men who come out in the gay world do so before the age of twenty-one. In contrast, only a fourth of lesbians come out this early. The majority of lesbians come out between the ages of twenty-one and twenty-nine but a substantial minority (about 15 percent) do not come out until they are thirty or older (Kimmel, 1978). Most are introduced to the gay world by friends or sexual partners. Some discover it through reading books, magazines, or newspapers, and some through correspondence or contact with homosexual organizations or representatives of such organizations (Saghir & Robins, 1973).

About half of all lesbians who come out to the gay community also come out to members of their immediate family. Only around a third of gay men come out to their families. Outside of family circles, however, lesbians are less likely to come out to employers, fellow workers, and neighbors but slightly more likely to tell at least some heterosexual friends about their homosexuality than are gay men (Bell & Weinberg, 1978).

For homosexual women the significance of coming out in the gay community is as great as it is for homosexual men. It not only aids in the confirmation of their homosexual identity but also leads to a redefinition and reevaluation of what it means to be homosexual. For both men and women, the earliest clues to their emerging homosexual identities are distinct feelings of "being different." Many people initially have no label or cognitive category to use in understanding how they are different until they encounter (through the media, books, friends, or other sources) the term "homosexual" and some definition of it. A thirty-year-old lesbian recalls her introduction to the concept of homosexuality:

The first time I heard about homosexuality was at the age of 15. I came across the word in a book and looked up the definition and found that it suited me. I was still having crushes and strong attractions to girls and this reinforced strongly my feelings about myself. (Saghir & Robins, 1973, p. 233)

Finding a word, a label, a category for oneself when the only identity that is there before is one of "being different" is, for many, an uplifting and profound experience. But for others, if that word or category is "lesbian" or "homosexual," the newfound identity may turn out to be unwelcome:

She spent many hours at the library looking up every reference she could find on the subject. There wasn't much: a few books about the male homosexual, with bare mention of the female. But as she skimmed rapidly through the pages, her stomach muscles began to tighten; she gritted her teeth and fought back tears. She had been feeling that she at last belonged, that there were other human beings in the world that she could relate to. But her elation was short-lived. What she had thought of as love, this desire that came from the purest of motives, was really despicable and degenerate, at least according to these books. The love she felt for Sandra, though never expressed, was a perversion, a sign of psychopathology, a crime against nature and a sin against God. The people she had wanted to know about, wanted to meet and relate to, were crude and disgusting. The joy of self knowledge, so dearly bought, had turned into a very sick joke. Her new self image was destroyed. (Martin & Lyon, 1972, p. 26)

The gay community provides an opportunity for redefinition by example of the word "lesbian" as well as of the word "homosexual." The woman who comes out sees that lesbians are not all "perverted," "psychopathological," "degenerate," or "crude" but are, rather, much like other women (Bell & Weinberg, 1978; Saghir &

Robins, 1973), with the obvious exception that they are sexually and emotionally attracted to women rather than to men. Indeed, one of the primary functions of the community is to support and reinforce the positive aspects of being homosexual (Monteflores & Schultz, 1978).

Sexual and Social Partnerships.   The institutions of any community are created and maintained to support the needs and desires of those who populate that community. Because women (gay or straight) are socialized to value sex primarily in the context of love and affection whereas males are more often shaped to value sex for the sake of sex, it is not surprising that the sexual patterns of gay women differ substantially from those of gay men. These differences are, in turn, reflected in the nature of the institutions associated with the gay female community.

There are, for example, substantially fewer gay female than gay male bars (Harry, 1974). The bars that exist for lesbians function primarily as gathering places for drinking, dancing, and socialization rather than as marketplaces for selecting partners for anonymous sex. Lesbians attend bars much less frequently than do homosexual men and, although some (around 20 percent) cruise for sexual partners, most (around 80 percent) go for entertainment. If a cruising lesbian picks up a sexual partner, she is likely to take her to her own residence and spend the night or full weekend with her. Recall that the majority of gay men studied spend a few hours or less with their partners (Bell & Weinberg, 1978).

Regardless of locale, lesbians cruise substantially less than do gay men. Virtually none cruise public streets, beaches, parks, or T-rooms and there are no gay baths devoted specifically to lesbian clientele (Bell & Weinberg, 1978). Lesbians more often seek sexual partners in the context of school, work, parties, social gatherings, and homosexual organizations and are more likely than their male counterparts to search for partners with whom they may establish more than just a sexual relationship. More than many gay men, they seek relationships accompanied by some degree of emotional commitment and at least a hope of relative permanency (Martin & Lyon, 1972; Saghir & Robins, 1973). Just as do heterosexual women, most lesbians consider sex more fully satisfactory when it occurs in the context of an emotional bond or commitment (Hedblom, 1973). Gay community members foster such searches for relationships by providing settings in which lesbians may meet other similarly inclined women (Nyberg, 1976). Additionally, many lesbian social support groups exist with the goal of providing mutual social and emotional support for lesbian community members.

Socialized to value emotional commitment as a prerequisite for sexual involvement, lesbians tend to have far fewer different homosexual partners than do gay males. For example, in the comprehensive study of Bell and Weinberg (1978), the average gay male studied reported having sex with over 250 different men but the average lesbian reported fewer than 9 different sex partners. Virtually every other study comparing gay males and lesbians (e.g., Saghir & Robins, 1973; Schafer, 1977) has obtained similar findings. Some related findings concerning differences in the nature of lesbian and gay male sexual partnerships are summarized in Table 11–7.

It is clear that the sexual and social partnerships of lesbians differ substantially from those of gay males. Lesbians are much more likely than are gay males to establish stable and lasting relationships with lovers. Many of these partnerships

Table 11–7.

Summary of some reported differences in the sexual activities and partnerships of lesbians and gay males.

Compared with Gay Males, Lesbians Are	
More Likely to:	**Less Likely to:**
Feel some affection for their partners	Have sex with strangers
Have sex more than once with their partners	Pay their partners for sex
See their partners again socially	Receive pay from partners for sex
Associate with their partners socially	Have sex in public places
Share personal information with their partners	Engage in group sex
Establish lasting relationships with their partners	Engage in homosexual voyeurism
Live with their sexual partners	
Be in love with their partners	
Consider their relationships "coupled" (enduring or permanent)	
Demand sexual fidelity from their partners	

SOURCE: Findings compiled from Bell & Weinberg, 1978; Saghir & Robins, 1973; Schafer, 1977.

endure for three or more years. If the relationships do terminate, they do so for reasons quite similar to those involved in the break-up of heterosexual relationships and of gay male relationships (Bell & Weinberg, 1978, p. 95):

I met somebody else who was more compatible and more interesting and more gratifying all around.

I couldn't take being used anymore. I felt like a meal ticket.

Her insane jealousy. She made a terrific scene in front of my insurance salesman. I told her I wouldn't tolerate that from anyone. I was embarrassed. He knew what was going on. I never saw him or her ever again.

VIEWS OF HOMOSEXUALITY

It is probably safe to say that no topic in the field of human sexuality is capable of provoking the amount and intensity of public and professional debate and controversy that has swirled around homosexuality. We will conclude this chapter by briefly reviewing some of the major views that exist concerning the nature of homosexuality. First, let us consider public views.

Public Attitudes and Beliefs

Several large-scale surveys leave little doubt that many Americans disapprove of and have fairly negative beliefs concerning homosexuality. For example, representative findings from studies in the late 1960s indicated that at that time most Americans thought of homosexuality as deviant, as detrimental to society, harmful to the nation (third behind communism and atheism), and harmful to American life. Underlying their attitudes were beliefs that homosexuality is an illness, a crime, or a sin. Homosexuals were seen as abnormal, perverted, mentally ill, and in need of psychiatric help. There was little support for legislation to remove legal sanctions against homosexual conduct (Weinberg & Williams, 1975).

In one of the most comprehensive studies of the 1970s it was apparent that few attitudinal changes had occurred at the public level (Levitt & Klassen, 1974). In this study, four of five Americans regarded homosexuality as obscene and vulgar and considered it always or almost always wrong regardless of whether two people loved each other. Over half thought of homosexuals as sick but capable of cure and supported legal prohibitions of homosexual behavior. Most thought that homosexuals could not be trusted as teachers or youth leaders, in government jobs, or as ministers, court judges, or physicians. Homosexuals in general were viewed as seducers of children, corrupters of fellow workers, and male homosexuals in particular as potential menaces to women when unable to find homosexual partners.

The available evidence (Millham, San Miguel, & Kellog, 1976; Nyberg & Alston, 1977) suggests that these negative attitudes have changed little in recent years in spite of increased public discussion of homosexuality by gay spokespersons, the widely publicized case of gay Air Force Sergeant Matlovich, and publicly announced changes in the views of psychiatrists (Barr & Catts, 1974) and psychologists. Antihomosexual attitudes appear to be firmly entrenched in our society and are most prominent among males, those with traditionally conservative attitudes regarding all aspects of sexuality, those with little education, the religiously devout, the elderly, those with the least contact with homosexuals, and, of course, those who consider themselves heterosexual (Farrell & Morrione, 1974; Lumby, 1976; MacDonald & Games, 1974; Morin & Garfinkle, 1978; Snyder & Spreitzer, 1976).

All studies reveal that a prominent element in public beliefs about homosexu-

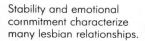

Stability and emotional commitment characterize many lesbian relationships.

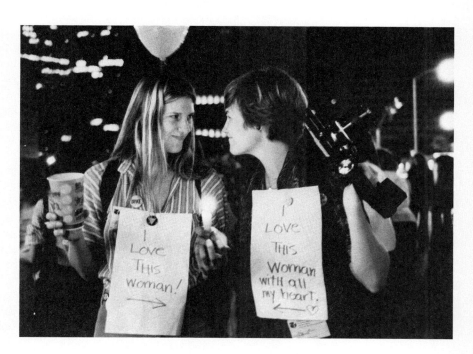

als is the idea that they are somehow "sick," "mentally ill," "abnormal," or "maladjusted." Interestingly, 11 percent of homosexual men surveyed by Weinberg and Williams (1975) also shared the belief that homosexuality is an illness. Let us now examine the issue of whether homosexuality is associated with pathology.

Homosexuality as Pathology

Until the late eighteenth century, the medical community thought of homosexuality and all other forms of nonprocreative sex in much the same way as did the general populace—as sinful and immoral. Under attack from several fronts, traditional religious views of homosexuality as sinful were rescued and bolstered by medical opinion that homosexuality is both a cause and a result of mental or emotional illness (Bullough, 1974). This *medical model* of homosexuality as illness held sway through at least the first two thirds of the present century. Recently, however, the medical model of homosexuality has been seriously challenged as traditional assumptions concerning the nature of mental illness and homosexuality have been more closely scrutinized (Szasz, 1965). For a fascinating account of the evolution of contemporary medical views of homosexuality, see Bullough (1974).

There has been a tremendous amount of research into the relationship(s) between homosexuality and psychological adjustment but in the present context it is possible to do little more than summarize some of the more significant findings and tentative conclusions of this research (see Gonsiorek, 1977; Morin, 1977; and Rosen, 1974 for more thorough reviews). The findings obtained and conclusions reached by investigations of homosexuality and adjustment are somewhat contradictory and depend upon the manner in which the research was conducted.

Many studies (see Gonsiorek, 1977; Rosen, 1974) have involved analyses of case history materials and other information about patients undergoing psychoanalysis or other forms of psychotherapeutic treatment. The findings obtained in such investigations provide evidence in support of the contention that homosexuals are indeed disturbed and maladjusted individuals. But the fallacy in this reasoning should be apparent. Patients undergoing psychotherapy are, by definition, people who are suffering from some sort of adjustment difficulties. To conclude from such findings alone that homosexuals are poorly adjusted or sick is equivalent to studying college students in therapy and concluding that all college students are sick and maladjusted.

To be sure, some homosexuals are poorly adjusted. But are they more so than heterosexuals or is the incidence of maladjustment higher among homosexuals than heterosexuals? Investigations comparing the relative degrees of adjustment found in nonpatient and noninstitutionalized samples of homosexuals and heterosexuals have provided mixed results but suggest that, in general, homosexuals differ little from heterosexuals in terms of adjustment (Gonsiorek, 1977). For example, it has been found that homosexuals and heterosexuals differ little in terms of defensiveness, personal adjustment, self-evaluation (Thompson et al., 1971), guilt (Haynes & Oziel, 1976), anxiety (Siegelman, 1972), and many other dimensions thought to be indicative of pathology or adjustment (Adelman, 1977; Ferguson & Finkler, 1978; Hooker, 1965a; Ohlson & Wilson, 1974; Reiss, Safer, &

Yotive, 1974; Saghir & Robins, 1973). Some investigators (e.g., Freedman, 1975) have even argued that gay men and women are better adjusted than their heterosexual counterparts.

It would be erroneous to conclude from these data that there are no differences whatsoever between homosexual and heterosexual samples in terms of variables related to adjustment. Some studies (e.g., Bell & Weinberg, 1978; Siegelman, 1978; Weinberg & Williams, 1975) have reported what might be regarded as evidence of poorer adjustment among some groups of homosexuals. For example, Weinberg and Williams (1975) found that homosexual men report lower levels of happiness, faith in others, and trust in others than do heterosexual men. Similar findings were obtained by Bell and Weinberg (1978) in their recent comprehensive study of male and female homosexuals. It appears, however, that relatively poor adjustment is characteristic of only some groups of homosexuals. Siegelman (1972, 1978), for example, reported that only highly effeminate homosexual men were less well adjusted than heterosexual men, and the poorly adjusted in the Bell & Weinberg (1978) study were those most regretful of even being homosexual ("dysfunctionals") and those who found themselves sexually and socially isolated from other people ("asexuals"). Those with full and active lives ("functionals") and with relatively permanent and happy partnerships ("close-coupled") were as well, if not better, adjusted than heterosexuals.

In conclusion, the available evidence does not support the proposition that homosexuality is an illness. Just as there are many ways to be heterosexual, there are many ways to be homosexual (Bell & Weinberg, 1978), some of which are and some of which are not associated with poor adjustment. In response to such findings (and pressure from gay liberation activists), in 1973 the American Psychiatric Association voted to remove homosexuality as a psychiatric disorder from its *Diagnostic and Statistical Manual of Mental Disorders*. In the recently revised manual (American Psychiatric Association, 1980), only the diagnostic category "ego-dystonic homosexuality" appears. The term is applied to those individuals whose homosexual arousal and preferences are accompanied by serious internal conflict and distress. Homosexuality itself is no longer classified as a psychiatric disorder. Shortly following the 1973 American Psychiatric Association action, the American Psychological Association issued the following statement (Conger, 1975, p. 633):

Homosexuality per se implies no impairment in judgment, stability, reliability, or general social or vocational capabilities.

Further, the American Psychological Association urges all mental health professionals to take the lead in removing the stigma of mental illness that has long been associated with homosexual orientations.

Thus, among professionals there is a growing tendency to regard homosexuality not as pathology but as an "alternate sexual life-style" that is neither more nor less "normal" or "natural" than is heterosexuality (Davison, 1976).

SUMMARY

Homosexual behaviors are sexual responses to or sexual contacts with others of one's own gender. Homosexuality is a sexual orientation in which people identify themselves as homosexuals—as being sexually attracted to and preferring same-sex individuals as sexual partners.

About half of all men and a third of all women recall engaging in homosexual contacts prior to reaching adolescence. Following the onset of adolescence, between 25 and 30 percent of all men have at least one overt homosexual experience that leads to orgasm. Between the onset of adolescence and age forty-five, between 10 and 15 percent of women reach orgasm through at least one homosexual contact. About 3 percent of men and 2 percent of women have exclusively homosexual histories throughout their lives, and another 3 percent of each sex have predominantly homosexual histories mixed with only incidental heterosexual experiences. Heterosexuality and homosexuality are best thought of as existing on a continuum where the sexual life of a person may be characterized in terms of the balance between heterosexual and homosexual contacts. Homosexual practices include all the sexual acts that might take place between a man and a woman except penile-vaginal penetration. Although some do, most homosexuals do not mimic stereotypic masculine or "active" and feminine or "passive" roles in their sexual activities.

The estimated 3 to 5 million men in the United States with homosexual identities are found in all educational, occupational, social, religious, age, and racial-ethnic categories. Between 10 and 20 percent of homosexual men marry at some time during their lives but the marriages are short-lived, less happy, and involve less coitus than those of heterosexual men. Homosexual men tend to be less religiously devout and more politically and socially liberal than are heterosexual men. The gender identities of homosexual men are firmly male but in their gender roles a minority display exaggerated feminine mannerisms. Similarly, some display hypermasculine characteristics. Most, however, are indistinguishable from heterosexuals in appearance or mannerisms. The social institutions of the gay male community (bars, baths, T-rooms) provide an almost unlimited supply of sexual partners and it is not unusual for gay men to have sex with over five hundred men. Almost all gay men express desires for stable committed relationships with another man.

The 1 to 3 million lesbians in the United States are found in all demographic categories. Up to a third of lesbians marry at some time but their marriages are of relatively short duration, described as unhappy, and coital frequency is low. Compared to heterosexual women, lesbians are less religiously devout, more liberal, and more likely to reside in large cities. Most lesbians have distinct female gender identities. Some assume and enact masculine gender roles in appearance, dress, and mannerisms. Most, however, are distinctly feminine in gender role and indistinguishable in this respect from straight women. The social institutions of the lesbian community are less varied and less sexually oriented than are those of the gay male community. Lesbians have substantially fewer sex partners and form more stable and committed relationships than do gay men.

Public attitudes are firmly against homosexuality and homosexuals are widely thought of as deviant, perverted, detrimental to society, and sick. In 1973 the American Psychiatric Association removed homosexuality from its listing of mental disorders. Many professionals now regard homosexuality as an alternate sexual life-style that is neither more nor less normal or natural than is heterosexuality.

SUGGESTED READINGS

Bell, A. P., & Weinberg, M. S. (1978). *Homosexualities: A study of diversity among men and women.* New York: Simon & Schuster.

Hoffman, M. (1968). *The gay world: Male homosexuality and the social creation of evil.* New York: Basic Books.

Kinsey, A., Pomeroy, W., & Martin, C. (1948). *Sexual behavior in the human male.* Philadelphia: Saunders. (See Chapter 21.)

Kinsey, A., Pomeroy, W., Martin, C., & Gebhard, P. (1953). *Sexual behavior in the human female.* Philadelphia: Saunders. (See Chapter 11.)

Martin, D., & Lyon, P. (1972). *Lesbian/woman.* New York: Bantam.

Masters, W. H., & Johnson, V. E. (1979). *Homosexuality in perspective.* Boston: Little, Brown.

CHAPTER OUTLINE

CHAPTER 12

VARIATIONS IN SEXUAL BEHAVIOR

Human behavioral diversity is nowhere more evident than in the realm of sexual expression and this is as true today as it has been since the beginnings of recorded history (Marmor, 1971). At the same time, it is clear that all societies and cultures have established their own codes and norms for acceptable forms of sexual conduct (Taylor, 1970). Usually these codes have been based on assumptions that the forms of sexual behavior practiced by the majority of the people are the only biologically "natural" modes of sexual expression. Behaviors that conform to such norms are labeled as normal and natural and those which vary from the norms are stigmatized as abnormal, unnatural, deviant, perverted, or aberrant.

The use of terms such as "abnormal" and "unnatural" in reference to sexual behavior implies the existence of universal and timeless agreement as to what forms of behavior are normal and natural. But conceptions of normal sexual behavior sometimes differ markedly from one culture to another (Ford & Beach, 1951) and from one era of history to another (Marmor, 1971). For example, kissing almost always accompanies sexual interaction in our society yet was considered by the Thonga of Africa as eating each other's saliva and dirt (Ford & Beach, 1951). Thus, what is considered abnormal in one time and place may be considered normal in yet another time and place. Consequently, there is a trend toward dispensing with highly stigmatizing and absolute-sounding terms such as "abnormal," "deviant," "perverted," and "aberrant" when referring to sexual practices that differ to some degree from the prevailing norms. Because they have not yet acquired the stigmatizing power of some of the others (although they eventually may), the terms "variation" and "variance" are now widely used in preference to such negative value-laden labels as those mentioned above.

Note, however, that while we use the rather nonevaluative terms "variation" and "variance" in this chapter, we do *not* consider all of the behaviors we discuss equally acceptable. Our own position is similar to that of others (Byrne & Byrne, 1977; McCary, 1978) and is based on the concepts of harm, consent, and privacy. *We consider acceptable any sex-related behavior that (1) causes no unwanted distress for the participants, (2) is engaged in with the full rational consent of the participants, and (3) takes place in privacy and out of sight and sound of unwitting and unwilling observers. We consider unacceptable all behaviors that do not meet each of these criteria.*

Complete sexual activity episodes may be characterized as consisting of three phases: (1) the stimulation of sexual arousal, (2) the behaviors motivated by sexual arousal, and (3) the culmination of sexual activity in orgasm. Sexual variations may be conveniently classified according to whether atypicality appears in phase 1 or phase 2. For example, phase 1 variations such as fetishism and pedophilia involve being sexually aroused by nonnormative erotic stimuli such as shoes and children. Phase 2 variations such as voyeurism and exhibitionism involve normative sources of sexual arousal (usually adult females) but atypical modes of sexual behavior (peeping and exposing). The discussion that follows is organized according to whether the behaviors in question involve variations in the stimulation or behavioral phases of the sexual activity sequence.

Though convenient for discussion, such a division is not totally satisfactory for at least three reasons. First, some variations involve atypical elements in both the stimulation and behavioral phases. Sadomasochism, for example, represents both an atypical stimulus for arousal (pain or the thought of pain) and atypical behavior in which the person achieves gratification by inflicting or receiving pain. Second, in some cases, separately designated variations appear simultaneously in the same person. For example, sadomasochism (primarily a behavioral variation) often involves one or more fetishistic elements (primarily an erotic stimulus variation). Third, rape and sexual assault are often motivated by other than sexual needs and must be discussed somewhat separately. Let us first examine some of the more prominent variations in types of erotic stimuli, then turn to variations in sexual expression, and finally to rape and sexual assault.

VARIATIONS IN TYPE OF EROTIC STIMULUS

Our society expects that beyond puberty most males and females will be erotically responsive and sexually attracted primarily to people of the other sex of about the same age. In some cases, however, variant patterns of erotic response and preference develop and it is with such patterns that we are concerned in this section.

Fetishism

The term **fetishism** is most frequently used when some inanimate object (gloves, shoes) or body part (hair, foot) that is neither a primary (genital) nor a secondary (breasts) sex characteristic is capable of evoking strong sexual arousal in an individual. It should be emphasized that the potential range of stimuli to which sexual responses may become attached is virtually limitless and the point at which sexual excitement in response to a particular object becomes a fetish is somewhat unclear. Usually, the extent to which the object is preferred as a substitute for a living sexual partner or the partner's genitals is used as a rough guide. Paul Gebhard (1969) has expressed this succinctly in the following passage:

I envision the whole matter of fetishism as a gradated phenomenon. At one end of the range is a slight preference; next is a strong preference; next is the point where the fetish item is a necessity to sexual activity; and at the terminal end of the range the fetish item substitutes for a living sexual partner. Nearly all humans have preferences as to the physical or sartorial attributes of their sexual partners. Hence I feel that statistical normalcy ends and fetishism begins somewhere at the level of strong preference. This is nicely exemplified by one man who had his first recognition of his own fetishism when he realized he had ignored a beautiful girl to court a plain girl with a particular hair style. The next stage, that of necessity, would be the case of a man who is impotent unless his partner wears a certain type of shoe. The ultimate stage is the man who habitually dispenses with the female and achieves orgasm only with the shoe. (pp. 72–73)

As suggested by Gebhard's analysis, most fetishes are found in males and reported cases of female fetishists are extremely rare (Stoller, 1977; Storr, 1964). Common fetish items may be conveniently divided into two classes. In one, the fetish is some sort of *inanimate object* and, in the second, it is some body part or characteristic of potential or actual sexual partners. The latter type of fetish is appropriately referred to as *partialism*.

Partialisms are often difficult to distinguish from the usual range of preferences expressed by people for certain physical characteristics in their partners. For example, most people are familiar with the terms "breast man," "ass man," and "leg man," which are often used in self-reference by men who find particular parts of the female anatomy more sexually exciting than others. These preferences fail to qualify as fetishes, however, unless a man becomes so preoccupied with the size of a woman's buttocks, the length or color of her hair, or the shape of her legs that he no longer sees her but instead sees only her buttocks, hair, or legs as his preferred sexual object.

In some inanimate fetishes, the erotic response is stimulated primarily by the material from which the object is made rather than by the type of object. A good example is a rubber fetish in which a person is aroused by rubber, and whether it

Partialism is a type of fetish that involves extreme preoccupation with a certain part of the body.

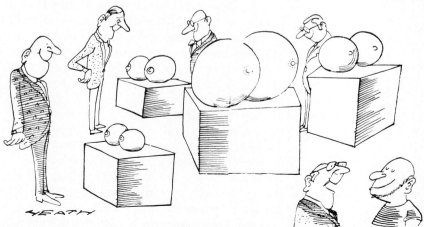

"You know what they want and you give it to them."
SOURCE: © 1983 Punch/Rothco.

is in the form of boots, gloves, coats, or other items is of little importance. In others it is the particular type of article itself that is of primary importance rather than the material from which it is made. The potential list of items is virtually endless but the most common objects are female clothing and footwear, particularly high heel shoes and boots. High-heeled shoes and high boots are frequently associated with sadomasochism and, as we shall note later, some types of fetishism and sado-masochism appear to be closely related phenomena (Gebhard, 1969).

What do fetishists do with such objects? Often fetish items are fondled, smelled, tasted, rubbed against the skin, gazed upon, or merely visualized in fantasy in order to heighten sexual arousal. Sometimes they are applied directly to the penis in masturbation (Marshall, 1974) or ejaculated upon following masturbation (Mathis, 1972). In some instances fetish objects may be used as adjuncts to coitus as in the case of a man who could not engage in intercourse with his wife unless she wore silk stockings and high heel shoes (Mathis, 1972).

When associated with autosexual behaviors exclusively, the items are often used only once and then discarded, destroyed, or hoarded. In part because of this, the fetishist often must resort to theft in order to acquire a sufficient supply of the fetish object. In addition to solving the supply and demand problem, the danger and excitement associated with stealing acts to increase the arousal value of the objects. Furthermore, to the extent that a particular fetish item, such as female panties, is used as a substitute for or symbol of an actual person, an item which actually belongs to and has been worn by a particular woman is more desirable than those that are purchased new. Thus, it is not surprising that a male's fetishism is often discovered as a result of his arrest for stealing garments from clotheslines, laundromats, or other locations. Examples are a twenty-one-year-old university student caught stealing trousers that he would use in masturbation and a fifteen year-old boy discovered hoarding over one hundred pairs of panties that he had stolen, ejaculated upon, and stored away in a trunk (Mathis, 1972).

What are the origins of fetishes? Although there are no fully satisfactory answers to this question, at least three factors seem to be of importance. First, it seems clear that there must be some sort of *conditioning experience* in which pleasure or sexual arousal is associated with the fetish object or items similar to it (McGuire, Carlisle, & Young, 1965). We have already described in Chapter 4 how Rachman (1966) was able to condition sexual arousal to boots in the laboratory by systemati-cally and repeatedly pairing photos of sexually stimulating nude females with photos of women's boots. In "real life" the original conditioning experience is often an accidental one. This is nicely illustrated by a case reported by Oswald (1962) of a thirty-two-year-old military recruit who became highly sexually aroused by tying himself up in black shiny rubber. The fetishistic behavior was traced to an early experience in which a group of boys tied a ground cloth over his head and manually stimulated him to orgasm. Following that experience, his primary mode of sexual expression became masturbation after "tying himself up with rubber groundsheets, a rubber hood and ropes. He came for treatment partly because he feared he might encompass his own death, as he had recently had difficulty in releasing himself" (Oswald, 1962, p. 201).

In the latter case, as well as others (Bebbington, 1977), it appears that only one intensely arousing experience is responsible for the fetish. Still other cases indi-cate, however, that fetishes can also develop over rather long periods in which less intense but nevertheless pleasurable experiences are repeatedly associated with a particular object. For example, the seemingly innocent praise of a mother for her son when he stroked her dress or complimented other women on their dresses was the apparent origin of the son's dress fetish in a case reported by Johnson (1953).

A second contributing factor in fetishism appears to be the *sexual symbolic value* of the object itself. That is, the most common fetish items are usually associated in some way with the body and seem to symbolize part or all of a human sexual partner (Epstein, 1975; Gebhard, 1969). Consider, for example, the panty fetish of a seventeen-year-old boy described by McGuire and his associates (1965). The fetish apparently originated when the boy was sexually aroused by seeing a girl clad only in her underwear and following this experience began to masturbate to the fantasy of scantily clad women. Eventually the memory of the original girl faded as did images of the women in his fantasies, leaving only the symbolic panties as the sexual stimulus.

Finally, it is often suggested (Coleman, 1976; Gebhard, 1969; Mathis, 1972) that extreme fetishism occurs only in the context of *sexual maladjustment*. That is, masculinity and potency doubts, fears of rejection by sexual partners, and sociosexual (heterosexual or homosexual) ineptness are all overcome through the fetishistic substitution of a nonthreatening, readily available object for human sexual partners.

We should emphasize that neither the above nor other (Gebhard, 1969) "explanations" taken singly or together can fully account for the origins of fetishism. Often the conditioning experience, if any, is obscure, as in the case of an individual whose fetish item was an automobile exhaust pipe (Bergler, 1947); or the sexual symbolic value of the object is unclear, as in cases of rubber fetishism (Epstein, 1975); or a pattern of sexual maladjustment is not obvious, as in the case, already noted, of a man's insistence that his wife wear high heel shoes, hose, and a garter belt during coitus (Mathis, 1972).

Fetishistic Transvestism

The term **transvestism** literally refers to cross-dressing, or wearing the clothing of the opposite sex. But the term itself is somewhat ambiguous because people may cross-dress for a number of reasons (Gebhard, Gagnon, Pomeroy, & Christenson, 1965). For example, some male homosexuals occasionally cross-dress, or "go in drag," for the purpose of attracting male sexual partners or simply to parody women or have fun as a "drag queen." Others may cross-dress as part of their roles as professional female impersonators in nightclubs. Transsexuals, or those whose gender identities are at variance with their anatomical sex, frequently cross-dress so that at least their clothes, if not their genitals, are consistent with their identities as males or females.

In its most accepted usage (Bentler, 1976; Buhrich & McConaghy, 1977b; Gebhard et al., 1965; Stoller, 1977), however, the term "transvestism" refers to the practice of wearing clothes of the opposite sex for the purpose of sexual gratification. As such it is, at least in part, a fetishistic behavior in which the transvestite (almost always a male) responds sexually to women's clothing, but only when he is actually wearing them or putting them on.

Although the popular view of a transvestite is that of the "drag queen" who parodies feminine dress and behavior as shown here, most transvestites are in fact heterosexual men who cross-dress for sexual gratification.

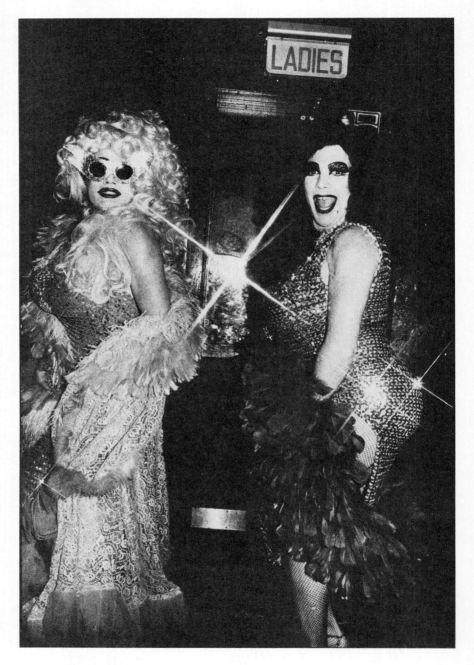

Like other fetishes (Gebhard, 1969), fetishistic transvestism occurs in degrees. Some men may merely experience enhanced sexual responses when wearing female clothing while others may be unable to become aroused unless they are cross-dressed. Similarly, some transvestites find wearing only one type of female garment (for example, panties or bras) sexually exciting while others initially react to only a single garment but eventually turn to complete cross-dressing for arousal (Stoller, 1977). Donning the female apparel may trigger orgasm with no additional stimulation, or it may serve as a prelude to masturbation or coitus.

Most fetishistic transvesites are men whose sexual preferences are heterosexual. They are sexually aroused by females (and by wearing their clothing), are often married, have clearly male gender identities, and have no desire for surgical reassignment as females (Benjamin, 1967b; Bentler, 1976; Buhrich & McConaghy, 1977a; Stoller, 1967, 1977). Although the origins of transvestism are not fully understood, as with other fetishes, sexually gratifying early experiences are often involved. The following case of a biologically normal married man in his twenties with children illustrates this well (Stoller, 1977, p. 210):

When he was four years old (his stepmother) dressed him in girl's clothes to punish him for getting dirty. . . . She did this several times subsequently, and within two years he had arranged with a neighbor girl to dress him up regularly during their after school play. The dressing-up died away for several years, but at age 12, he did it once again, almost casually. On starting to put his stepmother's panties on, he suddenly became intensely sexually excited and masturbated for the first time. For several years thereafter, he would only put on his stepmother's underwear and either masturbate or spontaneously ejaculate. Then, in mid-teens, he began taking underwear from the homes of friends' sisters, and in a year or so increased this activity to stealing women's underwear wherever he could find it. . . . He was attracted to girls and went out on dates, but being shy, he had less sexual experience than some of his friends.

He proposed to the first girl with whom he had a serious affair, confessed his fetishistic cross-dressing to her, and was surprised and relieved when she not only was not upset but assisted him by offering her underwear and by purchasing new pairs for him as he wished. Starting within a year after marriage, he found it more exciting to put on more of his wife's clothes than just her underwear, and now he prefers dressing completely in her clothes and having her assist him in putting on makeup and fixing his wig.

He feels completely male and is accepted by all who know him as a masculine man. He does not desire sex transformation. He has never had homosexual relations and is sexually attracted only by women's bodies.

As unusual as it may seem, parental initiation of cross-dressing is often discovered in the childhood history of transvestites (Stoller, 1967). Such experiences (often encouraged and rewarded by parents and relatives) may become emotionally as well as sexually gratifying and are further reinforced by sexual pleasure conditioned to cross-dressing if the boy masturbates while cross-dressed (Woody, 1973).

In many instances the sexual arousal produced by cross-dressing declines or disappears with age (Buhrich & McConaghy, 1977a; Meyer, 1974) but the act of cross-dressing continues to provide emotional gratification. The cross-dressing man is not only "comfortable" but also strongly identifies with his feminine appearance, while still retaining his male gender identity. Because their gender identity as males remains intact, such men are not transsexuals. But, since they no longer become sexually aroused through cross-dressing, neither are they fetishistic transvestites. The term "transgenderism" is sometimes used to characterize the behavior of these men (McCary, 1978).

Pedophilia

Pedophilia is a sexual variation in which an adult (almost always male) is erotically aroused by and derives gratification from sexual contacts with prepubescent children. Because adult-child sexual relations are serious legal offenses and among the most highly stigmatized forms of sexual expression, most of what we know about such activities comes from studies of convicted offenders. These studies, though limited by the fact that they focus only on those who have been tried and convicted of a sexual offense, have revealed the imprecision of the term "pedophilia" (from the Greek word meaning "lover of children"). That is, there are a variety of reasons why a man might engage in sexual contacts with children and, as we shall see, not all men who do so actually prefer children over adults as sexual partners as the term seems to imply (Cohen, Seghorn, & Calmas, 1969; Gebhard, et al., 1965). Thus, successful therapy programs for pedophiles must focus on the individual characteristics of the men involved (Kremsdorf, Holman, & Laws, 1980; Laws, 1980; Quinsey, Chaplin, & Carrigan, 1980).

Most adult-child contacts, whether heterosexual or homosexual, involve little more than fondling, genital exhibition, or genital manipulations. In heterosexual contact, attempts at coitus are rare, and even more rare are those in which penile-vaginal penetration is actually accomplished. This is, in part, due to the relatively small size of the prepubescent vagina but also because, for many men, the contacts represent "regressions" to or continuations of patterns of prepubertal sex play. That is, "mature" coital relationships with adult women are not simply displaced to sexually immature girls. In homosexual contacts, which are also often regressions to sex play activities, the most common act involves manual-penile stimulation usually done to rather than by the boy. Fellatio occurs in less than half the contacts and penile-anal penetration is extremely rare (Gebhard et al., 1965).

The usual image of the "child molester" is of a senile "dirty old man" lurking in the shadows and accosting unsuspecting young girls or boys. In fact, however, the most common situation involves a male between the ages of thirty and forty and a child twelve years old or younger who is known to the man. In over half of the cases, the adult and child know each other as friends, relatives, or casual acquaintances and little or no force or violence is involved. Nearly half of the contacts occur in the home of the adult, that of the child, or in a shared residence such as an apartment house. Only a fourth occur in the out-of-doors and the remainder take place in autos, theaters, or at schools. Almost a third of the heterosexual offenders are married and another 30 percent were once married but are separated, divorced, or widowed at the time of the contact. Smaller proportions of those who make homosexual contacts are or ever have been married (Gebhard et al., 1965).

In spite of the commonalities noted above, there is great diversity among adult men involved in sexual contacts with prepubescent children (Cohen et al., 1969; Gebhard et al., 1965; Groth & Birnbaum, 1978; Rossman, 1973b).

Heterosexual Pedophiles. Some men, for a variety of reasons, actually seem to have a clear interest in or preference for sexually immature girls. They have never developed or maintained relationships with adult women because of shyness or feelings of inferiority when around mature females. In many cases they are sadly lacking in sociosexual skills and simply feel more comfortable and confident when interacting with young girls. Often they have engaged in extensive and gratifying prepubertal sex play in which young girls become potent sex stimuli. In some instances they are also attracted to adult women but seek less threatening contacts with underage females (Levin, Barry, Gambaro, Wolfinsohn, & Smith, 1977). In still others, fragile, unstable, and unsatisfactory relationships are established with adult women but a preference for little girls remains, as illustrated in the following case of a married man in his thirties:

His wife was the first adult woman with whom he had had sexual relations, and from the beginning to the present, these have been joyless, with little erotic pleasure, and marred by his difficulty in getting an erection. . . . His wife's body never appealed to him because it is an adult female's; he avoids seeing her because to do so provokes feelings ranging from uneasiness to disgust. . . . Several times a year, he has found himself suddenly, unexpectedly, intensely excited and preoccupied with wanting a prepubertal girl to fondle. He has never experienced such excitement with, or thinking about, an adult woman. When he can get close to such a little girl, he seeks only to massage her body and fondle her genitals; he has never attempted penetration. On a few occasions, he has had a cooperative child touch his penis but, because of fear, he has never permitted this to advance to ejaculation. When he leaves the child, he masturbates. When trapped into needing an erection with his wife, he fantasizes fondling a little girl. (Stoller, 1977, pp. 201–202)

Even "normal" adult men evidence some sexual reaction to nude female children (Freund, McKnight, Langevin, & Cibiri, 1972) but the heterosexual pedophile is often much more responsive to little girls than to adult women (Atwood & Howell, 1971; Freund et al., 1972). Perhaps, because of this interest in prepubescent females, the pedophile's sexual history is often one of repeated child contacts and multiple arrests for such behaviors (Freund et al., 1972; Gebhard et al., 1965).

There are, however, some heterosexual pedophiles who show little evidence of enduring preferences for female children as sexual partners. These are men who have (at one time at least) achieved and maintained some semblance of an adult heterosexual relationship. Their contacts with young girls, then, are considered to be retreats to "immature" forms of sexual functioning. Often such retreats are impulsive acts that follow threats to their masculinity or disruptions of their adult sexual relationships. A frequent precipitating factor is the man's discovery that his wife or girlfriend is having an affair with another man (Cohen et al., 1969). The impulsive rather than premeditated nature of the contacts dictates that most often the man and girl involved are not acquainted.

Even though these men have established what superficially appear to be "normal" heterosexual peer relationships, their social, occupational, and marital adjustments are usually marginal at best. They do not handle the stresses of adult life well and often turn to alcohol for escape. Thus, intoxication is frequently associated with the child contacts. With the exception that the "victim" was known to the man, the following case of a twenty-seven-year-old married man is representative of such offenders:

After a rather restrained premarital life this shy and dependent young man married a girl who was more aggressive than he. She held a job, spent money freely, and went out frequently without her husband, leaving him at home to care for their child. He was periodically unemployed and felt perpetually jealous and inferior; the marriage continued to deteriorate. In a moment of depression he tried suicide. Not long thereafter while he was alone at home watching television some neighborhood children came in. One, a girl of ten, sat next to him and, according to him, hugged him. He became sexually aroused (coitus with his wife had become scant) and ultimately took her into the bedroom and attempted coitus. (Gebhard et al., 1969, p. 78)

As suggested by this example, deprivation of adult sexual contacts is sometimes involved in contacts with young girls. Sexual and affectional deprivation may, of course, occur for many reasons and certainly not all men who are deprived turn to children. Usually some impairment of judgment is involved among those who do. Thus, as many as 30 percent of those who initiate sexual contacts with children are temporarily or chronically impaired by alcohol, intellectual retardation, psychosis, or senile deterioration (Gebhard et al., 1965).

Homosexual Pedophiles.   Some homosexual pedophiles show a preference for prepubescent boys over prepubescent girls, adult females, and adult males as sexual partners. Their preferences for young boys are often based on their lack of ease with adults, the rather easily evoked emotional and sexual responsiveness of the young, and conditioned sexual attraction to the physical attributes of children (hairless bodies, smooth complexion, for example). This conditioning often occurs as a result of extensive childhood homosexual play. Thus, they are more sexually aroused by and attracted to young boys than to young girls or to adults of either sex (Freund & Langevin, 1976). Such preferences are reinforced and strengthened by postpubertal masturbatory fantasies and daydreams centered on young boys (Gebhard et al., 1965).

While these men sometimes have rather extensive histories of homosexual contact with other adult males, their interests in young boys are not usually substitutions of boys for adult men (Bernard, 1975). The preference for boys is often quite specific, suggesting a clear distinction between homosexuality and homosexual pedophilia:

Homosexuality and homosexual pedophilia are not synonymous. In fact it may be that these orientations are mutually exclusive, the reason being that the homosexual male is sexually attracted to masculine characteristics whereas the heterosexual male is attracted to feminine characteristics, and the sexually immature child's qualities are more feminine than masculine. . . . It appears, therefore, that the adult heterosexual male constitutes a greater sexual risk to underage children than does the adult homosexual male. (Groth & Birnbaum, 1978, pp. 180–181)

Some men's contacts with young boys reflect not an enduring preference for or attraction to youthful partners but a turn to such relationships in response to stress, drunkenness, sexual deprivation, or intellectual deficiency (Gebhard et al., 1965; Groth & Birnbaum, 1978). These men are most often exclusively heterosexual in their adult relationships and married. Their contacts with prepubertal boys are impulsive and unlikely to be repeated. Their adult heterosexual satisfaction is usually marginal in the quantitative as well as qualitative sense. The following example of a twenty-nine-year-old divorced man is representative:

He offered a 10-year-old neighbor boy a ride, drove to a wooded area, and forced the boy to fellate him. He then gave the boy a dollar, offered to buy him some pizza, and drove him home. . . . Ted's wife had a 4-year-old son from a previous marriage and bore him a daughter a year after their marriage. He states that their marital and sexual adjustment was good for the first year, but that after the birth of their daughter his wife went to work nights, and "that's when it all went downhill. She found somebody at work she liked better. I felt rotten." Within a year, Ted's wife separated from him and his first sexual offense occurred. (Groth & Birnbaum, 1978, p. 177)

Most pedophiles are rather moralistic and conservative men whose early histories are characterized by unsatisfactory sociosexual experiences and limited exposure to adequate sex education and even pornography (Goldstein, Kant, Judd, Rice, & Green, 1971). Most of them feel quite guilty about their sexual contacts with children (Gebhard et al., 1965). A much smaller, but more widely publicized, group of men make sexual contacts with children as part of a larger pattern of searching for new and varied sexual thrills. They seem to function without regard to societal controls, experience little or no guilt concerning their actions, and use any convenient warm-blooded animal, human or otherwise for sexual gratification (Gebhard et al., 1965).

Such men are frequently indifferent to the sex of their child partners and may, through the use of great force, inflict severe injuries on them. They usually have histories of other sex offenses as well as longstanding patterns of antisocial behavior (Cohen et al., 1969; Gebhard et al., 1965). They frequently patronize child prostitutes or, in some instances receiving national publicity in recent years, entice children into sexual acts by offering them toys or other rewards. For example, two men (ages forty-six and fifty-two) were arrested in Providence, Rhode Island, in 1977 for running a sex club called "Teen Challenge" for boys and girls between the ages of nine and thirteen. Meetings involved heterosexual and homosexual contacts between the children as well as between the children and the men. The children who performed well were rewarded with BB guns, bicycles, and other prizes (*Manhattan Mercury* [Kansas] Associated Press, February 17, 1977). Even though they constitute only a small proportion of those who use children as sex objects, such men usually attract much publicity and provoke great societal outrage.

What effects do sexual contacts with adults have on children? There are no clear answers to this question since research addressing the issue is relatively scarce. In fact, little is known about the actual incidence of such contacts and it seems probable that most adult-child sex relations go unreported (Tsai & Wagner, 1978). It has, however, been estimated that between 20 and 35 percent of all children experience sexual approaches from or contacts with adults before puberty (Kinsey et al., 1953; McCaghy, 1971). The amount of erotica and literature devoted to the topic suggests that such contacts are more widespread (at least in fantasy) than one might expect (Rossman, 1973a). As indicated earlier, most of these contacts involve little more than fondling, genital touching, or genital exhibition.

Though physical injury to the involved child is extremely rare (Katzman, 1972; Kinsey et al., 1953), it is generally assumed that most children are sexually and emotionally traumatized by such experiences. To be sure, many children are frightened or mildly disturbed by their contacts with adults. The degree of disturbance ranges from that which might be evoked at the sight of a spider to extreme terror and physical illness. Others are only mildly embarrassed and some are pleased and erotically aroused (Kinsey et al., 1953). Among those who are severely disturbed, the long-range effects include guilt, depression, mistrust of men, and sexual dysfunction (Tsai & Wagner, 1978). Among the important determinants of the child's reaction to such contacts are the reactions of parents and legal authorities. The anger and hysteria of those who discover that the child has had such contacts may disturb the child more than the contacts themselves (Kinsey et al., 1953). It has also been shown that the trauma experienced by victimized children is greatest when force and coercion are involved and when the "partner" is substantially (ten years or more) older than the child (Finkelhor, 1979). Furthermore, multiple contacts and those that continue over a long period are likely to lead to substantial distress for victims (Tsai, Feldman-Summers, & Edgar, 1979).

Incest

Sexual contacts between people who are close relatives are referred to as **incest**. Incest is forbidden by social taboos or legal codes in virtually every known society (Ford & Beach, 1951) even though definitions of which relatives are included in the codes vary from one society to the next (Sagarin, 1977). Even in the United States, relatives with whom sexual contacts are defined as incest differ somewhat from state to state. For example, in all fifty states the incest taboo extends to members of the nuclear family (siblings, parents and children) and to other close relatives including uncles, aunts, nephews, nieces, grandparents, and grandchildren. In another third of the states, sexual intercourse between first cousins is incestuous and half the states ban marriages between first cousins (Hunt, 1974).

The Incest Taboo.   Why is incest so universally forbidden and met with horror and revulsion? The question has prompted a great deal of speculation (Lester, 1972) and two major types of theories have been advanced. The first is based on *biological* considerations and the argument that *genetic inbreeding* increases the risks of inheritance of undesirable traits (Lindzey, 1967). Most inherited undesirable characteristics are carried by recessive, rather than dominant, genes, and inbreeding increases the likelihood that such genes will exert a negative effect on the resulting offspring. There are two basic explanations of how these biological considerations function to make incest almost universally taboo. First, it is thought, a society's awareness of the genetic risks inherent in incest would logically cause it to find some way to prohibit incest. Second, some speculate that highly inbred populations would be unlikely to survive because of high rates of infant mortality, physical defects, or other deficiencies (Lindzey, 1967); thus, those societies which do survive would be the ones that make incest taboo. The available evidence does suggest that the risks of such defects are greater in offspring resulting from parent-child, sibling, and first-cousin incest than in those born of nonincestuous relationships (Adams & Neel, 1967; Schull & Neel, 1965). It is, of course, unlikely that primitive societies were aware of such possibilities, which in their case makes the first explanation unlikely. Survival failures due to natural selection—the basis for the second explanation—can occur without any such awareness, however (Lester, 1972).

A second major line of theorizing has focused on *psychosocial factors* and the notion that incest is taboo because it seriously disrupts family relationships and creates intense rivalry and jealousy among family members. There are several versions of this theory (see Lester, 1972) and the relevant evidence is mostly indirect. Although serious family conflict and disruption are often associated with incest, it is unclear whether such difficulties are the stimulus for or the result of incestuous relationships or both (Gebhard et al., 1965; Maisch, 1972). Extensions of the psychosocial explanation include arguments that incestuous sexual and marital arrangements interfere with the establishment of cooperative ties among different families, tribes, and clans that might act to the economic, protective, and social advantage of individual groups as well as the larger society (Lester, 1972). Whatever its origin, the incest taboo has been with us for a long time and violations of this ancient code are usually met with considerable contempt and punishment.

Incest Incidence and Participants.   Because it is considered among the most despicable of acts, the incidence of incest is difficult to determine. Much of what is known is based on studies of men convicted of and institutionalized for incest. Since the well educated and economically advantaged possess the resources to avoid legal intervention and publicity when incest occurs, institutionalized populations are heavily overrepresented by the poorly educated and poor and are therefore difficult to generalize from (Amir, 1972; Tsai & Wagner, 1978). It should be understood, however, that incest occurs across all social and educational levels and is not entirely a lower-class phenomenon (Hunt, 1974).

In light of these research difficulties, it is not surprising that estimates of the prevalence of incest vary considerably from one study to the next (James & Meyerding, 1978). Hunt's (1974) national survey (of mostly middle- to upper-class people), however, revealed that around 9 percent of females and 14 percent of males had, at one time or another, experienced some sort of heterosexual or homosexual contact with a relative. In a sample including higher percentages of lower-class individuals, Finkelhor (1979) found around a fourth of both sexes reporting incest experiences. When corrected for failures to report, Hunt's figures suggest that 15 percent of males and 11 percent of females have experienced incestuous contacts. Among the males reporting incest experience of any kind, over a fourth of the contacts were with sisters and two thirds were with female cousins. The remaining experiences (less than .5 percent each) were with daughters, brothers, uncles, aunts, nieces, male cousins, and sisters-in-law. Females with incest experience most frequently had such contacts with brothers (39 percent), followed by male cousins (35 percent), sisters (8 percent), uncles (6 percent), and fathers (5 percent). Extremely small percentages of girls (less than .5 percent) experienced contacts with sons, grandfathers, female cousins, brothers-in-law, or stepfathers.

The vast majority of males and females had six or fewer incestuous contacts and for many (a third of the males and half of the females) the contacts occurred prior to puberty in the form of childhood sex play. Only around 10 percent of all brother-sister contacts included coitus and less than a third of males involved with female cousins engaged in coitus. Female contacts with male cousins included coitus in only 5 percent of the cases. Less than .5 percent of the male contacts with aunts, nieces, or sisters-in-law and female contacts with uncles or stepfathers involved coitus (Hunt, 1974). Hunt's findings are in agreement with those of others (Finkelhor, 1979; Gebhard et al., 1965; Kinsey et al., 1953), indicating that the most prevalent forms of incest in the general population involve siblings or cousins. Most research on incest, however, has focused on father-daughter relationships since they are more likely than others to come to the attention of and be dealt with by legal authorities and social agencies.

Father-daughter incest almost always occurs in the context of a seriously disorganized and unhappy family situation (Gebhard et al., 1965; Maisch, 1972; Weinberg, 1955). Usually in his late thirties or forties, the father is often a rather dependent and shy man who is socially incompetent and has a poor occupational record. His only real locus of authority is in the home and he may exert tyrannical control over family members (Maisch, 1972). Although highly moralistic and conservative concerning sexual matters, he often appears to be preoccupied with sex (Finkelhor, 1979; Gebhard et al., 1965).

Because of his frequent unemployment, he is often at home alone with the children since his wife (who is likely to be a rather unstable person herself) is forced to work in support of the family. In nearly 75 percent of the cases the husband-wife sexual relationship is unsatisfactory as a result of the wife's absence, disinterest, or illness (Maisch, 1972). During the inevitable marital stress resulting from such situations, the husband turns to his daughter for affection and sex. Often, the incestuous relationship is initiated when the daughter begins to mature sexually (Maisch, 1972). The potency of the combined effects of marital dissatisfaction and a daughter's sexual maturation as a stimulus to incest is revealed in many cases:

A man forty-one years old at the beginning of incest, his marriage had been full of tension for some years and he had no satisfactory sexual relationship with his wife. He began sexual activities with his daughter a year after her menarche: "She had always been quite reserved and always dressed and undressed alone. I only ever saw her dressed, all the same I could see that she was already quite well developed!" (Maisch, 1972, p. 177)

Father-daughter incestuous relationships frequently continue for a rather long time, often lasting three or more years (Gebhard et al., 1965; Maisch, 1972). Incestuous contact is usually premeditated and initiated by the father and rather passively tolerated by the daughter. Only small proportions of the involved daughters either actively and violently resist their father's advances or unequivocally and actively initiate the contacts themselves. The surprising duration of incestuous relationships results from a number of factors, including the daughter's fear of her powerful father, emotional dependence on him, lack of knowledge concerning her rights, and general feelings of shame and embarrassment that prevent her from exposing her father. Much less frequently involved are her own sexual motives, financial rewards, and actual romantic attraction to her father (Maisch, 1972).

The termination of incestuous father-daughter relationships most frequently occurs because of changes that occur in the daughter. As she grows older and seeks more and more extrafamily social contacts (including boyfriends), her father may be driven by jealousy to attempt to increase his control over her. Increasingly aware of her rights and plagued by conflict and guilt, the daughter becomes more resistant to her father's controls and demands and seeks to terminate the relationship. How does she do so? Sometimes she simply leaves home but more often she reports it to her mother, some other family member, a friend, or more rarely to the police (Maisch, 1972; Womack, 1975).

The Aftermath of Incest.   Although there are undoubtedly some incidents of incest that conclude with few, if any, ill effects for those involved (Mathis, 1972), many outcomes are not so fortunate. Often the results are disastrous for the victimized daughter, the family unit, and the offending father.

The discovery and prosecution of incest by legal authorities frequently provokes a crisis in what is already a seriously disorganized family. The offending father may be imprisoned, leaving the remaining family members with severe financial difficulties. Even if imprisonment does not occur, public scorn and ridicule may lead to social isolation of the family, and relocation to another community where the "secret" is safe may become necessary. Existing intrafamily tension and hostility may heighten to intolerable levels and culminate in the dissolution of the family unit (DeFrancis, 1969).

Although relieved by the termination of incest, the daughter faces the immediate emotional burdens of guilt, shame, bitterness, and lowered self-esteem (DeFrancis, 1969). In response, some who have been thus victimized become hostile, rebellious, and sexually promiscuous (Ferracuti, 1972). Many prostitutes report histories of incest (James & Meyerding, 1978).

Over the longer term, victims of father-daughter incest continue in adulthood to experience feelings of guilt and shame stemming from their knowledge that they contributed to the continuation of incest by maintaining secrecy and may have experienced some sexual pleasure from what they recognized as socially repugnant behavior. Feelings of depression and inferiority may further complicate matters for these women in their adult life. Among other outcomes are fear and mistrust of men as well as sexual dysfunction manifested in nonresponsiveness, lack of pleasure from sex, and flashbacks to the incestuous contacts during intercourse. Poignant examples of such reactions are reported by Tsai and Wagner (1978):

I liked it, but I hated myself and my father for it.

I felt guilty since I didn't fight as hard sometimes because it felt good to me.

I really feel inferior to other people ... it's hard to feel good about yourself when you're constantly carrying something with you that can't be talked about.

I don't trust any men—they have to earn my trust.

When loving you has been used against you when you're small, you make the association that people who love you mistreat you and you set up barriers.

I can't stand for men to touch me or even come near me; I get numb and nauseated.

I can get aroused but I just want to get it over with.

When sexual experiences bring back associations with my dad, there's always this feeling of guilt, humiliation, anger, resentment, and bitterness. (pp. 421–424)

Fortunately, group therapy with adult incest victims shows great promise of alleviating such negative residuals (Tsai & Wagner, 1978).

Gerontophilia

Gerontophilia is a sexual variation in which a young person is erotically aroused by and manifests a clear preference for elderly persons as sex objects. True preferential desires among the young for aged sexual partners are rarely reported and little is known about their dynamics (Mathis, 1972). Clearly, males or females with such preferences are not bound by the usual norms of physical attractiveness, which place a high value on youth. It has been suggested (Gebhard, 1975b) that some men who turn to elderly women for sexual gratification do so because of sexual insecurity and failure to function adequately with women at their own age levels. Still others may seek aged sexual partners out of sexual desire for parent-like figures (Mathis, 1972). We should emphasize that even though they are often regarded as unusual, there are usually few, if any, gerontrophilic elements involved in those May-December pairings that are based on truly affectionate bonds or financial motives.

Necrophilia

Necrophilia is an extremely rare sexual variation in which a person is attracted to and derives sexual gratification from corpses. Not surprisingly, necrophilia almost always occurs in the context of severe mental or emotional disturbance. It almost always occurs in men and it is generally agreed (Mathis, 1972; Stoller, 1977) that sexual attraction to and preference for dead bodies represents the ultimate extension of a man's desire for nonresistant, nonthreatening, and totally subjugated sexual partners. The necrophile sees himself as totally inept sexually and often hates as well as fears live women (Mathis, 1972; Stoller, 1977). Thus, the only "safe" woman is a dead one:

KT was an embalmer by trade. . . . KT had been fired from his job only two times. Upon the first occasion he had incited the rage of the owner of the establishment when he had been discovered fondling the breasts of a young girl who had just been brought in. . . . His next and final apprehension came almost two years later when he was working in a small town in the southeast. He was discovered having intercourse with a female corpse which he was preparing to embalm. He was severely beaten by the other employees—so severely that hospitalization was necessary. (Mathis, 1972, p. 202)

In less extreme cases, men with necrophilic preferences sometimes pay for the services of prostitutes who agree to simulate corpses (Krafft-Ebing, 1965) or request their sexual partners to act as if they were dead. Any movement by the woman may destroy such men's sexual interest. Understandably, their partners are often horrified:

This morning our daughter phoned—in hysterics. It seems her wedding night was a nightmare. Her husband asked her to take a very cold bath before coming to bed. He suggested that she soak in a tub for about half an hour. When she came to bed he asked her to close her eyes and be perfectly still. Then he said, "You may as well know that I am a necrophiliac . . . I can only make love to dead women or women who look as if they are". . . . Our daughter fled in panic, packed her bags and checked into another room. She is at the moment in a state of shock and under a doctor's care (Ann Landers Advises, January 4, 1976).

Bestiality

Bestiality refers to the *preferred* use of nonhuman animals as sex objects. Although true bestiality is rare, survey studies (Hunt, 1974; Kinsey et al., 1948, 1953) suggest that 5 to 8 percent of males and 2 to 3 percent of females experience some sort of sexual contact with animals during their lives. Such contacts usually occur during early adolescence and are more common among those reared on farms than those reared in cities. For example, Kinsey and his colleagues (1948) reported that between 40 and 50 percent of farm boys have sexual contacts with animals and as many as 17 percent of male adolescents who live on farms reach orgasm in their relations with animals. The animals with which rural males most often have sexual contact are calves or sheep even though virtually every type of farm animal, including chickens, ducks, and geese may be involved (Kinsey et al., 1948). The most frequent kinds of male contacts with mammals are vaginal coitus, manipulation of the animal's genitals, or oral stimulation of the boy's genitals by the animal (Hunt, 1974; Kinsey et al., 1948).

Females are most likely to have sexual contacts with household pets such as dogs and cats. Most involve only general body contacts with manipulation of the animal's genitals and oral-genital stimulation by the animals less frequent. Actual female coitus with animals is extremely rare but does occasionally occur (Kinsey et al., 1953). Although rare in reality, human female sexual relations with animals are not uncommon as the subject matter of mythology, folklore, pornography, and male fantasy (Kinsey et al., 1953).

VARIATIONS IN SEXUAL EXPRESSION

We have seen how the vicissitudes of life may shape people's erotic response potentials in molds that do not fully match the expectations and demands of the larger society. In yet other cases a people's erotic responses may be viewed as falling mostly within normatively acceptable ranges while their sexually motivated behavior is expressed in a variant and often socially unacceptable manner. In this section we will briefly examine some of the most frequent variant forms of sexual expression.

Voyeurism

Virtually all heterosexually oriented men and, perhaps to a lesser extent, women are erotically aroused by the sight of nudes of the opposite sex or by viewing heterosexual activity. In **voyeurism**, however, an individual (usually a man) derives an unusually great amount of sexual pleasure from *secretly* viewing sexual acts or nudes of the opposite sex.

Most often the voyeur (commonly called a Peeping Tom after the legend of Lady Godiva) endeavors to peer through windows (or other openings such as holes drilled in walls, doors, or floors) to secretly observe women undressing or engaged in some type of sexual activity. He does so without the consent of the observed parties (or the law) and the danger and excitement that this entails adds to his sexual arousal. Indeed, the "true" peeper may go to great lengths and run great risks in pursuit of a good sexual view. Requiring some agility and fleetness of foot, peeping is a young man's activity. It often necessitates scaling fences or trees, balancing on window ledges, and running foot races with irate husbands, neighbors, or police (Gebhard et al., 1965).

Obviously, peepers place a greater value on sexual looking than does the average man, who may occasionally take advantage of a viewing opportunity but who is unwilling to assume great risks in doing so. Who are these men and why do they sometimes prefer and obtain greater pleasure from peeping than from socially and legally acceptable forms of sexual activity? Little is known about the underlying motivations for compulsive voyeurism although several "explanations," including defense against castration anxiety, fixations on infantile sexual impulses, incestuous wishes, impaired instincts, and learning experiences, have been offered (Smith, 1976). What is known is derived mostly from studies of convicted peepers, the most comprehensive of which was conducted by Gebhard and his associates (1965).

In over 90 percent of the cases studied by Gebhard and his colleagues, the women chosen as voyeuristic objects were strangers to the men. At first conviction the average man was about twenty-four years of age and never married, although nearly a third of those convicted of peeping were or had been married at some time. Most of the men showed no evidence of serious mental or emotional disturbance, impairment due to drugs or alcohol, or intellectual deficiency.

The most striking characteristic of convicted peepers is a bleak and deficient history of sociosexual development. As adolescents, they have few heterosexual petting partners, are shy with females, and have strong feelings of inferiority and fears of rejection. As a result of their heterosexual ineptness, fear, and timidity, they turn to peeping for sexual gratification. Through peeping they avoid the expected trauma of personal heterosexual encounters and gain some personal sense of superiority and power over their unknowing "victims." Frequently, masturbation accompanies peeping, further enhancing its sexual excitement value for the peeper (Gebhard et al., 1965; McGuire et al., 1965).

Although most habitual peepers can be characterized by the heterosexual inadequacies described above, there are some men who do not make a habit of peeping but do so impulsively when an opportunity presents itself. Such men primarily react to situational opportunities under conditions in which their self-controls may be impaired by alcohol or low intelligence rather than by compelling personal needs.

Most peepers pose no physical danger to their victims, but some may follow their peeping with rape. It has been suggested (Gebhard et al., 1965) that those who enter buildings in order to peep or deliberately attract the female's attention by tapping on windows, leaving notes, or telephoning are more likely to become rapists than those who do not.

Exhibitionism

Exhibitionism occurs when a person, for purposes of personal sexual arousal or gratification, deliberately exposes his or her genitals to the opposite sex under conditions in which the exposure is socially inappropriate. Almost all exhibitionists ("flashers," "flag wavers") are male. Genital exposure that is accidental, occurs in the course of petting or coitus, or takes place in socially appropriate circumstances such as nudist camps or nude swimming is not exhibitionism.

Of all sexual offenses, exhibitionism accounts for more arrests than any other (Rooth, 1973). At the time of their first convictions, most exhibitionists are about thirty years of age. Nearly a third are married and close to another third were married at one time but are separated, divorced, or widowed at the time of the offense (Gebhard et al., 1965). While the circumstances surrounding acts of exhibitionism are diverse, some commonalities exist. For example, exhibitionists almost always expose themselves to women who are strangers. Over 90 percent of the targets are strangers, and the remainder are acquaintances, friends, or relatives.

Most often, exposure occurs out-of-doors and sometimes in quite crowded public locations. Some men drive around in their autos and, when likely targets are located, they open the car door and display their genitals. Still others may stand at open windows and expose themselves from their own residences (Gebhard et al., 1965). These behavior patterns, in conjunction with the fact that many exhibitionists repeat their acts again and again in similar or identical locations, place them in great jeopardy of being identified and apprehended. It has, in fact, been suggested that many such men desire to be caught (Mathis, 1972; McCary, 1978; Stoller, 1977).

In most cases, the exhibitionist's penis is erect and a few may even ejaculate upon exposure. Some masturbate while exhibiting and still others may exhibit, flee, and then masturbate (Gebhard et al., 1965). Most authorities (e.g., Gebhard et al., 1965; Mathis, 1972; Stoller, 1977) agree that the typical exhibitionist does not display his genitals as a gesture of sexual solicitation. The display itself is the sexual act from which gratification is obtained. The man hopes to elicit some reaction from the woman, be it surprise, embarrassment, anger, fear, or other responses. Further sexual contact is not usually desired and the man will generally exhibit from a distance of no less than six feet from his target. Little gratification is received if the woman shows no response and most men will flee if she shows any sexual interest (Stoller, 1977). Exhibitionists rarely touch or physically assault their "victims" and exhibitionism accompanied by rape is extremely rare (Mathis, 1972). Many victims are, however, highly psychologically disturbed by their experiences (Finkelhor, 1979).

At least two major categories of exhibitionists have been identified (Gebhard et al., 1965; Witzig, 1968). First are those men who for one reason or another have grave doubts and concerns about their "manliness" or "masculinity" in the sexual

Many exhibitionists expose themselves to the public from an open window or balcony of their own residence.

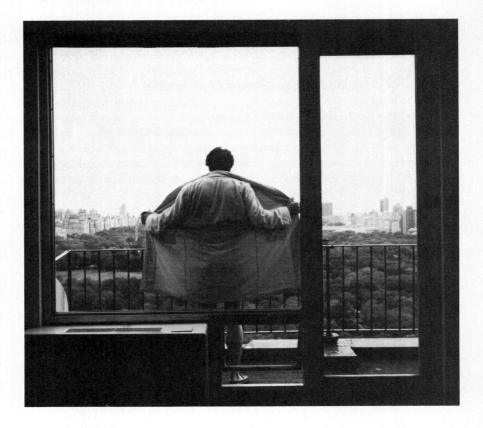

or nonsexual arenas of their lives. These men are insecure and uncomfortable in their relationships with others, particularly females, and are limited and late in their heterosexual development. They have few premarital petting and coitus partners and their heterosexual skills are poorly developed. Even when married, coitus with their wives is infrequent and unsatisfactory—many experience erectile difficulties—and much of their sexual expression is limited to solitary masturbation. They feel oppressed by women and relatively helpless and inept in their presence. In these cases, their exhibitionism seems to be motivated by a desire to affirm to themselves and to the world that they are, indeed, masculine. It is their way of crying out, "Look, I am a man" (Gebhard et al., 1965).

The following example is typical:

This married man in his 40s has always been shy with women, and after 16 years of marriage still is passive around his wife. During their infrequent intercourse (every 6 weeks to 2 months) he has difficulty getting or maintaining an erection. While his wife constantly bullies him, he does not complain, believing that she has a right to do so. In the last five years, he has succumbed to the urge to exhibit his penis to passing girls or women. This occurs on the street, in the daytime, under circumstances when he realistically runs great risk of arrest. In fact, he does this in the neighborhood where he lives, not even going to strange areas or cities.

He will stand to the side of a street and show his exposed penis to women passing in cars or to women walking on the other side of the street. He has an erection at these times. If he believes he was not noticed, he will shift his position or otherwise attempt to get their attention and when he has done so, he will not flee when he senses they are upset and might call for help.

On one occasion, he exposed himself to two teenage girls, who began chuckling and advanced toward him as if interested; this is the only time he has precipitously left the scene. He has been arrested six times and has already spent time in prison. His reputation is ruined, his family is humiliated, and his professional status is in terrible disrepair. Nonetheless, he says he will probably repeat the act. (Stoller, 1977, p. 203)

In these men, exhibitionism seems to stem from a truly compulsive urge. Often such urges are triggered by some emotionally stressful event such as being rejected or ridiculed by women or by experiencing some occupationally related failure. Exhibitionists of this sort usually feel guilty and ashamed following acts of exposure and those who truly desire to eliminate their exhibition often benefit greatly from behavior modification (Evans, 1968; Maletzky, 1974; Rooth & Marks, 1974).

A second category of exhibitionists includes men whose social controls and judgment are temporarily or chronically impaired by alcohol, intellectual deficiency, or emotional disturbance (Gebhard et al., 1965; Witzig, 1968). Included here are drunks who expose themselves for the misguided purpose of solicitation, as a drunkenly humorous gesture, or as an expression of contempt and hostility. Also included are the intellectually deficient, whose exposure results from lack of awareness of the socially disapproved nature of their acts or from futile attempts at sexual solicitation (Coleman, 1976).

Frottage

Frottage is a variant form of sexual expression in which a man *(frotteur)* obtains sexual pleasure by rubbing or pressing against women. The behavior usually takes place in crowded locations such as elevators, buses, and subways. The man will seemingly inadvertently make contact with women's legs or buttocks with his flaccid or erect penis. It is thought that men who engage in frottage have great difficulty in establishing coital relationships with women due to fears of their own social and sexual inadequacy.

Klismaphilia

Though little is known about its origin or dynamics, **klismaphilia** refers to deriving erotic pleasure from receiving or giving enemas. Pleasure associated with receiving enemas is probably related to the erotic sensitivity of the anus and rectum and the fact that early in life enemas are often administered by concerned and loving mothers (McCary, 1978). The resulting pleasure and the affectional association may tend to eroticize the experience for some individuals.

RESEARCH HIGHLIGHT

Eliminating Unwanted Variant Sexual Behavior Through Behavior Modification

Many of the variant forms of sexual expression discussed in this chapter are illegal or otherwise problematic for those who engage in them. Individuals involved in pedophilic, voyeuristic, exhibitionistic, or other variant forms of sexual behavior often seek (or are forced to seek) professional assistance in eliminating their problematic behaviors. Although many forms of assistance are available (Coleman, 1976), the preferred mode of intervention in many cases is some type of behavior modification that focuses specifically on elimination or modification of the undesired behavior itself. One such intervention procedure, covert sensitization, pairs, in the imagination, scenes of the pleasurable but unwanted behaviors with aversive or unpleasant scenes in an effort to diminish the gratification received from the unwanted behaviors.

Maletzky (1974) reports the successful use of a modified form of covert sensitization to eliminate exhibitionistic desires and behaviors in ten men. The men were seen individually and induced to vividly imagine and visualize exhibitionistic scenes. At the point when their sexual pleasure was escalating, the "therapist" introduced suggestions of aversive experiences and held an uncapped bottle of a foul-smelling chemical (valeric acid) under their noses. The men were then led to vividly imagine escape from the exposing situation and the noxious odor was removed. The following excerpt is representative of such imaginary, therapeutic adventures:

You see this great looking girl walking on your right. You slow down to get a better look—she's blonde, about 16, and really stacked. You can see her breasts under her tight blouse, and her skirt is so short you can see her legs all the way up! You start to get excited just by looking and turn the car around to follow her. Now she's on your left, and you slowly pull up to her as you start to play with yourself and your penis starts to get harder and stiffer. You can't help but think about touching and fondling her, and you just ache to be naked with her [valeric acid introduced], to see her be surprised and happy at how big and hard your penis is. But as you stop the car and start to take it out, that bad smell comes back and that sick feeling in the pit of your stomach. You really get turned off as your stomach turns over and over and pieces of your supper catch in your throat. You try to gag them back down but you can't; big chunks of vomit gush out of your mouth, dribble down your chin, and go all over you. . . . The blonde can see you now, all soft and vomiting all over yourself, and she is starting to get your license number! . . . you've got to get out of there! [valeric acid removed] You quickly clean yourself off and drive away, rolling down the windows to get some fresh air. . . . you drive away, glad that you're out of there. (Maletzky, 1974, pp. 35–36)

As may be seen in the figure here, after several sessions in which imagery of exposure situations was paired with aversive imagery and the foul odor, overt (actual) and covert (exposure urges or fantasies) exhibitionistic behaviors were both dramatically reduced and these effects were still apparent at the twelve-month followup period. This study, as well as others (Bandura, 1969), clearly demonstrates the usefulness of behavior modification techniques in the elimination of unwanted variant sexual behavior.

Frequencies of covert and overt exhibitionistic behavior immediately before, immediately after, and 12 months after treatment.

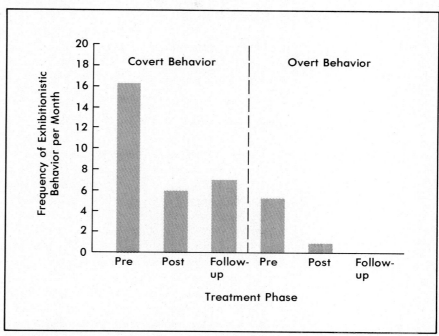

SOURCE: Data from Maletzky, 1974.

Nymphomania and Satyriasis

Nymphomania and **satyriasis** are terms used to refer to the behavior of women and men, respectively, who exhibit extraordinarily high sexual appetites and levels of sexual activity. In such people sexual demands and activities seem to dominate and often interfere with all other life concerns. "True" nymphomania and satyriasis are probably quite rare, but the terms are often used by people who view their own partners as having unusually strong sexual drives. Some men, for example, might view a woman who desires intercourse two to three times a week as a nymphomaniac while others might view such desires as average or below average. In reality, it is probably the insatiability and compulsivity of sexual needs and activities that define a person's behavior as variant or not. Nymphomania or satyriasis often is associated with the need of the individual to confirm her or his own attractiveness and value as a woman or a man in response to a negative self-concept (Mathis, 1972).

Sadomasochism

The term **sadomasochism (S & M)** refers to variant forms of sexual behavior in which sexual arousal and gratification are obtained through inflicting or receiving pain. The word is derived from **sadism** and **masochism**, which are in turn derived, respectively, from the names of the French author the Marquis de Sade and the Austrian novelist Leopold von Sacher-Masoch. The Marquis de Sade wrote extensively of his erotic fantasies and acts in which he obtained sexual pleasure by whipping, beating, or otherwise inflicting pain on his sexual partners. Sacher-Masoch, on the other hand, extolled the sexual pleasures of being physically and psychologically mistreated by his lovers. Our use of the single term, sadomasochism, reflects the general belief (Gebhard, 1969) and the available evidence (Spengler, 1977) that persons who are aroused by sadistic activities (inflicting pain) are usually aroused by masochistic activities (receiving pain) as well.

Although it may be difficult to comprehend how the two might become closely linked in sadomasochism, pain and sexual arousal often go hand in hand (or perhaps more precisely put, paw in paw) in nonhuman mammalian species (Ford & Beach, 1951; Maple, Erwin, & Mitchell, 1974). The precoital activity of skunks, minks, domestic cats, and other animals includes a considerable amount of violence, which sometimes results in severe wounds to the "lovers." In humans, mild pain administered through tickling, biting, and scratching is a rather common part of sexual interactions and often adds to sexual excitement. Kinsey and his associates (1953), for example, reported that over 50 percent of both sexes experience some erotic response from being bitten by their sexual partners. In addition, over 10 percent of women and 20 percent of men in the Kinsey studies reported some erotic response to sadomasochistic fantasies or stories. More recently, Hunt (1974) reported that sexual pleasure is experienced through inflicting pain by about 5 percent of men and 2 percent of women and through receiving pain by about 3 percent of men and 5 percent of women. Furthermore, even though the origins of the linkages are obscure, it now seems clear that under some circumstances (Malamuth, Feshbach, & Jaffe, 1977) sexual and aggressive motives become closely linked (Barclay, 1970, 1971b).

In sadomasochism, however, the pain-sex associations are so strongly formed that administering and receiving pain become integral or even essential parts of sexual acts. How are such associations formed? First, it has been suggested that *conditioning experiences* in which strong sexual arousal is paired, perhaps unintentionally, with giving or receiving pain are involved. For example, Gebhard (1965) reported the development of sadomasochistic desires in a man following an adolescent experience in which he was having a fractured arm painfully set without anesthesia. While comforting the boy, an attractive nurse caressed him and held his head against her breast, creating a powerful association between pain and erotic arousal.

Second, sadomasochism is often found in a context of powerful *feelings of guilt, shame, and disgust concerning sexual expression*. For the sadist, sexual arousal and behavior become possible only if he or she is able to punish and express contempt for the other person for engaging in such despicable behavior. For the masochist, receiving punishment and degradation expiates any guilt that might result from any sexual activities that occur (Coleman, 1976; Gebhard, 1969).

In still other cases, a third factor may be involved. Relatively *severe psychopathology* combined with rigid and puritanical attitudes toward sex are often found in so-called sadistic murderers. Almost always committed by men and, although constituting less than 1 percent of all homocides (Swigert, Farrell, & Yoels, 1976), sadistic sexual murders attract a tremendous amount of publicity and generate extreme disgust and horror in most people. Sometimes, as was supposed in the case of Jack the Ripper, sexual satisfaction is derived from the murder alone or from mutilation of the corpse. In other instances, killing is followed by sexual intercourse with or, as in the case of the Boston Strangler, masturbation and ejaculation upon the corpse (Mathis, 1972).

As is often true of taboo or variant forms of sexual behavior, most of what we know about sadomasochists and their sexuality comes from studies of limited samples of people. Included here are those who seek treatment (Mathis, 1972), those who attempt to attract sexual partners by placing ads in newspapers or belong to S & M clubs (Spengler, 1977), and those who, like de Sade and Sacher-Masoch, record their sexual fantasies and activities (Greene & Greene, 1974).

Even from such limited data, however, some generalities have emerged. For example, it now seems clear that relatively few sadomasochists are exclusively sadists or exclusively masochists (Gebhard, 1969; Spengler, 1977), in part because sexual partners are difficult to find and out of necessity two sadists or two masochists may be forced to alternate between their sadistic and masochistic roles. The available evidence indicates that about a third of sadomasochists prefer the sadistic role, another third the masochistic role, and another third are truly versatile and equally comfortable in either role (Spengler, 1977).

Sadomasochistic desires and preferences are about equally prevalent in those who are heterosexually, homosexually, and bisexually oriented. Furthermore, relatively few surveyed sadomasochists (16 percent) express preferences exclusively for sadomasochistic activity, with the remainder preferring a mixture of sadomasochistic and nonsadomasochistic activity. Most sadomasochists fully or partially accept their preferences as pleasurable and "normal" (Spengler, 1977).

Sadomasochistic activity usually takes place in the context of a carefully scripted ceremony or ritual. Pain per se is not pleasurable and, as with most people, accidental pain is truly antisexual for the sadomasochist. Often a theatrical drama is enacted in which the masochist presumably has done something wrong and the sadist metes out punishment. Punishment may take many forms but often includes restraint with ropes or chains (bondage), beating and whipping (discipline), painful torture, or degrading acts such as urinating (urolagnia) or defecating (coprolangnia) upon the wrongdoer. Sexual arousal and orgasm may take place during punishment, the punishment may simply serve as arousing foreplay prior to more conventional behavior, or the participants may be aroused by contemplating the pain after it has ceased (Gebhard, 1969).

Such dramas sometimes involve an impressive array of fetish items and props or paraphernalia including torture devices, hoods, handcuffs, and specialized uniforms (Gebhard, 1965). The prevalence of various forms of punishment and fetish items as reported by a sample of over two hundred surveyed sadomasochists (Spengler, 1977) is indicated in Table 12–1.

If all of this seems a bit gruesome and cruel, it is important to realize that even though sadomasochistic relationships involve pain and humiliation, the acts often, paradoxically, take place in an overall context of affection and tenderness. The goal in consensual S & M relationships is not to produce lasting and serious injury but to relate sexually in a way that is mutually pleasurable and satisfying.

RAPE AND SEXUAL ASSAULT

Although they differ somewhat from state to state, most legal definitions of **rape** generally refer to an act of coitus that is performed without the consent of the woman. The charge of rape may be made when the woman's consent has been bypassed through the use of force, threat of force, or deception, or if she is unable to provide rational consent because of unconsciousness, sleep, intoxication, or mental retardation. Coitus under such conditions is usually classified as *forcible rape*. Coitus with a female below the legal age of consent (usually sixteen) is a separate category of offense referred to as *statutory rape*. In any case, some degree of actual or attempted penile-vaginal penetration (however slight) must occur before rape or attempted rape may legally be determined to have occurred (Amir, 1971). Some states, however, have broadened their definitions of rape to include

Table 12–1.

Types of sadomasochistic practices and fetish items and the percentage of over 200 sadomasochists surveyed who reported employing them.

Sadomasochistic Practice	Percentage	Fetish Items	Percentage
Whip	66	Leather	50
Cane	60	Boots	50
Bonds	60	Jeans	19
Anal manipulations	26	Uniforms	16
"Torture" apparatus	27	Women's clothing	14
Nipple torture	9	Rubber	12
Needles	6		
Clothespins clamps	7		
Hot objects	7		
Coprophilia	5		
Knives or razor blades	4		

SOURCE: Data from Spengler, 1977.

A shop display of paraphernalia sold to some sadists and masochists for use in their sexual activities.

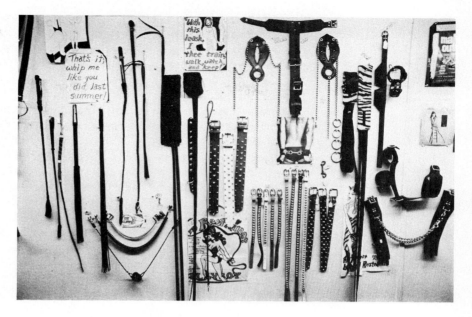

oral, anal, and other forced sexual contacts (*Sex and the Law*, September 1979). It is with forcible rape that we are concerned in this section and particularly with those rapes that occur through the use of physical force or threats of such force.

Until recently, a man could not be legally accused of raping his wife because permanent consent to coitus was considered as an integral part of the marital contract (Brownmiller, 1975). Several states, however, now have laws allowing a wife to charge her husband with rape. In December 1978 an Oregon man became the first to be prosecuted for raping his wife. He was acquitted. Since then, at least one conviction has been obtained. Women may be (but rarely are) charged with rape by assisting a man in raping another woman. In those rare cases in which a woman forces her sexual attentions on a man she is usually charged with "sexual assault." In one such case, an eighteen-year-old man reported being tied to a chair for three days and forced at gunpoint to submit to the "sexual advances" of a thirty-two-year-old woman. The woman was charged with kidnapping, first-degree criminal assault, and a firearms violation (Knight-Ridder News Service, December 14, 1978).

Incidence and Circumstances of Rape

According to the Federal Bureau of Investigation, there were over 82,000 reported rapes in the United States in 1980 (FBI, 1981). Even though this figure indicates the occurrence of one rape every 6.4 minutes, it is likely that far more rapes take place than are actually reported. Because of the feelings of embarrassment and guilt it evokes in the victims and their fears of retaliation from their assailants (FBI, 1981), rape is probably the most underreported violent crime. (The responses of victims to rape are discussed in more detail later.) Even though various estimates (Amir, 1971; Griffin, 1976; Offir, 1975) place the "true" incidence of rape at five to twenty times higher, it is impossible to arrive at any reliable estimate of the actual unknown instances of rape or any other crime (Amir, 1971). It is clear, however, that the incidence of reported rape has increased substantially (more than 100 percent) over the last decade so that, according to FBI (1981) reports, in the early 1980s, out of every 100,000 women in the United States, 155 were raped (85 in large cities, 40 in smaller cities, and 30 in rural areas).

Of all rapes and attempts reported, over three fourths are completed. In 1980, 49 percent of reported rapes resulted in the arrest of the assailant(s), with the highest arrest rates occurring in rural areas, followed by relatively small cities and then large metropolitan areas. Most of those arrested were between the ages of eighteen and twenty-two, and over half (54 percent) were under age twenty-five. Slightly over half (51 percent) were white and 48 percent were black (FBI, 1981).

Our knowledge of the details of rape is limited to those rapes that come to the attention of legal authorities and the extent to which this knowledge may be generalized is open to much debate (Brownmiller, 1975). Nevertheless, some commonalities have emerged from the research. First, it appears (Amir, 1971; MacDonald, 1971; Gager & Schurr, 1976) that most women who report a rape say that their attacker was a stranger. For example, Amir (1971) and MacDonald (1971) reported, respectively, that 52 and 60 percent of rapes were committed by men who were unknown to their victims. While these figures are consistent with society's view of the rapist as a stranger lurking around a dark corner, many reported rapes are committed by men who know their victims as casual acquaintances, close neighbors, close friends or boyfriends, family friends, or relatives (Clark & Lewis, 1977). Even when they do not know each other, rapists and their victims live in the same general neighborhood in over 75 percent of the cases (Amir, 1971).

Over half of all reported rapes occur in the residence of the victim or that of the offender and another 10 to 15 percent occur in other inside locations such as vacant houses, housing projects, commercial establishments, and churches. The remaining one fourth to one third take place out-of-doors or in automobiles (Amir, 1971; Brownmiller, 1975; Macdonald, 1971). Regardless of location, the vast majority (70 percent or more) of forcible rapes are premeditated rather than impulsive, spur-of-the-moment assaults (Gebhard et al., 1965). This is particularly true of pair or group rapes (accounting for up to 10 percent of rapes), in which two or more offenders select and assault a single victim (Amir, 1971; Brownmiller, 1975; Groth & Birnbaum, 1979).

By definition, forcible rape involves the use of force. But force can be applied in many ways and in varying degrees. In his study of rape in Philadelphia, Amir (1971) distinguished between the use of nonphysical (coercion and threats, intimidation, threat with weapons) and physical forms of force. All of the rapes studied involved some form of nonphysical force and fully 85 percent of all rape victims were subjected to physical force and violence to varying degrees. Nearly 30 percent of all the rapes reported involved some degree of "roughness," with the attacker holding or pushing the victim. Mild beatings (slapping) occurred in 22 percent of the cases before and in 3 percent of the cases after the rape. Brutal beatings, which included kicking and repeated pummeling with fists, were involved in 20 percent of reported rapes. About 12 percent of the women raped were choked into submission by their assailants. Not surprisingly, extreme force and violence occurs more frequently when the victim and offender are strangers (Amir, 1971). Serious physical injury to rape victims in Denver from 1970 to 1972 occurred in less than 10 percent of the cases and it is estimated that less than 1 percent of all murders are associated with sexual assaults (Selkin, 1975).

Even though serious physical injury does not always accompany rape, victimized women are often forced to perform acts that are experienced as degrading and humiliating. In one of the few detailed studies of the sexual acts involved in rapes, Holmstrom and Burgess (1980) documented the fact that more than penile-vaginal intercourse is often involved. Of the 112 raped women in this study, 95 percent reported being forced to engage in intercourse. In addition, however, at least some women reported being forced to engage in fellatio, anal intercourse, cunnilingus, nude dancing, homosexual behavior while the rapist watched, manual stimulation of the rapist's genitals and anus, oral stimulation of the rapist's anus, and a variety of other acts. Some women reported that the rapist(s) urinated on them, inserted objects into their vaginas, bit or burned their breasts, or ejaculated on them. The degrading and humiliating nature of rape for its victims is clearly illustrated by excerpts from the experiences of one woman who was raped by a pair of men:

Angie's two assailants drove south on the freeway to another town. The driver parked on a deserted road in a wooded area. They put handcuffs on her and held the screwdriver to her. Each had sex with her. Then they made her stand in between them while they punched at her. Then they had her lie on the hood of the car. There was a kind of ritual to it. They had her assume various positions, one man would watch and one would have sex, and so on. They also had matches that they lit and threw at her. They stood her up and had sex, had her perform fellatio, had anal intercourse with her. After penetration, the men masturbated and then put the semen on the victim. (Holmstrom & Burgess, 1980, p. 433)

Rapists

As we indicated previously, most convicted rapists are in their late teens or early twenties. Nationally, a slight majority are white (FBI, 1981), although in some urban areas heavily populated by blacks, the majority of reported rapes are committed by blacks (Amir, 1971; Brownmiller, 1975). Perhaps 50 percent of men who rape have been drinking prior to the offense (Rada, 1975) even though the influence of alcohol is an important element in only one third or less of forcible rapes (Gebhard et al., 1965). Even though they come from all socioeconomic levels, most convicted rapists are unemployed or involved in unskilled or skilled labor (Amir, 1971; Kirk, 1975) and somewhat less intelligent as measured by standard IQ tests than are non–sex offenders (Karacan, Williams, Guerrero, Salis, Thornby, & Hursch, 1974; Ruff, Templer, & Ayers, 1976). From 30 to 40 percent are married and at least another 25 percent have been married but are separated, divorced, or widowed at the time of the offense (Gebhard et al., 1965). Finally, many have extensive histories of nonsexual criminal convictions (Gebhard et al., 1965).

Beyond these "social bookkeeping" bits of information, little is actually known about rapists and the motives underlying their actions. In their attempts to understand the dynamics of rape, however, researchers have developed at least two lines of thought. One of these (Cohen et al., 1969; Gebhard et al., 1965; Groth & Birnbaum, 1979; Rada, 1978) has focused on attempts to identify *typologies of rapists* and is based on the assumption that rape results from individual psychological disturbances of a chronic or temporary nature. The second treats rape as a byproduct of *sex-role socialization patterns* (Brownmiller, 1975; Gager & Schurr, 1976). Underlying this view is the assumption that Western societies socialize men to dominate and control women, sometimes with the use of sex. Let us examine these two perspectives.

Rapists as Psychological Types.   On the basis of studies of convicted sex offenders, several investigators (e.g., Amir, 1971; Gebhard et al., 1965; Cohen et al., 1969) have attempted to classify rapists in terms of what appear to be commonly observed individual patterns of causal dynamics. For example, noting that acts of rape involve both sexual and aggressive features, Cohen and associates (1969) suggest that at least four types of rapists may be identified.

The first is the *displaced-aggression* type of rapist. For this man, the act of rape is primarily aggressive, and sexual intent, feelings, or gratification are minimally present or absent:

The sexual behavior is used to physically harm, to degrade, or to defile the victim in the service of this aggressive intent. The acts are experienced by the offenders as the result of an "uncontrollable impulse" and almost always follows some precipitating, disagreeable event involving a wife, girlfriend, or mother. . . . Sexual excitation is often absent or only minimally present. The offender must masturbate in order to get an erection and in a large number of cases, he cannot reach orgasm. It is readily apparent that the sexual behavior is not meant to gratify an intense sexual desire but rather is serving an aggressive motive. (Cohen et al., 1969, p. 250)

Referring to this as "anger rape," Groth and Birnbaum (1979) emphasize the anger and rage that motivates the rapist.

The second in this typology, the *compensatory* type of rapist, uses aggression primarily in the service of sexual needs. In most cases such offenders are extremely passive and submissive and obsessively concerned with feelings of sexual inadequacy for which the rape compensates. If the victim resists or struggles vigorously, such offenders usually flee:

The offender is always in a state of intense sexual excitation and often has an orgasm in the simple pursuit of the victim or upon making some physical contact. The recurrent fantasy in such offenders is that the victims will yield, submit to intercourse, in which he will be especially virile and so pleasing to the victim that she will become enamoured of him and invite him to repeat the sexual acts. (Cohen et al., 1969, p. 250)

This type of offender may also be characterized as a "power rapist" who uses the sexual attack as a means of asserting power and dominance over his victims (Groth & Birnbaum, 1979).

Sex-aggression-diffusion rapists, the third type, display a mixture of sexual and aggressive desires. Sexual arousal seems to merge with aggressive arousal so that sexual desires cannot exist without accompanying aggressive desires:

. . . he projects such feelings [sexual-aggressive desires] onto his victim and sees her struggles and protestations as seductive—"Women like to get roughed up; they enjoy a good fight." Such perceptions are made in the context of very brutal assaults. . . . all . . . relationships, with . . . women, show this same quality of an eroticization of aggressive behavior. (Cohen et al., 1969, p. 250)

Groth and Birnbaum (1979) refer to this pattern as "sadistic rape" in which sexuality and aggression fuse with the result that sexual pleasure is derived from physical abuse of the victim. Such men are often very loud, assertive, and "hyper-masculine" and when they rape, they often become very brutal and vicious.

Impulse rapists, the fourth group in the Cohen typology, appear to act out of impulse in an opportunistic manner. Often rape takes place as an afterthought following robbery or burglary. Neither sexual nor aggressive motives play a prominent role in such rapes, which seem to be simply an expression of the offender's predatory nature (Cohen et al., 1969).

Other investigators (e.g., Gebhard et al., 1965) have identified yet a fifth category of rapists who appear to be pleasure oriented and largely devoid of concern for social norms. These *amoral delinquents* or *antisocial personalities*

. . . simply want to have coitus and the females' wishes are of no particular consequence. They are not hostile toward females, but look upon them solely as sexual objects whose role in life is to provide sexual pleasure. If a woman is recalcitrant and will not fulfill her role, a man may have to use force, threat, weapons, or anything else at his disposal. . . . [This type of rapist] regards women as mere pleasantly shaped masses of protoplasm for sexual use. (Gebhard et al., 1965, p. 200)

Although systematic data relevant to these typologies are relatively scarce, it is apparent that the motives underlying acts of rape are multiple and generally represent complex configurations of sexual and aggressive needs as well as deficient or ineffective socialization in terms of acceptable modes of heterosexual interactions. Many convicted rapists appear to be irritable, hostile, angry, and suspicious men who are unpredictable in both action and deed (Rader, 1977).

One important characteristic that seems common to most rapists is that they are considerably *more sexually aroused by rape* and sex-aggression fantasies and stimuli than are nonrapists (Abel, Barlow, Blanchard, & Guild, 1977; Barbaree, Marshall, & Lanthier, 1979). Some are also *less aroused by nonaggressive sex* and sex cues than are nonrapists (Abel, Blanchard, & Becker, 1978). Thus, one of the seemingly most effective treatment programs for rapists focuses on modification of sexual arousal patterns, as well as on development of heterosexual skills, improvements in self-control, and hostility reduction (Abel et al., 1978).

Rapists as Products of Sex-Role Socialization Patterns.   In contrast to attempts to identify types of rapists with respect to patterns of personal and social pathology, some researchers (e.g., Brownmiller, 1975; Gager & Schurr, 1976; Griffin, 1976) argue that rape is primarily the outcome of sex-role socialization practices. Standard rearing practices in our culture emphasize aggression, power, and dominance as desirable male characteristics and passivity, weakness, and submissiveness as desirable female characteristics. Extended to the sexual sphere, to be "masculine" is to be sexually aggressive and dominant and, from this perspective, rape is viewed as one important expression of power and dominance over women (Sanday, 1981). The sexual aspects of rape are deemphasized in this theoretical approach and rape is commonly characterized as a violent rather than a sexual act (Brownmiller, 1975; Gager & Schurr, 1976; Weis & Borges, 1973).

In her thought-provoking and insightful historical and cultural analysis of rape, Susan Brownmiller (1975) has described how the interacting effects of superior male physical strength, attempts to control paternity by controlling female sexuality, and a variety of other factors have acted in concert to create a view of women as sexual property whose chastity and monogamous fidelity are of paramount importance. One way for a man to assert his power and dominance over other men is to defile the other's property—rape his women. In exchange for protection from wholesale rape women were expected to accept the domination of one man and remain continuously sexually accessible to that man exclusively. Brownmiller argues that the same forces are involved in contemporary relationships between men and women and that rape or the ever-present danger of rape is one way in which men maintain control over women as well as over other men. The elimination or at least reduction of rape as a serious social problem would require reworking our sex-role socialization practices:

Once we accept as basic truth that rape is not a crime of irrational, impulsive, uncontrollable lust, but is a deliberate, hostile, violent act of degradation and possession on the part of a would-be conqueror, designed to intimidate and inspire fear, we must look toward those elements in our culture which promote and propagandize these attitudes, which offer men, and in particular, impressionable, adolescent males, who form the potential raping population, the ideology and psychologic encouragement to commit their acts of aggression without awareness, for the most part, that they have committed a punishable crime, *let alone a moral wrong.* (Brownmiller, 1975, p. 439)

The proposition that rape is exclusively an aggressive act committed by psychologically "normal" men socialized to consider women as chattel is a compelling one but just as difficult to examine empirically as notions that all rapists are men suffering from some emotional disturbance. Given the available evidence that not all men rape and that at least some rapes involve a strong sexual element, it seems reasonable to consider rape as *both a sexual and an aggressive gesture growing out of individually as well as culturally conditioned needs and motives.*

Rape Victims

Virtually no female, regardless of age or physical appearance, is immune to rape. Victims range in age from young infants to very old women. The majority of rape victims, however, are between the ages of ten and twenty-nine, and the most frequent target of rape is a female in her late teens or early twenties (Amir, 1971). Perhaps because of their ages, relatively few (about 25 percent) are married. Another fourth are above the age of legal marriage but still single, and most of the rest (about 40 percent) are females who are below the usual ages for marriage

(Amir, 1971). Because rape occurs most often in such settings, women who live in urban lower-class neighborhoods with high crime rates are more subject to rape than any other class. Many, then, are black lower-class females (Amir, 1971; Brownmiller, 1975). This profile of the statistically "typical" rape victim should not obscure the fact that any woman of any age, marital status, ethnic group, socio-economic bracket, educational level, or occupational group is a potential target of rape.

All rapes or attempted rapes involve interaction between the victim and offender. Victim behavior in rape has been the subject of a great deal of controversy but, unfortunately, a limited amount of research. One of the most hotly debated issues concerning rape is the possible role of the victim as a precipitator of her own rape (Amir, 1971; Brownmiller, 1975; Weis & Borges, 1973). The controversy is based, in part, on the paradoxical juxtaposition of two erroneous beliefs concerning female sexuality. Existing side by side are widespread culturally shaped beliefs that women neither enjoy nor seek out sexual activity but at the same time secretly (perhaps unconsciously) wish to be raped (Burt, 1980). We have disposed of the first of these beliefs in previous chapters, particularly Chapters 4, 5, and 8, and noted in addition in Chapter 8 that, even though some women have fantasies of being seduced by a man's use of at least mild pressure, virtually no women have any desires to be sexually assaulted.

Nevertheless, it is sometimes argued that some women are subtle coconspirators in their own attacks in that their rape desires expressed through word or deed actually precipitate sexual assault. That is, a woman who dresses in a "sexy" fashion, allows a man who is not her husband in her home, walks alone at night, ceases sexual interaction with a man short of intercourse, or does not violently resist a rapist at all possible costs is merely "asking for and getting what she deserves" when she is raped. Such attitudes are fairly widespread and found not only in potential or actual rapists but also in many law enforcement officials, medical personnel, and court officials (Field, 1978). For example, late in 1978 a Utah judge reversed a jury's unanimous guilty verdict against a man accused of rape. Speaking of the white victim, the judge's comments are revealing: "She was sitting in a bar with a black man in a flimsy dress, taking his affection, eating his food, drinking his drinks—there's a whole lot to be said here about mutual consent" (Associated Press, December 27, 1978). Tragically, many rape victims themselves accept this same mythology regarding the manner in which they responded to the rapist and reacted to the rape (Burt, 1980).

Rape Trauma Syndrome.   Burgess and Homstrom (1974) have convincingly demonstrated that rape is a traumatic experience for women, the aftereffects of which may persist for months or even years. They have described a *rape trauma syndrome*, which is a consistent two-phase pattern of emotional reactions a woman experiences after a rape or attempted rape.

The first, or *acute, phase* begins immediately following the rape and may persist for several weeks. During the first few hours after the rape some women experience what is described as an "expressive reaction" involving crying and expression of fear and anger. Others manifest a "controlled reaction," in which they appear unusually calm, composed, and subdued. These initial reactions eventually resolve into longer-term feelings of jumpiness, humiliation, anger, embarrassment, and desires for revenge. Particularly evident are feelings of guilt and self-blame in which many women torment themselves endlessly with questions and self-retributions concerning what they had done to cause the rape: "I shouldn't have let him in"; "I shouldn't have let him buy me a drink"; "I shouldn't have worn that low-cut blouse."

Following the acute phase is a *long-term reorganization phase* lasting up to several months or years in which a woman's life may be seriously disrupted. During this period, some rape victims move several times, change their telephone numbers, refuse to go to work, and develop phobic fears of places resembling the location of the attack. Some develop aversions to or fears of sexual contact, and sexual relationships with husbands or boyfriends become severely disrupted (Feldman-Summers, Gordon, & Meagher, 1979). At all times following the rape, a woman's chances for successful adjustment are enhanced by emotional support from significant persons (husband, parents, friends) in her life (Wortman, 1978).

Fortunately, many communities are creating rape crisis centers to which rape victims may turn for emotional support, medical and legal advice, and assistance in dealing with hospital and police personnel who are sometimes callously suspicious of women's rape claims. It is also fortunate that, largely due to the efforts of feminists, the police, hospitals, courts, and state legislatures are becoming more sensitive and sympathetic to the plight of rape victims. For example, in most cases it is no longer permissible to introduce a woman's previous sexual history in court trials of rape cases.

Preventing Rape.   What should a woman do to avoid sexual assault? This is not an easy question to answer since many of the more "obvious" precautions involve inconvenience, severely restrict a woman's freedom of movement, or seem to foster a sense of interpersonal distrust (Gager & Schurr, 1976). Nevertheless, some basic precautions should be taken:

- Keep doors and windows locked with secure devices at all times.

- Keep chain locks latched when opening doors.

- Do not admit male strangers to dwelling for any reason if you are alone.

- Do not go out alone on dark or deserted city streets.

- Keep car doors locked at all times and drive with windows up if possible.

- Check rear seat of car before getting in.

- Do not hitchhike or pick up hitchhikers.

- Do not be embarrassed or reluctant to run, scream, and request assistance if you suspect you are being followed by a potential assailant.

What should a woman do if she is attacked? Again, the answer to this question is not an easy one to provide. There is no way to predict how an assailant might react to any specific type of victim behavior. The physical odds are clearly in the favor of rapists and if they think they can complete their assault without being caught, most will usually proceed (Huntington, 1975). In his study of *completed rapes*, Amir

Learning self-defense can prove a valuable precaution to take in protecting oneself against sexual assault.

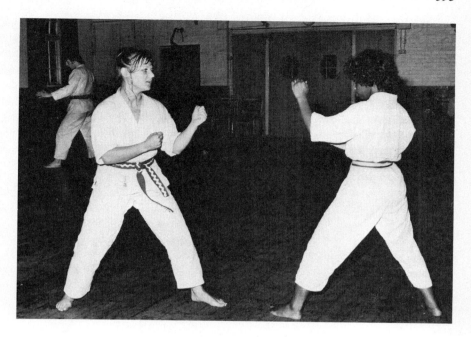

(1971) reported that 55 percent of rape victims displayed submissive behavior involving verbal protests, 27 percent screamed or tried to escape, and 18 percent strongly resisted by kicking, biting, hitting, or throwing objects. Some suggest that in order to avoid serious physical injury, a woman should submit to the rape without strong resistance. Submission provides no guarantee against injury, however, since of all those brutally beaten in Amir's study, nearly a third had reacted submissively. Two thirds of the brutal beatings occurred when the women resisted and fought violently.

If a woman decides to resist, she should do so immediately and vigorously, for those who first act submissively and then resist are often savagely beaten by their assailants (Selkin, 1975). Her actions should be designed to aid in her escape rather than to wreak havoc on her attacker. She should scream, kick, scratch, bite, and hit forcefully. Women who do so are more likely to avoid actual rape than those who simply talk or plead with their attacker (Bart, 1981). Self-defense classes for women are now being offered in many communities and concerned women are advised to seek their assistance.

SUMMARY

Even though all cultures have developed codes and norms of acceptable sexual conduct, there have always been people within those cultures whose sexual behavior differs in some way from that of the majority. Because they are less value laden than some others, the terms "sexual variation" and "sexual variance" are often used in reference to those behaviors that depart from normative forms of sexual behavior.

One major classification of sexual variations includes patterns of erotic response and attraction to atypical stimuli and objects. Fetishism is a sexual variation in which people have strong erotic responses to inanimate objects or body parts not usually considered sexual stimuli. Fetishes are thought to originate in powerful or repetitive conditioning experiences pairing sexual arousal with some object which is symbolic of a human sexual partner. Sexual maladjustment may predispose a person to the development of fetishes. Fetishistic transvestism is a variation in which sexual gratification is achieved through cross-dressing. Fetishistic transvestites are usually heterosexual men with firmly established male gender identities.

In pedophilia, an adult male is erotically attracted to prepubescents. Some have generally failed to establish sexual relationships with adults of either sex. Others do not truly prefer children as sex objects but turn to such contacts in response to stresses encountered in sexual functioning with adults. Some pedophiles make sexual contacts with children as part of a larger pattern of pleasure seeking without regard to societal controls. Incest is sexual contact between close relatives. The most frequent form of incest is between brothers and sisters, although father-daughter incest has received the most attention. Father-daughter incest usually occurs in the context of a seriously disorganized family situation and the emotional impact on the involved daughter is frequently debilitating. Gerontophilia, necrophilia, and bestiality are rare variances in which people are erotically attracted to those much older than themselves, to corpses, and to animals, respectively.

Variations in sexual expression include sexually motivated behaviors that are atypical. In voyeurism a man's primary source of sexual gratification comes from secretly viewing nude females or females involved in sexual activity. Most voyeurs ("peeping Toms") are men who, because of deficient sociosexual development, shyness, and strong masculinity doubts, cannot establish close personal relationships with women. Exhibitionists achieve sexual gratification by exposing their genitals to women under inappropriate circumstances. Like voyeurs, exhibitionists have serious doubts about their masculinity and seem to try to affirm to themselves and the world that they are men by offering the evidence through genital exposure.

In frottage, a man obtains sexual pleasure by rubbing his penis against the bodies of unsuspecting women. Klismaphalia is obtaining sexual pleasure by giving or receiving enemas. Nymphomania and satyriasis are conditions of inordinately high sexual drives in women and men, respectively.

Sadomasochism is obtaining sexual gratification through inflicting (sadism) or receiving (masochism) pain. The development of sadomasochism is thought to result from powerful or repetitive conditioning experiences linking pain and sexual arousal. Feelings of guilt, shame, and disgust concerning sexuality may predispose a person to sadomasochistic desires such that sexual gratification is seen as permissible only if it is accompanied by punishment.

Rape is sexual activity forced upon a woman without her consent. Rapists may be thought of in at least two ways: (1) as men who rape due to personal psychological disturbances or (2) as "normal" products of a socialization system that trains men to be sexually aggressive, demanding, and dominant. It is reasonable to regard rape as growing out of individually as well as culturally conditioned needs and motives. Many people hold a cynical view of rape and insist that a woman cannot be raped unless she really wants to be. Thus, in rape cases, it is not uncommon for the victim to be treated much like an offender. Yet rape is a traumatic event for women and leads to such feelings as fear, guilt, and distrust of men which may persist for many months or years. Several precautions may be taken to avoid rape or to escape from an assailant once an attack has begun.

SUGGESTED READINGS

Brownmiller, S. (1975). *Against our will: Men, women, and rape.* New York: Bantam.

Gebhard, P. H., Gagnon, J. H., Pomeroy, W. B., & Christenson, C. V. (1965). *Sex offenders.* New York: Harper & Row.

Mathis, J. L. (1972). *Clear thinking about sexual deviations.* Chicago: Nelson-Hall.

Masters, R. E. L. (1962). *Forbidden sexual behavior and morality.* New York: Julian Press.

PART 5

PROBLEMS IN SEXUALITY

CHAPTER OUTLINE

CHAPTER 13

SEXUAL DYSFUNCTIONS AND TREATMENT

There is nothing "natural" about the way people express themselves sexually. From infancy on, people learn how they ought to think, feel, and behave sexually (Harlow & Harlow, 1965). Yet the messages they receive about sex are mixed. Some experiences lead them to associate sexual activity with joy and relief and others to associate sex with humiliation, shame, and frustration.

Everyone starts out as a sexual being. William Masters (1975) has observed that most boys are born with an erection and those who are not develop one shortly after birth. Girls are equally sexual; virtually all of them lubricate within the first six hours of life. As reported by Yates (1978),

... masturbation culminating in climax may occur as early as the first months of life. The baby girl is the most enthusiastic and proficient. With unmistakable intent, she crosses her thighs rigidly. With a glassy stare she grunts, rubs, and flushes for a few seconds or minutes. If interrupted, she screams with annoyance. Movements cease abruptly and are followed by relaxation and deep sleep. This sequence occurs many times during the day, but only occasionally at night. The baby boy proceeds with distinct penis throbs and thrusts accompanied by convulsive contractions of the torso. After climax, his erection (without ejaculation) quickly subsides and he appears calm and peaceful. Kinsey reports that one boy of eleven months had ten climaxes in an hour and that another of the same age had fourteen in thirty-eight minutes. (p. 12)

In infancy, all individuals have *some* experiences that ensure that, forever after, they will possess the *potential* to be profoundly sensual. The infant lies cuddled in its mother's arms, nursing as she murmurs to it. The infant inhales her scent, feels her radiating warmth, nuzzles her soft skin. The infant's father tosses it up in the air, nuzzles it, applies baby oil to its damp, chapped genitals. These pleasurable experiences provide a basis for the infant's later sexual functioning. Most infants, however, also have other experiences that make them anxious about sexuality.

Hay (1978) has noted that early on, parents convey their unease about their infant's budding sexuality:

By the time you read about baby care in all the books, magazines, pamphlets, and charts, you assume you know what to expect when attempting to do the most necessary and routine infant care tasks.

However, the first time you actually perform one of these tasks all by yourself, you may find yourself reacting differently to your baby's nakedness than you expected you would. The genitals that seemed so benign (even cute) earlier, may now seem quite intimidating. How could such disproportionately large organs not have made this same impression on you when the nurse was there showing you how to do this same task. You recall the bath and diaper demonstrations given in your prenatal care classes, and you realize, perhaps for the first time, that the doll that was used for the demonstration didn't have genitals.

Now there are these creases, nooks, folds, and orifices to contend with. You are responsible for getting them clean and dry. You have to get into all these creases—behind, in between, underneath—or else your baby will get diaper rash, and worse, infection. You have to smooth powder or smear lotion over every soft and sensitive centimeter of your baby's bottom or you will cause your baby great

An infant's early sensual experiences, such as being held and cuddled by its mother, help establish patterns for future sexual functioning.

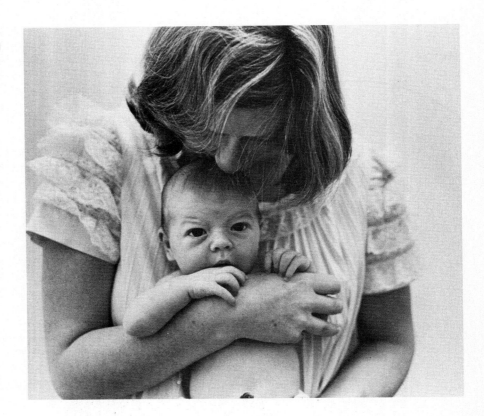

pain and discomfort, even permanent damage. But you can't help but wonder, as you actually handle those new swollen parts that are so much redder and fuller than the rest of this tiny, birdlike creature, if you are performing a lewd and lascivious act. You know you should be gentle and loving as you handle your baby's genitals, but you try not to be too *gentle and loving. (pp. 6–7)*

As children get older, the mixed messages continue. Some parents reassure their children that their bodies are beautiful. Others convince their children that their bodies are too scrawny or too fat, or too something—that their sex organs are shriveled, ugly, or smelly.

Some children receive clear sexual information. Some parents teach their children to name *all* of their body parts, penis and clitoris as well as eyes, nose, fingers, and toes. (Sometimes girls have a little trouble *finding* their clitoris, much less identifying it. Yates (1978) recommends that parents identify their daughter's clitoris by touch or use a mirror to show its location.) Other parents label their children's sex organs in the vaguest terms: "Did you hurt yourself 'down there'?"

Some parents find it easy to tell their children how to behave sexually. Most parents, though, have a hard time coming right out and saying how they feel. When they want their children to quit putting food in their hair or to stop tormenting their brothers, they do not hesitate to tell them clearly and forcefully what they expect. But they treat sexual matters very differently. Most parents do not openly admit how they feel: "I don't want you to masturbate at all," or "Oh, sure I tell you not to masturbate (because that is what good parents are supposed to do), but I'll be secretly pleased if you do (because that's what *real* boys do)," or "All the authorities say masturbation is OK and I have to say it's OK too, but I don't really mean it!" Instead, they send their messages in code. When sexual issues arise, they nervously smile and snicker or stop dead in their tracks; their faces redden, their lips tighten, they give their children withering looks. Children know they have done something terrible, but often they are not quite sure what.

Most Americans agree that it is parents, not the church or the school, and certainly not friends, who should teach their children about sex. The problem is, of course, that most parents are too shy or misinformed to do much sex educating. Thus, if you ask people where they actually learned about sex, the answer is clear—from their friends, who did not know anything either (Commission on Obscenity and Pornography, 1970).

The media, parents, and friends communicate a variety of confusing messages: Sex is wonderful, but nice people don't do it. A real man is tender and loving—and controlled and tough. A real woman is passionate and yielding—and aloof. One should be light-spirited sexually, but a single sexual misstep can ruin you. It is from this kaleidoscope of experiences—clear and confused, and delightful and painful—that people's sexual attitudes, feelings, and behavior emerge. Sometimes the results are **sexual dysfunctions**, or difficulties in sexual functioning.

In this chapter, we focus on some of the things that can go wrong with sexual functioning. First, we will discuss sexual dysfunctions in specific detail. No one knows exactly how many people experience sexual dysfunctions. According to Masters and Johnson (1970), however, "A conservative estimate would indicate half the marriages (in this country) are either presently sexually dysfunctional or imminently so in the future." Second, we will discuss generally how sex therapy programs are designed to treat sexual dysfunctions. And finally, we will briefly outline specific treatments employed to remedy vaginismus, erectile dysfunctions, and ejaculatory problems.

SEXUAL DYSFUNCTIONS

Since people are all unique, there are an infinite number of things that can delight or frustrate them about their sexual lives. Some people are acutely uncomfortable if they have to initiate sex but they are fine once things get started. Some people like to lie around all day Saturday caressing their partners. Others assume "Slam-bam-thank-you-ma'am" is the natural order of things. Are these liabilities or assets? It depends on one's definition. There are several things, however, that most couples agree can constitute sexual dysfunction. (Even here there can be disagreement. A dean from a Southern college once asked why "impotence" should be considered a sexual dysfunction. "Wasn't it," he questioned, "a blessing from God?") Let us first consider the major male sexual dysfunctions.

Male Dysfunctions

A man's sexual functioning can be intensified or blocked at several stages. According to Helen Singer Kaplan (1974), in order for a man to function normally, he must (1) desire his partner erotically, (2) be capable of getting and sustaining an erection, and finally (3) be capable of experiencing an orgasm. Desire/arousal/ orgasm—these are the critical steps in sexual response. Men may develop sexual problems at any of these points.

Sexual Apathy.   Without the first critical step—desire—sexual response is impossible. In previous eras **sexual apathy**, or lack of sexual desire, in men was rarely mentioned. In the Victorian era, when men were supposed to want sex and women were not, the man who was rarely interested in sex could convince himself that he was just "considerate." In our more sexual era, such men are more likely to conclude that they have a sexual problem.

There are a wide array of reasons why men feel little or no sexual desire (Kaplan, 1979; Reckless & Geiger, 1978): they may, for example, be afraid of establishing too close a relationship with anyone, they may be exhausted "workaholics," or they may be depressed. Recently, sex therapists have begun to encounter more and more men with such problems. Researchers are beginning to devote substantial effort to discover the best way to stimulate sexual interest where there is none. Thus far, though, clinicians have not been too successful in instilling interest in disinterested men.

Erectile Dysfunction (ED).   For most men, erectile dysfunction is a devastating experience. "Impotence," the term traditionally used to signify the inability to attain an erection, also means a lack of power, strength, and vigor—the antithesis of all that we consider masculine (Zilbergeld, 1978). Most clinicians disapprove of the term because they feel it is insulting and inaccurate. The partners of men with ED are usually devastated by the experience, too. They often feel humiliated ("What's wrong with me that I can't turn him on?") as well as frustrated.

With some men, erectile dysfunction results from lack of desire for their partners. Without desire, they find it impossible to become aroused. Generally, however, **erectile dysfunction (ED)** men experience difficulty with the second stage in the desire/arousal/orgasm sequence—they desire their partners but find it difficult to achieve or maintain an erection nonetheless. Kaplan (1974) has described a typical case:

The patient was a handsome and successful 30-year-old businessman who had been divorced two years before. . . . His wife left him because she fell in love with and wished to marry a close friend of the family.

The divorce was very traumatic for the patient. He became depressed and was left with deep feelings of insecurity. He kept ruminating about why his wife had left him, and whether he was inferior to the other man.

Eight months after the separation he went to a party and met an aggressive woman who wanted to have sex with him right there. On her urging they went to an upstairs room (which did not have a lock) and attempted to have intercourse on the floor. He became excited and erect, but for the first time in his life, lost his erection. He tried to regain his erection to no avail.

He reacted with alarm to his experience. He felt depressed and extremely humiliated and embarrassed. He never saw the woman again. One month later, he tried to make love to another woman but again lost his erection when the memory of his previous failure intruded into his mind. From then on the problem escalated. (pp. 128–129)

There are two forms of ED. A man with *primary erectile dysfunction* has *never* been able to maintain an erection long enough to have sexual intercourse. A man with *secondary erectile dysfunction* could, at one time in his life, achieve and maintain an erection but now, for some reason, has trouble doing so. Secondarily dysfunctional men vary in when their erectile problem occurs. Some have totally lost the ability to achieve erection. Others can attain erection, but they lose it when they attempt intercourse or in the midst of intercourse. Some men are functional in one situation but not in others. For example, one man had no trouble responding to pickups but found it impossible to function with his wife.

Sooner or later, almost all men find themselves caught up in a sexual situation and discover that their penis will not rise to the occasion, or they experience an initial erection that then disappears in the middle of their activities. This is such a common occurrence that most men do not even think of it as a problem—it is just one of the facts of life. Only if a man has persistent erectile failures should he be considered dysfunctional. Masters and Johnson (1970) classify a man as dysfunctional if he has erection problems 25 percent of the time in his sexual encounters.

Erectile dysfunction may have *organic, functional,* or *psychogenic* (psychosocial) causes (Kelly, 1961). Organically caused ED—ED that has its origins in anatomical defects in the central nervous or reproductive system—is rare. Functional ED is somewhat more common. It occurs occasionally, when excessive use of alcohol or narcotics, circulatory problems, early undiagnosed diabetes, aging, stress, or physical exhaustion interferes with sexual functioning.

Psychogenic problems probably account for about 50 to 85 percent of all cases of ED (Harper, 1965). The brain stimulates the neural centers of the spinal cord which control erection. Emotional inhibitions can interfere with this process. If men feel too much guilt or anxiety to abandon themselves to their sexual feelings, or if they feel pushed into having sex yet are not at all sure they can come through, they are likely to experience erectile failure (Kaplan, 1974; Zilbergeld, 1978).

Premature Ejaculation.   A man may also have difficulty with the last stage in the desire/arousal/orgasm sequence. Two problems may occur in orgasm: either premature or retarded ejaculation. Discussion of the latter follows this consideration of premature ejaculation. The most common male sexual dysfunction, especially among young men, is premature ejaculation. Of the men studied by Kinsey and his associates (1948), most seemed to be exceedingly swift in progressing from penetration to ejaculation. Some ejaculated at the slightest provocation, often when they merely *thought* about entering their partners. A substantial number reached a climax within ten or twenty seconds after beginning sexual intercourse. Seventy-five percent reached orgasm within two minutes of initiating sexual relations. Is this a problem? In 1948 Kinsey and his colleagues did not think so:

It is curious that the term "impotence" [sic] should ever have been applied to such rapid response. It would be difficult to find another situation in which an individual who was quick and intense in his response was labeled anything but superior, and that in most instances is exactly what the rapidly ejaculating male probably is, however inconvenient and unfortunate his qualities may be from the standpoint of the wife in the relationship. (p. 580)

Now, over thirty years later, views have changed. Today, most clinicians would consider Kinsey's "superior man" to be a premature ejaculator.

What exactly *is* premature ejaculation? Sex therapists have had a hard time settling on a definition. Some argue that if a man has an orgasm within thirty seconds after entering his partner's vagina, his ejaculation is "premature." Others believe that a man should be able to last for at least ten thrusts before ejaculation. LoPiccolo (1978) felt that a man should be able to last for four minutes. (But what if he and his partner *both* have orgasms earlier than that?) Masters and Johnson (1970) labeled a man as premature if he reaches orgasm before his partner does more than 50 percent of the time. (But what if she *never* has an orgasm?) Today, probably most clinicians would agree that **premature ejaculation** is ejaculation that occurs too soon for the man's or his partner's satisfaction because he cannot voluntarily control it (Zilbergeld, 1978; Kaplan, 1974).

Clinicians have observed that men with ejaculatory control react very differently from premature ejaculators during a sexual encounter. Men with ejaculatory control usually focus intently on their sexual feelings. Little by little, they have learned to identify the physical sensations of increasing excitement and how to intensify or tone down sexual arousal at will by varying the timing or the depth of their thrusting. The premature man has not learned to do this. Instead of focusing on his sensations, he tries to "distract" himself, biting his lips, digging his fingernails into his palms, thinking about other things, in a vain effort to control his responses ((Lazarus, 1978). Actually these "distractions" increase his problems. He never learns to calibrate his sexual feelings or to control his level of excitement. He plunges ahead and then, all of a sudden, realizes that he is about to have an orgasm.

By the time of this realization, his responses are out of control; there is nothing he can do to delay ejaculation.

How do men and women react to prematurity problems? It varies. There are a few men who believe, with Kinsey and his colleagues, that prematurity is natural and take their problem in stride. Most do not. As portrayed in the following description (Lehrman, 1970), generally prematurity is intensely upsetting for both men and women:

Many home remedies are tried, such as an enforced regime of not touching the male genitals during sexual foreplay; then, when the woman's sexual tension is very high, he'll plunge in and cause a pathetic interaction: She will be thrusting desperately to get some satisfaction before he ejaculates, and he will just as desperately be trying to distract himself—by thinking of unrelated matters—in order to keep from ejaculating. This self-defeating interplay, frustrating to both because the highly excited woman forces the male to ejaculate while he is actually suppressing his enjoyment in order not to, finally leads the couple to avoid sex. Nothing, of course, will make the premature ejaculator ejaculate more prematurely than long periods of continence between sex exposures. And so the problem is compounded. (pp. 34–35)

Retarded Ejaculation.   Some men have no trouble becoming aroused and maintaining a firm erection. Yet, although they urgently desire orgasmic release, they cannot ejaculate while their penis is in their partner's vagina. This form of sexual dysfunction is known as **retarded ejaculation**. One such case was described by Kaplan (1974) as follows:

The patient had left his wife and four children when he became infatuated with another woman. His ejaculatory inhibition had its onset after this woman, for whom he had sacrificed his marriage and family and risked his financial and professional status, left him for another man because she was "bored and dissatisfied" with him. The patient reacted to this rejection with an intense agitated depression, which prompted him to seek psychoanalytic treatment. The acute emotional reaction abated after some time. However his ejaculatory dysfunction persisted; he was unable to ejaculate intravaginally with any partner. (p. 337)

Retarded ejaculation is a relatively rare form of sexual inadequacy and seldom has a physical cause. There are, however, several psychological reasons why men find themselves unable or unwilling to ejaculate while in their partner's vagina (Kaplan, 1974). Some men love their partner but are afraid unconsciously to "soil" her. Some men secretly, or not so secretly, resent their partner and "punish" her by withholding affection. Some men are afraid of fathering a child. Still others worry about their performance (Razani, 1978).

Female Dysfunctions

As with men, sexual response in women can be intensified or blocked at any of several stages (Kaplan, 1974) in the desire/arousal/orgasm sequence. In order for a woman to function normally, (1) she must desire her partner erotically, (2) she must become aroused and lubricate, and (3) she must be capable of experiencing an orgasm from clitoral or clitoral-vaginal stimulation. Fischer (1973) found that 66 percent of women prefer clitoral to vaginal stimulation. The various components of sexual response in women are surprisingly independent—a woman can be intensely aroused, yet never reach orgasm. Or a woman can fail to become aroused, remaining dry and tight, yet reach orgasm. Something can go wrong at any of the stages in the desire/arousal/orgasm sequence.

Sexual Apathy.   As we noted earlier, at one time many people believed that "nice" women should not be interested in sex. Then, sexual apathy, or lack of desire, was not considered to be a problem, but the natural state of affairs. In this more sexual era, however, more and more women are coming to clinics for help in overcoming sexual apathy.

Clinicians believe that there are a variety of reasons—psychological and physical—why women might not desire sex. They may, for instance, have been brought up to believe that nice girls should not be interested in sex. They may be exhausted. They may be depressed. As is true for men with sexual apathy, clinicians have not been very successful in instilling desire in sexually apathetic women. Currently researchers are beginning to devote substantial effort to finding new techniques for dealing with this difficult problem (see Kaplan, 1979).

Sexual Unresponsiveness (SU).   This sexual dysfunction affects a woman in the arousal stage of the desire/arousal/orgasm sequence. **Sexual unresponsiveness** refers to the inability of a woman to become sexually aroused as indicated by a lack of vaginal lubrication. In day-to-day language, this problem is often called "frigidity." However, many therapists argue that scientists should avoid this term, as it is both insulting and inaccurate.

A few SU women have problems with the first stage in the desire/arousal/orgasm sequence—they simply do not desire their partners. Thus, it is not surprising that they have difficulty becoming aroused. Many women, however, *do* desire their partners but nonetheless have great trouble becoming aroused—that is, they have difficulty lubricating. They do not develop an "orgasmic platform." (The muscles and tissues surrounding the vaginal inlet do not become engorged with blood.) We will consider the underlying causes of sexual unresponsiveness subsequently, along with causes of orgasmic dysfunction.

Orgasmic Dysfunction.   Some women experience erotic feelings, lubricate copiously, and show genital swelling. Their difficulty lies not in becoming aroused, but in reaching orgasm; in other words, they experience **orgasmic dysfunction**. One woman described the problem this way:

I have never yet come, so having sex usually ends up a little sour. I have been very excited and feeling very good when the man I'm with comes—which is the end of really active, exciting lovemaking—but still I feel very depressed, unloved, and I feel like crying, sometimes I have cried (though I usually tried not to, so I wouldn't upset my lover). It's hard to describe how bad and totally alone and ignored this makes me feel. (Hite, 1976, p. 116)

Another made the following observation:

*It's like being the only person with the cake with no frosting—you feel you're
missing something but you're not sure what. (Hite, 1976, p. 115)*

There are two forms of orgasmic dysfunction: A woman with *primary orgasmic
dysfunction* has never been able to achieve an orgasm through any activity. A
woman with *secondary orgasmic dysfunction* is variable in her sexual response—
sometimes she is orgasmic and sometimes not (Kaplan, 1974). Both Kinsey and his
colleagues (1953), in their early survey, and Hunt (1974), in his more recent study,
found that only about half of the married women in the United States achieved
orgasm 90 to 100 percent of the time during their sexual encounters. By 1972, only
53 percent of women were experiencing orgasm with any regularity (Hunt, 1974).

A woman's sexual difficulties—sexual unresponsiveness or orgasmic dysfunction—may have *psychogenic* or *organic* causes (Ellis, 1961). According to Masters
and Johnson (1970), the problem is rarely a physical one. Only about 10 to 20
percent of women's sexual dysfunctions have a physical cause. These include
disorders of the nervous system, hormonal imbalances, inflammation or lesions of
the internal or external genitalia and surrounding areas, or injuries to the genitals.

Almost always, it is psychological problems that prevent women from abandon-
ing themselves to sexuality and lead to sexual unresponsiveness and orgasmic
dysfunction. Sometimes, women dislike their partners:

*Some women . . . respond to gentle partners; others are "turned on" by commanding
ones. . . . Some women require complete devotion and become very excited only if it
is apparent that their partners are strongly aroused by them. Others are bored by
their eager lovers, preferring the unattainable partner who must be seduced and for
whose attention they must compete with other women. (Kaplan, 1974, pp. 357–358)*

Many women express their unconscious (or not so unconscious) anger at their
mates by refusing to respond to them (McGuire & Steinhilber, 1970). Barbach
(1975) described one such case:

*Sarah had been well trained to wait on men and she was good at it. She was a
good seamstress, a good cook, and a caring and selfless companion, but she ended
up resenting her partner and the fact that he thought he could repay her by making
love to her. Without even realizing it, she found herself thinking, 'You think you're
so hot, I'll show you. I won't have an orgasm. (p. 49)*

Sometimes, the problem is really a cultural one. Since the Victorian period, a
double standard has existed. Men were allowed, if not encouraged, to be sexual.
Women were supposed to save themselves for marriage and not be too sexual
thereafter. Today, remnants of the double standard still exist (see Baker, 1974;
Ehrmann, 1959; Kaats & Davis, 1970; Reiss, 1960; Schofield, 1965; and Sorenson,
1973.) As a consequence, many women find it extremely difficult to think of
themselves as sexual beings. One investigator observes: "Psychologists have put a

The attitude that any display of sexuality is unacceptable in women dates back to Victorian times and may still account for the ambivalence many women feel about their sexuality.

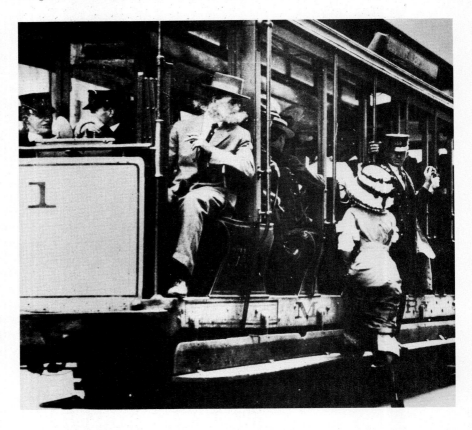

psychological label [frigid] on women who are unable to do as adults, what they were brought up to be unable to do" (cited in Barbach, 1975, p. 32).

Sometimes, the problem is really a technical one. As we noted earlier, the penis and the clitoris are the primary sites of sexual pleasure. If the woman's clitoris is not adequately stimulated (either directly or indirectly), there is little chance she can reach orgasm. Yet, many couples fail to adequately stimulate the clitoris during intercourse. They rely entirely on penile thrusting, which, of course, provides only indirect stimulation of the clitoris. Often this is not enough:

As Dr. Sanford Copley put it, when interviewed on the television show "Woman," this indirect stimulation of women could be compared to the stimulation which would be produced in a man by the rubbing of the scrotal skin (balls), perhaps pulling it back and forth, and so causing the skin on the upper tip of the penis to move, or quiver, and in this way achieving "stimulation." Would it work? Admittedly, this form of stimulation would probably require a good deal more foreplay for the man to have an orgasm. You would have to be patient and "understand" if it did not lead to orgasm "every time."

Masters and Johnson's theory that the thrusting penis pulls the woman's labia, which in turn pulls the clitoral hood, which thereby causes friction on the clitoral glans and thereby causes orgasm sounds more like a Rube Goldberg scheme than a reliable way to orgasm. (Hite, 1976, p. 168)

How do most couples react to such problems? People always view a man's sexual problems as a disaster. Their reactions to a woman's lack of responsiveness or orgasm are much more varied. Some women casually accept the fact that they lack erotic feelings. Many, however, feel inadequate, disappointed, frustrated, resentful, and angry (Nelson, 1974). A few men are secretly pleased by their wives' lack of interest. They may think they have finally found a "good woman." Some simply accept the situation. Many men, however, are upset: "If she loved me she'd respond." "If I were a 'real man', I'd know what to do." They put pressure on their mates to perform, which only increases the problem.

Dyspareunia.   A few women suffer from **dyspareunia**, or "painful intercourse." When they attempt to have intercourse, they may feel a sharp pain, twinges of discomfort, or simply ache. The pain may be felt around the clitoris and vaginal entrance, in the vagina, cervix and uterus, or deep in the pelvis. Not surprisingly, women with dyspareunia shrink from intercourse.

Often dyspareunia has a physical cause (Abarbanel, 1978). Polyps, cysts, and tumors of the reproductive system may make intercourse painful. An episiotomy, an incompletely performed abortion, or rape (expecially gang rape) may produce scar tissue in the vaginal opening, the movement of which is painful. If a woman has a vaginal infection, the walls of her vagina may become irritated. Some women produce insufficient vaginal lubrication during intercourse. This is often a special problem for many women in the postmenopausal period; the mucous membrane of the vagina becomes fragile and thin and women also fail to secrete sufficient lubrication for easy penile intromission. Vaginal creams are frequently prescribed in such cases (Rubin, 1966). Sometimes, too, the vagina is irritated by the chemicals contained in contraceptive foams, creams, jellies, or suppositories. Some women are allergic to the rubber or plastic in condoms and diaphragms or to the harsh chemicals in commercial douches. Usually, a physician can treat such problems.

Dyspareunia can also be psychogenic. Women who are frightened about some aspect of intercourse, for example, may react to their fear by tightening their vaginal muscles, thus causing intercourse to be painful. In such cases, sex therapy is helpful (Abarbanel, 1978).

Vaginismus.   Whenever the partner of a woman with **vaginismus** tries to penetrate her, the muscles surrounding her vaginal entrance involuntarily begin to spasm. Naturally enough, the attempted intercourse becomes exceedingly painful. Intercourse is usually impossible. Here is one therapist's description of her client's experience:

Sally was a virgin when she married and when she went to her physician for her pre-marital exam, he informed her about what to expect with intercourse. He told her it would feel like a steel rod being shoved into her vagina and that it would be very painful. Her reaction was to develop vaginismus and dyspareunia. . . . Since she expected sex to be a painful experience, she tensed her vaginal muscles to help guard against the anticipated hurt. Ironically, her attempt to protect herself from the pain actually caused it. (Barbach, 1975, p. 32)

Sometimes, vaginismus has a physical cause. Any physical problem that makes intercourse painful can lay the groundwork for the vaginismic response.

Generally, however, vaginismus is psychogenic (Frank, 1948; Kaplan, 1979; Masters & Johnson, 1970). Some women feel guilty about sex. Other women are so badly informed that they assume that intercourse will be painful. They are so frightened that they develop the very reaction that ensures it will be—vaginismus. Still other women are vaginismic because they are afraid of becoming pregnant. Sometimes women who have been raped develop vaginismus.

Masters and Johnson (1970) found that dysfunctional men's wives often develop vaginismus. The men attempt intercourse again and again only to fail. Eventually, the women begin to "lock out" their partners.

Needless to say, vaginismus usually has a devastating effect on a couple's relationship. Many vaginismic women are humiliated and frustrated by their problem. Their partners, naturally enough, feel frustrated and rejected. Marriages of many years' duration remain unconsummated as a result of vaginismus (Dawkins & Taylor, 1961; Fuchs, Hoch, Paldi, Abramovici, Brandes, Timor-Tritsch, & Kleinhaus, 1978).

SEX THERAPY PROGRAMS

Masters and Johnson's *Human Sexual Inadequacy* (1970) sparked a revolution in the treatment of sexual problems. In the decade since their pioneering effort, sex researchers have developed a wide array of techniques for helping people overcome sexual problems (e.g., Annon, 1976; Barbach, 1975; Heiman, LoPiccolo, & LoPiccolo, 1978; Kaplan, 1974; or Zilbergeld, 1978.)

The American Association of Sex Educators, Counselors, and Therapists (AASECT) has established guidelines for the training of sex counselors and therapists (AASECT, 1973) and certifies those sex therapists who meet its standards. Persons seeking the names of qualified professionals in their part of the country should contact AASECT, 5010 Wisconsin Avenue, N.W., Suite 304, Washington, D.C., 20016.

Of course, sex therapists use a wide variety of techniques for dealing with sexual dysfunction. Zilbergeld, for example, focuses on techniques *individuals* can use to improve their sexual functioning while Masters and Johnson focus on improving *couples'* sexual functioning. Let us consider these two approaches.

Individually Oriented Therapies

Treatment programs designed to improve sexual functioning at the individual level have several facets (Zilbergeld, 1978). Some of the most important are briefly described here.

Setting Goals. When people think about improving their sex lives, they tend to think in very general terms. They would like sex to be "better" somehow, "more exciting." For sex therapists, such goals are too vague. They encourage clients to decide *precisely* what it is about their sex lives that they would like changed. One such precise goal, for instance, might be: "I want to be able to come right out and refuse to engage in oral sex." Therapists try to reduce these desired major changes to a series of precise and manageable subgoals. Clients can then begin to tackle these subgoals, one at a time.

Body Images.   Many people are not very comfortable with the shells they inhabit. Many are too shy even to look at themselves nude. When they do, reluctantly, they conclude that their bodies just do not "stack up." Compared to some of the fantastic myths they may have accepted as to how "real men" or "real women" are *supposed* to look, they have a point. No one can measure up to those standards.

Zilbergeld (1978) observed that "penises in fantasy land come in only three sizes—large, gigantic, and so big you barely get them through the doorway." A penis is or should be "two feet long, hard as steel, and can go all night" (pp. 23–24). Such penises are frequent inhabitants of the fictional world of erotica of the type found in Henry Miller's (1962) *Tropic of Capricorn*. Little wonder, then, that with sexual heroes like Miller's as their models, many men feel they fail to "measure up" physically (Zilbergeld, 1978).

Women are exposed to comparable idealized images and many fear that they, too, are physically inadequate. Shere Hite (1976) asked women "Do you think your vagina and genital area are ugly or beautiful? Do they smell good or bad?" Here is a sampling of the replies she received:

I think my vagina is beautiful, rich, fertile—I especially like my black pubic hair. The smell is at times erotic and this turns me on—but I don't believe in not bathing to keep the smell.

It's ugly—lots of extra flabby skin, all wrinkled and flapping.

Ideally, genitals are beautiful and smell sensuous. But really they are bad looking and sometimes stink.

Lovely, fascinating, curious, mysterious, despite self-examination.

I sense that men think that while they're blessed with a wondrous organ, women are cursed with something downright repulsive. (pp. 237–240)

The combination of myth and ignorance is powerful. People grow up thinking it is enormously important to be beautiful but suspecting that, somehow, they just do not measure up. Indeed, many people are so self-conscious about their bodies that they spend enormous amounts of time and energy, during a sexual encounter, trying to arrange their bodies artfully so that only the best parts show. Some people even insist on making love with all the lights out. As people become more comfortable with their bodies, their sexual pleasure increases.

Therapists' first task, then, is to help their clients become more comfortable with their own bodies. Hartman and Fithian (1972) suggest clients take off their clothes, stand in front of a full-length mirror, and carefully examine their bodies, looking at them from all angles—standing, kneeling, sitting with legs spread wide apart. Next, they are to explore their nipples, breasts, and genitals and try to see themselves as their lovers see them. Generally, people are pleasantly surprised to discover that their bodies are far more appealing than they expect them to be. That discovery is often an immediate boon to sexual responsiveness. Of course, a few people discover they look worse than they expected. But even then, a careful examination of what they *really* look like gives them a realistic idea of what they need to work on next.

RESEARCH HIGHLIGHT

The Body Image

Ellen Berscheid and her colleagues (1972, 1973) contacted 62,000 men and women, ranging in age from seventeen to sixty-five and over. They selected a sample of 2000 of the men and women who filled out their questionnaires. Their sample, chosen to approximate national distributions, consisted of 50 percent men and 50 percent women. Within each sex, 45 percent were twenty-four years old or younger, 25 percent were between twenty-five and forty-five, and the rest were forty-five or older. The researchers asked people how satisfied they were with various parts of their bodies.

The table below indicates how the national sample of men and women responded. Overall, most were fairly satisfied with their appearance. Both men and women were self-conscious about their weight. Perhaps because excess weight tends to settle in the mid-torso area—abdomen, buttocks, hips and thighs—people who were embarrassed about their weight were generally dissatisfied with these particular body parts. Almost half of the women worried about the size of their hips. A third of the men worried about having a "spare tire."

Only half of the men and women were "quite" or "extremely" satisfied with the size and appearance of their chest or breasts and sex organs.

The rest were less content. The respondents' written comments indicated the depth of their concern (Berscheid et al., 1973):

When your first gynecologist says to you, out of the blue, "Do you feel unfeminine because of your small breasts, dear" you begin to think they're a bit on the small side. (p. 121)

Since everyone has started going braless, two years ago, I find that my breasts, which are too big for my body, attract undue attention; I'm extremely self-conscious about them. (p. 121)

One man observed,

When I was an adolescent, I had the misfortune to see a sex manual which showed male and female pubic hair distributions. Horrors—my own pubic hair was the perfect model of the feminine pubic pattern—and still is! (p. 121)

Relaxation.　When people are keyed up, frightened, or distracted, they cannot concentrate on pleasurable sensations. Thus, therapists' next step is to teach them how to relax (Heiman, LoPiccolo, & LoPiccolo, 1976; Wolpe, 1966). Deep muscle relaxation exercises, outlined below, are an effective relaxation technique.

In performing these exercises, clients are to begin by doing whatever they normally do when they want to relax. They might turn on soft background music. They might take a warm bath. Then they are to find a comfortable place to lie down (a reclining chair or a bed, perhaps), lean their heads back against the pillows, close their eyes, let their arms and hands hang loose, and relax.

How Satisfied or Dissatisfied People Are with Body Parts

Overall Body Appearance	Quite or Extremely Dissatisfied		Somewhat Dissatisfied		Somewhat Satisfied		Quite or Extremely Satisfied	
	Women 7%	Men 4%	Women 16%	Men 11%	Women 32%	Men 30%	Women 45%	Men 55%
Face								
hair	6	6	13	14	28	22	53	58
eyes	1	1	5	6	14	12	80	81
ears	2	1	5	4	10	13	83	82
nose	5	2	18	14	22	20	55	64
mouth	2	1	5	5	20	19	73	75
teeth	11	10	19	18	20	26	50	46
voice	3	3	15	12	27	27	55	58
chin	4	3	9	8	20	20	67	69
complexion	8	7	20	15	24	20	48	58
overall facial attractiveness	3	2	8	6	28	31	61	61
Extremities								
shoulders	2	3	11	8	19	22	68	67
arms	5	2	11	11	22	25	62	62
hands	5	1	14	7	21	17	60	75
feet	6	3	14	8	23	19	57	70
Mid Torso								
size of abdomen	19	11	31	25	21	22	29	42
buttocks (seat)	17	6	26	14	20	24	37	56
hips (upper thighs)	22	3	27	9	19	24	32	64
legs and ankles	8	4	17	7	23	20	52	69
Height, Weight and Tone								
height	3	3	10	10	15	20	72	67
weight	21	10	27	25	21	22	31	43
general muscle tone or development	9	7	21	18	32	30	38	45
Sexual Characteristics								
chest/breasts	9	4	18	14	23	24	50	58
size of sex organs	1	6	2	9	18	19	79	66
appearance of sex organs	2	3	5	6	18	19	75	72

SOURCE: From "The Happy American Body: A Survey Report" by Ellen Berscheid, Elaine Walster, and George Bohrnstedt in *Psychology Today*, November 1975. Copyright © 1973 by American Psychological Association. Reprinted by permission.

Then they are ready to begin the relaxation exercises—to systematically tense, then relax, their bodies' major muscle groups, one by one. First, they tense a group of muscles; this makes it easy to recognize just how tension is experienced in those muscles. Then they relax those same muscles. This procedure makes it easy to identify tense versus relaxed states, and to relax quickly. After the exaggerated tension of the exercises, relaxation feels better than ever.

They begin systematically to tense and relax their bodies. They press the back of their head firmly against the pillows to notice the sensations of tension, pressure, and strain. They relax and let their head sink softly into the pillow. They tense their foreheads, wrinkling them into a deep, angry frown to feel the tension. They relax to feel their forehead become smooth while concentrating on the feelings of relaxation. They tense the muscles around their eyes and squeeze their lids as tightly together as possible. Feeling the tension in their eyebrows, eyelids, and nose, they then relax, to feel the tension flowing away.

They then proceed to tense and relax the following muscle groups (Heiman et al., 1976, p. 46):

- Lips and jaws

- Neck and chin

- Hands, by clenching them

- Wrists and forearms, by extending them and bending the hands back at the wrists

- Shoulders, by shrugging them

- Chest, by taking a deep breath and holding it, then exhaling

- Back, by arching the back up and away from the support surface

- Hips and buttocks, by pressing buttocks together tightly

- Thighs, by clenching them

- Lower legs, by pointing the toes and curling toes downward

When people are done with the deep muscle relaxation exercises, they are told to pause for a moment, enjoy their relaxation, then get up slowly, stretching their whole body. Once people are relaxed, they are in optimum condition to make love.

Touching.   Children can get totally absorbed in sensual experience. They caress silky fabrics. They inhale a variety of smells with gusto, and bite, nibble, and lick any objects they encounter. They suck one thumb while gently caressing their faces with the other hand. By adulthood, however, many people have learned to equate sensuality with sin, an association that interferes with sexual responsiveness.

Zilbergeld (1978) has developed a series of exercises designed to help people relearn the delights of the sense of touch. To begin developing their enjoyment of touching and being touched, people apply body lotion, oil, or powder to their bodies. They then continue by exploring their bodies—stroking their toes, feet, and inner thighs, their entire bodies. They vary the types of strokes and pressure, trying light touches, circular movements, and firm pressures, to see what they like.

Masturbation.   Kinsey and his colleagues (1948, 1953) defined masturbation as "self-stimulation which is deliberate and designed to effect erotic arousal." Hunt (1974) found that 94 percent of the women he interviewed masturbated. This does not mean, however, that they felt comfortable about masturbation. Hunt asked his sample of two thousand men and women whether they agreed with, disagreed

Table 13–1.

Attitudes of men and women of various ages toward masturbation.

"Masturbation is wrong"	Age of Respondents				
	18–24	**25–34**	**35–44**	**45–54**	**55 & over**
Percentage agreeing					
Men	15	16	27	28	29
Women	14	17	27	33	36
Percentage disagreeing					
Men	80	81	67	67	63
Women	78	77	68	55	52
Percentage with no opinion					
Men	5	3	6	5	8
Women	8	6	5	12	12

SOURCE: Adapted from Hunt, 1974.

with, or had no opinion on the statement "Masturbation is wrong." Their replies are shown in Table 13–1.

It is evident that people, especially older people, are not quite sure what they think about masturbation. They generally have mixed feelings about it, yet still engage in it. But, therapists argue, unless men and women have an intimate knowledge of their own bodies—what they like and what they do not, what arouses them and what does not—they will have difficulty communicating this information to a partner.

When "J" (1969) and "M" (1971) recommended masturbation as a way to learn about one's sexuality, it shocked people. Now, a decade later, almost all sex therapists recommend that men and women masturbate in order to get into intimate touch with their bodies, and few people object.

Barbach (1975), Heiman et al. (1976), LoPiccolo and Lobitz (1978), and Zilbergeld (1978), as well as others, offer a number of suggestions concerning therapeutic masturbation. Initially, people are urged to engage in *focusing*— attending to their sensual feelings. They first set the scene, with, say, candles or incense, music, and dimmed lights, and relax into a sexual mood. They then begin to explore their bodies. During this exploration they are to focus only on their bodily sensations. At first this is difficult. Because most people have been trained not to pay attention to their sensual feelings, their minds may wander and they may start to daydream. If that happens, the prescribed procedure is simply to bring their attention back to the body. Focusing helps people get back in touch with their feelings. Having developed the ability to focus, they are ready to explore the various self-pleasuring techniques that are available.

According to Barbach (1975), masturbation is an easy way for women to learn about their sexuality. Supporting this contention is the finding of Masters and Johnson (1966) that, in women, masturbation produces more rapid, more intense, and more dependable orgasms than does sexual intercourse. Hite (1976) asked approximately two thousand women, "What is the importance of masturbation?" Her respondents reported that they derive a variety of benefits from masturbation.

Some women saw it as a learning experience:

It's a way to explore one's sexuality without the self-consciousness of having someone there. (p. 15)

Masturbation gave me the knowledge I could achieve orgasm. (p. 14)

Some women also felt masturbation helped them have better sex with those they felt closest to:

Masturbation teaches you to know your own body, and to gratify it, which leads to increasing your sense of independence and may also increase your ability to relate to someone else; being able to tell someone else what gives one pleasure can do a lot for a relationship. (p. 15)

Other women saw it as a means to independence and self-reliance:

It gives me control over my body because I don't have to be dependent on another person for sexual fulfillment. Because this is possible I have control over my relationships. (p. 15)

And many women described it as pure pleasure—important in its own right:

The importance of masturbation is for you to be able to love and care for yourself totally, an expression of self-sufficiency and completeness. (p. 17)

It helps me calm down, feel warm (I get very cold at night), go to sleep, work out my fantasies, and meet the sexual needs of the day. (p. 17)

It lets you satisfy yourself best, when you really, really want to get into having an intense, very heavy, strong orgasm. (p. 18)

Barbach (1975) suggests a variety of techniques in which nonorgasmic women might stimulate themselves sexually:

Use oil, saliva, or the natural lubrication of the vagina to keep the genital tissues moist so that no irritation develops. Explore by stimulating the area with various types of strokes and pressures. What do very light feathery touches feel like? How about harder rubbing? Try massaging the clitoral area with your fingertips by making gentle but firm circular motions. Some women like to stimulate the glans of the clitoris directly while others find this area too sensitive for direct stimulation and prefer to massage the areas directly surrounding the clitoris above, below, or to the sides. Find out what feels best for you. Many women rub one finger back and forth over the clitoris with varying speeds and intensity. Or the clitoris could be massaged between the forefinger and middle finger massaging also the whole area by stroking up and down the clitoral shaft. Many women enjoy having their fingers or something else in their vagina while the clitoris is being stroked. (p. 96)

As we noted in Chapter 8, some women bring themselves to orgasm in still other ways—by exerting muscular tension on their thighs and buttocks, by rubbing the genitals against pillows, clothing, or other objects, by running water directly on the clitoris, or by using a vibrator.

Barbach (1975) also recommends use of the **Kegel exercises**. The Kegel exercises were discovered accidentally by physician Arnold Kegel (1952) in the course of treating a forty-two-year-old woman who had been suffering from frequent loss of urine for several years. A physical examination revealed that her **pubococcygeus (PC) muscle**—the muscle that runs alongside the vaginal orifice—was weak and she did not know how to contract it. Kegel gave her an exercise program to strengthen it. During her last visit, the patient mentioned in passing that not only had the exercises cured her ailment, they had also dramatically improved her sex life.

Kegel studied several thousand women and came to the same conclusion. He observed:

Whenever the perivaginal musculature is well developed . . . sexual complaints are few or transient. On the other hand, in women with a thin, weak pubococcygeus muscle . . . expressions of indifference or dissatisfaction regarding sexual activity were frequently encountered. When a more careful history was taken, the symptoms revealed a definite pattern. . . . In the patients' own words: "I just don't feel anything"; or "I don't like the feeling"; or "The feeling is disagreeable." . . . Following restoration of the pubococcygeus muscle, numerous patients incidentally volunteered the information: "I can feel more sexually"; and some experienced orgasm for the first time. (Kegel, cited in Kline-Graber & Graber, 1978, p. 228)

Clinicians are still debating as to whether or not the exercises are helpful. Probably they are the most useful if the woman's PC muscle has poor tone, or has been stretched in childbirth.

The exercises are relatively simple. A woman's first step is to learn to identify the pubococcygeus muscle. She can do this easily by urinating and voluntarily interrupting the flow of urine. It is the PC muscle that stops the flow. The Kegel exercises consist of flexing the PC muscle ten times in a row, six times a day at the beginning and, over time, working up to longer periods. The objective, as in any form of exercise, is to strengthen the muscle through repeated use. Some women find that if they voluntarily tense and relax the PC muscle during masturbation or intercourse, it increases their excitement levels (Kline-Graber & Graber, 1978).

As described in Chapter 8, men masturbate in a variety of ways. Most grip the shaft of their penis firmly and move their hand rhythmically over it in a "milking" motion. Others rub the penis against a pillow, a towel, or the bed covers.

In the views of Zilbergeld (1978) and LoPiccolo (1978), masturbation is an important way for men to learn about themselves. By masturbating they can not only learn about their sexual preferences but also acquire skills that are useful in sexual relations, including techniques for preventing or overcoming erection problems and for developing ejaculatory control. And, of course, they can have an intrinsically satisfying experience.

All of the techniques discussed above enable individual men and women to become more knowledgeable about and more comfortable with their own sexuality. Therapists have also developed techniques to enable partners to develop the same knowledge of and sense of ease with each other.

Couple Oriented Programs

The most prominent therapists—Hartman and Fithian (1972), Kaplan (1974), LoPiccolo and LoPiccolo (1978), and Masters and Johnson (1970)—have evolved the therapy programs that are most commonly used with couples.

Some therapists believe that a team consisting of a man and woman as cotherapists works best. Some people feel that no man can thoroughly understand female sexuality, and vice versa. Many clients prefer to have a same-sex therapist, because they feel he or she will be sympathetic in interpreting their feelings to their partner (Lehrman, 1970; Masters & Johnson, 1970). Masters and Johnson (1970) require couples to live in a treatment center for two weeks. Other therapists assume it is more effective, and certainly less expensive, to live at home while learning how to integrate sexuality with their everyday lives. Most programs of couple therapy involve several steps, which we will describe here.

The Sex History. The therapists' first step is to try to obtain some sense of the couples' sexual attitudes, feelings, and experiences. Thus, the couple is asked to provide a detailed sex history. What, exactly, does this mean? One procedure used in compiling the sex history—that developed by Heiman et al. (1976)—is described here by way of example.

First, therapists try to understand their clients' early attitudes and feelings about affection, closeness, trust, male-female relationships, and sex. They chronicle their early sexual experiences. Questions asked of a couple include, for instance: What were attitudes toward sex in your home? Were you allowed to ask questions about sexual topics? Were your parents affectionate with each other? With you? What were your sexual experiences? At what age do you first recall having pleasurable genital feelings? When did you first experiment with masturbation? What were your dating experiences?

Then clients are asked about their current situation. The first questions focus on the couple's attitudes and beliefs: To what extent is sex integrated in their lives, or strictly set aside? What are they capable of changing? What areas would be difficult or impossible to change? Next come questions about sexual behavior: What is the couple's relationship like? How well do they communicate? What is their sexual relationship like? Finally, therapists interview the couple about their sexual problems, attempting to diagnose *exactly* what is going wrong in their sexual encounters.

Learning to Communicate. When it is difficult to do something, people tend to convince themselves that it is not really necessary to do it. It is very difficult for most people to talk to their partners about their sexual feelings. Many people expect their partners to have ESP and to know exactly how they feel about sex and what sexual activities and behaviors they like. They think of all this as obvious. But it is not. There are simply no techniques or behaviors that all men and all women find arousing.

Recently, the *Village Voice* interviewed New Yorkers about what makes a man or a woman "a good lover." There was no consistency in readers' answers. Some men liked women who were assertive. Others preferred women who were shy. Some women liked men who were sexual experimenters, who tried a variety of

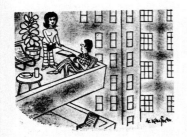

"Look at the corner apartment on the 12th floor. That's what I want you to do to me."

In order to have a good sexual relationship, communication is essential.

SOURCE: Reproduced by special permission of *Playboy* magazine. Copyright 1978 by *Playboy.*

positions as well as oral and anal sex. Others liked men who were "not into anything kinky." The conclusion: There is no such thing as "a good lover." The things that are intensely erotic for one person are repulsive or boring for another. If one is to have a good sexual relationship, communication is essential.

Barbach (1975) and Zilbergeld (1978) have observed that sometimes men and women's reluctance to talk to their partners is more than a mere reluctance to speak openly about sex. Some people are afraid to bring up the things that bother them in their day-to-day encounters, but their smoldering guilt and resentment poison their sexual relations.

Some people are afraid that if they tell one another honestly how they feel, they might hurt or be hurt. ("Jim would be humiliated if I told him I've been faking orgasm all these years." "Ethel would be devastated if I simply said straight out that the reason I hate cunnilingus is that her vagina smells just *awful*.") The irony is that usually men and women's "secrets" are no secret at all; usually their partners already have an inkling of precisely how they feel. When such feelings are brought out in the open, the most usual reaction is relief.

Therapists stress that all sexual disorders are shared disorders; both partners contribute to the problem and both are responsible for overcoming it (LoPiccolo, 1978). LoPiccolo has found that "most patients suffering from sexual dysfunction are woefully ignorant of both basic biology and effective techniques." For example, one woman's sexual anxieties began when she noticed that her clitoris disappeared when her husband stroked it. This, she concluded, proved she was repelled by their lovemaking. Of course, if anything, this fact "proved" just the opposite. The clitoris normally retracts during the plateau phase of arousal (Masters & Johnson, 1966).

The therapists spend some time, then, giving clients written material, showing them films, and discussing sexual facts with them. Some people are afraid to ask their partners for anything for fear of being turned down. Others are afraid of intimacy. They worry that if they expose their inner feelings, they will be vulnerable to their partners. Still others feel that although the *status quo* may be miserable, at least they are familiar with it. It feels safe.

All therapists, then, spend a considerable amount of time persuading their clients to talk honestly and openly with one another. It is the only way to ensure good sex (Zilbergeld, 1978; Barbach, 1975).

Sensate Focus, or "Pleasuring." The next step in therapy is "sensate focus" (if a client is participating in Masters and Johnson's program), or "pleasuring" (if in Kaplan's program). Dysfunctional couples often are "spectators" during lovemaking. Instead of getting swept up in their own sensory feelings, they observe their own and their partner's reactions with cold detachment. Thus, part of therapy is to help couples get "in touch" with their senses. Of course, all the senses—sight, smell, hearing, and tasting included—are important in lovemaking, but the core of sensate focus is the sense of touch.

In programs such as Masters and Johnson's (1970), one of the partners is designated as the giver of pleasure. The givers try to stroke, fondle, and massage their partner's body in any way that they think will cause delight (Downing, 1972). They are instructed *not* to touch their partner's breasts or genitals in this first session. In the early stages of sex counseling, many couples are so uneasy about their own sexuality that it is impossible for them to relax if they think their partner might touch these areas. Masters and Johnson (1970) observe:

For most women, and for most men, the sensate focus sessions represent the first opportunity they have ever had to "think and feel" sensuously and without the need to explain their sensate preferences, without the demand for personal reassurance, or without a sense of need to rush to "return the favor" . . . or without pushing for orgasm. (p. 73)

The following is an account of one man's reactions to the touching exercises:

Jack, a man in his forties who had come for therapy with his wife, agreed to try the touching exercises only after he was convinced that they would help in the treatment of his erection problems. The first time he and his wife snuggled, he became disappointed and then furious because he didn't get an erection. He strongly believed that the purpose of any kind of physical contact was to arouse him so that he could have intercourse. He was then told that the snuggling was to continue and that he should do everything possible to prevent himself from getting an erection. There was to be no genital contact whatever. Jack was at a loss to understand what was going on but agreed to find out what this touching stuff was about. It wasn't easy for him, for he believed in all the male myths more strongly than most men, but he gradually got more comfortable with touching. Within a few weeks, he even admitted that he was enjoying the new physical closeness with his wife. . . . But the real surprise was what Jack said in a phone conversation six months after the end of therapy.

The chances that a couple will enjoy a satisfying sexual relationship will be greater if the couple can take pleasure in simply touching and being close to one another.

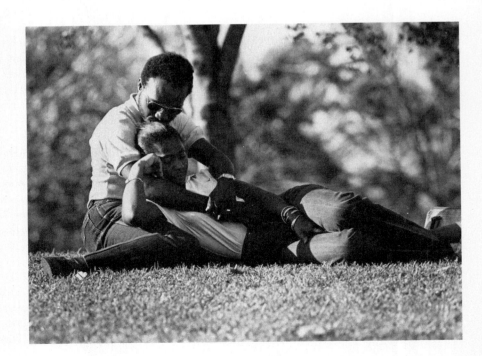

"I owe you a lot. Sex is fine, and that's great. But there's more. This closeness and cuddling stuff is really something. I never would have believed that I, of all people, would like it. Never even occurred to me to try it. Our lives are better because of it. I've gotten addicted to having my feet rubbed and licked and it's great." (Zilbergeld, 1978, pp. 123–124)

Exploring the Genitals. Once the couple are thoroughly comfortable with the sensate focus exercises, they are free to move on. They can begin to caress their partner's breasts and genitals during their pleasuring sessions. Once again, they can experiment, exploring various motions and pressures (see Chapter 10).

Many couples prefer to use lotions while doing these exercises. Some men and women find sexual fluids distinctly unsettling. They find vaginal lubrication, menstrual blood, or seminal fluid distasteful. Once they become used to rubbing each other with lotions, however, they often become equally comfortable with sexual fluids.

Nondemand Sexual Intercourse. Finally, couples are allowed to engage in sexual intercourse. They are urged to enjoy intercourse in and of itself and not to strive for orgasm. Such instruction usually reduces their anxiety enough so that both can reach orgasm. Paradoxically, it is often the case that the most efficient way to reach a goal is by not trying too hard to reach it.

Thus far, we have written as if heterosexual couples are the only ones with sexual problems. Of course this is not the case. Those who are interested in the sex therapy techniques that have been developed for gay and lesbian couples should refer to Masters and Johnson (1979) and McWhirter and Mattison (1980).

TREATMENTS FOR SPECIFIC DYSFUNCTIONS

Specific dysfunctions such as vaginismus and erectile dysfunction are often treated by means of special approaches. Let us examine some of these.

Vaginismus

The treatment for vaginismus is surprisingly simple. The therapist begins by providing women with some basic sex education. Sometimes that is all it takes to get women to relax sexually.

In the next step, "systematic desensitization," relaxation is the primary goal. The woman is asked to imagine that her lover is approaching her and is encouraged to relax. When she can enjoy such fantasies without feeling uneasy, she is encouraged to picture herself lying in bed with him, to envision him approaching her with an erection, and finally to imagine she is actually having intercourse. She progresses from each fantasy to the next only as she is able to attain total relaxation. When she is completely relaxed and comfortable with all these fantasies, she is ready for the vaginal dilation exercises.

The next step is to extinguish the woman's vaginismic response. The physician begins by inserting a wire-thin catheter in her vagina. Generally, this is easily tolerated. Slowly, larger and larger catheters are introduced. The last catheter introduced is the circumference of an erect penis. Some women are advised to keep a catheter in the vagina overnight in order to expedite the deconditioning process.

Clients may follow the same procedure at home. First, they gently insert their own finger (or their partner's finger or a tampon) into their vagina and let it remain there until they become comfortable. Then they move to two or more fingers (Fuchs et al., 1978). Soon the vaginismic spasms disappear and penile penetration is possible.

Erectile Dysfunctions

Naturally enough, men with erection problems often approach sexual encounters with trepidation. They are worried that they will not be able to get an erection or, worse yet, that they will get one, only to lose it at a crucial moment. And their fears are justified. Once they start to worry about their performance, they ensure their own failure.

Thus, therapists start by giving men special exercises designed to increase their confidence that they can develop an erection, lose it, and regain it. Men are told to focus in on their penis and move their hand rhythmically back and forth over their penis until they have a firm erection. Once they have a firm erection, they are instructed to stop, think about something else, and let their erection disappear. Once their penis is soft, they can start to masturbate again. They repeat this exercise again and again and in so doing provide themselves with a graphic demonstration that an erection lost can easily be regained (Masters & Johnson, 1970).

Slowly the tasks escalate. Men are told to try the same exercise, but this time while fantasizing about having sex with a partner. Next, they are to repeat the same exercise, but while fantasizing losing and then regaining an erection. Finally, they are to practice masturbating while imagining the "worst that can happen"—losing their erection.

Once men can gain and lose an erection at will when alone, they are ready to practice controlling their erection when they are with their partners. Again, the man soon discovers that a loss of firmness is never permanent; there are more erections where the last one came from.

On about the tenth day of Masters and Johnson's program, a couple is instructed to make a first attempt at intercourse. They practice an exercise designed to allay the man's fear that he may lose his erection when he enters his partner's vagina or begins thrusting. She strokes his penis until he has a fairly firm erection. Then she places herself in the female-superior position, with her partner on his back (see Figure 10–3, p. 297). Some men lose their erections when they stop focusing on their sensations and begin searching for their partner's vaginal entrance. By the time they find it, it is too late. Thus, she inserts his erect penis into her vagina, holds it there firmly, and begins to move slowly back and forth. The couple repeats this exercise several times.

Then the couple is ready to move on. This time the woman is instructed to remain relatively still while the man thrusts. Eventually, these "simultaneous pelvic pleasuring" exercises lead to orgasm. According to Masters and Johnson (1970), these procedures are successful with 60 percent of men with primary erectile dysfunctions and 74 percent of men with secondary erectile dysfunctions.

Some men prefer technological solutions to erectile problems. They may, more specifically, look for chemical solutions. Although the search for an aphrodisiac is as old as history, none has been found (see Chapter 4). For example, the well-known Spanish fly is not just ineffective, it is dangerous. It causes acute irritation of the intestinal and urinary tract. Its use sometimes leads to painful erection (priapism) or death. Testosterone injections may be helpful in those rare cases where men have a severe hormone deficiency, but such cases are rare. In general, it is totally ineffective.

Other men search for mechanical solutions to their problems—and such solutions are available. In recent years technicians have developed two types of *penile implants*. In one, a surgeon implants one or two silicone rods in the penis. This gives a man a permanent semierection, making his penis firm enough to insert into the partner's vagina during intercourse but not so erect that he is embarrassed in other situations. This implant does not impair a man's erotic sensation or his capacity for orgasm and ejaculation.

A more complicated hydraulic model exists—the Inflatable Penile Prosthesis. Inflatable cylinders are inserted in the penis, a reservoir of fluid is placed under the abdominal muscles, and a pumping mechanism is lodged in the scrotum. When a man wants to have an erection, he simply presses on a bulb in his scrotum. The fluid in the reservoir inflates the cylinders in his penis and erection is immediate. To return his penis to its normal state, the man simply presses the bulb in his scrotum once again and the fluid returns to the reservoir, deflating the cylinders. Once again, the implant does not interfere with orgasm or ejaculation.

Obviously, sex therapists do not recommend that people try to solve their emotional problems chemically or mechanically. Penile implants offer some hope for men who have no other hope—men suffering from diabetes (50 percent of men with diabetes have erectile problems), neurological disorders, accidental injury, complications following surgery, or other organic problems. But for most men, implants are more trouble than they are worth. Surgery is always risky, and most men find the implants embarrassing, ineffective, uncomfortable, and disappointing.

Premature Ejaculation

The aim of treatments for premature ejaculation is to teach men how to gain control over orgasm. They are designed to help men (1) focus in on their penis, (2) learn slowly, in step-by-step fashion, to gauge exactly how close they are to the point of ejaculatory inevitability, and (3) increase or decrease their level of arousal at will.

Focusing. Most men who experience premature ejaculation have great trouble really focusing on their feelings. Their mind keeps wandering. They keep warning themselves not to get too excited: "Slow down! Don't come! Oh no!" They try to distract themselves in the hope that this will slow ejaculation down. Actually, such distractions sometimes increase their problems. They never learn to calibrate their feelings. Thus, therapy for these men begins with the focusing exercises described earlier.

Start-Stop Masturbation.   As noted, masturbation can serve as a valuable exercise in control. The therapist tells men to focus their thoughts on their penis and, with a dry hand, slowly to begin to masturbate. They are to keep track of their arousal level. When they become very excited and feel they are approaching the point of orgasm, they are to stop masturbating. They must, however, continue focusing on their penis to notice exactly how it feels as their erection subsides, in about two to three minutes. When they no longer feel that their ejaculation is imminent, they are to begin to masturbate again.

This start-stop masturbation exercise gives men practice sensing just how aroused they are. Once they learn that, they are ready to progress to more difficult tasks. For example, they are instructed to try the preceding exercise using lubrication, which is sometimes more arousing, while varying the type of stroke, while relaxing or tensing their pelvic muscles, or while fantasizing, or not, about sex.

Learning to Control Arousal Level.   To gain further control over premature ejaculation, men are told to masturbate for fifteen minutes, without stopping and without ejaculating. They are told to allow themselves to become very excited, and then to make subtle changes to decrease their level of arousal. Some adjustments they may make include slowing down their pace, decreasing the pressure of their thrust, being careful not to stimulate the head of the penis, focusing on the shaft instead, or changing the type of stroke—for example, using shorter strokes or circular motions (Zilbergeld, 1978). They can also try relaxing or tensing their pelvic muscles and seeing what effect that has. They are encouraged to try all of these methods in order to discover what works best and then to perfect these techniques.

Once men have mastered these basic exercises, they are ready to practice these exercises with their partners. The man begins by lying on his back. His partner begins to stimulate his penis (Figure 13–1). As he focuses on his penis, he usually becomes increasingly excited. When he feels he is reaching the point of ejaculatory inevitability, he asks his partner to stop. She does so *immediately*. Once men feel they have good control under these conditions, they are ready to move on.

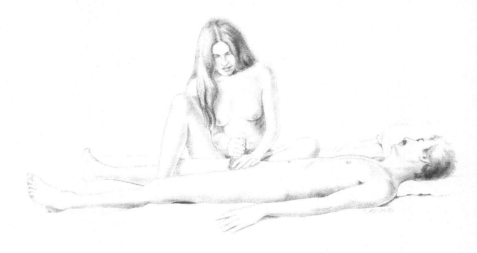

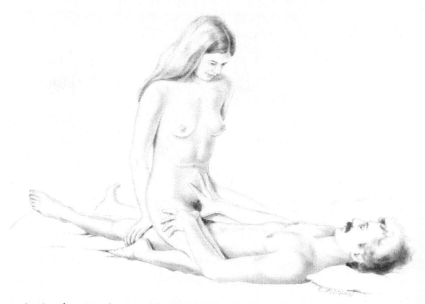

Again, the man lies on his back. His lover sits on his legs as shown in Figure 13–2. She caresses his penis until he has an erection. She begins to rub his penis gently around the outside of her vagina and in her pubic hair. If this becomes too exciting for her partner, she stops and waits until he has gained control of his ejaculatory processes. Then the man slowly inserts his penis in his partner's vagina. She remains totally still. The man's only task is to focus on his sensory feelings. If he begins to lose his erection, his partner contracts her pelvic muscles a few times or moves ever so slightly. This is usually enough to keep the man's erection firm.

Once the couple feels comfortable with these exercises, they can try some others. For example, the next time the man or woman inserts the man's penis into her vagina, she begins thrusting slowly. The man can tell her how fast to go. Then he can begin to move slowly. Gradually the couple can increase their pace, employing subtle adjustments whenever necessary, to slow things down and even stop for awhile, if need be, to prevent ejaculation. Finally, the couple is encouraged to explore different positions.

The "Squeeze Technique."   Masters and Johnson (1970) use an additional technique—the squeeze technique—in the treatment of premature ejaculation. They point out that a woman can dampen a man's arousal simply by grasping his penis where the head and shaft join and squeezing, as illustrated in Figure 13–3. (Also see Lazarus, 1978.) Problems of premature ejaculation appear to be solved by this method. Indeed, Seman (1956) reported a 100 percent success rate and Masters and Johnson (1970) a 98 percent success rate using the squeeze technique.

Retarded Ejaculation

Kaplan (1974) recommends that therapists use "systematic densensitization" techniques to eradicate the retarded ejaculator's phobia about ejaculating in his partner's vagina. Initially, men are instructed to engage in sex play with their partners.

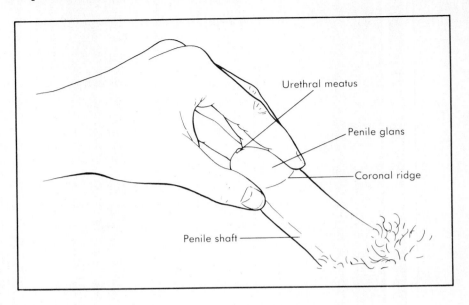

At the end of a sexual encounter they should try to achieve orgasm in whatever way they can. For example, some very inhibited men can only reach orgasm if they fantasize about their partner while masturbating to climax in the bathroom behind locked doors. In such cases, the man would engage in foreplay with his partner, go to the bathroom, lock the door, fantasize, and masturbate to orgasm. Then he would try to achieve orgasm with the door partially open and, once he is able to do that, with his partner actually looking on. When the couple feels comfortable with this, they progress to more difficult tasks. Can she stimulate him to orgasm? Can she stimulate him to climax in close proximity to her vaginal entrance? Can he enter her vagina a moment before he is about to ejaculate? Step by step, the couple works up to the point where the previously retarded ejaculator is able to enter his partner's vagina at fairly lower levels of excitement, thrust as he pleases, and climax within her vagina. How successful is such deconditioning? Masters and Johnson (1970) report that 60 percent of retarded ejaculators can be cured.

SUMMARY

There is nothing "natural" about the way people express themselves sexually. From infancy on, people learn how they ought to think, feel, and behave. Most people have some sexual experiences that are profoundly rewarding and others that are devastating. It is from these experiences—delightful and painful—that people's sexual attitudes, feelings, and behavior emerge. Sometimes the outcomes include various sexual difficulties or dysfunctions. The major male sexual dysfunctions are: (1) sexual apathy, (2) erectile dysfunctions, (3) premature ejaculation, and (4) retarded ejaculation. The major female sexual dysfunctions are: (1) sexual apathy, (2) sexual unresponsiveness, (3) orgasmic dysfunction, (4) dyspareunia, and (5) vaginismus.

A variety of sex therapy programs have been developed to assist people in overcoming sexual dysfunctions. Individually oriented therapies stress goal setting, improving body images, learning to relax, touching exercises, and masturbation. Couple oriented therapies are based on individual needs as revealed by sex histories and involve training in communication, sensate focus or pleasuring, genital exploration, and non-demand sexual intercourse.

Special approaches have been devised for treating specific dysfunctions such as vaginismus, erectile dysfunction, and premature and retarded ejaculation.

SUGGESTED READINGS

Barbach, L. G. (1975). *For yourself: The fulfillment of female sexuality.* New York: New American Library.

Heiman, J., LoPiccolo, L., & LoPiccolo, J. (1976). *Becoming orgasmic: A sexual growth program for women.* Englewood Cliffs, N. J.: Prentice-Hall.

Kaplan, H. S. (1974). *The new sex therapy.* New York: Brunner/Mazel.

Masters, W. H., & Johnson, V. E. (1970). *Human sexual inadequacy.* Boston: Little, Brown.

Zilbergeld, B. (1978). *Male sexuality: A guide to sexual fulfillment.* Boston: Little, Brown.

CHAPTER OUTLINE

MAJOR SEXUALLY TRANSMITTED DISEASES
Gonorrhea
Non-Gonococcal Urethritis
Syphilis
Genital Herpes
Granuloma Inguinale (Chronic Venereal Sore)
Lymphogranuloma Venereum (LGV)
Chancroid ("Soft Chancre")

SEXUALLY OR NONSEXUALLY TRANSMITTED DISEASES
Acquired Immune Deficiency Syndrome (AIDS)
Vaginitis
Cystitis
Genital Warts
Pubic Lice (Crabs)

CHAPTER 14

SEXUALLY TRANSMITTED DISEASES

Sexually transmitted diseases (STD), or **venereal diseases (VD)**, are those that are contracted primarily through intimate sexual contact. The incidence of STDs is at epidemic proportions in the United States.* The most prevalent infectious disease in the United States is the common cold. But gonorrhea, genital herpes, and nongonococcal urethritis (NGU) are close behind, followed by syphilis. According to the Centers for Disease Control, in 1981 there were around one million *reported* cases of gonorrhea and 31,000 reported cases of syphilis. Since physicians generally report only 30 to 50 percent of the cases of gonorrhea they encounter, the Centers estimate that there were between 2 and 6 million cases of gonorrhea and 120,000 cases of syphilis in 1981 (Centers for Disease Control, 1982). The Centers do not yet report statistics on the incidence of genital herpes or NGU. However, estimates of the incidence of new cases of genital herpes range from 200,000 to 1 million per year.

All of this does, indeed, sound like an epidemic. For a number of reasons, STDs have been particularly difficult to control. One reason is that no immunizing vaccines are presently available to combat their spread. As we will see, however, when detected, most STDs can be cured. Yet people who develop symptoms are often reluctant to seek immediate medical attention. Some continue to be active sexually and may infect one or more other people before seeking treatment. Their reluctance to seek treatment may stem from many sources, including fear of social stigma, fear of the reactions of regular sexual partners who expect sexual fidelity, and fear that the fact that they are sexually active will become known (Rosebury, 1971). Let us now turn to a brief examination of some common and some uncommon sexually transmitted diseases.

*The authors gratefully acknowledge the collaboration of Dr. Mark Edwards, Rockefeller University, on this chapter.

MAJOR SEXUALLY TRANSMITTED DISEASES

In this chapter we will address a series of questions: (1) What are the most common and some of the less common sexually transmitted diseases? (2) What are the causes, symptoms, and modes of transmission of sexually transmitted diseases? (3) How are the sexually transmitted diseases treated and, if they are untreated, what are the consequences? (4) What can be done to prevent or reduce a person's chances of contracting sexually transmitted diseases? At the outset, we must emphasize that diagnosis and treatment of sexually transmitted diseases should be attempted only by or under the supervision of qualified physicians.

Gonorrhea

Gonorrhea ("the clap," "the drip," "a dose"), a bacterial infection that is contracted sexually, is described as early as the Old Testament (about 1500 B.C.). Hippocrates (400 B.C.) speculated that gonorrhea resulted from excessive indulgence in the "pleasures of Venus" (the goddess of love). Galen (200 A.D.) erroneously believed that gonorrhea is caused by an involuntary loss of semen. It was Galen who gave the disease its name—from *gonos*, the Greek word for "seed," and *rhois*, the Greek word for "flow." Finally, in 1879, Albert Neisser identified the kidney-shaped bacterium, the gonococcus, which is now named *Neisseria gonor-*

In this poster from the 1920s, people's fears of contracting sexually transmitted diseases were used in an attempt to limit their sexual activities.

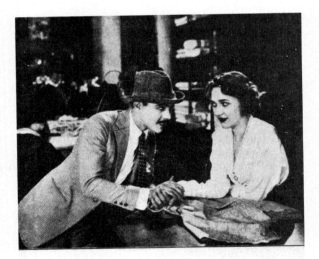

"Pick-up" acquaintances often take girls autoriding, to cafès, and to theatres with the intention of leading them into sex relations. Disease or child-birth may follow

Avoid the man who tries to take liberties with you He is selfishly thoughtless and inconsiderate of you

Believe no one who says it is necessary to indulge sex desire

Know the men you associate with

rhea. Gonorrhea may affect the throat, the genital and urinary organs, and the anorectal region.

It would save many people much embarrassment if people *could* pick up gonorrhea from toilet seats, doorknobs, or swimming pools. But this is nearly impossible. Usually, the only way a person can contract gonorrhea is by having direct sexual contact with an infected person. *Neisseria gonorrhea* lives best in warm moist environments—in the moist linings of the mouth and throat, the genitals, or the anorectal regions—the areas that are involved in oral, genital, or anal sex. Outside these areas, the organisms die within minutes to hours.

People who have sexual contact with an infected partner do not always get gonorrhea. The risk of infection is less than 100 percent; however, if people have sexual contact several times with an infected person, their chances of becoming infected increase.

Symptoms.   Generally, *men* begin to notice something is wrong three to five days after a sexual encounter with an infected partner. Symptoms can appear as early as one day or as late as two weeks after infection. The first symptom is a thin, clear mucous discharge, which flows out of the opening of the penis. Within a day or two, the discharge turns thick and creamy. It is usually white, but it can be yellow or yellow-green. The opening of the penis may become swollen and stand out from the glans. Some uncircumcised men find that their glans is red and irritated. There is an even more obvious symptom—most men feel an intensely painful, burning sensation when they try to urinate. The urine may contain a little blood. Some infected men also notice that their lymph glands in the groin are tender. The symptoms of gonorrhea are usually so painful that most men immediately consult a physician and are treated with antibiotics.

If for some reason the disease is left untreated, it may infrequently spread and have serious complications. Infection and inflammation, accompanied by abscesses, may spread up the urogenital tract. Any of the following may be affected: the penis, Cowper's ducts and glands, the prostate gland, the seminal vesicles, the bladder, the ejaculatory ducts, the vasa deferentia, and the epididymes. As the infection spreads throughout the man's urinary and genital tract, he usually experiences intense pain. He may also become sterile in rare instances.

Anorectal and oral gonococcal infections are frequent results of anal and oral sex with an infected partner. Anorectal infection may be asymptomatic (without symptoms) or may produce burning sensations and discharge. If these symptoms are not treated, they may eventually subside and the man may become an asymptomatic carrier of gonorrhea, infecting subsequent partners. Oral gonococcal infection is often asymptomatic but occasionally may infect the throat, producing pharyngitis, or the tonsils, producing tonsillitis.

Unfortunately, 50 to 80 percent of *women* who get gonorrhea do not notice any symptoms. For many women, the first hint they may have that they are infected is when their partner discovers infection in himself. Obviously, it is critically important for men who discover they are infected to inform all of their sexual contacts.

In women, gonorrhea usually gains its initial foothold in the cervix. Within a few days, pus begins to seep out of the cervical opening. Few women notice this discharge, which may be green or yellow-green. Since the cervix lies high in the vagina, most women do not notice any symptoms. As infection of the cervix

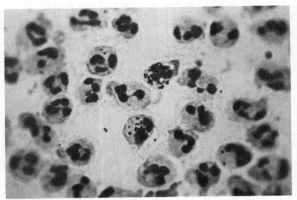 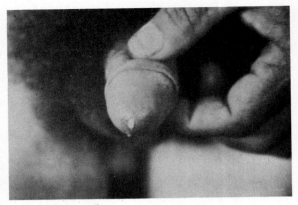

(Left) *Neisseria gonorrhea,* the causative organism of gonorrhea. (Right) Among the symptoms of gonorrhea in men is a pus-filled discharge from the penis.

continues, the vaginal discharge may become heavier. This discharge should not be confused with a normal discharge, which is clear or white and nonirritating. Sometimes the urethra and its opening become infected. Women may feel a burning pain when they urinate.

If gonorrhea is untreated, it may spread rapidly to other parts of the woman's body, with a serious complication peculiar to women—pelvic inflammatory disease (PID). In PID, the gonorrhea organism spreads to all of the following: Bartholin's glands and ducts, the bladder, the uterus (where it may cause menstrual problems), and the fallopian tubes. As the infection spreads, women may begin to have fevers, headaches, and backaches and experience severe abdominal pain, nausea, and vomiting. They may rarely become sterile. Approximately 20 percent of untreated gonorrhea in women results in PID and 15 percent in sterility (Schofield, 1979).

A pregnant woman can transmit gonorrhea to her newborn child. As the fetus passes down the birth canal, it can become infected. That is why, by state law, when infants are born, the physician must put silver nitrate drops or antibiotic solutions in their eyes to prevent blindness that may result from eye contact with the gonorrheal bacteria.

Treatment.   Generally, a physician can tell if a man has gonorrhea simply by examining his genitals and doing a microscopic examination of his discharge. With a woman, laboratory tests are usually necessary. To make a diagnosis, the technician swabs the patient's throat, tonsils, cervix, and anus, and wipes the swabs onto a growth medium. If, after twenty-four to forty-eight hours, *Neisseria gonorrhea* are present, the bacteria will have multiplied and their colonies will be visible. These bacteria are then chemically tested to confirm their identity.

In most instances, gonorrhea can be cured by giving infected individuals an injection of penicillin into the muscle of the buttocks. Recently, though, a strain of *Neisseria gonorrhea* has emerged which is resistant to the action of penicillin. The total number of gonorrhea cases in the United States that are caused by this strain is still low. However, the presence of this organism in the United States points out the necessity of proper medical diagnosis, treatment, and follow-up examination. If the gonococcus is resistant to penicillin, or if the patient is allergic to penicillin, the physician can prescribe tetracycline tablets or other appropriate antibiotic treatment.

Non-Gonococcal Urethritis

Non-gonococcal urethritis (NGU), also called nonspecific urethritis (NSU), is an inflammation of the urethra that is not caused by gonorrhea. The symptoms include a thin, clear, or somewhat creamy discharge from the penis and mild pain during urination. The discharge resulting from NGU is thinner and clearer and the pain during urination less severe than with gonorrhea. NGU is transmitted sexually and symptoms appear within two to three weeks following infection. All of the exact causes are not fully agreed upon but the organisms *Chlamadia trachomatis* and *Uriaplasma ureolyticus* are thought to be involved. NGU is commonly diagnosed in the United States. Tetracycline is often the treatment of choice since NGU does not respond to penicillin. Some cases of untreated NGU may lead to complications such as PID.

Syphilis

Syphilis is one of the most serious sexually transmitted diseases, the first symptoms of which are small painless sores at the point(s) where the causative organisms enter the body. If untreated, syphilis may lead to very serious consequences and even death.

Syphilis has a long history. In the tropical rain forests of Africa, prehistoric men and women suffered from yaws, a close relative to syphilis. There are descriptions of syphilis-like diseases in ancient Chinese, Indian, Hebrew, and Greek writings. Egyptian mummies have been found that reveal unmistakable signs of the disease. Since the time of Columbus, nations have blamed each other for the disease. The French called syphilis "the Italian disease," Italians called it "the French disease," and the English sometimes called it "the Spanish disease."

Great historical figures have been infected by syphilis—kings, popes, doctors, scientists, poets, artists, and dancers. Victims include biblical figures—Abraham and Sarah, the Pharaoh of Genesis, Miriam, David and Bathsheba, and Job; political figures—Julius Caesar, Cleopatra, Herod, the emperor Tiberius, Charles V of France, Peter the Great, Frederick the Great, Napoleon, King Edward VII, Lord Randolph Churchill, Mussolini, Hitler, Pope Sixtus IV, Columbus, Henry VIII, Ivan the Terrible; and fine arts figures—Boswell, Beethoven, Keats, Schubert, Nietzsche, Gauguin, Strindberg, de Maupassant, van Gogh, and Oscar Wilde.

In 1981 approximately 31,000 cases of syphilis were *reported* in the United States (Centers for Disease Control, 1981). This probably represents 15 to 50 percent of the cases that actually occurred.

Treponema pallidum (T. pallidum), the bacterium that causes syphilis, has a thin, delicate spiral-shaped appearance. The organism can rapidly penetrate the membranous linings of the urogenital, anorectal, and oral areas or skin that has been scraped. Unless the organism remains within these warm, moist areas of the body, it soon dies. Thus, the primary way to contract syphilis is *by* oral, genital, or anal sex. The spiral shape of the organism enables it to propel itself easily and it may distribute itself throughout the body.

Unless halted by effective treatment, syphilis goes through four different stages: primary, secondary, latent, and late (or tertiary). Let us now examine the symptoms associated with each stage.

Primary Syphilis.   The incubation period for syphilis can range from ten days to three months. Usually, three or four weeks after men and women are infected, they develop one or more chancres (pronounced "shankers"). In men the chancre usually appears on or about the penis. In women, it usually appears on the cervix or the vagina. This explains, once again, why women are often unaware that they have contracted the disease. However, chancres may also appear on the labia, tongue, lips, or anus. Often only one chancre appears. When the chancre first appears, it is a painless, dull red lump about the size of a pea. Sometimes it is covered by a yellow or gray crusty scab. The chancre usually persists for three to six weeks. During this period, it is extremely infectious. At this stage, men and women may have some additional symptoms—headache, mild nausea, painless enlargement of the lymph glands, or pain in the joints. Eventually, the chancre will disappear. Sometimes at this point people who have been worried that they *may* have syphilis breathe a sigh of relief. They decide that they did not have syphilis after all or that they are cured. Often, however, they are not cured. The disease continues to the secondary stage and the infected individuals continue to transmit it to their sexual contacts.

Secondary Syphilis.   A man or woman may show no symptoms for weeks or months. Then, suddenly a rash appears. Syphilitic rashes vary in appearance. Sometimes they are merely pink or brown spots that one can barely see. Sometimes they are rubbery, hard, raised bumps. The rash may involve the face, palms of the hands or soles of the feet, the chest, the back, arms, and legs. On the warm, moist areas of the body such as that between the buttocks, the rash may be wet and

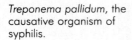

Treponema pallidum, the causative organism of syphilis.

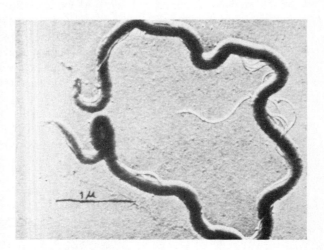

1 μ

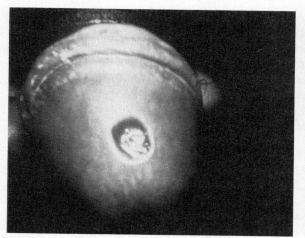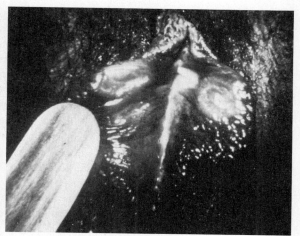

Syphilitic chancres on the penis and on the labia.

oozing. The fluid which oozes from the rash is extremely contagious. The rash may also appear on lips, tongue, tonsils, throat, and vocal cords. Not surprisingly, infected men and women may notice that they have developed a mild sore throat and a husky voice. In many cases, lymph glands become enlarged.

Some men and women have other symptoms. They lose their eyelashes and eyebrows; their hair looks "moth-eaten." They suffer from a general feeling of ill health, experience headaches, nausea, loss of appetite, pain in the muscles, joints, and bones, and a persistent fever.

Within two to six weeks, however, the rashes clear and the symptoms disappear. Once again, infected people are in danger of convincing themselves that they never had anything ("It must have been an allergy to chocolate") or that they have been cured. In fact, the disease often enters the next stage—the latent stage.

Latent Syphilis.   If secondary syphilis is not treated, the disease enters a period of latency that may last for many years, during which there may be no symptoms. Latent syphilis can be diagnosed by the demonstration of a positive blood test for syphilis. The mechanism by which *T. pallidum* becomes latent is unknown. Following the first year of the latency stage the disease is no longer as infectious; however, a pregnant woman can still pass it on to a fetus. About two out of three untreated people live the rest of their lives without any further problems and symptoms never recur. The remaining one in three develops the complications of late syphilis.

Late (Tertiary) Syphilis.   After the secondary stage, syphilis may lie dormant for months or for as long as fifty to sixty years and then, suddenly, erupt without warning. Any part of the body may end up being attacked or seriously damaged. Here we will consider only some of the most common problems that develop.

In so-called benign syphilis, the infected person develops *gummas*, large destructive gummy ulcers, on the affected organs. The skin, muscles, digestive organs, liver, lungs, eyes, or endocrine glands may be affected. These gummas may lead to the degeneration of the organs on which they appear. Or, the skull, bones, and joints may be permanently damaged by the gummas. *Cardiovascular syphilis* attacks the heart and blood vessels, producing damage that is sometimes fatal. In *neurosyphilis* the brain and the spinal cord are affected. This produces neurological disorders including insanity and paralysis. (A shuffling gait was once the mark of an advanced syphilitic.) Neurosyphilis is usually fatal. In short, in the tertiary phase, syphilis may damage almost any organ in the body. Once tissues have been seriously damaged, repair is virtually impossible.

Congenital Syphilis.   During pregnancy, some mothers inadvertently pass syphilis on to their unborn children. Such children are then born with congenital syphilis. How can this happen? The infected mother transmits syphilis to her unborn child through the small blood vessels of the placenta. Before the fourth month of pregnancy, the placenta is not well developed; thus, the syphilis organisms cannot reach the fetus. If a mother is treated for syphilis before her fourth month, her child will usually not develop congenital syphilis. After the fourth month, the mother can infect her child. If syphilis is detected and treated during this period, however, both the expectant mother and her child will be cured. For this reason, doctors often routinely give expectant mothers blood tests for syphilis several times during their pregnancy.

Treatment.   Diagnosis can be made by physical examination of the pregnant woman and a blood test for antibodies indicating the presence of the organism. The physician may also examine fluid from the primary chancre for *T. pallidum* organisms.

Syphilis can be treated with a variety of antibodies. Most comonly, penicillin is injected into the muscle of the buttocks. If an infected person is allergic to penicillin, he or she can take tetracycline tablets instead.

Genital Herpes

Herpes is thought to be the second most common sexually transmitted disease in the United States. Unfortunately, physicians are not yet required to report the disease, so the United States Public Health Service can only guess at the frequency. Estimates of the prevalence of genital herpes were as high as 200,000 to 500,000 new cases in the United States in 1981 (Leo, 1982).

Genital herpes is caused by the virus *Herpes simplex*. There are two closely related *H. simplex* viruses: Type 1, which is usually responsible for cold sores, and Type 2, which usually causes genital herpes. Type 1 can occur genitally and Type 2 orally, however; this reversal might occur, for example, as the result of infection during oral sex.

Although genital herpes is often transmitted during sexual relations, it may also be spread by other means. Once men contract the disease, their symptoms are more pronounced than are women's. Herpes can infect either the anorectal, urogenital, or oral areas of the body—those areas involved in sexual encounters.

What does genital herpes look like? At first, small soft blisters appear on the infected areas. Soon afterwards, the blisters break open and form itchy, painful open sores. After four to five days, the sores become less painful and begin to heal by themselves. The person may also feel enlarged lymph glands in the groin while washing, and sometimes urination is painful.

Because *H. simplex* is a virus, antibiotics are not helpful in treatment. Furthermore, because the virus can become latent by entering nerves, it is difficult to treat with any agent. Symptoms can recur as a result of stress, such as final exams, financial problems, pregnancy, or unusual happiness or excitement.

The absence of active lesions on the surface of the skin or membranous lining of the oral, genital, or anorectal cavities means that viral agents are not present on the surface and the person cannot transmit the disease. However, prior to the eruption of active lesions there may be a tingling or itching sensation and virus particles may be present, rendering the person infectious. Therefore, the disease can be transmitted from the time immediately preceding the appearance of sores, *which is virtually impossible to anticipate*, until the sores are gone.

For women, the fact that herpes may reappear under stress is a special problem. If a pregnant woman develops lesions at the time of delivery, a physician will deliver the child by cesarean section. If the child were to pass through the birth canal, it would become infected, with disastrous consequences: severe brain damage or death of the newborn infant. While often discussed as a possibility, a causal relationship between cervical cancer and infection with genital herpes virus is not established.

Cures for *Herpes simplex* are being actively sought. The first effective treatment (not cure) is a drug called acyclovir, which is available by prescription. A drug called 2-deoxy-D-glucose also seems to shorten the average duration of an attack and to prevent recurrence. The substance is presently undergoing testing and is not yet licensed for medical use. The scientific and medical communities are actively seeking more effective treatments, cures, and preventive vaccines for genital herpes. In 1983 both British ("Scientists Find," June 13, 1983) and United States ("Claim of Cure," June 24, 1983) scientists claimed to have discovered effective cures. Their claims, however, have not yet been verified and, in any case, the drugs would not be available for some time. (Up-to-the-minute information about herpes can be secured from HELP [Herpetics Engaged in Living Productively], HELP-ASHA, Box 100, Palo Alto, California 94302).

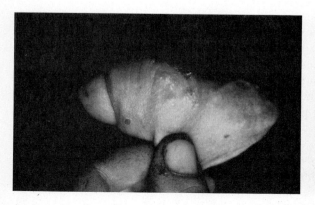 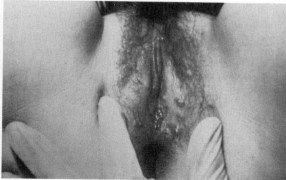

Herpes simplex-2 lesions of the male and female genitals.

Granuloma Inguinale (Chronic Venereal Sore)

Granuloma inguinale is a sexually transmitted disease caused by an infectious agent known as *Calymmatobacterium granulomatis*. It is most common in tropical climates and may be transmitted sexually. The first symptoms appear three days to six months after infection. A blister or lump appears on the sexual organs, anus, groin, or thighs. At first the blister is painless. However, it soon develops into a raised, open sore that bleeds easily. As this painful ulceration spreads, the area becomes vulnerable to infection by other bacteria. Once again, men's symptoms are far more obvious than are women's. Diagnosis is fairly simple. The infecting organism is identified from smears taken from the raw areas. The most effective antibiotics for treating granuloma inguinale are tetracycline and ampicillin.

Lymphogranuloma Venereum (LGV)

Rare and restricted primarily to the Southeast in the United States, **Lympho-granuloma venereum**, a disease caused by a microorganism called *Chlamydia trachomatis*, is most common in the tropics. The organism has some of the properties of a bacteria, some of a virus. LGV is a disease of the lymphatic system. During the infection, the invading *C. trachomatis* organisms are concentrated and destroyed in the lymph nodes, causing the lymph nodes to become swollen and painful. LGV is transmitted by vaginal, oral-genital, or anal intercourse. It is possible to spread it by other close contact as well.

   The incubation period for LGV may last from a few days to three weeks. The first symptoms of LGV may pass unnoticed. Infected people develop a small, pimplelike, painless sore on their sexual organs. The first obvious signs of the disease appear later, when the lymph glands in both sides of the groin become enlarged and tender. Headache, fever, chills, and considerable pain follow. If LGV is left untreated, the infection may spread to the anus and rectum and can result in rectal damage. LGV infection of the lymph vessels in the vagina or penis can block the normal flow of lymph fluid to produce genital elephantiasis—massive growth of the sexual organ.

   Diagnosis of LGV can be made by blood tests. Treatment consists of giving the infected person sulfa or broad-spectrum antibiotics such as tetracycline.

Chancroid ("Soft Chancre")

Chancroid is found rarely in the United States but is more common in the Far East and the tropics. **Chancroid** is caused by the bacillus *Corynebacterium vaginalis* and is usually transmitted by vaginal, oral-genital, or anal intercourse. The bacteria enter through small cuts or scratches in the skin.

   Men's symptoms are usually more pronounced than are women's. Women are sometimes "carriers," passing on the disease to their male partners, unaware that they themselves are infected. A few days after infection, several small sores appear on the sexual organs. At first, the sores look like raised bumps, surrounded by a red border. They soon develop into pus-filled pimples, forming painful sores that resemble the syphilitic chancre. Soon, the pustules burst and spread. In 50 percent of untreated cases, the chancroid bacteria infect the lymph glands in the groin. The glands become hard, enlarged, and painful. Physicians can usually diagnose chancroid by taking a culture of the sores. Treatment consists of orally administered tetracycline.

SEXUALLY OR NONSEXUALLY TRANSMITTED DISEASES

There are a variety of diseases affecting the genital and reproductive systems that may be transmitted sexually or by other means. Let us briefly examine the most common of these.

Acquired Immune Deficiency Syndrome (AIDS)

Acquired Immune Deficiency Syndrome (AIDS) is the name given to a recently reported complex of health problems in which victims develop a serious loss of their natural immunity against disease. The immunity loss leaves patients with AIDS vulnerable to a number of diseases that might not otherwise be a threat. The most common of these "opportunistic" diseases are a rare form of cancer called Kaposi's sarcoma and a form of pneumonia called *Pneumocystis carinii*. AIDS is a very serious disease with death resulting in up to 50 percent of the cases, depending on the opportunistic disease contracted. To date there is no known cure or effective vaccine for the disease (Centers for Disease Control, March 1983).

About 95 percent of the victims of AIDS are males, around 75 percent of whom are homosexual or bisexual. Others at risk for AIDS are intravenous drug abusers, Haitian entrants to the United States, and persons with hemophilia (Centers for Disease Control, March 1983). However, some women, children, and others not in the above groups have also contracted AIDS, which suggests that no person is completely beyond risk of contracting the disease (Fisher, 1983).

There are no clear-cut symptoms of AIDS. However, many victims experience fever, loss of appetite, weight loss, fatigue, and enlargement of lymph nodes over a period of months before the onset of specific opportunistic diseases (Centers for Disease Control, 1983).

Because it is such a deadly illness, an intensive search for the cause of AIDS began immediately after the disease was identified. Most investigators suspected that some sort of virus was involved that may be transmitted through blood, semen, and other bodily fluids (Fisher, 1983). In May 1984, Dr. Robert Gallo of the National Cancer Institute and his many collaborators reported four studies that seemed to confirm this suspicion. They reported that a newly identified subgroup of the human T-cell leukemia virus family, named HTLV-III, is the probable causative agent. The HTLV-III virus and antibodies to the virus were isolated in a large percentage of AIDS patients and those showing early signs of the disease (Marx, 1984). This important discovery opens the way for the development of specific tests to identify the virus and blood or other fluids that may be contaminated by the virus. Added to this is the possibility of developing a vaccine to protect high-risk persons against the disease. For now these are future goals that are being pursued intensely (Marx, 1984).

What can be done to avoid contracting AIDS from sexual activities? There are no specific preventive steps. However, because the incidence of the disease ap-

RESEARCH HIGHLIGHT

Preventing Sexually Transmitted Diseases

Earlier in this chapter we referred to the prevalence of STDs as nearing epidemic proportions. Many approaches to reducing the spread of STDs have been used, but most have been relatively ineffective. Perhaps most ineffective are attempts to prevent sexual activity among young, unmarried people. A second approach has been to make information concerning symptoms of STDs easily available, to provide free treatment, and to require physicians to report some kinds of STDs to public health officials. In reality, many cases go unreported. This, of course, short-circuits efforts to identify and treat those who have had sexual contact with others with STDs. However, even if treated, infected people are likely to transmit their infection to one or more other people.

In recent years there has been a renewed interest in developing methods to prevent the transmission of STDs among sexually active people. Preventive action may be taken before, during, and after sexual contacts. Summarized below

are steps that individuals may take to lessen the probability of their contracting an STD in the course of a sexual encounter. They are not 100 percent effective but are better than no preventive measures at all. (Boston Women's Health Book Collective, 1976; Hart, 1977).

Before Sexual Interaction
1. *Communication:* Sexual partners should be candid concerning recent exposure to or current infection with any STD. Effective diagnosis and treatment should precede any sexual contact if either is the case.

2. *Genital examination:* A man's penis, scrotum, anus, buttocks, and surrounding areas should be visually examined for warts, sores, reddened areas, and other signs of infection. His penis may be "milked" from base to glans and the urethral opening examined for the presence of cloudy discharge.

A woman's vulva, anus, and buttocks should be visually examined for warts, sores, reddened areas, and other signs of infection such as thick,

white, yellow or yellow-green vaginal discharges.

Sexual contact should be avoided if signs of infection are noted.

3. *Genital disinfection:* The external genitals may be washed with soap and water prior to sexual contact. The effectiveness of this method may be limited since many infecting organisms reside inside the male urethra. The value of vaginal douching is thought to be minimal.

During Sexual Interaction
1. *The condom:* Though not perfect, the value of condoms for preventing STD transmission has long been recognized. To be effective, a condom must be put on the erect penis *before* any sexual contact begins.

2. *Vaginal foams, creams and jellies:* Many of the available contraceptive foams, creams, and jellies for intravaginal use provide *some* protection against STD transmission.

After Sexual Interaction
1. *Genital disinfection:* Immediately following sexual contact, washing the genitals with soap and

water may provide some protection. Vaginal douching with an approved medicated preparation may also have some preventive value.

2. *Urination:* Urination following sexual contact may provide some protection for men. STD organisms may be flushed from the urethra and the acidity of urine is hostile to some organisms.

3. *Medication:* Some drugs applied directly to a man's penis or introduced into the urethra after sexual contact provide some protection against gonorrhea. Others may be introduced into the vagina to protect women. These are not generally available to the public in the United States.

When the risk of infection is high, physicians may prescribe tetracycline or other antibiotics in small doses for use immediately after contact. The use of these drugs should always be supervised by a physician.

pears to be greatest among those (particularly gay males) who have multiple sexual partners, a more cautious life-style in which only one or a few people are sexual partners has been suggested as one step toward prevention (Fisher, 1983). Of course, if a diagnostic test is developed, the possibility of widespread screening for the virus may emerge.

Vaginitis

Vaginitis is a general term referring to inflammation and infection of the vagina and is, perhaps, the most common genital disease in women. The vaginal lining secretes a protective mucuslike substance that normally is slippery and appears clear or slightly milky. When dry, the discharge may have a yellowish appearance. Sexual arousal increases the amount of these secretions.

Normally, vaginal secretions are slightly acidic. The acidity (pH) of water is 7.0, that of vinegar is 5.0, and, under normal conditions, that of the vagina is between 4.0 and 5.0. This slightly acidic vaginal environment prevents the overgrowth of a number of microorganisms (fungi, bacteria) that routinely live in the vagina. Sometimes, however, the vaginal pH shifts toward alkaline (basic), allowing the microorganisms to multiply rapidly and irritate and infect the vaginal walls. A variety of factors seem to increase women's susceptibility to such infections. Among them are exhaustion, poor diet, frequent douching, antibiotic treatments, pregnancy, contraceptive pill use, diabetes, and other conditions that disturb the vaginal environment. The three most common types of vaginal infection are discussed here.

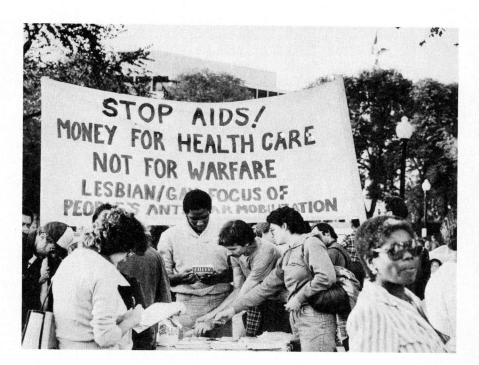

Members of a gay political organization demonstrate for government funding to combat AIDS, a sometimes fatal disease that most frequently afflicts male homosexuals.

Candida Albicans (Candida).   ***Candida albicans*** is a yeast that is sometimes transmitted sexually. Normally, harmless quantities of *Candida* are present in everyone's mouth, skin, vagina, and rectum. When a woman's system is in balance, *Candida* is kept in check. When a woman's system is out of balance and becomes less acidic (more alkaline) than usual, *Candida*, which grows best in a very *mildly* acidic environment, begins to multiply. The woman develops a slight vaginal discharge. This discharge is thick, white, and curdlike, looks like cottage cheese, and may smell like baking bread. There is intense vaginal itching, and the vagina becomes dry and red. Sexual intercourse is painful.

Candida is relatively easy to diagnose. The examining physician will see thick cheesy patches on the vaginal walls of the infected woman. Diagnosis may be confirmed by microscopic examination of the discharge for the presence of yeast organisms. Treatment usually consists of the use of vaginal suppositories of mystatin (Mycostatin). Symptoms usually disappear within two to three days, but treatment should be continued for up to a month since *Candida* organisms are quite hardy. In severe cases, the cervix, vagina, and vulva are painted with gentian violet, a dye that inhibits the growth of *Candida*.

Trichomonas Vaginalis (Trich).   ***Trichomonas vaginalis*** is a microscopic, single-cell, pear-shaped parasite that can be found in both men and women. It grows best in an alkaline environment and can survive on damp objects for several hours. Thus, a woman can become infected from contact with a toilet seat, a towel, or a washcloth that has been used by another infected person. (This is one of the few diseases you *can* catch from a toilet seat.) Most often, however, it is contracted through intercourse—men serve as carriers. At least 50 percent of all women have trich organisms in their vaginas.

Many women with *Trich* have a thick, foamy vaginal discharge. It may be white, green, or gray, and has a foul odor. The discharge irritates the vagina and the vulva, which become bright red and itchy. *Trich* can also cause urinary infections. Doctors usually treat *Trich* with an oral dose of metronidazole (Flagyl). Or, if the woman prefers, at the direction of her physician, she can insert vaginal suppositories of metronidazole high in her vagina each night before going to sleep.

Nonspecific Vaginitis (NV).   **Nonspecific vaginitis** is a term used to refer to vaginal infections not specifically caused by *Candida* or *Trichomonas* organisms. The walls of the vagina may appear cloudy, puffy with fluid, and covered by a thick coat of pus. The discharge may be white or yellow and possibly streaked with blood. Symptoms sometimes include lower back pain, cramps, and swollen lymph glands in the groin and abdomen. Treatment is usually with sulfa creams or suppositories (Vagitrol, Sultrin, or AVC cream) or with metronidazole.

Cystitis

Cystitis is an infection of the bladder. Nearly every woman contracts a bladder infection sooner or later. Intestinal bacteria, such as *Escherichia coli (E. coli)*, which are present in the digestive tracts of men and women, inadvertently get into the bladder through the urethra. Cystitis may be transmitted by sexual intercourse and is so common among newlywed women that the term "honeymoon cystitis" is sometimes used to describe it. During intercourse, the bacteria enter the urethral opening and travel to the bladder. Women are especially susceptible to cystitis because they have substantially shorter urethras than do men.

The symptoms of cystitis may appear suddenly. The woman begins to feel that she has to urinate every few minutes. When she does urinate, it burns intensely. Treatment is usually with a sulfa drug such as sulfadiazone sulfisoxazole (Gantrisin), or sulfamethoxazole (Gantanol).

Genital Warts

Genital warts *(Condylomata acuminata)*, growths on the genitals that are caused by a virus, are fairly common. They can be spread in a variety of ways—including sexual intercourse. One to three months after contact with an infected person, the warts appear around the cervix and vagina, or on the penis, or anus. When small, the warts look like the little pieces of hard, raised skin. Eventually, they become very large and take on a cauliflowerlike appearance. If the warts are in a moist area, they flourish.

The usual treatment for warts is the application of podophyllin, a caustic preparation of a dark red resin from the mandrake plant. This must be done only under medical supervision, for the substance is potentially toxic if used incorrectly. For large warts, surgical removal is often necessary.

Pubic Lice (Crabs)

Phthirus pubis, or **pubic lice**, infest the pubic hair. Adult lice are about the size of a pinhead. They appear as yellowish gray or rust-colored specks. Under a microscope, a louse looks very much like a crab, with three pairs of claws and four pairs

Genital warts of the vulva.

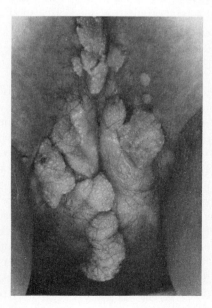

Figure 14–1.

Pubic louse (crab).

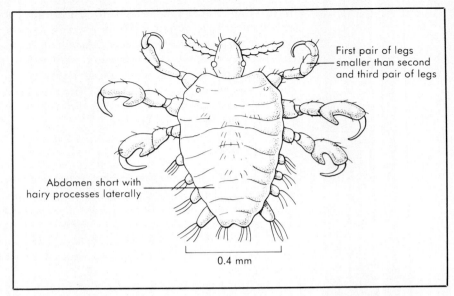

First pair of legs smaller than second and third pair of legs

Abdomen short with hairy processes laterally

0.4 mm

of tiny legs, as shown in Figure 14–1. Often, lice are sexually transmitted. One may, however, acquire them from contact with infested clothing, bedding, towels, or toilet seats.

Like mosquitoes, lice feed on blood. Thus, their primary symptom is intense itching, which results from bites. Adult lice and their eggs (nits) can be killed quite easily if one applies gamma benzene hexachloride (Kwell), which comes in the form of a prescription cream, lotion, or shampoo, to the infected area and as a precaution to all other hairy parts of the body. A-200 pyrinate, a preparation that can be purchased without a prescription, may also be used. All clothing and bedding must also be thoroughly washed or cleaned.

SUMMARY

Sexually transmitted diseases (STDs), or venereal diseases (VDs), are those diseases that are or may be contracted through intimate sexual contact.

Gonorrhea is the most common of the STDs and is caused by gonococcal bacteria. The primary symptoms in the male are a white or yellowish discharge from the penis and a burning sensation during urination. Around 80 percent of women infected with gonorrhea show no overt symptoms. Gonorrhea is treated successfully with a large injection of penicillin.

Non-gonococcal urethritis is an inflammation of the urethra in either sex that is not caused by gonorrhea. Tetracycline treatment is usually quite effective.

Syphilis is a bacterially transmitted disease, the first symptom of which is a painless sore during the primary stage at the point or points where the bacteria enter the body. Penicillin treatment will successfully cure syphilis at this stage. If left untreated, the disease enters a secondary stage during which the primary symptom is a rash on many parts of the body. If untreated at this time with penicillin, the disease enters a latent stage during which all overt symptoms disappear and it may be diagnosed only by a blood test. It may appear, if untreated, once again many months or years later as late-stage or tertiary syphilis in which various body organs are attacked, leading to death.

Genital herpes is caused by the Type 2 *Herpes simplex* virus and the primary symptoms are painful blisters on the affected organs—usually the genitals. There is no cure for herpes, although the early symptoms usually disappear, possibly to reappear on future occasions.

Granuloma inguinale, lymphogranuloma venereum, and *chancroid* are STDs more common in the tropics than in the United States. Each may be successfully treated with antibiotics.

A number of diseases may be sexually or nonsexually transmitted. *Acquired Immune Deficiency Syndrome (AIDS)* is a recently identified disease in which a victim's natural immunity to many specific diseases is seriously reduced. It often leads to death and there is currently no effective cure for AIDS. It is thought to be caused by the HTLV-III virus and is most often found in sexually active gay males. Limiting oneself to one or only a few sexual partners may be the most effective way to avoid contracting AIDS from sexual contact.

Vaginitis is inflammation and infection of the vagina that may be caused by a number of factors, the most common of which are *Candida albicans*, a yeast that is sometimes transmitted sexually, and the *Trichomonal* parasite that may be transmitted sexually, causing *Trichomonas vaginalis*. Nonspecific vaginitis refers to vaginal infections not specifically caused by *Candida* or *Trichomonal* organisms. All of these forms of vaginitis may be successfully treated with medicated vaginal suppositories.

Cystitis is an infection of the bladder caused by bacteria. A frequent urge to urinate and a burning sensation during urination are the most frequent symptoms. Treatment is usually with sulfa drugs.

Genital warts are growths on the genitals caused by a virus that may be transmitted sexually. Treatment is usually with a caustic solution that destroys the warts or, more rarely, by surgical removal of the warts.

Pubic lice, or "crabs," are parasites that infect the pubic hair, causing intense itching. Treatment consists of the application of specific solutions that kill the lice.

SUGGESTED READINGS

The Boston Women's Health Book Collective (1976). *Our Bodies, Ourselves*. New York: Simon and Schuster.

Gay Community Services Center. *Gay V.D.: Facts for women and men*. For a copy, send 20 cents to 1614 Wilshire Blvd., Los Angeles, CA 90017.

Grower, J., & Grace, D. (1971). *The ABC's of VD*. Englewood Cliffs, N.J.: Prentice-Hall.

Rosebury, T. (1971). *Microbes and morals: The strange story of venereal disease*. New York: Viking.

Rozan, S. & Liehawitz, M. *Politics of gonorrhea*. For a copy, send 25 cents to Louise Rice, 65 Chestnut Street, Cambridge, Mass. 02139.

PART 6

THE INTERPERSONAL AND SOCIAL CONTEXTS OF SEXUALITY

CHAPTER OUTLINE

CHAPTER 15

LOVE AND ATTRACTION

Recently, we asked our students what they meant by love. We received a surprising array of answers:

Love is caring for someone almost as much as you care for yourself.

Love is the cement of a socioeconomic union.

Love: It involves complete honesty, trust, acceptance, concern for another person.

Love is total absorption in another person. She becomes the focal point in your life. Practically all of your important decisions are made with her in mind. When you are with her, you are happy even if you aren't doing anything. You would do anything for her.

Love = wonderful feeling, everything goes right (you're on Cloud 9). Feeling of sharing, giving and receiving in turn.

Love hurts. When in love your feelings become more emotional and sensitive and it's very easy for even little things to hurt you.

LOVE

In *A New Look at Love*, Elaine Hatfield and G. William Walster (1978) reviewed what a number of writers including Sigmund Freud (1933), Reik (1944), and Foucault (1978) have had to say about love. They concluded that for most people, there are two distinctly different kinds of love—passionate love and companionate love. They offered the following definition of **passionate love**:

A state of intense longing for union with another. Reciprocated love (union with the other) is associated with fulfillment and ecstacy. Unrequited love (separation) with emptiness; with anxiety or despair. A state of profound psychological arousal. (p. 9)

Companionate love they viewed as quite different. Companionate love appears to have much in common with liking; it is "the affection people feel for those with whom their lives are deeply intertwined" (p. 9). The primary difference between liking and companionate loving is in the depth of feeling and the degree of involvement with the other person. Let us review what is known about these two very different forms of love.

Passionate Love

Both mind and body make a unique contribution to emotional experiences. (See, for example, Schachter, 1964; Hatfield and Walster, 1982.) Both must be in harmony if people are to have a true emotional experience. Our perceptions of what it is appropriate to feel determine what emotion—love or hate, desire or disgust, anger or fear, grief or joy—we feel. Physiological factors determine whether or not we feel any emotion at all.

Cognitive Determinants of Love.   People's assumptions about what they *should* be feeling in a specific situation have a profound impact on what they do feel. By adolescence, people's culture, their family, and their own experiences give them some clear ideas as to what emotions it is appropriate for them to feel in various situations. They know that they should feel elated when something unexpectedly good happens and depressed when things fall apart. According to Schachter (1964), people's assumptions as to what they should feel are critically important in determining what they do feel.

American society offers many images of passionate love. As a consequence, people are primed to label a wide variety of experiences as passion. For example, Ellen Berscheid and her colleagues at the University of Minnesota asked college students: "What is passionate love?" They obtained strikingly different answers. Most of the students assumed that passionate love is an intensely pleasurable state. They associated love with the joy of loving and being loved, with security, with the pleasure of finally having someone's understanding, with sexual fulfillment, with excitement, having fun, and so on. "Painful things *could* happen," they shrugged, "but that's rare." Other students' descriptions were not so enthusiastic, however: "Love is terrible." "I never want to fall in love again!" They associated passionate love with sexual longing, loneliness, uncertainty, confusion, anxiety (would they be loved in return, or laughed at?), frustration, jealousy, anger and violence, and pain. For some students, then, passionate love is virtually synonymous with agony. Indeed, the original meaning of passion was agony—as in "Christ's passion."

So while passionate love means pleasure for some, others equate it with pain. These very different ideas of passion profoundly affect people's emotions and, ultimately, the ties they make in the name of love.

Physiological Determinants of Love.   In addition to a cognitive element, all emotions have a second, indispensable component—intense physiological arousal. Joy, anger, passion, and hate all give themselves away by their telltale symptoms—a flushed face, rapid breathing, a pounding heart, and trembling hands.

Delightful experiences such as talking with someone who loves and understands us, finding an island of security in an unstable world or excitement in a boring one, and making love are physiologically arousing. Extremely painful experiences like anxiety and fear, sexual frustration, jealousy, anger, and total confusion are arousing too. Thus, under the right conditions, either joy or anguish (or a combination of the two) should have the potential for intensifying passion. Scientists have accumulated considerable support for the contention that both mind and body are critically important in shaping emotions. People's minds determine what specific emotion they feel. Their bodies determine whether or not they feel any emotion at all. (See Hatfield & Walster, 1982, for a review of this literature.)

Companionate Love

Psychologists have devoted much effort to discovering why individuals like and experience companionate love for the people they do. Their findings have led them to theorize that two important factors may be involved: reinforcement and equity.

Reinforcement Theory.   Theorists such as Baron and Byrne (1977), Thibaut and Kelley (1959) and Homans (1974) cite the principle of reinforcement in order to explain why people are intensely attracted to some people and repelled by others. They contend that people like those who reward them and dislike those who punish them. People generally feel some tenderness for those who make them feel good about themselves—those who like their looks and their style, who are always ready with funny jokes or an outrageous adventure, and who make them feel needed. People resent others who offer them helpful hints on how they might improve their personalities, for their own good, of course, or who are crabby, boring, deceitful, and generally disagreeable.

At first glance, one's reaction to this "law of attraction" might be: "So what? We figured that out long ago!" Reinforcement research, however, leads to some conclusions that are not so obvious. First, scientists have found that people come to like people who are merely *associated* with pleasure and to dislike those who are merely *associated* with pain. For example, when skiers are sitting in a mountain cabin, drinking a fine wine, relaxing after a hike in the snow, they may feel a rush of affection for friends who just happen to be around. Conversely, when college students have a splitting headache, are rushing to finish a term paper that is overdue, and are frustrated because their apartment is overflowing with dirty dishes, moving crates, and cat hair, they may well feel a little angry at the unfortunate friend who just happens to drop by.

Social psychologists have collected considerable evidence for the contention that life is not really fair—that people are influenced not by others' good or bad *intentions*, but rather by what life with them is really like, whether it is their doing or not. William Griffitt (1970) tested the notion that people's reaction to others is tinged with traces of their feelings about the environments they inhabit. He asked college students to read a description of an anonymous stranger (sometimes said to be quite similar, sometimes quite dissimilar, to themselves) and to indicate how

Companionate love is marked by a sense of reinforcement, in which each person derives satisfaction and self-esteem from the other.

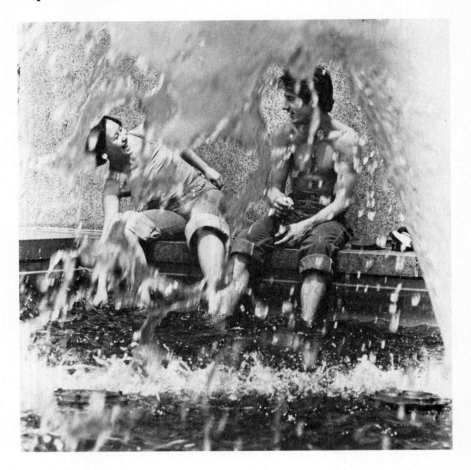

they felt about the other. Half of the students met in a cool, calm environment; the others met in an uncomfortably hot room. Students ended up liking the stranger a great deal more when they "got acquainted" with him or her in comfortable surroundings than when they got acquainted in a hot, sticky, close environment.

Maslow and Mintz (1956) tested the same hypothesis by inviting men and women to look at photographs of other men and women. Half of the students met in a pleasant room with soft lighting, elegant draperies, beautiful paintings and sculpture, and plush chairs. The others met in a grimy, shabbily furnished room with harsh, overhead lighting, dirty, torn window shades, stark, drab walls, and battered, overflowing tin ashtrays.

The researchers predicted that when their subjects met in the attractive room, they would feel at ease and their good cheer would generalize to anything they were asked to judge. When they were in the ugly room, they would feel angry and depressed and their negative mood would generalize to the things they were asked to judge. They were right; those who met in the cheerful room were far more positive about the photographs than those who met in the ugly room.

Equity Theory.   Most people long for their love relations to be special. They may be willing to agree that in the workaday world people are "selfish" and spend most of their time seeking that which makes them happy and shunning that which does not. When it comes to love, though, almost everyone feels that, somehow, things should be different. If it is "true love," so the mythology goes, people will care more about their partners than themselves. They will act selflessly and never be concerned with what is in it for them. And, of course, people expect their lovers to feel a similar surge of selfless devotion.

It is easy to see why people long to *believe* that love relationships are special relationships that transcend social exchange. The yearning for unconditional love is a primitive one. All of us would like to believe that, even if we lost our looks, our minds, or, worse yet, our jobs, we would continue to be loved passionately (Fromm, 1956; Murstein, 1976; and Rubin, 1973). But, as Elaine Walster (Hatfield) and her colleagues observed in *Equity: Theory and Research* (1978), the accumulating evidence forces psychologists to be more realistic.

Men and women who insist that they are capable of dispensing love with no thought of return are simply deceiving themselves. Those who expect such selfless love from their partners most assuredly are deceiving themselves. In fact, the more men and women are able and willing to give another, the more they can expect in return. Let us consider the evidence that leads psychologists to these conclusions. Couples will not even enter into a relationship, much less stay in it, unless it is profitable to *both* of them. Blau (1968) contends that dating individuals end up with the mate they "deserve." If people expect to keep an affair going, they must make their partner "an offer he or she can't refuse." The more desirable people are, the more desirable the partners they can attract; the less desirable they are, the more likely it is that they have to settle for less desirable "leftovers." Thus, Blau argues, principles of equity insure that people get what they deserve in the relationship market.

Research supports the contention that the more equitable a romantic or marital relationship is, the more viable it will be. For example, Sara Kiesler and Roberta Baral (1970) invited college men in to see how well they could do on a "new" intelligence test. The men were tested under two conditions. In the high self-esteem condition, each man was led to believe that he was doing unusually well. The experimenter smiled and nodded and mentioned how extraordinarily well he was scoring. In the low self-esteem condition, each man was led to believe that his IQ score was embarrassingly low. The experimenter made it apparent that he was displeased with his performance—he frowned, looked away, and muttered that other men had performed far better.

Each student was given the test individually. During a break in testing, the experimenter and the student took a coffee break in a nearby canteen. There, they bumped into a friend of the experimenter—a college woman who was actually an actress. The woman's attractiveness was systematically varied. Sometimes, she was very appealing, with becoming makeup and fashionable clothes. Other times, she was very unimpressive, with no makeup, heavy glasses, her hair pulled back with a rubber band, and a clashing and sloppily arranged skirt and blouse. After the couple was introduced, the experimenter excused himself to "run an errand." This gave the couple a chance to chat privately.

What the experimenter was *really* concerned with, was how interested the men were in the woman. If they offered to buy coffee or a snack for her, ignored her when she said she should get back to work, requested her phone number, or asked her for a date, they were given points on an index of "romantic behavior." Kiesler and Baral found strong support for the contention of equity theory that the more self-confident men feel, the more attractive a woman they will feel entitled to. The men whose self-esteem had been raised behaved most romantically with the attractive woman. Those whose self-esteem had been lowered behaved most romantically toward the rather dowdy woman. In this case, birds did seek out romantic partners "of a feather."

Couples can be well *matched* from the standpoint of equity in a variety of ways. For example, the handsome man (who is not especially dependable) may prefer a woman who is as beautiful and as irresponsible as himself, or he may decide to pursue a woman who is far plainer, but is far more dependable than he is. Bernard Murstein and his colleagues (1974) provide a compelling description of the way such complex matching might operate:

A handsome man is seen with a woman of mediocre attractiveness. "I wonder what he sees in her?" may be the quizzical question of a bystander. Quite possibly, she possesses compensating qualities such as greater intelligence, interpersonal competence, and wealth than he, of which the bystander knows nothing. . . .

Another case of compensatory exchange might be indicated if an aged statesman proposed marriage to a young beautiful woman. He would probably be trading his prestige and power for her physical attractiveness and youth. (pp. 3–4)

There is evidence to support the contention that people do engage in such complicated balancing and counterbalancing in selecting mates. For example, in one study Elaine Hatfield, Mary Utne, and Jane Traupmann (1979) contacted college men and women, newlyweds, and elderly couples and asked them to assess their relationship: *How much did they (and their partner) contribute to the relationship?* How good-looking, sociable, loving, understanding, considerate, helpful, "easy to be with," and so forth was each partner? What did each get out of the relationship? In light of their answers to these questions, then, the following question was put to the respondents:

Considering what you put into your relationship, compared to what you get out of it . . . and what your partner put in, compared to what (s)he gets out of it, how would you say your relationship "stacks up"?
+3. I am getting a much better deal than my partner.
+2. I am getting a somewhat better deal.
+1. I am getting a slightly better deal.
* 0. We are both getting an equally good . . . or bad . . . deal.*
−1. My partner is getting a slightly better deal.
−2. My partner is getting a somewhat better deal.
−3. My partner is getting a much better deal than I am.

This provided a measure of how equitable the men and women perceived their relationship to be.

Three and one half months to a year later, they tracked down the couples and asked what had become of their relationship. As expected, the relationships that both partners perceived as equitable (as indicated by a score of 0) were the most stable. At the time of the second interview, the men and women in those relationships were most likely to still be going together and were most confident that they would still be together a year or five years hence. The men and women who felt they were being cheated in their relationships (those scoring -1 to -3), and who presumably had every reason to hope that something better would come along, were naturally quite pessimistic about the future. Interestingly enough, however, so were the men and women who knew that they were getting far *more* than they deserved from their relationships (those scoring $+1$ to $+3$). They had every reason to hope the relationships would last, but they were not very optimistic about their chances. A review of existing research (Hatfield, 1982) suggests that men and women who feel fairly treated in their relationships are happier and more satisfied and have a more sexually satisfying and more stable relationship than do other couples.

Now that we have discussed what passionate and companionate love are, we will proceed to examine how most people meet the individuals they eventually end up loving—passionately, companionately, or both.

BECOMING ACQUAINTED

"How can I meet some women? In my classes, the sex ratio is 9 men: 1 woman" (engineering major at the University of Wisconsin, Madison). "How can I meet some men? Half of the men I meet are married" (young woman in Atlanta). "How can I meet some men? I'm tired of hanging out in gay bars" (young man in Atlanta).

Obviously, the first step in a love affair is to meet some appropriate partners. Strangely enough, the importance of this first step is generally underrated by men and women who are the most anxious to meet suitable dates or mates. They do not recognize how important it is to arrange their lives so that they *routinely* bump into eligible partners.

Although adolescents tend to forget that association breeds attraction, generally their parents do not. Some parents wheedle, cajole, or bribe authorities to sell them houses in the "right" neighborhoods, admit them to the "right" clubs, and their children to the "right" schools—just so their children can meet and marry the "right mates." Goode (1959) pointed out that most societies are more realistic than our own; they simply assume that if young people are allowed to associate, they will, by hook or by crook, find some way to have sexual relations. Parents know that they must strictly control whom their children meet if they want to have any control over whom they marry. For example, he noted, in Polynesia princesses are strictly chaperoned and separated from "undesirables." In contrast, youngsters of run-of-the-mill status are allowed to participate in considerable love play.

The *propinquity* proposition states: "Other things being equal, the closer two people are located geographically, the more likely it is that they will be attracted to each other." There is solid evidence that people are reluctant to search very far for a partner—they almost always end up dating and marrying those who happen to be around on a day-to-day basis (see Berscheid & Walster [Hatfield], 1978).

Geographic proximity increases the likelihood that two people will form a relationship.

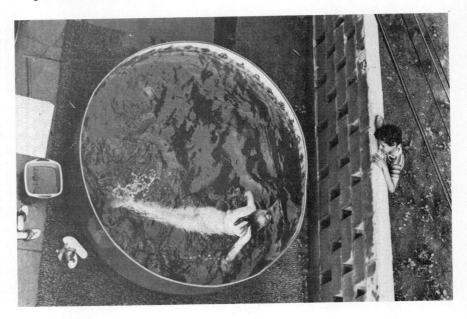

Leon Festinger and his colleagues (1950) conducted one of the more interesting studies demonstrating the relationship between proximity and friendship choice. They examined the development of friendships in a new apartment complex. The housing development consisted of small apartments arranged in U-shaped courts; all the apartments except the end ones faced onto a grassy area. The two end apartments in each court faced onto the street. Festinger (1951) arrived at the intriguing conclusion that to a great extent architects can determine the social life of the residents:

It is a fair summary to say that the two major factors affecting the friendships which developed were (1) sheer distance between houses and (2) the direction in which a house faced. Friendships developed more frequently between next-door neighbors, less frequently between people whose houses were separated by another house, and so on. As the distance between houses increased, the number of friendships fell off so rapidly that it was rare to find a friendship between persons who lived in houses that were separated by more than four or five other houses. . . .

There were instances in which the site plan of the project had more profound effects than merely to determine with whom one associated. Indeed, on occasion the arrangements of the houses severely limited the social life of their occupants. . . . In order to have the street appear "lived on," ten of the houses near the street had been turned so that they faced the street rather than the court area as did the other houses. This apparently small change in the direction in which a house faced had a considerable effect on the lives of the people who, by accident, happened to occupy these end houses. They had less than half as many friends in the project as did those whose houses faced the court area. The consistency of this finding left no doubt that the turning of these houses toward the street had made involuntary social isolates out of the persons who lived in them. (pp. 156–157)

There were other architectural features that had an important impact on the residents' social life. Any architectural feature that brought people into proximity with other residents tended to increase their popularity. It was found, for example, that the residents of the apartments near the entrances and exits of the stairways made more friends than other residents. Similarly, the residents of the apartments near the mailboxes had unusually active social lives. It appears, then, that if people want to meet men and women, they should snap up that dormitory room or apartment in that "impossible" location—near the lunchroom (where the clatter of dishes would drive anyone crazy), on the floor where all the parties are held, near the piano room—in the midst of all the hubbub. And they should avoid like the plague that little room off in a corner or that cozy little cottage tucked away on an isolated beach.

Proximity is an important factor, not just in determining who meets whom, but even in determining who marries whom; a person's search for the ideal mate often ends with the boy or girl next door. Sociologists routinely find that the closer people live, or work, or play with someone, the more likely they are to end up marrying that individual. Clarke (1952) interviewed more than four hundred couples at the time they applied for marriage licenses. He found that, at the time of their first date together, 37 percent of the couples were already living within eight blocks and 54 percent within sixteen blocks of each other. The number of marriages decreased steadily and markedly as the distance between the couple's homes increased. Further corroboration of the importance of propinquity in mate selection comes from Abrams (1943), Katz & Hill (1958), and Kennedy (1943). As Kephart (1961) has observed: "Cherished notions about romantic love notwithstanding, it appears that when all is said and done, the "one and only" may have a better than 50–50 chance of living within walking distance!" (p. 269).

There are probably several interlocking reasons why people are so likely to end up falling in love with an individual close at hand. First, the opportunity for meeting is excellent. Americans simply have a better chance to meet someone from next door than someone from Saudi Arabia. If people never meet, they cannot very well discover they like one another.

Second, psychologists have found that, familiarity—in and of itself—generally breeds liking. For example, Zajonc (1968) has shown that repeated exposure to *anything* generates positive feelings. The more people see others, the more they like them. Zajonc provides the following example of such an exposure process taken from an Associated Press article on February 27, 1967, from Corvallis, Oregon:

A mysterious student has been attending a class at Oregon State University for the past two months, enveloped in a big black bag. Only his bare feet show. Each Monday, Wednesday, and Friday at 11:00 a.m. the Black Bag sits on a small table near the back of the classroom. The class is Speech 113—basic persuasion. . . . Charles Goetzinger, professor of the class, knows the identity of the person inside; none of the 20 students in the class do. Goetzinger said students' attitudes changed from hostility toward the Black Bag, to curiosity and finally to friendship. (p. 1)

Zajonc cites much experimental evidence that mere exposure breeds liking. He argues that such a process occurs, in part, because people are programmed to evaluate unfamiliar people and things negatively (something unfamiliar is potentially dangerous). Repeated exposure informs them that these people and things are not dangerous, so they can relax and respond positively.

A third reason why people so often end up marrying the boy or girl next door is that American neighborhoods tend to be segregated along racial, ethnic and social class lines. Thus, people are most likely to find a partner similar to themselves close to home (Berscheid & Walster [Hatfield], 1978).

There is one final reason why those close to home are the most likely prospects for love—we "just happen" to bump into them. Some men and women are willing to openly advertise that they are looking for a lover. They put an ad in the *Village Voice* or the *Kansas City Star* and that is that. We have all seen such ads: "M, devastatingly handsome, professional, looking for F to share an afternoon, and maybe my life." "F, looking for man 40 to 60; good sense of humor." "M seeking adventurous, unconventional, playful male. Only college educated need apply. Send photo." But most people are extremely shy about admitting that they are searching for romantic and sexual partners. Many people are so fearful of being identified as unpopular, that they are terrified to be seen alone, even when they want to be. For example, there is a ready market for books that counsel men and women in how to overcome the shame of dining alone: "Begin by going to restaurants where you're sure you won't know anybody." "Take a book" (Napolitane & Pellegrino, 1977; La Barre, 1977).

So how do people ever find someone? Hatfield and Walster (1978) offer some specific hints on how to go about looking for someone to love. Essentially, they suggest that people get intensely involved in some job or activity that "just happens" to bring them into continual contact with potential lovers. Generally, people search for partners while pretending they are doing something else. This is one

Though many people hesitate to admit that they are looking for a romantic partner, others are quite open about stating what they want.

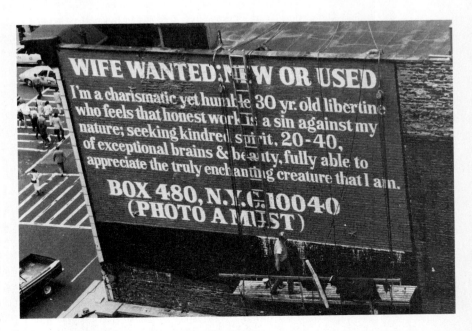

reason why those people they keep bumping into—in their neighborhood, at school, or at work—are the people they are most likely to get involved with.

Once people have met an array of potential friends and lovers, they are faced with a second problem. How do they then go about deciding who and what they want in a mate?

DATING AND MATING PREFERENCES

People who are desperately searching for someone to love often claim they would "settle for anyone." They do not mean it. Researchers have found that such people, when asked to list all their acquaintances and then indicate which of them they would be willing to date, consider a startlingly small percentage of their acquaintances to be "eligible."

Rosenblatt (1974), an anthropologist and social psychologist, has pointed out that most Americans cannot even imagine some of the relationships that are common in other parts of the world. He illustrates:

For example, few Americans would consider an extramarital sexual relationship with someone under the age of ten or over the age of 90, and few would consider a permanent intense affair carried out by mail or only during the Christmastime holidays of each year. When people step out of bounds they ordinarily step into the boundaries for stepping out of bounds. (pp. 83–84)

Every culture sets standards as to who is appropriate to marry. Without even thinking about it, people filter potential partners through a fine mesh screen of desired qualities: He can't be too young. She can't be too tall. They can't be too poor. Most people are not even aware of how many potential partners they unthinkingly reject. The rigorousness of these primary screenings became painfully evident to computer dating companies when they began to calculate how many people they would have to enroll in their programs if they were to do the barest minimum of matching—for example, match up couples who live in the same town, are of the opposite sex, may want partners of the same socioeconomic class, religion, and educational level, are roughly the same height, and are of about the same age. One computer company calculated that it would need more than a million subscribers just to match on the basis of these few traits.

Demographic Characteristics

Sociologists have collected voluminous evidence that Americans do faithfully follow cultural dictates in selecting a mate. Let us examine some of these.

- *Age.* The average woman marries at twenty-one, the average man at twenty-three (U.S. Department of Commerce, Current Population Reports, 1971). In six out of seven American marriages, the groom is as old as, or older than, the bride. In two out of three marriages, the difference in ages is less than five years (Udry, 1974).

- *Race.* In the United States, the proportion of marriages which occur across racial lines is extremely small. Even today, only about one tenth of 1 percent of marriages are interracial (Heer, 1966; Jacobson, 1959).

- *Social class.* Men and women marry partners whose families closely resemble their own in family income and occupational status (Centers, 1949; Rettig & Pasamanick, 1959).

- *Education.* Men and women almost always marry partners whose educational level is virtually identical to their own (U.S. Census of Population, 1960).

- *Religion.* Almost all people marry partners of the same major religious group—Protestant, Catholic, or Jewish (Udry, 1974). In a study of marriages in New Haven, Connecticut, sociologists found that 97.5 percent of Jews, 94 percent of Catholics, and 74 percent of Protestants married partners from their own religious group (Hollingshead, 1950).

Personal and Behavioral Characteristics

Although people may start their search for a partner by seeking a "culturally acceptable mate," they all hope for much more. Many people seem to start out wanting, and really expecting, an unrealistic degree of perfection in their partners. Unfortunately, few individuals end up getting all those things they "just have to have." Neubeck (1969) points out that in a single love relationship, the chances of a couple feeling that all of their basic personality needs are being fulfilled are slim. There is some support for Neubeck's contention. In a study of 453 engaged or recently married persons, Bergler (1948) found that only 18 percent felt their emotional needs were "extremely" or "well" satisfied by their mates. The vast majority of men and women felt unloved, or lonely, or misunderstood.

So people cannot have everything. But then what *should* they look for in date or mate? Hatfield and Walster (1978) give the following advice:

Give up the fantasy that you are entitled to an almost perfect mate. This fantasy is a destructive one. The "Standard American Male" and the "Standard American Female," equipped with all the virtues, simply do not exist. People come in a variety of packages, each with its unique blend of strengths and weaknesses.

What you should be looking for, then, is someone whose particular pattern of traits interlocks nicely with your own. You can select one of two—or maybe even a dozen—things you feel are critical to have in a mate. But then you have to quit. You must resign yourself to the fact that any partner is going to possess a multitude of less appealing traits. We're not telling you to give up your dreams; rather, we're encouraging you to become more aware of your own humanity and the delightful variety of partners, partly perfect and partly flawed, available to you.

One caution: Since you can only expect to get a few of the characteristics you want in a mate, you should think very carefully about what things are most important to you in a partner. Your society says the man you marry must be of your race and socioeconomic class, and must be physically attractive, must want to get ahead professionally, and must be good at sports. That's something it cares about—but do you? Your mother says the woman you marry should be polite, neat, reliable, and put up with your Aunt Maude's quirks. That's something she cares about—but do you?

If you've not had very much experience, it is, of course, difficult for you to know exactly what you like and dislike in a partner. Be patient. The only sure way to discover what you care about is via experience. When you've had a chance to become deeply involved with many kinds of men and women, you'll discover that, with certain kinds of lovers, everything seems to go so well ... while with others, life is impossible. When in doubt, ask yourself, "Is this the kind of person I want? Or is this the kind of person I've been told I should want?" (pp. 152–153)

ATTRACTING SEXUAL PARTNERS

When we asked students in our human sexuality classes "What attracted you to the person you're in love with right now?" they gave us answers like these:

He has a grin that can kill you.

She is so gentle with me. She really cares and wants me. She took me home and made me a part of her family. She made love to me with her whole self. She was totally absorbed in me.

I'm intrigued with his looks, his "hard guy attitude"—besides being very physically attracted to him. I also love his tenderness and strength—besides being very physically attracted to him.

A special spark in her personality. She is a real bitch. I love it. Independent and smart!

Let us consider some of the traits that more systematic research has shown to make a man or woman appealing.

Physical Attractiveness

Anthropologists usually delight in pointing out how much cultures differ from one to another. There is at least one cultural universal, however—in all societies, beautiful women and handsome men are appealing (Ford & Beach, 1951). But what constitutes physical attractiveness?

The question of what is physically attractive and why is one that has fascinated novelists, poets, and street-corner pundits for centuries. Unfortunately, the popularity of the question is not reflected in the definitiveness of the available answers.

A few intrepid analysts (e.g., Bain, 1868) attempted to advance theories of beauty in hopes of bringing order to the chaos, but without conspicuous success. Darwin (1952) surveyed the concepts of beauty of various tribes and societies throughout the world and he concluded that there is no universal standard of beauty. Modern analysts agree (Berscheid & Walster, 1974).

Even today, authors of serious treatises on beauty are inevitably reduced to gaping at the dazzling variety of characteristics which humans, in various historical periods and societies, have considered to be beautiful and sexy. Let us review what little is known about the traits that are considered to be physically attractive in humans.

RESEARCH HIGHLIGHT

What Do People Want?

Recently, Jane Traupmann (1978) and Mary Utne (1978) interviewed several hundred dating couples, newlyweds, and elderly couples in order to find out what they wanted from their relationships. They began by conducting a series of intensive in-depth interviews in order to get a sense of what each couple's intimate relationship was like and what kinds of things were important to them. They found the array of things intimates thought were important to their relationship remarkable in its variety—ranging from "a sense of humor" to a "love of dry fly fishing." Finally, they set out to winnow out their list, and learn what a random sample of couples felt they wanted out of their relationships.

Most men and women could agree that all of the following were critically important in choosing a date or a mate:

Personal Concerns

Social Grace: Being sociable, friendly, and relaxed in social settings.

Intellect: Being intelligent and informed.

Appearance: Being a physically attractive person; being concerned for physical appearance and health; giving attention to such things as clothing, cleanliness, exercise, and good eating habits.

Emotional Concerns

Liking and Loving: Liking one's partner and showing it. Feeling and expressing love for one's partner.

Understanding and Concern: Knowing one's partner's personal concerns and emotional needs and responding to them.

Acceptance: Accepting and encouraging role flexibility; letting one's partner try out different roles occasionally—for example, letting the partner be a "baby" sometimes, a "mother," a colleague or a friend, an aggressive as well as a passive lover, and so on.

Appreciation: Openly showing appreciation for the partner's contributions to the relationship; not taking one's partner for granted.

Physical affection: Demonstrating affection by touching, hugging, and kissing.

Sex: Participating in the sexual aspect of the relationship; working to make it mutually satisfying and fulfilling. Sexual fidelity; living up to or being faithful to one's agreements about extramarital relations.

Security and Freedom: Committing oneself to one's partner and to the future of the relationship together. Respecting a partner's need to be a free and independent person; allowing one's partner to develop as an individual in the way that he or she chooses—for example, allowing the partner freedom to go to

Other Societies. Ford and Beach (1951) examined more than two hundred primitive societies. They were unable to find *any* universal standards of sexual attractiveness. They found enormous cultural differences as to the particular bodily organs or characteristics that are considered critical determinants of beauty. For some societies, the shape and color of the eyes are of critical importance; for others, the features of primary interest are height and weight. In still others, what really matters is the size and shape of the external sexual organs—the penis and the labia major and minora. To complicate matters still further, even if two societies do agree as to which bodily parts are important, they rarely agree as to what

school or not, to work at the kind of job or career he or she likes, to pursue outside interests, to do things alone or with other friends, or simply to be alone sometimes.

Day-to-Day Maintenance: Contributing time and effort to household responsibilities such as grocery shopping, making dinner, house cleaning, and car maintenance.

Finances: Contributing income to a "joint account."

Sociability: Being a partner who is easy to live with on a day-to-day basis; that is, being someone with a sense of humor, who is not too moody, does not get drunk too often, and so on. Being a good companion; suggesting interesting joint activities as

well as participating in joint activities one's partner might suggest. Telling one's partner about the day's events and special concerns; being interested in hearing about one's partner's concerns and daily activities. Fitting in; being compatible with one's partner's friends and relatives; liking them and trying to make them like you.

Decision Making: Taking a fair share of the responsibility for making and carrying out decisions that affect both partners.

Remembering Special Occasions: Being thoughtful about sentimental things, such as remembering birthdays, anniversaries, and other special occasions.

Opportunities Gained and Lost
Opportunities Gained: Chance to be married. Marriage gives many people the opportunity to partake of the many life experiences that depend on being married (for example, having the chance to be included in "married couple" social events, having children, having someone to count on in old age).

Opportunities Foregone: Marriage necessarily requires people to give up certain opportunities in order to be in this relationship (for example, the opportunity to date others, have a career, travel, and so forth) (Hatfield, et. al. [1982]).

constitutes beauty in those portions of the body. For example, in some societies like our own, a thin woman is assumed to be more attractive than a plump one; the reverse is true in most others.

Table 15–1 presents an overview (Ford & Beach, 1951) of the characteristics that various societies consider to be marks of beauty. Let us look at some of these societal preferences more closely.

Bronislaw Malinowski (1929) observed that for the Trobrianders, a Western Pacific people, and for many others, *facial appearance* is the primary standard of physical attractiveness:

Table 15–1.

Societies showing preference for selected female traits.

Ford and Beach found that societies differ greatly in what they consider female beauty. Data from other researchers make it clear that there is also considerable disagreement on what constitutes male beauty.

Trait	Number of Societies
Plump body build Abelam, Chiricahua, Chukchee, Ganda, Hidatsa, Maricopa, Nama, Pukapukans, Ramkokamekra, Siriono, Tarahumara, Thonga, Wogeo	13
Medium body build Apache, Hopi, Pima, Sanpoil, Thompson	5
Slim body build Chenchu, Dobuans, Ila, Masai, Palaung, Tongans	5
Broad pelvis and wide hips Chukchee, Hopi, Kwakiutl, Maricopa, Siriono, Wogeo	6
Narrow pelvis and slim hips Yakut	1
Small ankles Kwakiutl, Lengo, Tongans	3
Shapely and fleshy calves Ila, Kwakiutl, Maori, Tongans, Wogeo	5
Elongated labia majora Dahomeans, Kusaians, Marquesans, Nama, Ponapeans, Thonga, Trukese, Venda	8
Large clitoris Easter Islanders	1
Long and pendulous breasts Azande, Ganda	2
Large breasts Alorese, Apache, Hopi, Kurtatchi, Lesu, Siriono, Thonga, Trukese, Wogeo	9
Upright, hemispherical breasts Manus, Masai	2

SOURCE: Ford & Beach, 1951.

It is a notable fact that their main erotic interest is focused on the human head and face. In the formulae of beauty magic, in the vocabulary of human attractions, as well as in the arsenal of ornament and decoration, the human face—eyes, mouth, nose, teeth, and hair—takes precedence. (pp. 295–296)

However, cultures differ markedly in what sorts of faces are assumed to be good looking. Most peoples consider a light skin to be attractive. However, the Pima (North American Indians) and members of several other societies prefer dark-skinned individuals. Skin color is also important in two Western Pacific societies, the Dobuans and the Wogeo. The Dobuans consider albinos to be particularly repulsive. For the Wogeo, things are even more complicated—light-skinned natives prefer light-skinned mates; dark-skinned natives prefer dark-skinned ones.

In most societies, people feel that a woman with a plump *body build* is more attractive than a slim one. For example, Ford and Beach (1951) report that the Siriono in South America assume a desirable sex partner should be young and fat. A woman should have big hips, large but firm breasts, and a deposit of fat on her sexual organs. "Fat women are referred to by the men with obvious pride as *ereN ekida* (fat vulva) and are thought to be much more satisfying sexually than thin women, who are summarily dismissed as being *ikaNgi* (bony). In fact, so desirable is corpulence as a sexual trait that I have frequently heard men make up songs about the merits of a fat vulva...." (pp. 86–88).

Sexual characteristics are important determinants of attractiveness in many cultures. In a few cultures, the size and shape of the woman's breasts determines whether or not she is sexually attractive. The preferred shape varies; some peoples prefer small, upright breasts. The Wogeo feel that breasts should be firm with the nipples still facing outwards, not turning to the ground. A young girl with pendulous breasts, "like a grandmother," is pitied. Other peoples like long and pendulous breasts.

Some peoples equate "attractive external genitals" with "sexual attractiveness." In some societies, elongated labia majora are considered sexually attractive. Young girls are advised to pull the clitoris and the vulvar lips in order to enhance their value as sexual partners.

Before puberty, girls on Ponape in the Western Pacific undergo treatment designed to lengthen the labia minora and to enlarge the clitoris. Old impotent men pull, beat, and suck the labia to lengthen them. The girls put black ants in their vulva so that their stinging will cause the labia and clitoris to swell. The girls must repeat these procedures until the desired results are obtained.

Most people insist upon cleanliness as a means of ridding the body of foul and repulsive odors. In some societies a perfume is used to cover up offensive body odors. The Wogeo, for example, use aromatic leaves to combat the odor of perspiration. Many peoples, both men and women, anoint the skin with scented oils to increase their sexual attractiveness. In many societies, men and women wear sweet-smelling flowers either on the body or in the hair. Cayapa men use sweet-scented herbs to attract women; Western Apache girls wear aromatic plants to attract boys.

Our Own Society.   Different societies find it impossible to agree as to who is beautiful and sexy, but within a given society there is reasonable consensus. Americans show surprising agreement in their evaluations of others' beauty. Supreme Court Justice Stewart once said of pornography that he could not define it, "but I know it when I see it." When asked "What is beauty?" Americans would echo his statements. They may have trouble defining it, but they know it when they see it.

For example, one team of social psychologists asked college students to examine the photographs of college women. They found that the students—both men and women—were in striking agreement as to who was beautiful and who was not (Kopera, Maier, & Johnson, 1971). A study was conducted in Great Britain in which a national daily newspaper asked readers to rank the "prettiness" of twelve photographs of women's faces. The thousands of readers who responded, even though they ranged in age from eight to eighty and were from markedly different social classes and regions, had similar ideas as to what is beautiful (Illiffe, 1960).

Luckily, for the vast majority of us, although there is substantial agreement as to what is beautiful, there is not *complete* agreement. The poetic hope that everyone will be found beautiful by someone also seems to be true. For example, Cross and Cross (1971) reported: "The most popular face in the sample was chosen as best of its group of six by 207 judges but there was no face that was never chosen, and even the least popular face was picked as *best* of its group (of six portraits similar in age, sex, and race) by four subjects" (p. 438).

According to the folklore, men and women are supposed to have markedly different standards of beauty—and everything else. For example, women are supposed to prefer delicate, ladylike women, while men are supposed to prefer earthy, sexy ones. And, the folklore continues, women are supposed to be a pushover for pretty boys, while men value rugged good looks. The preceding studies indicate that this stereotype is not true. Men and women show surprising agreement as to what is good looking and what is not.

Americans agree as to what constitutes good looks—overall. But what happens when we examine beauty in greater detail? What *is* a "good-looking" man or woman?

Nancy Wiggins and her colleagues (Wiggins, Wiggins, & Conger, 1968) conducted a systematic study of what men think is beautiful and sexually appealing. The psychologists prepared 105 silhouettes of nude women. One silhouette had a "Golden mean" sort of figure—average-sized breasts, buttocks, and legs. The remaining silhouettes' breasts, buttocks, and legs were systematically varied in size. For example, some silhouettes had large (+2), moderately large (+1), standard

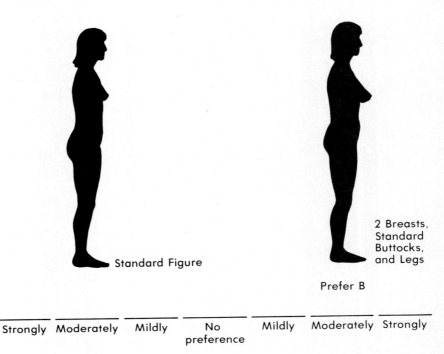

Standard Figure

2 Breasts, Standard Buttocks, and Legs

Prefer B

Strongly Moderately Mildly No preference Mildly Moderately Strongly

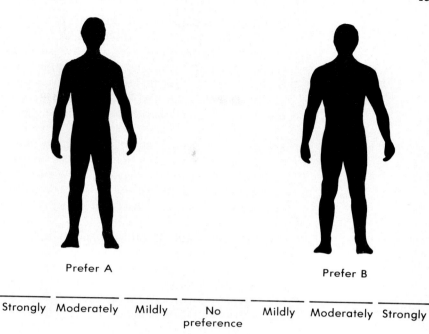

Prefer A   Prefer B

| Strongly | Moderately | Mildly | No preference | Mildly | Moderately | Strongly |

(0), moderately small (-1), or small (-2) breasts. The silhouettes' legs and buttocks were varied in the same way. (An illustrative pair of silhouettes is shown in Figure 15–1). College men were asked to look at the figures, two at a time, and indicate which one they liked best.

Most men judged the women with medium-sized breasts, buttocks, and legs to be far more attractive than those women in whom any of these features was unusually small or large. The most popular figure had medium legs, medium to slightly small buttocks, and slightly large breasts.

What about women? What do they think is sexually appealing? Paul Lavrakas (1975) constructed nineteen different male figures on graph paper, combining the same-sized head with different-sized arms, legs, and torsos (see Figure 15–2). He then paired the figures in all possible ways and photographed the pairs on 35 mm slides. He asked seventy women from the ages of eighteen to thirty to rate each pair. Overall, women preferred men with a medium-wide upper trunk, a medium-thick lower trunk, and thin legs—a look that has been labeled the Robert Redford tapered "V-look." The most disliked build had either a thin upper trunk or a wide lower trunk, the "Alfred Hitchcock pear-shaped look" (see Figure 15–2).

Importance of Beauty. Young people often say they do not care about beauty. For example, when psychologists asked college students how important looks, personality, intelligence, and character were in a date, men and women alike insisted that personality was what really counted, followed by character and then by looks. Intelligence brought up the rear (Tesser & Brodie, 1971). Scientists find that in real life, however, beauty is often all that matters on a first date (Walster et al., 1966; Berscheid et al., 1971; Huston, 1973; Curran & Lippold, 1975).

Recently Murstein (1976) proposed a "stimulus-value-role" theory of marital choice. He theorized that, at first glance (in the "stimulus" stage), all we *can* know about a person is what kind of first impression the person makes. We know what the person looks and sounds like, what other people say about the person, and not much else. Murstein pointed out that the stimulus stage is of crucial importance:

For, if the other person does not possess sufficient stimulus impact to attract the individual, further contact is not sought. The "prospect" in question might make a potentially exemplary, compatible spouse, he might manifest value consensus and superb role compatibility with the perceiver. But the perceiver, foregoing opportunities for further contact, may never find this out. (pp. 116–117)

Communicating Attraction to Others

What is the best way to communicate attraction to others? The advice psychologists give depends on how comfortable people feel with prospective dates. Are they shy, with little experience? If so, they have to start at the beginning, learning the very elementary skills of social interaction—perhaps, for example, simply to say hello to others. Are they outgoing and friendly, with a great deal of experience? If so, they can begin experimenting with more complex interactions.

Shyness.   Zimbardo (1977), a Stanford psychologist, conducted a long-term study of shyness. He asked nearly five thousand people two questions: "Do you presently consider yourself to be a shy person?" and "If you answered no, was there ever a period in your life during which you considered yourself to be shy?" Zimbardo found that more than 80 percent of the people he talked to admitted that they had

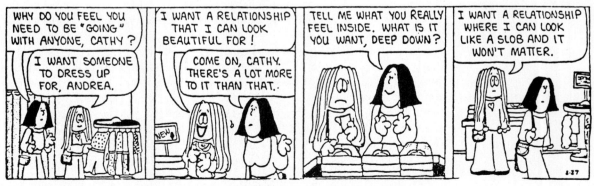

At least in the early stages of a relationship, physical attractiveness is a highly desirable quality in a romantic partner.

SOURCE: Copyright 1979, Universal Press Syndicate. Reprinted with permission. All rights reserved.

Table 15–2.

Shy people report less sexual experience than those who are not shy.

Experience	Percentage Reporting Experience	
	Not Shys	**Shys**
I have masturbated	81	66
I have petted	87	73
I have had intercourse	62	37
I have had oral sex	60	39

SOURCE: Data from Zimbardo, 1977.

been shy at some point in their lives. Of these, over 40 percent considered themselves shy at the time they were surveyed. Psychologists have found that 54 percent of men and 42 percent of women admit that they have trouble with dating (Shmurak, 1973).

Shy people feel it is risky to start a conversation, to invite someone out, to begin a sexual interaction. They are very unsure of themselves. ("Perhaps she was joking when she said, 'Interested in a movie sometime?'" "Perhaps he was looking at my friend when he said, 'Would you like to dance?'") They fear they may say or do the wrong thing. When faced with such painful imaginings, what do shy people do? Do they take the risk and forge ahead or withdraw? Generally, they do nothing. Zimbardo observed that the shy suffer inordinately in sexual encounters. They have less experience than most, as Table 15–2 indicates, and they admit they enjoy sex less.

Overcoming Shyness. Shyness researchers, such as Philip Zimbardo in America and Michael Argyle (1975) in England, have devised specific step-by-step programs to teach people to be more outgoing. Essentially, their programs break the process of getting to know others into a series of small, manageable steps. As a shy person practices the early steps and becomes comfortable with those, it becomes easier and easier to move on to more difficult encounters. The shy are asked to make a contract with themselves. What is it that they desire? To have some men friends? Women friends? In order to attain these large goals, they need to break them down into a series of smaller goals and work on those. Smaller goals, for instance, might be set as follows:

1. To learn to say hello to the people they pass on the street or see in their classes.

2. To practice striking up conversations with people in grocery stores, laundromats, classrooms, buses, and finally, at parties.

3. To practice keeping a conversation flowing—first in safe circumstances, later in more difficult dating situations.

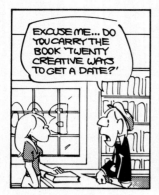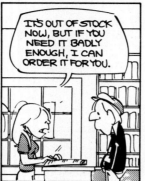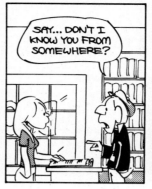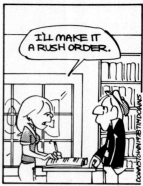

For some people, getting acquainted is the most difficult step in forming an intimate relationship.

SOURCE: © 1979 Tim Downs.

4.   To learn to say goodbye—to make it clear that they have enjoyed talking to their partners, that they have to go, but that they want to see them again.

5.   To practice asking others for dates, starting small and gradually progressing. Shy daters are usually extremely fearful of rejection. Thus, they are advised to start out by asking others to group activities—"A group of us are going to the movies. Why don't you come along?" Later on they can progress to single dating.

Once people have a date, what then? Christensen and Arkowitz (1974, 1977) work with college students who have had no dating experience in their entire lives. They teach students minimal dating skills. They work to improve the poor dater's skills in three areas: ideas, emotional reactions, and behavior. When it comes to ideas, nondaters are too critical of themselves (Bandura, 1969); they tend to discount their successes and brood about their failures (Miller & Arkowitz, in press; Glass, Gottman, & Shmurak, 1976). Nondaters also have to learn to be more relaxed emotionally as well as learn a few basic behavior skills (MacDonald, Lindquist, Kramer, McGrath, & Rhyne, 1975; Twentyman & McFall, 1975; Argyle, 1978).

Their clients begin by *practice* dating. Men and women who volunteer for the program agree to date anyone else in the program. The object is not romance, but learning how to date. They may start out on a coffee date, coaching each other about what to say. They then go out to a movie with a group of students. Next may come a number of full-fledged dates with their fellow volunteers. Finally, they are ready to go out with someone they really care about. They can check back with the group for further coaching.

Once people have found they are interested in and have done their best to interest another, how can they tell if they have succeeded? How can they determine whether the other is interested and they should continue to pursue the relationship or the other is not and they should abandon it? This is the next subject we will consider.

Interpreting Others' Attraction to Oneself

Obviously, one way people can find out how others feel about them is to ask. Sometimes, however, people are too shy to ask. Or they ask but their partners are unable or unwilling to say how they feel. What then?

Scientists have found that people give away their feelings in a wide variety of ways (see Argyle, 1975; Cook & McHenry, 1978.) For example, Goffman (1971), in *Relations in Public*, pointed out that we all possess a subtle repertoire of techniques—formal gestures, postures, and so on—for indicating whether or not we are with others. He calls these "tie signs." A man holding a woman's arm is a blatant tie sign. Romm Harré (1977) added that we possess an equally large repertoire of *un*tie signs. These signs, which broadcast a state of enmity, a wish to be seen to be *not* together, may be, for example, "pointedly gazing at different window displays, shrugging off a tentative placating hand with a sharp upward and sideways movement of the shoulder girdle" (p. 343). What are some of the other tie and untie signs we use?

Eye contact.   When people are chatting with others, they normally look at them, on and off, for short periods. Michael Argyle (1967) found that people glance at casual acquaintances from 30 percent to 60 percent of the time. But if they really like someone, they tend to glance at them—they "check in" to make sure everything is all right—far more often than that (see Argyle, 1967; Exline, 1972). Rubin (1970) found that lovers spend more time gazing into one another's eyes than do others.

Body Posture.   Sir Francis Galton was a slightly eccentric Victorian psychologist. He was, like many other stiffly repressed Victorians, intrigued by the idea that he might be able to tell who had succumbed to love or who was having an illicit extramarital affair by observing some telltale signs of love.

Galton (1884) conceived of an ingenious way to invade his friends' privacy, as described below:

The poetical metaphors of ordinary language suggest many possibilities of measurement. Thus, when two persons have an "inclination" to one another, they visibly incline or slope together when sitting side by side, as at a dinner table, and they then throw the stress of their weights on the near legs of their chairs. It does not require much ingenuity to arrange a pressure gauge with an index and dial to indicate changes in stress, but it is difficult to devise an arrangement that shall fulfill the three-fold condition of being effective, not attracting notice, and being applicable to ordinary furniture. I made some rude experiments, but being busy with other matters, have not carried them on, as I had hoped. (p. 179)

Research supports Galton's contention that people's posture is a tip-off to their feelings. People snuggle toward someone they love and stiffly arch their bodies away from those they do not (Berscheid & Walster [Hatfield], 1978).

Often without being aware of it, men and women use body language to communicate their interest in another person.

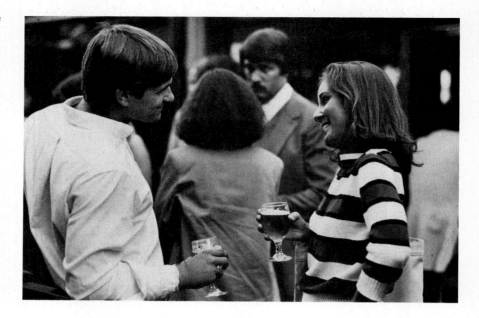

Distance.   Observers can learn a lot about how people feel about others by noticing how close or how far away from each other they stand. The person who shyly walks close to others, takes every excuse to accidentally graze their hands or backs, or who bumps up against others probably feels warm toward them. People who keep striding on ahead of their mates, forcing them to rush to keep up, are sending a message too—they would like a little distance for a while (Berscheid & Walster [Hatfield], 1978).

Thus far, we have discussed nonverbal indicators that scientists are very sure are associated with liking. Scientists have chosen a single behavior—amount of eye contact or distance—and have carefully worked to pin down that behavior's relationship to interpersonal attraction. Some researchers have been willing to go out on a limb, however, and speculate about the complicated patterns of behavior that reveal how people feel about others. Their speculations are interesting, but the careful documentation that they are correct does not yet exist. For example, Albert Scheflen (1975) described various "signs" of courtship behavior, specifically, those indicating courtship readiness, positioning for courtship, and invitation to courtship. Here we will briefly characterize these signs.

Courtship Readiness.   People who are beginning to flirt with the idea of a sexual encounter quickly give themselves away. The bags around their eyes and their ugly jowls miraculously disappear. Their eyes brighten. They blush (or grow pale). Their posture improves; they suck in their potbellies. Their leg muscles become firmer. (Think of all the "beefcake" or "cheesecake" ads depicting an arrogant model staring defiantly, his or her pelvis slung forward, legs apart—a stance designed to sell cigarettes, beer, and sex.) The sexually interested begin preening.

Aroused women might stroke their hair, glance at their makeup in the mirror, or sketchily arrange their clothing. Aroused men might comb or stroke their hair, fidget nervously with their ties, button and readjust their coats, or pull up their socks. These body language signs all combine to say, "I'm interested. Are you?"

Positioning for Courtship.   At any college mixer, sorority or fraternity dance, or local singles bar, one can observe men and women moving unconsciously through an informal mating dance. Sometimes, when men and women seem simply to be chatting—albeit a little self-consciously—arguing about the latest drug scandal in Washington, charter flights to Europe, or the weather, in fact, argues Scheflen, they are doing much more. If they are attracted to one another, they are deftly arranging and rearranging their bodies in ways that send a clear message to others: "We're together. This is our territory. Keep out!" They lean toward each other and place their chairs or extremities in such a way as to block off aisles.

Of course, sometimes men or women are eager to send the opposite message: "I'm trapped! Save me!" Such reluctant partners unconsciously position themselves quite differently. They gaze longingly at the ceiling, or glance distractedly about. They twist their bodies away from their partner toward any larger group. They squirm and shuffle their feet.

Actions of Appeal or Invitation.   Men and women often seduce one another by inviting body language. A man may stroll over to a woman's table and gaze at her— just a second too long. In response, she might direct flirtatious glances at him, gaze at him a little too long, cock her head attentively, or nervously cross and uncross her legs, thereby revealing part of her thigh. Her appeal may be as shy as exposing her wrist or palm, or as bold as aggressively thrusting her breast forward, or slowly stroking her fingers along her thigh or wrist. In response to such "hot" communications, a man might loosen his tie, or move in closer than he normally would.

It seems, then, that psychologists have a great deal to tell us about how people go about meeting appropriate partners, how people go about interesting others, and how people can tell if others are or are not interested in them. But such dating formulas are only a start. Most family therapists argue that the exciting thing about intimate relations is that people can explore—confide things in one another that they have never dared reveal before and try things they have never tried—and that makes love delightfully unpredictable.

SUMMARY

Psychologists have concluded that there are two distinctly different kinds of love— passionate love and companionate love. Passionate love is defined as "a state of intense absorption in another." Sometimes passionate lovers are those who long for their partners and for complete fulfillment. Sometimes they are those who are ecstatic at finally having attained their partner's love, and momentarily, complete fulfillment. It appears that both cognitive factors and physiological factors are critical determinants of whether or not people feel passionately in love. Peoples' minds determine what specific emotion they feel. Their bodies determine whether or not they feel any emotion at all.

Companionate love is defined as "the affection people feel for those with whom their lives are deeply entwined."

Psychologists have a fairly good idea why people love the people they do. They cite the principles of reinforcement and equity in order to explain why people are attracted to some people and repelled by others.

How do most people meet the people they will eventually end up loving? It appears that propinquity breeds attraction. Other things being equal, the closer two people are located geographically, the more likely it is that they will be attracted to each other. There is solid evidence that people are reluctant to search very far for a partner. They almost always end up dating and marrying those who happen to be around on a day-to-day basis.

Every culture has standards as to whom it is appropriate to marry. Sociologists find that Americans generally choose partners who are similar to themselves in a variety of demographic characteristics including age, race, social class, education, and religion. Psychologists find that Americans try to select partners with the personal characteristics they admire. As reported in the Research Highlight, Traupmann and Utne interviewed several hundred dating couples, newlyweds, and elderly couples in order to find out what they wanted from their relationships. They found that couples agreed that a variety of personal concerns, emotional concerns, day-to-day concerns, and opportunities gained or lost (twenty-five in all)—were critically important in their relationships.

Though defined differently from one society to the next, physical attractiveness is a potent sexual attractant. Communicating attraction is often difficult due to shyness. Various training programs have been developed to assist people in overcoming shyness and dating difficulties. Determining whether others are attracted to oneself can also be difficult. Obviously, one way people can find out how others feel about them is to ask. Sometimes, however, people are too shy to ask. Or if they are willing to ask, their partners are unable or unwilling to say how they feel. What then? Scientists have found that people give away their feelings in a wide variety of ways: They look at such "tie" and "untie" signs as eye contact, body postures, and the distance people stand from others. People can use such signals to decode how others feel about them.

SUGGESTED READINGS

Argyle, M. (1975). *Bodily communication*. New York: International Universities Press.

Duck, S., & Gilmour, R. (Eds.) (1980). *Personal relationships*. Vol. 1, *Studying personal relationships*. London: Academic Press.

Duck, S., & Gilmour, R. (Eds.) (1981). *Personal relationships*. Vol. 2, *Developing personal relationships*. London: Academic Press.

Duck, S., & Gilmour, R. (Eds.) (1981). *Personal relationships*. Vol. 3, *Personal relationships in disorder*. London: Academic Press.

Duck, S. W. (Ed.). (1982). *Personal relationships*. Vol. 4, *Dissolving personal relationships*. London: Academic Press.

Hatfield, E., & Walster, G. W. (1978). *A new look at love*. Reading: Mass.: Addison-Wesley.

Reik, T. (1944). *A psychologist looks at love*. New York: Farrar and Rinehart.

Zimbardo, P. (1977). *Shyness*. Reading, Mass.: Addison-Wesley.

CHAPTER 16

THE CULTURAL, RELIGIOUS, AND LEGAL CONTEXTS OF SEXUALITY

The patterns of human sexual behavior that have been the main focus of earlier sections of this book are those that are most characteristic of American and other Western societies. Even within this rather limited context, the differences among people and various subgroups of people in sexual practices, attitudes, and beliefs are striking. These variations provide ample testimony that, within the limits imposed by anatomy and physiology, human sexuality may be molded into many forms.

But the various forms taken by human sexuality are not haphazardly or randomly determined. They are shaped and regulated by a number of psychological and social factors. Among the most important of these shaping factors are *culture, religion,* and *law.* In this chapter we provide a brief overview of various ways in which human sexuality is influenced and regulated by the cultural, religious, and legal context in which it occurs. Let us begin with a consideration of the cultural context of human sexuality.

THE CULTURAL CONTEXT OF SEXUALITY

The world's peoples are generally organized into societies that are characterized by differing cultures. A **society** is "an enduring cooperating, self-reproducing group of individuals with organized patterns of interrelationships" (Beach, 1978, p. 7). The **culture** of a society is its "shared patterns of belief, thought, speech and action" (p. 7). The culture of any society is reflected in many ways—in its dressing and eating habits, in its social and political structure, and, of importance here, in its patterns of sexual beliefs, attitudes, practices, and regulations.

Most of what we know about cultural variations in sexuality comes from the research of anthropologists. Though the methods used by anthropologists are many and varied (Marshall & Suggs, 1972), major contributions have been made by at least two types of investigations. First, some investigators spend time living in and recording what information they may obtain concerning a society's sexuality (Malinowski, 1929; Marshall, 1972; Messenger, 1972). A second major source of data is information contained in the Human Relations Area Files originally compiled by Yale University as a repository of facts about many cultures. In their now classic work, Clellan S. Ford and Frank A. Beach (1951) relied on these files to survey the sexual practices, beliefs, and attitudes of 190 societies around the world. Both of these types of investigations make it abundantly clear that cultural influences permeate all aspects of sexuality.

Our discussion of cultural factors is organized around three major dimensions of sexuality. First, we consider some of the ways in which culture shapes beliefs, attitudes, and practices relevant to the *biological aspects* of sexuality. Second, we examine cultural variations in *erotic codes*. Finally, we discuss cultural differences in various types of *sexual behavior*.

Culture and the Biology of Sex

Although there is no reason to suspect that the fundamental biological aspects of sexuality differ systematically from culture to culture, the beliefs, attitudes, and meanings attached to the biological "facts" vary across cultures. Three areas in which wide cultural variations are found are conception, pregnancy, and menstruation.

Conception.   On East Bay, one of the Melanesian islands of the Southwest Pacific, views of conception follow an agricultural model. Semen from the man is regarded as the seed and the womb of the woman as the garden soil. Secretions from the womb (uterus) are thought of as providing necessary moisture and nutrients for the growth of the fetus. Since repeated intromissions of semen (repeated plantings) are thought to lead to multiple births, ejaculation in the vagina during pregnancy is carefully avoided (Davenport, 1978).

Among the Ashanti of Ghana, it is believed that conception occurs in the womb when ejaculate from the man mixes with the blood of the woman. The mother's blood is thought to become the blood of the child and the father's semen to contribute the spirit and life force of the child (Davenport, 1978).

Both the East Bay and Ashanti views somehow link coitus with conception. But some societies, at least in the past, have not seemed to have fully recognized such a link. For example, some of the aborigines of Australia and the natives of the Trobriand Islands once thought that pregnancy resulted when a "spirit child" entered the womb and was nurtured there until birth. Intercourse was thought only to make it easier for the spirit to enter or to open up the womb to provide space for the fetus to grow. Both of these groups now have at least a rough understanding of the coitus-conception relationship. Indeed, it is possible that the earlier reported beliefs were mostly ways of expressing a mystical side of conception in the way that some people in our own society describe children as part of God's work (Davenport, 1978).

Pregnancy.   Most societies, including the United States, have certain beliefs and practices associated with pregnancy. Some of these beliefs concern the advisability of coitus during pregnancy. Recommendations in the United States have varied substantially over the years. Usually based on beliefs concerning the medical safety of the pregnant woman or the fetus, recommendations have ranged from advice that coitus be avoided throughout pregnancy to advice that coitus is acceptable until shortly before delivery. Contemporary views are that recommendations should be tailored to the medical and psychological needs of the individual woman and her partner (Masters & Johnson, 1966). As noted above, on East Bay intercourse during pregnancy is generally avoided. Beliefs that multiple ejaculations in the vagina result in multiple births lead to especially strong avoidance of ejaculation into the vagina of a pregnant woman. In contrast, the Mangaians (of the Cook Islands) encourage continued intercourse during pregnancy because it is thought both to be more pleasurable and to make for an easier birth (Marshall, 1972).

Probably all human societies have beliefs and practices that are linked to attempts to control the sex and well-being of the fetus and to prevent abnormal births. Some of these concern the activities of the pregnant woman. For example, in certain societies if a pregnant woman desires a male child, she will engage in some masculine activity. In others, to prevent ugliness or malformations in the unborn child, she will avoid looking into the faces of animals. Or desiring an easy and safe birth, she will eat mostly slimy and viscous foods to ease the passage of the child at birth. In some cultures hooped ropes and vines are avoided to prevent the umbilical cord from becoming entangled about the baby's neck (Davenport, 1978).

All of these practices, of course, are based on the assumption that the mother's experiences affect the unborn fetus. The father's experiences are sometimes implicated as well and he may carefully avoid situations or events that may harm the developing fetus. In a practice known as the **couvade**, reported among the Basques and South American Indians, the father goes through a ritual sympathetic labor as the mother goes through the actual labor of childbirth. Because of assumed mystical connections between the father and both the mother and the child, this is thought to increase the likelihood of an uncomplicated delivery (Davenport, 1978; Ford & Beach, 1951).

Menstruation.   People's understanding of menstruation is subject to many culturally shaped beliefs, attitudes, and practices. In addition to viewing menstruation as debilitating to women in many ways (Bullough & Bullough, 1977), most societies, including our own, limit intercourse during menstruation. This is often because menstrual discharge is regarded as disgusting or even as polluting or dangerous to men (Ford & Beach, 1951). As a result, men may carefully avoid a menstruating woman and she may even be isolated until her period is over.

Pre-Christian Hawaii was a culture with strong menstrual avoidance. Menstruating women were confined to their quarters, which were carefully avoided by men. Because these quarters were thought to be always polluted by menstruation, men never entered this part of the dwelling. Contact with anything associated with menstruation contaminated men, the only solution to which was a ritual purification (Davenport, 1978). In some Papua New Guinea societies, contact with menstrual discharge is viewed as a cause of illness, debility, and even death for men. Women are thought never to be totally free of contamination. Men and women live highly segregated lives and men have intercourse with their wives reluctantly, infrequently, and then only for reproductive purposes. Finally, in some cultures, menstruating women must refrain from gardening and food preparation lest they ruin the crops or pollute the food (Davenport, 1978).

These examples illustrate substantial diversity among cultures in beliefs and attitudes connected with the biological aspects of sexuality. In addition, however, they reveal some of the ways in which sexual behaviors are regulated by such beliefs and attitudes. When and under what circumstances sexual intercourse is permitted, how menstruating and pregnant women are treated, and how to create or avoid pregnancy are all dictated to a certain extent by cultural patterns. Let us now examine cultural differences in erotic codes—that is, outlooks regarding the nature of sexuality and what is viewed as sexually stimulating.

Culture and Erotic Codes

Every culture has its own erotic code consisting of (1) an overall view as to whether sexuality is something positive to be pursued or something negative to be avoided and (2) an inventory of cues that are regarded as erotic. In this section we examine some of these codes.

Good Sex and Bad Sex.   Different cultures around the world have widely varying overall outlooks on sexuality. Some are extremely negative and some extremely positive (see Research Highlight), but most probably fall between these extremes (Ford & Beach, 1951). The basis for the outlook of those cultures that regard sexuality negatively is usually a belief that sex is linked with sin or with ill health. The culture of Inis Beag described in the Research Highlight is one example of how the Christian tradition carried to extremes may negate all of sexuality. Health beliefs may have the same effect. For example, at one point in history on Yap Island in the Pacific, sexual intercourse was thought to cause weakness and susceptibility to disease among men at all times and among women during pregnancy. These beliefs were accompanied by a strong negative attitude toward and suppression of sexuality. Similarly, many other cultures associate sex with various supernatural beliefs. Members of these cultures engage in intercourse in constant fear of sorcery or the wrath of various spirits (Davenport, 1978).

In most cultures, including our own, sexuality is embedded in a complex network of positive and negative feelings. For the Gusii of Kenya sexuality is expressed in combination with hostility and conflict. Women are expected to resist men's sexual demands and men to overcome the resistance through force, perhaps causing some physical pain. On the other hand, the women are often overtly seductive and intercourse closely resembles a ritualized rape (Davenport, 1978). The Trukese of the Pacific view sexual expression as natural and gratifying, yet a substantial amount of pain and frustration accompanies sexual intercourse and foreplay. Biting, scratching, jabbing, and hair pulling are normal components of intercourse and, as among the Trobrianders (Malinowski, 1929), the battle scars of love are taken as signs of sexual success (Ford & Beach, 1951).

Erotic Cues.   Every culture has its own views regarding what is erotic and attractive and what is not. *Physical characteristics* are important in all societies, but

RESEARCH HIGHLIGHT

Sex-Negative and Sex-Positive Cultures

Inis Beag:
A Sex-Negative Culture

Inis Beag is the name used by John C. Messenger (1972) to refer to a small island society off the coast of Ireland. Inis Beag is remarkable for its sexual restrictiveness and resulting sexual "ignorance." It is an extreme example of a culture that regards almost all sex as bad.

So negative are the feelings about sex that few women understand the physiological significance of menstruation or menopause and menstruation is regarded as shameful and disgusting. Men believe that intercourse is injurious to their health and women that it is an ordeal that they must endure. The people admit no knowledge of such sexual activities as tongue kissing, manual stimulation of the penis by females, oral breast stimulation, fellatio, cunnilingus, premarital, extramarital, or postmarital intercourse, or homosexuality.

Nudity is carefully avoided, even during bathing. Seamen are known to have drowned, having avoided learning to swim because it involved scant clothing. Men and women keep their underwear on during intercourse.

When it occurs, marital sex is always initiated by the man and only the male superior face-to-face position is used. The man reaches orgasm as soon as possible and then falls asleep. Female orgasm is virtually unknown, doubted to exist, or considered deviant if it occurs. Much of this sexual repression seems to have its origins in teachings of the Catholic church. It is instilled early in children by direct instruction or punishment.

Mangaia:
A Sex-Positive Culture

Contrasted with the restrictive and negative approach to sex in Inis Beag are the attitudes of the residents of Mangaia, one of the Cook Islands of the South Pacific (Marshall, 1972). Mangaia is an extreme example of a culture that regards almost all sex as good.

The biological aspects of sexuality are fully accepted as natural and genital nudity is acceptable in children—for girls up until around age five and for boys until around age twelve when the glans is exposed by the ritual of superincision. Young children masturbate and may play at copulation but only in private. Around age twelve or thirteen, both boys and girls receive direct sexual instruction. For boys this instruction takes place as part of superincision rites. Superincision is an extremely painful operation in which the penis is cut lengthwise along the dorsal (top) side exposing the glans of the penis. The boy is now considered "a man" and is instructed by an older male "expert" in the ways of pleasing a woman. He learns of cunnilingus, breast stimulation, and how to bring a woman to orgasm during intercourse several times before he has his own orgasm. This is followed by "on-the-job training" by an older experienced woman with whom he has his first actual practice in intercourse.

At about the same age girls receive sexual instruction from older women and often have their first intercourse with an older man. The young Mangaians then actively seek each other out and intercourse becomes an every-night affair. Virility and skill are demanded of the young man. He is expected to be able to continue active in-and-out thrusting for fifteen to thirty minutes while his partner moves her hips "like a washing machine" and reaches orgasm two or three times. Most Mangaian boys have ten or more different sexual partners between the ages of thirteen and twenty and the "nice" girl has three or four. The eighteen-year-old boy is said to have intercourse every night of the week and to have about three orgasms each night. By age forty-eight this drops to two or three nights per week with one orgasm per night. Under conditions of sexual "deprivation" (travel, illness, or death of spouse) extramarital sexual activity is widely tolerated. The Mangaians do, indeed, live in a sex-positive culture.

the particular features that are regarded as attractive vary widely. In most societies it is generally true that the physical beauty of women is more important than that of men. A man's attractiveness more often is determined by his skills and success than by his physical appearance (Ford & Beach, 1951).

General body build is important in most cultures. The majority of societies studied by Ford and Beach (1951) seem to consider plumpness and even what we might call obesity in women as attractive. In addition women with a broad pelvis and wide hips are generally preferred. For example, the Siriono men prefer a woman who is fat, has large hips and breasts, and a deposit of fat on her vulva. In contrast, however, the Masai value slimness, roundness of form, delicacy, and small upright breasts in their women. For some, as noted earlier, the appearance of the external genitals are determinants of erotic attractiveness. The Nama and Thonga of Africa consider elongated labia majora to be attractive and Easter Islanders value a large clitoris. These structures are sometimes pulled and manipulated in order to increase the attractiveness of young girls (Ford & Beach, 1951). Still others pay little attention to genitals but focus on the appearance of head and face—eyes, mouth, nose, teeth, and hair—as do the Trobrianders (Malinowski, 1929).

The *sight of sexual organs* is everywhere thought of as having the potential to arouse sexual desire. At the same time, all societies have evolved rules of modesty that dictate how sexual organs are to be covered. The rules vary greatly but most cultures require that the genitals of adults be covered in all but intimate situations (Davenport, 1978). Where different standards exist for men and women, it is usually the women who are required to cover their genitals. An exception is Aoriki in the Solomon Islands; the women go entirely naked until after marriage and childbirth while after puberty men's genitals must be covered (Davenport, 1978).

In many societies people are required to use only minimal genital coverings. A small patch of material may cover only the pubic area of women or, as in Papua New Guinea, men may be required only to cover the head of the penis with a small, brightly colored gourd held in upright position with a strap around the waist. Even in societies where men and women go entirely naked throughout their lives, as do the Kwoma of the Pacific, there are rules that limit viewing the female genitals. Men are forbidden to stare at a woman's genitals and women are expected to walk and sit in such a way that the vaginal opening is never exposed (Davenport, 1978; Ford & Beach, 1951).

Deliberate exposure by a woman of her genitals is a common form of sexual invitation in only a few societies. For example, among the Kurtatchi of the Pacific, a woman desiring intercourse with a man will simply lie down in his presence with her legs apart. However, if she exposes her genitals, even accidentally, she is inviting sexual assault by any passing man (Ford & Beach, 1951).

As in our own society, these modesty customs are often manipulated to convey sexual meanings. Dress and behavior may be designed to provide arousing glimpses of erotically significant parts of the body. Many other stimuli also serve to provoke sexual desire. The use of oils, lotions, and fragrances from leaves and flowers to attract and arouse sexual partners is widespread. The dances of many cultures deliberately stimulate sexual desires, as do songs, musical tunes, and poetry. As in our culture, sexual allusions and jokes are used widely in conversations to convey sexual meaning. Sharing of particular gifts is often a form of sexual invitation. Finally, in many cultures desirous lovers resort to love magic—some

Virtually every culture has rules that govern modesty, although there is considerable variance in what is considered permissible.

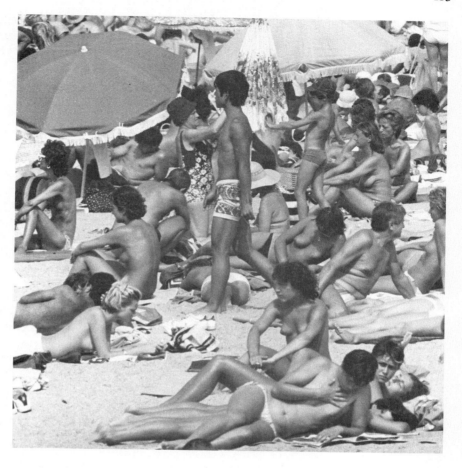

supernatural means of attracting a sexual partner. Even though the specifics of what, how, and when various erotic cues come into play differ widely, clearly every culture has its own list of stimuli thought to arouse and sustain sexual interest (Davenport, 1978; Ford & Beach, 1951).

Culture and Sexual Behavior

Cultural differences in beliefs, attitudes, and practices regarding the biological aspects of sexuality and erotic codes are reflected in wide differences in actual sexual behavior. We focus now on some of these differences in masturbation, heterosexual behavior, and homosexual behavior.

Masturbation.   Almost all societies take a rather dim view of masturbation among adults. Many regard it as an inferior form of sexual expression practiced only by those who cannot obtain a sexual partner. Others (many African societies) link masturbation to illness, while still other societies, such as Inis Beag, consider it sinful. There are, of course, exceptions such as the Lesu of New Ireland in the

Pacific who expect adult women to masturbate when they are aroused and lack a sex partner (Davenport, 1978; Ford & Beach, 1951). Attitudes toward masturbation by children, though, are often different. Many societies view masturbation by young children as natural. Such a stance is taken by those of East Bay and Mangaia. Even these societies, however, think of masturbation after puberty as less than desirable (Davenport, 1978).

Even though reliable data are difficult to obtain, it appears that at least some adults, particularly men, in most societies do engage in masturbation. For example, Trukese men reportedly masturbate in secrecy while watching women bathe (Ford & Beach, 1951). Masturbation appears to be less common among women but does occur in some societies even though it is generally disapproved. In contrast to the masturbation practices of American women, vaginal insertion of a penis substitute is often more common than clitoral manipulation. African Azande women use a phallus fashioned from a wooden root. Lesu women masturbate by sitting with one heel pressing against the genitals for stimulation but never use their hands (Ford & Beach, 1951).

Heterosexual Behavior.   All studied societies have regulations concerning who may participate in heterosexual activity with whom. Most of these regulations are tied to the age of the people involved and the relationships that exist among them.

Ford and Beach classified societies as ranging from restrictive to permissive regarding attitudes and practices related to heterosexual activities among unmarried youth. In the most restrictive societies adults attempt to deny children any form of sexual expression. Severe punishment follows any discovered masturbation or sex play and sex is never discussed in the presence of children. The Murngin of Australia remove children from the home at four or five years of age so that they will witness no adult sexual behavior. Others, such as the Abipone of South America strictly segregate boys and girls at all times prior to marriage. In spite of these restrictions, however, most children privately engage in sexual behavior before puberty ranging from masturbation to attempts at intercourse (Ford & Beach, 1951).

Even some of the more restrictive societies lift many of their prohibitions when children reach puberty. For example, among the Siriono of South America, premarital intercourse affairs among adolescents are quite common. Where the restrictions remain through adolescence they are typically more severe for girls than for boys, as in our own society (Ford & Beach, 1951).

Less restrictive societies have formal codes that are prohibitive to the young and unmarried but the codes are rarely enforced. Widespread sexual activity takes place in secrecy and is tolerated if not flagrant. Even though adults are fully aware of what is going on they often ignore private sexual involvements. For the Andamanese of Southeast Asia, premarital intercourse is common and tolerated as long as it is secret. If a girl becomes pregnant, however, the couple usually marries (Ford & Beach, 1951).

There are a large number of permissive societies with completely tolerant and accepting attitudes toward premarital sexual expression. Public sex play, including attempts at intercourse, are rather common in some societies. The Siriono start their children early with the parents stimulating the genitals of young boys and girls and providing them complete access to sex information. Children of the Lesu are free to observe adults (except their parents) engaging in intercourse. Adolescents are given full approval to engage in sexual intercourse. Trobriand children begin their sex lives between the ages of eight and ten. Approved sexual activities include masturbation, heterosexual and homosexual oral-genital stimulation, and heterosexual intercourse (Ford & Beach, 1951).

Ford and Beach (1951) define two general types of heterosexual partnerships. **Mateships** are relatively permanent sexual, social, and economic unions often recognized legally or religiously as marriage. **Liaisons** are less permanent unions based more exclusively on sex. Both types of partnerships are subject to differing regulations and practices from one culture to another.

Mateships may be **monogamous** (one man and one woman), **polygynous** (one man and two or more women), **polyandrous** (one woman and two or more men), or polygynous and polyandrous (two or more men and two or more women simultaneously). Though our own society legally recognizes only monogamous relationships, less than 16 percent of the societies studied by Ford and Beach (1951) could formally be designated as insisting on monogamy.

The vast majority of these multiple-mateship societies were classified as polygynous—permitting a man to have more than one mate at a time. In most of these arrangements all wives do not share equal status. The first wife may have authority over all others and even be the legal mother to all children born. Even so, in African polygynous societies the husband must pay equal attention to all wives and customarily spends his nights with each in rotation. Some of these societies permit only certain women as additional mates. Most commonly they are the sisters of the first wife. Other societies require a man to take as a wife the widow of his brother. Because of such restrictions and economic factors, only about half of the men in many polygynous societies actually have more than one wife at a time (Davenport, 1978; Ford & Beach, 1951).

Polyandrous societies in which one woman has two or more mates are rare. Among the Toda of India women marry the younger brothers of their first husband or some other man if no male siblings are available. Similar practices are found in Tibet. Marquesan women (Central Pacific), in contrast, marry other men who are not closely related to the first husband (Davenport, 1978; Ford & Beach, 1951).

Polygynous and polyandrous combinations are even more rare. The Kaingang of Brazil permit permanent sexual unions of multiple men with multiple women. Even there such relationships are rare and the majority of mateships are monogamous (Ford & Beach, 1951).

All societies limit the establishment of sexual liaisons. We have already described some of the customs regarding premarital liaisons and will limit our present discussion to those that involve at least one mated (or married) individual. Almost 40 percent of the societies studied by Ford and Beach approved of some type of extramarital sexual unions. In some societies both men and women are expected to engage in multiple affairs as long as all incest rules (discussed below) are followed.

Toda men and women of India are allowed extramarital partners. The polyandrous women may take several lovers as well as several husbands. The Siriono limit extramarital liaisons to siblings-in-law. A man may have sex with his wives' sisters, his brothers' wives, and the sisters of his brothers' wives. A woman has sexual access to the husbands of her sisters and to her husband's brothers. "Wife lending" or "wife exchange" is customary among the Chukchee of Siberia and the Eskimos of North American. Traveling men are granted sexual access to the wives of their hosts in exchange for reciprocal privileges (Ford & Beach, 1951).

Like our own, most societies studied by Ford and Beach disapprove of extra-marital liaisons. Many are more restrictive regarding married women than married men. Even so, some men and women in all societies do occasionally have such affairs and attempt to keep them secret. If discovered, those involved may be subjected to punishment ranging from mild to harsh (Ford & Beach, 1951).

All societies have some type of **incest taboo**, or prohibition of matings and sexual liaisons between certain relatives. Precisely which relatives are prohibited as sexual partners varies from one society to another. Some include only close relatives while others extend to relatives so distant as to severely restrict the number of approved partners available. Virtually all societies condemn parent-child and sibling sexual relationships. Most also extend the prohibitions to aunts, uncles, nieces, nephews, and first or second cousins. Punishment for violation of incest taboos range from admonishment to severe beatings (Davenport, 1978; Ford & Beach, 1951).

Homosexual Behavior.   Attitudes toward homosexual behavior and homosexuality vary widely from one culture to another. There are some societies like our own, in which all forms of homosexual behavior are condemned for any people. Some, on the other hand, approve of homosexual behavior among the young but not among adults. Still others fully approve of homosexual behavior for some people or under special circumstances.

Ford and Beach (1951) were able to obtain information about homosexual behavior in seventy-six societies and noted that in only around one third is this form of behavior totally taboo. Though some homosexual behavior inevitably occurs in these societies, it is usually in secrecy. The penalties for discovery range from ridicule to death. For example, Rwala Bedouins sentence male and female homosexual offenders to death.

The majority of the societies studied by Ford and Beach, however, approve of at least some forms of homosexual behavior. In some, an institutionalized form of homosexuality exists in which particular men dress and act like women and form sexual relationships with other men. Often, as among the Siberian Chukchee, such men are thought to possess supernatural powers and are held in high esteem.

In some societies homosexual behavior is expected among all men and boys. Siwan men of Africa, for example, lend their sons to one another for sexual purposes and both married and unmarried males are expected to have homosexual affairs. As part of his puberty rites each Karaki boy of New Guinea is initiated into anal intercourse by older bachelor males. He continues his passive role in anal intercourse for a year and then spends the rest of his unmarried life having anal intercourse with the new initiates. As a general rule, it appears that homosexual behavior is less likely to occur in women than in men in all studied societies. Moreover, homosexual behavior is not the predominant type of sexual activity in any society (Ford & Beach, 1951).

THE RELIGIOUS CONTEXT OF SEXUALITY

Inhabitants of Inis Beag regard almost all forms of sexual expression with distaste. Mangaians condone and even endorse premarital intercourse. Siwan men and boys are expected to engage in homosexual behavior and the Toda of India are allowed extramarital intercourse. In the United States almost all forms of nonmarital and some forms of marital sexuality are subject to disapproval. These widely varying attitudes and values regarding what is good or bad, right or wrong, moral or immoral in sexuality arise from many interacting sources. In Western societies such as our own, religion has been and is a major source of sexual values. In this section we briefly consider some of the ways in which sexuality is shaped by the religious context in which it occurs. Our primary focus will be on sexuality in Western cultures, particularly the United States.

The Judeo-Christian Tradition

Any discussion of sexual values and ethics in Western cultures must focus on what is known as the Judeo-Christian tradition. This is the religious foundation for most Western societies and is the basis for many contemporary sexual values, rules, and regulations. As implied by its name, this tradition is the joint product of the beliefs and teachings of Judaism and Christianity.

Judaism and Sexuality. The most important source of religious belief for Jewish people is the Old Testament of the Bible, written between around 800 and 200 B.C. The Old Testament has a great deal to say about sexuality and is also a major source of sexual values for Christianity.

The Old Testament approach to sexuality is basically a positive one, but only within the context of marriage. This approach is established in Genesis, the very first book. Here, the fundamental purpose of sex is clearly spelled out: "Be fruitful and multiply, and fill the earth and subdue it; and have dominion over the fish of the sea and over the birds of the air and over every living thing that moves upon the earth" (Gen. 1:27–28). That is, sex is good because it is necessary for reproduction and expansion of the human population. The type of relationship within which sexuality is expressed is also specified: "A man leaves his father and cleaves to his wife and the two become one flesh" (Gen. 2:24).

Thus, in Judaism the purpose of sex is procreation and it is to take place in the context of marriage. This rather positive view of marital intercourse contrasts sharply with the negative values placed on any other form of sexual expression. Any nonmarital, nonprocreative sex was severely condemned by the ancient Jews and still is by orthodox Jews today. Jewish laws were clear. Premarital and extra-marital intercourse were forbidden and the punishment for adultery was death. Homosexual behavior, masturbation, and bestiality were nonprocreative and punishment for such behaviors could include death (Lev. 20:10–19). Contraception and abortion were forbidden since they interfered with the only purpose of sex—procreation (Bullough & Bullough, 1977).

Christianity and Sexuality.   The emergence of Christianity is, of course, marked by the teachings of Jesus and of the followers he attracted. In fact, however, Jesus had very little to say specifically about sexuality. He did speak to the "sin of adultery" on a few occasions (Matthew 5; John 8) but did not elaborate a complete sexual ethic. For the most part, it appears that his views were quite similar to those found in Old Testament teachings.

Partly because of Jesus' relative silence regarding sexual matters, the formulation of Christian ethics of sexuality was left to New Testament writers and other theological scholars such as St. Paul, St. Augustine, and St. Thomas Aquinas. Reflecting a combination of his own views and those of Jesus, St. Paul provided the foundation of the Christian view of sexuality in his New Testament writings. St. Paul advocated **celibacy** primarily became of his belief in the "Second Coming" of Christ. He believed that in preparation for this event, people should spend time in prayer, worship, and spreading of Gospel. Marriage and sex were viewed as distractions from this task. Like the authors of the Old Testament, he saw marriage as the only context for sex and condemned all other forms of sexual expression as "sins of the flesh" (1 Cor. 7; Gal. 5).

St. Paul's views provided the framework for later Christian teachings and a basis for the **asceticism** that characterized the writings of the "fathers of the church" between around 150 and 600 A.D. Asceticism is a doctrine that indulging in bodily and material pleasures interferes with the attainment of the "higher" spiritual or intellectual values of life. Celibacy thus came to be viewed as a superior state to marriage and sexual expression.

This view was carried to extremes by St. Augustine (354–430 A.D.), one of the most influential of the church fathers. Following a youth of promiscuity and sexual indulgence, Augustine was converted to Christianity and condemned all sexual expression as sin. Writing in *The City of God* (after 412 A.D./1950), he proclaimed that even marital intercourse was tainted by the "original sin" of Adam and Eve. Intercourse was viewed as necessary for procreation but nonetheless a shameful act. This negative view of sexuality supplied the foundation for subsequent Catholic ideology and the basis for later (twelfth century) requirements persisting today that all clergy (priests, nuns) be celibate.

During the Middle Ages, St. Thomas Aquinas (1225–1274) emerged as the most influental interpretor of Catholic theology. Relying on divine revelation, "right reason," and "natural law," Aquinas essentially laid down the laws of Catholic sexual morality. According to his natural law of sexuality, the sole purpose of sex was procreation and all nonprocreative sex was sinful. Within marriage, procreative sex was permissible. All other nonmarital, nonprocreative sex was sinful. Nonmarital intercourse (fornication), extramarital intercourse (adultery), masturbation, nocturnal emissions, rape, incest, homosexuality, bestiality, and seduction violated God's natural law and were forbidden. A similar status was accorded contraception and abortion (Thomas Aquinas, 1267–73/1968).

Protestantism and Sexuality.   Until the sixteenth century Christianity and the Roman Catholic church were one and the same. Led by Martin Luther and John Calvin, the Protestant Reformation challenged many of the fundamentals of Catholic theology. For somewhat different reasons, both Luther and Calvin rejected the church's views of clerical celibacy, the virtues of chastity, and marriage. The emerging Protestant theologies regarded marriage and sex within marriage as a natural state of human affairs but retained the view that marriage was the only legitimate context for sex.

Under Protestantism, the family was exalted and any form of sexual activity that threatened the integrity of the family condemned. The Calvinist Puritans, many of whom fled England to the New World, evolved a strict code of sexual morality and ethics. Viewing people as inherently weak and sinful, the Puritans insisted upon strict self-discipline and imposed rigid codes and laws of sexual conduct. But sex within marriage was honorable and not viewed solely as procreative in purpose. The contraceptive prohibitions of the Catholic church were weakened in Protestantism and marriage was viewed as more than an arrangement for breeding.

Victorianism and Sexuality.   Though Puritan codes and standards of sexual conduct may seem somewhat rigid and repressive, they pale in comparison with those of England during the reign of Queen Alexandrina Victoria (1819–1901). During the Victorian era, most forms of sexual expression, even in marriage, were viewed with disgust and as potentially harmful. Victorian sexual morality was based not so much on Christian theology as on erroneous medical and scientific beliefs.

Semen was viewed as a vital life substance, the excess loss of which could be potentially damaging (see Chapter 8). Men were thought of as sexual "maniacs" and women as asexual. Moral men, it was believed, must constantly struggle to avoid semen wastage, and moral women must aid in this struggle by not provoking men's sexual urges. Even in marriage, sexual activity was to occur in moderation and nonmarital sex was strictly forbidden. Of course, masturbation, homosexual behavior, and other forms of sexual expression were condemned as well. Strict rules of public decency and propriety were formalized but the widespread hypocrisy of the upper classes in violating the rules is well known. Indeed, it is questionable whether the formal codes had a major influence on the actual sexual practices of any large segment of English or American society (Bullough & Bullough, 1977).

Western sexual morality has been strongly influenced by a blend of the Judaic and Christian theology that we have briefly outlined. Two themes are consistently evident in this Judeo-Christian tradition of sexuality. The first is the notion that the teachings of God, Biblical writers, and theologians are the only legitimate bases for sexual values. Second is the tendency to translate theologically derived values into *legalistic rules*. Legalistic rules are those that set forth in absolute terms what is right and wrong, allowed and disallowed, and in some instances how rule violations will be punished. As we shall see later in this chapter, many Judeo-Christian rules have been incorporated into our own legal codes of sexual conduct.

Situationism, Humanism, and Sexuality.   Theological legalism has been challenged in recent years both from within and outside of theology. From a Christian standpoint, Joseph Fletcher (1966) has been the leading proponent of what is known as situation ethics, or **situationism**. Situationists propose that moral and ethical decisions regarding sexuality as well as other matters be made not on the basis of absolute universal laws but on the basis of the characteristics of the situation a person finds himself or herself in. The guiding principle to be used is love and concern for the well-being of fellow humans. If decisions are based on this principle they are inherently moral and good. Thus, one's intentions in a particular situation determine whether a particular act is right or wrong regardless of the actual outcome of the act. For example, while the Judeo-Christian traditional point of view would insist that premarital intercourse is always wrong, situationism would say it is right if at least two conditions are met. First, another person must not be intentionally hurt or exploited by the sexual act. Second, the actual decision to engage in premarital intercourse must be motivated by love and concern for the welfare of those involved (Fletcher, 1966).

A second major challenge to traditional legalism is what is rather loosely called **humanism** (sometimes called the New Morality). As an approach to sexual ethics and morality, humanism rejects religious and supernatural sources as guidelines. Instead, humanism relies on the ability and obligation of the individual person to make his or her own sexual decisions and to take responsibility for them. The basic goal of life is seen as the pursuit of individual happiness but not at the expense of others. Faith is placed in the ability of people to make decisions guided by this goal rather than in theologically prescribed rules.

Situationism and humanism are, in part, the basis for what has been called the "New Morality" in contrast to the "Old Morality" dominated by legalistic and absolute rules of sexual conduct. Even though sexual values and attitudes have changed substantially during the last several decades, the New Morality has not replaced the Old Morality. Indeed, the voices of fundamentalist Christian morality arose loudly in opposition to situationism and humanism in the late 1970s and 1980s through groups such as the Moral Majority and others. Let us now consider some of the views of the Old (traditional) and New Moralities concerning specific sexual practices.

Religious Views of Sexual Practices

In this section we briefly examine how some common sexual practices are viewed within the context of Western religious values. Because many of these values are now being challenged by the views of situationists and humanists, our approach will be a comparative one. That is, we will compare the Judeo-Christian Old Morality with the New Morality that has recently emerged.

Heterosexual Intercourse. The Judeo-Christian tradition has always viewed marriage as the only legitimate context for sexual intercourse. Thus, premarital and extramarital intercourse are always wrong in the Old Morality.

The traditional opposition to premarital intercourse was originally based on concern over the welfare of unwanted children that potentially might result from intercourse. With the appearance of effective means of contraception, this objection has lost some of its meaning. However, since the traditional view also holds that the purpose of sex is procreation, even "protected" premarital intercourse is regarded as wrong. This position has been repeatedly reaffirmed by the Catholic leadership (Paul vi, 1968; Sacred Congregation for the Doctrine of the Faith, 1976).

In contrast to this "hard-line" approach, the New Morality would allow, but not necessarily encourage, premarital intercourse under certain conditions. If the decision is based on love and concern for all involved and another person is not harmed or exploited, premarital intercourse is allowable. The assumption is, of course, that people are able to evaluate their feelings accurately and to judge the potential harm that might result from the sexual act. Whether such assessments may be impassionately made by passionately involved couples is open to question. At any rate, neither situationists nor humanists condone impersonal, casual, or "promiscuous" sex.

Both the New and the Old Moralities view extramarital intercourse negatively. The Judeo-Christian view is that extramarital intercourse is sinful because it is an act of unfaithfulness to the laws of God. The New Morality takes a dim view of extramarital sex because it is seen as breaking the trust and commitment that should be involved in marriage. Extramarital relationships are seen as symptoms of problems in marriage and not to be absolutely condemned in all situations. Instead, restoration of love and commitment is encouraged so that the couple may establish a more satisfactory relationship, if possible.

Contraception.   The Roman Catholic and Orthodox Jewish opposition to "artificial" means of contraception and birth control remains steadfast. These so-called artificial means of contraception and birth control are any techniques other than periodic abstinence or the "rhythm methods" (see Chapter 3). For both of these groups, interference with conception or birth is seen as against natural law or the will of God, which is that the only purpose of sex be procreation.

The Catholic position is nicely summarized by Lynch (1968, p. 151):

Since [artificial means of contraception] interfere with the properly performed act of love in marriage, which intends the union of the sperm with the egg, these actions are contrary to the nature of the act and contrary to the nature of God's plan or the natural law and are, therefore, immoral or sinful.

In spite of this "official position" of the Catholic church, there is evidence that the majority of Catholics in the United States do use contraceptives of one kind or another (Westoff & Bumpass, 1973).

Most Protestants and relatively liberal Jews do not oppose the use of contraceptives. They recognize sex as serving purposes other than procreation. Within its proper context (marriage) sexual intercourse is acknowledged as a legitimate source of pleasure and expression of love. Furthermore, many argue that all children born should be wanted and that couples should be ready and willing to assume the responsibility of having and rearing children. The threat of a "population explosion" is sometimes cited as a moral basis for limiting family size as well. These groups join situationists and humanists, then, in arguing for the responsible use or non-use of contraceptives as determined by the specifics of the situation.

Abortion.   Abortion has become one of the most hotly debated issues of our time (see Chapter 3). For the most part it is an ethical debate and those who take either a pro or con stance are likely to be adamant in their views.

For the Roman Catholic church, the Orthodox Jews, and most conservative Protestant groups, abortion as a means of birth control is wrong. The Roman Catholic position is representative of the view of many who oppose abortion. Human life is regarded as beginning at the moment of conception and thus abortion is viewed as a premeditated termination of life, or murder. Logically it follows, of course, that Catholics must avoid and oppose the use of any contracep-

Two sides of the abortion controversy are expressed by marchers in this demonstration.

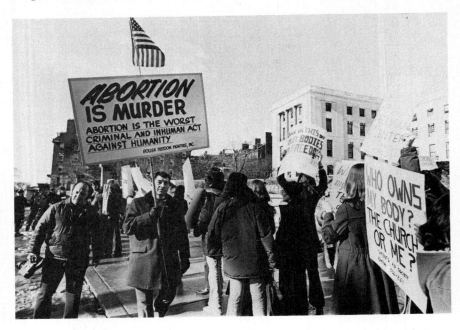

tives such as IUDs that terminate conception once it has occurred (Paul VI, 1968). "Right-to-life" groups generally adhere to the Catholic position that abortion is the same as murder.

The central assumption in this stance is that a fertilized ovum is a living human being from the moment of fertilization onward. Whether this assumption is "correct" or "incorrect" cannot be answered by scientific means. To be sure, the biological *potential* for human life is present in an embryo or fetus. But when does an embryo or fetus attain the status of living human being? This will be an issue of debate for some time and decisions at the individual level will remain a matter of personal faith and conviction.

Some liberal Protestant and Jewish groups accept abortion under some conditions. They condone therapeutic abortions performed to protect the physical or mental health of the woman or when the pregnancy results from rape or incest. Situationists argue that absolute rules or laws should not be imposed. Instead, the course of action that serves the greatest good should be followed. The quality of life that might face the unborn child, its mother, and other involved people should receive consideration. Yet another view is that abortion decisions should be left to the pregnant woman herself. Is it not her body and does she not have the right to determine what happens to it? Clearly, a consensus on this issue is unlikely to be reached in the near future.

Homosexual Behaviors and Homosexuality.   Historically, the Judeo-Christian tradition has been unbending in its condemnation of homosexual behaviors and homosexuality. From the Judeo-Christian point of view, homosexuality is unnatural (nonprocreative), nonmarital by definition, and against the will of God. According to some interpretations, the Old Testament documents the destruction by God of the city of Sodom for homosexual excesses. Others, however, question this interpretation (McNeill, 1976).

Regardless of the basis for it, most of today's Christian believers condemn homosexuality as sinful and unnatural. Biblical fundamentalists are particularly adamant in this stance. From some quarters, however, a somewhat different position has emerged. In a 1976 Vatican statement (Sacred Congregation for the Doctrine of the Faith, 1976), the Catholic church reaffirmed its insistence that *homosexual behaviors* are unacceptable but acknowledged that *homosexuality* (being homosexual) is not necessarily sinful. Homosexuals must simply accept celibacy as a sexual life-style. Various other Christian groups have expressed similar views.

More liberal theologians are even more accepting in their views of homosexuality. Indeed, the United Church of Christ and the Episcopal Church have ordained openly gay people as ministers or priests. Others argue that individuals' sexual orientation is irrelevant to their status as Christians. Instead, value is placed on the formation of relationships characterized by mutual love, respect, and commitment regardless of whether they are heterosexual or homosexual partnerships (Thielicke, 1964). Despite the tolerance of these views, however, many gays feel a sense of rejection by the Christian community (see Chapter 11). In many larger cities, congregations such as the Metropolitan Community Church have emerged to help fill the religious needs of gay Christians.

THE LEGAL CONTEXT OF SEXUALITY

Cultural and religious values define for societies what sexual activities are acceptable and unacceptable. In most societies these values are translated into rules of sexual conduct that may or may not be formally codified. Those discovered in violation of the rules may be subject to various "penalties" ranging from mild ridicule in some cases to death in others. Even when not discovered, violators often impose penalties upon themselves in the form of guilt feelings, doubts concerning their own "normality," or anxiety concerning possible detection by others. In modern societies, many sexual values and rules have acquired the status of legally enforceable laws. Our purpose in this section is to discuss the nature and some of the major features of sex laws in the United States.

The Nature of Sex Laws

It has been suggested that the United States probably has more laws regulating sex than any other country in the world (Slovenko, 1965). There are federal, military, state, county, and municipal laws that tell us what sex is legal and what is illegal. Because of the tremendous number of such laws and because they are constantly being changed, it would be impossible to compile a list that would not immediately be outdated. It is possible, however, to examine some of the bases for such laws and to categorize them into a few broad classes.

There is substantial debate concerning what the proper purposes of any laws might be (MacNamara & Sagarin, 1977; Packer, 1968; Slovenko, 1965). Historically,

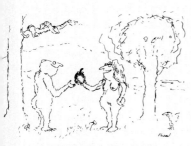

Although some people question the merit of such laws, there are many regulations that attempt to control sexual activity between consenting adults.

however, laws have been deemed necessary to (1) protect individuals, (2) protect the social order, and (3) preserve public morality (Slovenko, 1965).

In the realm of sexuality, laws to protect individuals include those against the use of force or coercion to obtain sexual gratification, against exploitation of the immature, and against sexual activities (for example exhibitionism) that might offend innocent bystanders. To preserve the family, which is considered the basic unit of the social order of society, there are laws against adultery. Similarly, laws against fornication were originally designed to help prevent out-of-wedlock births and to guarantee children a supportive family.

Perhaps the most controversial purpose ascribed to sex laws is that of preserving public morality. Morality is, in part, a matter of religion and it is a basic tenet of our constitution that religion and state should be separate. Nevertheless, from the Judeo-Christian tradition's insistence that sex is for procreation within the confines of marriage, we have (or have had) laws against homosexual behavior, oral-genital sex, anal intercourse, contraception, abortion, and other sex-related activities. Many such laws are being questioned by those who regard sex as a personal and private matter that should not be subject to legislation.

There are many potential ways that sex laws might be categorized, none of which are entirely satisfactory (MacNamara & Sagarin, 1977). However, three broad classes may be identified for the purpose of discussion. First are laws that apply to the sexual conduct of *consenting adults in private*. Included here are laws against fornication, adultery, oral-genital contacts, anal intercourse, and homosexual behaviors. Many authorities (Packer, 1968) think such laws should be eliminated. Second are laws against various *nonconsensual sexual acts* that involve force, coercion, or violence, exploitation of minors and others incapable of providing legal consent, and various public nuisance behaviors such as exhibitionism and voyeurism that occur without the consent of all involved parties. Finally there are laws against the *commercial use of sex* such as those prohibiting prostitution and the sale of obscene materials.

Some of the activities included in each of these categories are described in the following section. Note that the legal status of and penalties for these activities may vary from state to state. Note, too, that even though some of the laws may seem archaic and somewhat amusing, they define crimes and should be taken quite seriously.

The Law and Adult Consensual Sex

Most laws regulating the sexual activities of consenting adults in private are intended to keep sex within marriage, to limit sexual behavior to only those acts that are potentially procreative, and to preserve the integrity of the family. Clearly, such laws reflect the Judeo-Christian view of sexuality. Let us consider some of them.

Fornication. **Fornication** is a legal term referring to heterosexual intercourse between unmarried people. It is typically reserved for use in those instances that do not involve more serious violations such as rape, incest, or adultery. Many states have laws against fornication with penalties ranging from a small fine (ten dollars in Rhode Island) to imprisonment (three years in Arizona for *cohabitation* of unmarried men and women). Laws against fornication are being or have been dropped in many states. In states retaining such laws, prosecution is rare and tends to be selectively applied to the poor or racial minorities (MacNamara & Sagarin, 1977). It is perhaps fortunate that such laws are seldom enforced since the majority of American males and females violate them at some time in their lives (see Chapter 10). In this same context, we should also mention that *seduction* is illegal in some states. Seduction is a male's use of unfulfilled promises of marriage in order to have intercourse with a woman. Here females are considered victims and only males may be prosecuted, with penalties ranging from a few months to several years imprisonment (MacNamara & Sagarin, 1977).

Adultery. **Adultery** is heterosexual intercourse between two persons, at least one of whom is married to someone else. Adultery is a criminal offense in most states. In some it is only a misdemeanor punishable by fines. In others, however, it is a felony punishable by up to five years in prison. These penalties are rather tame compared to those of our Puritan forebears, who punished adulterers with death or branded the letter *A* on their foreheads. Adultery laws originated from a desire to protect the integrity of the family and, for many years, in New York adultery was the only offense considered sufficient grounds for divorce. Though few people approve of adultery, laws against it are rarely enforced and many think that they should be abolished (MacNamara & Sagarin, 1977).

Noncoital Heterosexual Behaviors. Laws dictate not only with whom one may have sex but also what sex acts are permissible. Many states, for example have statutes prohibiting even married couples from engaging in fellatio, cunnilingus, and anal intercourse. Of course, these same laws also apply to unmarried individuals. These prohibited behaviors are widely defined as "crimes against nature" and included under broadly and often vaguely written **sodomy** laws. The basis for considering such activities unnatural and crimes against nature is to be found in the Judeo-Christian tradition that the natural purpose of sex is reproduction and sexual behaviors that have no reproductive potential therefore violate the natural law.

The penalties for violations that these laws carry can be severe. For example, consensual sodomy in some states is a felony punishable by a fine of up to $5000 or up to twenty years in prison or both. Other states classify these behaviors only as misdemeanors and over a third of the states have repealed or reformed their sodomy laws (Boggan, Haft, Lister, & Rupp, 1975; MacNamara & Sagarin, 1977). Because of the increasing prevalence of these behaviors, particularly fellatio and cunnilingus, it is probably fortunate for most couples that the laws are rarely enforced against heterosexuals. Of course, most people conduct their sexual activities in private and discovery is unlikely. In practice, crime-against-nature and sodomy laws are most often invoked against gays (Boggan et al., 1975).

Contraception and Abortion. The traditional view that sex is for procreation has been reflected in laws that seek to control contraception and abortion. Until 1965, for example, laws existed to prevent the distribution of information concerning contraception even by physicians. Use of contraceptives was also prohibited by such laws. In *Griswold v. Connecticut* (1965) the Supreme Court invalidated the last remaining state law governing the use of contraceptives by married couples.

The court invoked the "right of privacy" in explaining its decision. In effect, it declared marital sexual activities to be private matters, at least concerning contraceptive practices. In a subsequent decision *(Eisenstadt v. Baird*, 1971), the court invalidated a Massachusetts law forbidding the distribution of contraceptive information to the unmarried.

Until the late 1960s all states had laws that severely restricted the rights of women to obtain abortions. Following various reforms in several states allowing abortion when the pregnancy resulted from incest or rape or threatened the physical or mental health of women, the U.S. Supreme Court declared unconstitutional all laws prohibiting abortion during the first trimester of pregnancy *(Roe v. Wade*, 1973). Abortions may, however, be regulated during the second and third trimesters. The ruling extended the right of privacy to decisions regarding abortion. As we noted in Chapter 3, subsequent rulings have established that a woman need not have the consent of her husband or parents to obtain an abortion and that the government need not provide funds to finance abortions. In combination with similar Congressional actions such as the 1977 Hyde Amendment, the decision on funding has had the effect of making legal abortions difficult for the poor and the young to obtain (Lincoln, Doring-Bradley, Lindheim, & Cotterill, 1977). Abortion is, of course, a highly emotional issue and so-called right-to-life and pro-choice forces will continue to battle in public, the legislature, and in the courts.

Homosexual Behaviors and Homosexuality.   In most of our states common homosexual acts are illegal. Laws that declare fellatio, cunnilingus, and anal intercourse unlawful apply regardless of the sex of the participants. As we noted above, though, most prosecutions for such "crimes against nature" or sodomy occur when people of the same sex, usually males, are involved. The penalties for convictions can be quite extreme, ranging up to twenty years of imprisonment. Homosexuality itself is not illegal. For one to be attracted to and to prefer same-sex people as sexual partners is no crime. In many jurisdictions, however, it is a crime actually to engage in sex with others of the same sex (Boggan et al., 1975).

It is relatively rare for someone to be arrested and prosecuted for engaging in specific homosexual acts because most take place in private. Arrests for homosexual behavior usually occur when the acts are performed in some public place such as a restroom, park, automobile, or theater. As we noted in Chapter 11, such places are common "cruising grounds" for gay males in some locales.

The majority of arrests, however, are made not for engaging in specific acts but for solicitation of such acts, loitering in public places, disorderly conduct, indecent exposure, or lewdness (Boggan et al., 1975). Most of these arrests occur when a police officer, acting as a decoy, hangs around a public restroom or other cruising ground for the purpose of enticing homosexuals to solicit sexual contacts. A second officer, observing the solicitation, makes the arrest and the decoy serves as a witness against the accused. Some argue that this practice is dangerously close to entrapment—inducing someone to commit a crime that they would not normally commit (Boggan et al., 1975; MacNamara & Sagarin, 1977). The practice is also controversial because it can be argued that police officers should be employed for the prevention of more serious crimes rather than spending time and money in the enticement of homosexuals (Slovenko, 1965).

More than a third of the states have now abolished or reformed laws that prohibit oral-genital and anal-genital sex when conducted by consenting adults in private. Thus many heterosexual and homosexual acts that were once illegal are now legal in these states. It is unlikely, however, that such changes will have much effect on the number of arrests and prosecutions of homosexuals since the majority are for solicitations in public places.

In 1976, the U.S. Supreme Court was provided an opportunity to declare unconstitutional all state antihomosexual laws. In upholding a state of Virginia law, however, it chose not to do so. Because of this decision, it is likely that further reform of these laws affecting homosexuals will be a legislative rather than a court process (MacNamara & Sagarin, 1977).

The Law and Nonconsensual Sex

Many authorities question whether it is the proper function of law to be concerned with the private sexual lives of consenting adults (MacNamara & Sagarin, 1977; Packer, 1968; Slovenko, 1965). Few, if any, question the role of law in regulating sexual activities that are performed without the informed legal consent of all participants. In this category are two classes of laws. First are those prohibiting the use of force or exploitation in sexual relations such as laws against rape and adult-minor sexual contacts. Second are laws pertaining to various "nuisance" behaviors such as voyeurism and exhibitionism that occur without the consent of at least one of the participants. Let us briefly examine each of these classes of laws.

Forcible Rape. In our extended discussion of the topic in Chapter 12, we noted the alarming increase in the number of forcible rapes reported during the last several years. From a legal standpoint, the most usual definition of **rape** is

the act of sexual intercourse with a female person not the wife of, or judicially separated from bed and board from, the offender, committed without her lawful consent. Emission is not necessary; and any sexual penetration, however slight, is sufficient to complete the crime. (Slovenko, 1965, p. 48)

Several aspects of this definition deserve attention. First, only a female can legally be a rape victim and only a man can be guilty of rape except when a woman assists a man in raping another woman. In this case the woman is an accessory to the crime. Second, in most jurisdictions a man cannot be guilty of raping his wife unless they are legally separated. This rather glaring exception to rape laws is changing in a few states, and in at least two cases men have been tried for raping their wives. The first, in Oregon, ended in acquittal and the second, in Massachusetts, resulted in the first conviction in the United States. Third, some penetration of the vagina by the penis must take place before a rape has legally occurred. Finally, it must be established that the woman did not willingly consent to have intercourse with the man.

Though the penalties for rape are among the most severe in the land, convictions in rape cases are rather difficult to obtain. In part, this is because many rapes go unreported or defendants are found guilty of lesser charges or are never apprehended (see Chapter 12). Another problem, however, and one that often becomes a major issue in rape trials, concerns the consent of the woman. Related to this, of course, is the inferred amount of force or coercion used by the defendant in accomplishing the act.

It must be concluded that the woman did not willingly consent to intercourse with the defendent and her previous sexual history with the defendant or other men is sometimes presented as evidence of her probable consent. In effect, some victims are put on trial by the humiliating and accusatory nature of the questions they must answer in court. Most states have now restricted presentation of the woman's sexual history and made it inadmissable as evidence. In some states, the amount of physical resistance shown by the victim is used as evidence relevant to her consent. Some courts require evidence of the utmost physical resistance (bruises, scars) while others recognize the very real possibility that some victims may show little physical resistance because of fear of additional injury or even death (MacNamara & Sagarin, 1977).

There are many directions that reform of laws dealing with rape might take. The American Law Institute (1962), for example, suggests a broadening of those conditions in which it can be said that a woman does not give legal consent to intercourse. This includes not only cases in which she submits by force or fear of injury but also those in which she is intoxicated, unconscious, otherwise mentally impaired, or falsely believes the man is her husband. Michigan law includes forced fellatio, cunnilingus, anal intercourse, insertion of objects other than the penis into the vagina or anus, and other types of sexual contacts, as well as forced penile-vaginal penetration, in its list of acts that are defined as varying degrees of rape.

Adult-Minor Sexual Contacts.   Although a few societies condone some form of adult-child sexual relations, most severely condemn such behavior. Most of our own states have laws against what is variously worded as carnal knowledge of a juvenile, statutory rape, contributing to the delinquency of a minor, or impairing the morals of a minor. These laws prohibit an adult male (usually over age 17 or eighteen) from having sexual intercourse with a female under the legal age of consent. From state to state the age of consent for females ranges from as young as twelve to as old as seventeen. These laws apply regardless of how old the female appears to be, how sexually mature she is, how much sexual experience she has, or whether she willingly or even eagerly consents to the intercourse. By definition, she cannot give legal consent (Slovenko, 1965).

The intent of these laws is to prevent the sexual exploitation of young females by older men. In reality, however, it is possible in some states for an eighteen-year-old male to be charged with statutory rape or one of the other listed offenses if he has intercourse with his sixteen-year-old girlfriend. This is a quite different situation from one in which a forty-year-old man has intercourse with a sixteen-year-old female. In order to differentiate such situations, some, including the American Law Institute (1962), suggest that an age differential should be specified in such laws. For example, if the female is under sixteen and the male is at least four years older, an offense might be charged.

Most states have, in addition to those noted above, laws against child molestation, indecent behavior with a child, or sexual abuse of a child. These prohibit adult sexual contacts or activities other than intercourse with the immature. The prohibited activities vary but may include genital and nongenital physical contact, solicitation, exhibitionism, or providing a child with pornography (Slovenko, 1965). In Chapter 12 we discussed some of these behaviors in detail. It is sufficient to note here that such acts may be subject to severe penalties (up to life in jail) and that the applicable laws suffer from many ambiguities. For example, definitions of "immaturity" are unclear and the prohibited acts are often not clearly specified. Nevertheless, most agree that some such laws are desirable and necessary.

Exhibitionism and Voyeurism. Most societies have rules and regulations regarding public exposure of body parts that are directly or indirectly involved in sexuality. Similarly, most societies demand that one's sexual activities be conducted in private and that others not observe such activities (Ford & Beach, 1951). In our own society, most jurisdictions have laws against genital exposure, public sexual activities, and viewing the sexual activities or sexual anatomy of others without their knowledge or consent.

In Chapter 12, we discussed exhibitionism as the public display of one's genitals to unwilling observers for purposes of sexual gratification. We also described some of the characteristics of those who do so (usually men) and the consequences of the acts. Here we are primarily concerned with the fact that such behavior is everywhere illegal in the United States. Convicted violators may face fines up to 5000 dollars and imprisonment up to five years or even indeterminate prison terms when "sexual psychopath" laws are invoked (Boggan et al., 1975; MacNamara & Sagarin, 1977).

Though the effects of such behavior on observer "victims" are usually limited to shock, surprise, fear, and sometimes even amusement, most people and authorities are in favor of laws regulating exhibitionism. There are, however, some problems with such laws. For example, the laws (usually against "indecent exposure") are often extended to apply to situations where the distinction between public and private is rather fuzzy. People have been convicted of indecent exposure for nude sunbathing in their backyards and for being nude in nudist camps. Another problem is that the laws often vaguely define the anatomy that cannot be displayed as "private parts." All are meant to include genitals and many include a woman's breasts, particularly the nipples. Thus, many "topless" dancers must use "pasties" or otherwise cover their nipples in many jurisdictions. In the case of topless or nude dancers, the willingness of the observers is usually not in question since most customers pay but the laws are often invoked anyway.

Voyeurs, or "peepers," are people (usually men) who receive sexual gratification by secretly viewing the opposite sex nude or the sexual activities of others without their consent. The penalties for voyeurism are usually light but may be extreme if the offender is prosecuted under sexual psychopath laws. Though it is unclear whether the usual peeper poses any serious threat to victims or society (MacNamara & Sagarin, 1977), most of us take for granted our right to privacy, particularly in sexual matters. Thus, most authorities see a continuing need for laws against voyeurism or peeping (MacNamara & Sagarin, 1977; Slovenko, 1965).

Exhibitionism and voyeurism are not only nonconsensual sexual behaviors but they also constitute a public nuisance and violate what many see as the moral sense of society. Many other sexual and sex-related behaviors share these characteristics and are likewise illegal in most locales. These include *transvestism* (cross-dressing for sexual purposes), *necrophilia* (having sex with corpses), *bestiality* (having sex with animals), *making obscene telephone calls*, and *frotteurism* (sexual touching of others without their consent). The penalties for such behaviors vary from state to state but most of the general public view laws against these activities as desirable (MacNamara & Sagarin, 1977).

The Law and Commercial Sex

The final class of laws that we will discuss are those that apply to the commercial exploitation of sexuality. More specifically, we will look briefly at laws dealing with prostitution and obscenity and pornography.

Prostitution.   **Prostitution** is generally defined as the exchange of sexual services for money. In its most recognized form, it involves a woman selling sexual services to a man. Less often it involves exchanges between two men and even less commonly a man selling his services to a woman. Prostitution is illegal everywhere in the United States except for a few counties in Nevada.

Often called the "oldest profession," prostitution has existed for centuries, sometimes in fully approved forms. In ancient Greek society, for example, prostitutes played a role in various religious rights and were institutionalized as "temple prostitutes." In medieval Europe prostitution was tolerated and in the Victorian era the British looked upon prostitution as a necessary evil that preserved the faithfulness of wives and the chastity of daughters.

In the United States prostitution takes various forms. In most large cities streetwalkers solicit customers on the streets or in bars. Groups of prostitutes may work in a brothel managed by a "Madam" who acts as a hostess and financial manager. Some massage parlors are small-scale versions of brothels in which, for an extra fee, the "massage" may include sexual intercourse or manual, or oral genital stimulation. Call girls are generally the highest class of prostitutes. They have rather select lists of clients, do not solicit from strangers, are highly paid, and are relatively safe from the police (MacNamara & Sagarin, 1977).

Male prostitutes who provide services for women are called **gigolos**. They are similar to call girls in that they provide companionship as well as sex for a female clientele that generally consists of wealthy middle-aged women. Men who sell their services to other men are referred to as hustlers. They are like female streetwalkers since they generally solicit strangers on the streets.

Most arrests and prosecutions for prostitution are actually for solicitation and usually involve streetwalkers. These arrests usually result either from periodic "sweeps" by the police in which prostitutes are rounded up or from solicitations enticed from prostitutes by police decoys. As we noted in connection with the arrest and prosecution of homosexuals, these practices are viewed by many as entrapment (MacNamara & Sagarin, 1977). It is rare for a prostitute's customer ("john") to be arrested. Convicted prostitutes are usually fined a rather small amount and then released to resume their activities. All other people who are involved in prostitution are also subject to prosecution in most jurisdictions. This

The Chicken Ranch, in Nye County, Nevada, is one of the few government-authorized houses of prostitution in the United States.

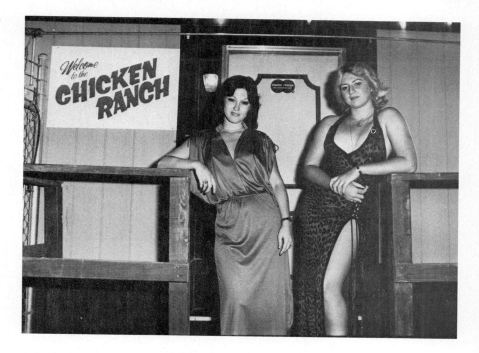

includes procurers (those who lure or coerce women into becoming prostitutes), pimps (those who solicit customers for prostitutes and share in their earnings), operators of houses of prostitution, and any others who contribute to prostitution (for example, cabdrivers or hotel clerks). As we noted above, however, most arrests and convictions are of the prostitutes themselves (Slovenko, 1965).

Laws defining prostitution as a crime are controversial. Enforcement is extremely difficult and involves amounts of money and police time that might, in the view of some, best be devoted to more serious crimes. It is also sometimes argued that prostitution is a victimless crime—one that does no legal harm to anyone and has no demonstrable victim. Thus, laws against prostitution may be seen as attempts at legal control of the morality of consenting partners—a questionable enterprise (Slovenko, 1965). Even though more serious crimes such as robbery, assault, and blackmail are sometimes associated with prostitution, it may be argued that this is so because prostitution is illegal. Some researchers believe that if it were decriminalized (penalties removed) and given the status of a legitimate business, perhaps some of the associated offenses and links with organized crime could be minimized (MacNamara & Sagarin, 1977). Indeed, an in-depth review of the issue resulted in the decriminalization of prostitution in Great Britain (Wolfenden, 1956). In the U.S., however, the American Law Institute (1962) recommends retention of laws against prostitution.

Pornography and Obscenity.   We have already noted the substantial amount of ambiguity that exists in sex laws and in the definitions of just what is illegal. This ambiguity is nowhere more apparent than in the area of regulations concerning pornography and obscenity. United States courts and legislative bodies have struggled with the related issues of whether to regulate explicit sexual materials and, if so, how to regulate such materials since the early 1800s.

In part, the major problem faced by the courts and lawmakers is one of definition. Though sometimes used interchangeably, the terms pornography and obscenity are not equivalent. **Pornography**, which is generally used to refer to materials (literature, art, films, etc.) that depict sexuality in a manner that is presumed to be sexually arousing, is not a legal term. Pornography is not illegal. **Obscenity** is a legal term that has been defined and redefined many times by lawmakers and the courts. The production, distribution, selling, and display of obscene materials is everywhere illegal in the United States.

But what is obscene? This question is at the heart of the legal issue since the U.S. Supreme Court *(Roth v. United States*, 1957) has ruled that obscenity is not protected by the First Amendment guarantee of freedom of speech and of the press and, by extension, of film, literature, and art. In the popular language, the word "obscene" refers to that which is foul, disgusting, lewd, and offensive. Following a number of earlier attempts, in 1973 *(Miller* v. *California*, p. 24) the Supreme Court provided the most recent legal definition of obscenity. It declared that the test for obscenity of materials is:

(a) whether "the average person, applying contemporary community standards" would find that the work, taken as a whole, appeals to the prurient interest, (b) whether the work depicts or describes, in a patently offensive way, sexual conduct specifically defined by the applicable state law, and (c) whether the work, taken as a whole, lacks serious literary, artistic, political, or scientific value.

This decision, in effect, returned the responsibility for defining obscenity to local communities using state laws. No national standard can now be said to exist. The major problem, as some see it, is that local community standards differ widely throughout the nation, and that what is obscene in a small rural community might not be in a large urban area. This situation has the potential for "prior censorship," in which an author, publisher, film producer, or artist might feel pressure to produce only material that would pass the most stringent test of obscenity. (Mac-Namara & Sagarin, 1977).

The need for laws regulating obscenity and pornography is usually justified by assuming that pornography is somehow harmful. Of major concern are the potential effects that pornography might have on children. There is, however, no evidence that children are affected in any way by such materials. Indeed, because of significant ethical and legal problems, it is now difficult, if not impossible, to investigate such concerns scientifically.

A second assumption is that exposure to pornography increases the probability of sex crimes. As we saw in Chapter 4, however, the scientific evidence does not support this claim. In fact, there are some data suggesting that sex crimes are less probable where explicit erotic materials are freely available. A third belief is that pornography is harmful simply because of its capacity to sexually arouse the average person. There is little doubt that explicit erotica does have a sexually arousing effect on most adults (see Chapter 4). Whether this is good or bad is, of course, a moral issue and one that science cannot answer. Whether sex laws should exist to regulate morals is as debatable here as in many other instances we have cited in this chapter.

SUMMARY

Human sexuality is influenced by the cultural, religious, and legal contexts in which it occurs. Each culture has its own views of the biological aspects of sexuality such as conception, pregnancy, and menstruation. The erotic code of a culture includes its view of sexuality as something good or bad and its inventory of cues that are defined as erotic and nonerotic. There are wide cultural variations in beliefs, attitudes, and practices associated with actual sexual behavior. Almost all societies take a rather dim view of masturbation in adults although some tolerate masturbation in children. It is likely, however, that some men and women do masturbate in every society. All societies regulate who may engage in heterosexual activity with whom. These regulations are tied to the ages of the people involved and to the relationships that exist among them. Though not the predominant form of behavior in any studied society, many societies are much more tolerant of homosexual behavior than is our own.

Most major religions have a great deal to say about sexuality. Western sexual values and beliefs have been strongly influenced by the Judeo-Christian tradition—a blend of Judaic and Christian teachings concerning sexuality. The central feature of this tradition is that it regards procreation as the primary purpose of sex and marriage as the only legitimate context for sex. From this standpoint, legalistic rules of what is right and wrong sexual behavior have evolved. Situationists and humanists object to the application of absolute rules to sexuality and suggest instead that sexual decisions be shaped by individual situations and personal concerns. Even so, our own society's views regarding heterosexual behaviors and many other aspects of sexuality continue to be strongly shaped by the Judeo-Christian tradition.

Cultural and religious values define for societies what sexual practices are acceptable and unacceptable. In most modern societies these values are translated into laws that carry penalties for violations. In our own society many sex laws are derived from Judeo-Christian theology. Laws that regulate the sexual conduct of consenting adults in private include those against fornication, adultery, oral-genital sex, anal intercourse, and homosexual behaviors, and those concerning sex-linked activities such as contraception and abortion. Many authorities think that these are private personal matters and should not be subject to public laws. A second class of laws regulates sexual activities that are performed without the legal consent of all involved participants. These include laws against rape, adult-minor sexual contacts, and "nuisance" behaviors such as exhibitionism and voyeurism. A final class of laws applies to the commercial exploitation of sexuality. Included are laws against prostitution and against obscenity and pornography. These are sometimes referred to as "victimless crimes" and many argue for the abolition of related laws.

SUGGESTED READINGS

Boggan, E. C., Haft, M., Lister, C., & Rupp, J. P. (1975). *The rights of gay people.* New York: Discus Books.

Bullough, V. L., & Bullough, B. (1977). *Sin, sickness, and sanity.* New York: Garland Publishing.

Cox, H. (Ed.) (1968). *The situation ethics debate.* Philadelphia: Westminster Press.

Ford, C. S., & Beach, F. A. (1951). *Patterns of sexual behavior.* New York: Harper.

MacNamara, D. E. J., & Sagarin, E. (1977). *Sex, crime, and the law.* New York: Free Press.

Marshall, D. S., & Suggs, R. C. (Eds.) (1972). *Human sexual behavior: Variations in the ethnographic spectrum.* Englewood Cliffs, N.J.: Prentice-Hall.

CONCLUSIONS

CHAPTER OUTLINE

CHAPTER 17

EMERGING TRENDS IN SEXUALITY

The last three decades have been witness to some dramatic changes in sexuality. Indeed, these changes have appeared to some so complete as to be revolutionary. In its most general usage, the term "revolution" refers to a complete or marked change through which traditional ways and thoughts are abandoned and replaced with new patterns.

In our own society, a sexual revolution would be reflected in changes that involve radical departures from the Judeo-Christian traditional view of sex. The two central features of this tradition are that (1) the primary if not sole purpose of sex is procreation and (2) the only fully legitimate form of and context for sex is heterosexual intercourse within marriage (see Chapter 16). Whether or not we are in the midst of a revolution that will overthrow these views is a matter of some debate (Gagnon, 1977). It is clear, however, that change is taking place and that change will continue in the future. Current and possible future changes involve both patterns of sexual behavior and the traditional linkage between sex and procreation.

SEX AND PROCREATION

Dramatic technological advances in recent years have made it increasingly possible to effectively separate sex from procreation. Innovations in contraceptive and reproductive technology have, in turn, affected sexuality in many ways. Let us examine some of these advances and possible breakthroughs of the future.

Contraception and Birth Control

It is probably safe to say that the development and introduction of the contraceptive pill during the 1950s has been one of the major factors in changing modern sexual attitudes and practices. The Pill made it possible to conveniently separate sex from conception and, in doing so, contributed to changes in sexuality. But the Pill and other contraceptive devices have their drawbacks, such as undesirable side effects, inconvenience, unreliability, and cost (see Chapter 3). We still search for the perfect contraceptive that is safe, convenient, reliable, inexpensive, and acceptable to users. What are some of the possibilities of the future?

Female Contraception.   With the exceptions of the condom and vasectomy, most contraceptive techniques are designed for women. Because of some of the disadvantages of devices such as the traditional Pill, the diaphragm, IUDs, and contraceptive foams (see Chapter 3), scientists continue to search for more satisfactory female contraceptives.

One of the disadvantages of hormonal contraceptive pills (the Pill) is that they must be taken daily in order to be effective. Potentially more convenient and less subject to error would be a longer-acting hormone that could be taken infrequently. One possibility under development and testing is long-acting injections of progesterone (the Shot) that provide protection for up to three months. Even though it is apparently very effective and in use in many foreign countries, the FDA has not approved Depo Provera, the trade name for the Shot, for use in the United States (Hatcher, Stewart, Stewart, Guest, Stratton, & Wright, 1980).

Also under investigation are under-the-skin implants that gradually release contraceptive hormones. Such implants may have the potential to provide contraception for up to five years or longer. A major problem is that the implanted capsules or pellets must be surgically removed (Hatcher et al., 1980). Other hormonal devices that show some promise include vaginal rings that secrete hormones that are absorbed through the vaginal wall, once-a-month hormonal doses, and even nasal sprays containing hormones. In addition, some scientists are searching for ways to immunize females against conception. This may work by inhibiting the implantation of a fertilized egg or stimulating the production of antibodies that destroy sperm. All of these techniques, however, are still in the experimental stage (Hatcher et al., 1980).

More effective mechanical contraceptives that avoid the side effects of hormones are also being developed. For example, a small sponge containing a spermicide may be inserted into the vagina to cover the cervix. It is easily inserted by the woman and may remain in place at all times except during the menstrual flow. At this time it is removed and washed and reinserted following menstruation. It acts both as a sperm barrier and spermacide. A small cervical cap made of rubber or plastic has been developed through the collaboration of a gynecologist and dentist. A custom-fitted cap about the size of a thimble is fashioned to cover the cervix. The cap is equipped with a one-way valve that allows menstrual flow out of the uterus but prevents semen and sperm from entering. The cap may be worn for long periods of time (McBride, 1980).

Sterilization has become an increasingly popular method of contraception. One disadvantage of sterilization is that virtually all procedures involve surgery and a relatively low probability of successful reversal (see Chapter 3). As an alternative to severing and tying the fallopian tubes, a relatively new procedure is undergoing testing in which the tubes are plugged with silicone. An instrument called a hysteroscope is inserted through the vagina and cervix into the uterus. The instrument is then used to pump liquid silicone into the fallopian tubes. The liquid solidifies and blocks the tubes. The procedure requires only about half an hour, may be done in a doctor's office, and involves no surgery or general anesthesia. There is also the possibility that reversal may be more successful than with conventional procedures ("Reversible Sterilization," 1979).

Male Contraception.   At this time the only truly effective methods of contraception for men with no serious side effects are the condom and vasectomy. The search for a safe, long-acting, convenient, and reversible male contraceptive, however, is an active one.

In 1979 the Chinese claimed to have developed a contraceptive pill for men that meets these requirements. The pill, called **gossypol**, contains derivatives from the cotton plant. It must be taken daily for a period of time (around three months) and less frequently at a maintenance level thereafter. It is said to work by suppressing sperm production. When he stops taking the pill, a man regains his fertility in about a year. The drug, however, causes weakness, nausea, stomach distress, and reduced appetite, which raises questions regarding its acceptability as a male contraceptive (Benditt, 1980; Maugh, 1981).

Another approach involves an implant that gradually releases hormones interfering with the production and growth of viable sperm. In animal tests, an implant containing the hormone prostaglandin has caused sterility for up to six months. This procedure has not been perfected for humans as yet ("And Birth Control Implant for Men Shows Promise," 1978).

Both testosterone and progesterone inhibit sperm production and both have been investigated as possible male contraceptives. Injections of such substances slowly produce sterility in men. There are, however, many side effects associated with these powerful hormones and it is unlikely that they will be approved for use in the near future (Hatcher et al., 1980).

It is doubtful that an adequate chemical contraceptive for males will become available soon. The major problem is that, in order to be effective, these substances must affect millions of sperm. In doing so, they also have a number of undesirable side effects. The search continues, however (Hatcher et al., 1980).

Procreative Alternatives

Advances in contraceptive technology have made it increasingly possible for heterosexual intercourse to occur without resulting in pregnancy and procreation. No longer must sex always or usually lead to procreation. On the other side of the coin, advances in reproductive technology have made procreation possible without intercourse. What are some of these advances and what developments might there be in the future?

Artificial Insemination.   Artificial insemination has been used successfully in animals for at least two hundred years. In this process, viable sperm are inserted into the vagina or cervix shortly before ovulation is expected and conception takes place as usual. The procedure is usually used in humans when a man's sperm count is low or he is otherwise sterile. In artificial insemination by the husband (AIH), several samples of the husband's ejaculate are collected and combined to make one sample with a higher sperm count. Artificial insemination by a donor (AID) may be used when the husband is sterile or for other reasons. It has been estimated that about 1 percent of all children born in the United States today are conceived through artificial insemination (Francoeur, 1974).

It is also possible to preserve sperm and semen by freezing. Thus, semen may be saved for possible future use by men who undergo vasectomies or medical treatments that might destroy or damage their own sperm. Several commercially operated sperm banks that provide such services are operational in the United States (Francoeur, 1974).

A highly controversial use of artificial insemination is in situations in which a woman is sterile but the couple wishes to have a child that is biologically the husband's. A *surrogate mother* might be paid or even volunteer to be artificially inseminated by the husband and then bear his child. Such procedures have been carried out in the United States. The controversy arises over possible legal and interpersonal questions concerning who is the mother of the child.

Ovum Transplantation (Test-Tube Babies).   The world's first so-called "test-tube baby" was born in 1978 to a British couple. Louise Brown was conceived outside her mother's body. An ovum was first removed from her mother Lesley Brown's ovary and fertilized in a culture dish with sperm from her father. After two and one half days of cell division, the fertilized egg was then implanted normally and the pregnancy was established. Following a fairly smooth pregnancy, the healthy baby was delivered by Caesarean section. At this writing, the healthy child has celebrated her sixth birthday.

Ovum transplantation is now a rather common procedure and one that is fairly widely available. It requires a great amount of skill that more and more medical specialists have developed. It offers some hope for those women who desire

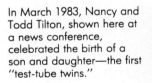

In March 1983, Nancy and Todd Tilton, shown here at a news conference, celebrated the birth of a son and daughter—the first "test-tube twins."

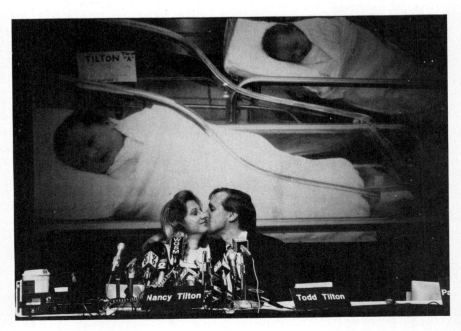

children but are infertile because of blocked, scarred, or otherwise nonfunctional fallopian tubes. Reproduction without intercourse is possible with this procedure. But it raises at least one difficult ethical and legal question. What is the status of the fertilized egg before it is transplanted to the woman's uterus? If the medical team judges the fertilized egg defective in some way are they free to discard it and terminate the procedure?

Looking ahead, we can see other potential controversies associated with ovum transplantation. As noted, surrogate mothering through artificial insemination creates questions surrounding who the real mother of the child is. The same issues may arise in another type of surrogate mothering. Suppose a woman other than the one who produced the egg could have the fertilized ovum implanted in her uterus. Who then is the "real" mother of the baby? Still another possibility is that a woman who cannot ovulate might "borrow" an egg from another woman to be fertilized by sperm from her own husband. The egg would then be implanted into her own uterus. Who is the biological mother in this instance—the woman who produced the egg or the woman who carried the child in pregnancy? Of course, the possibility of fertilization by sperm from a man other than a woman's husband also exists, as it does in artificial insemination by a donor.

Embryo Transplantation. **Embryo transplantation** is a procedure in which a developing embryo is removed from the uterus of one woman and transferred to the uterus of another woman, establishing a pregnancy in the second woman. Long used with livestock, the first successful embryo transplantation in humans was reported in the summer of 1983. Semen from an infertile woman's husband was used to artificially inseminate an ovum of a donor woman inside the donor woman's body. After around five days the fertilized egg was removed from the donor woman and placed in the uterus of the infertile woman, establishing a pregnancy. ("New Test Tube Research," 1983). This procedure, of course, raises many of the same controversies as does ovum transplantation.

Genetic engineering has now reached a stage where genetic scientists may modify and even create new life forms in the laboratory. Recombinant DNA technology makes it possible to remove and replace individual genes on chromosome structures. Combining ovum transplantation and genetic engineering technology, it may be possible in the future to select characteristics of people at the time of fertilization. One would hope, of course, that such undesirable characteristics as mental retardation, physical defects, and mental illness might be eliminated by such procedures. But who is to decide what characteristics are desirable and undesirable in human beings? Might not such technology be "misused" for social and political purposes as forecast by Aldous Huxley in *Brave New World*?

Advances in reproductive technology such as those described above do not and will not occur in a vacuum. Each brings with it a number of ethical and legal problems that require serious examination. Other potential breakthroughs loom on the horizon that promise still further possibilities (Francoeur, 1974). For example, *artificial wombs* in which a fertilized egg could be maintained until birth outside a woman's body are under study. **Cloning** is the reproduction of an organism from a single cell taken from that organism. In its simplest form this involves replacing the nucleus of an ovum with the nucleus of a body cell from a donor, resulting in an embryo that is a genetic duplicate of the donor. Cloning has received a large amount of publicity in recent years but, to date, has not been accomplished in humans.

FUTURE SEXUALITY

Throughout this book we have documented many ways in which sexuality has changed during the last several decades. We have seen rather dramatic changes in patterns of sexual behavior, attitudes about sexuality, and knowledge about sexuality. To be sure, there have been dramatic increases in our scientific knowledge about sexual functioning. Behaviorally and attitudinally the overall trend has been one of increased liberalization. What might we anticipate in the near future?

Predicting the future is risky business. Mostly we must rely on extrapolations from what appear to be current trends. But current trends can be deceiving. Some are simply short-lived fads that receive much publicity and others may be disrupted by major events such as technological advances, wars, or political and social upheavals. Undaunted by these potential hazards, we offer in the next few pages a few predictions that seem reasonable to us.

Heterosexual Patterns

In spite of the apparent reemergence of social and political conservatism in the United States during the late 1970s and early 1980s, we anticipate a continuation of the overall liberalization trend in heterosexual practices and attitudes. This should be evident both in nonmarital and marital heterosexual patterns.

Nonmarital Sex.   The prevalance of premarital intercourse has steadily increased during the last two decades (see Chapter 10). Almost all of the available evidence points to continuation of this trend (Gagnon, 1977; Hunt, 1974). It is likely that we will soon reach a point at which 85 to 90 percent of all males and females will have intercourse before marriage. The average age at which teenagers first have intercourse is now sixteen and nearly 80 percent of all teenagers have intercourse by the time they are nineteen (Alan Guttmacher Institute, 1981).

These increases in premarital intercourse have been accompanied by increased contraceptive use among the unmarried young. Unfortunately, however, the number of unwanted teenage pregnancies has continued to climb. This seems to be because many sexually active teenagers use relatively ineffective means of contraception such as withdrawal or contraceptive foam. Unless efforts to promote more effective contraceptive practices among unmarried teenagers are successful, we may expect to see continued rises in the prevalence of unwanted pregnancies, unwanted babies, teenage abortion, and teenage marriages with high probabilities of early divorce (Alan Guttmacher Institute, 1981).

In 1981 the Census Bureau reported that the number of unmarried couples cohabiting, or "living together," had tripled to over 1.5 million since 1970. Along with Census Bureau reports that people are postponing marriage to later ages or not planning to marry at all, this suggests that the prevalence of nonmarital sexual relations will continue to increase in the coming few years. Indeed, it seems clear that the unmarried are becoming more and more wary of traditional marriage and the relatively high divorce rate and seeking nonmarital heterosexual alternatives. The most likely of these alternatives to increase further appear to be nonmarital cohabitation and single living. It seems unlikely that some of the more exotic and unusual heterosexual partnerships such as "group marriage" and "communal marriage" will become much more prevalent (Gagnon, 1977; Hunt, 1974).

Marital Sex.   The nature of marriage has changed rather substantially during the last two decades. There has been a movement toward depolarization of gender roles. Many women are no longer content to assume the traditional role of "housewife," in which they are responsible for housework and child-rearing while their husbands hold jobs, make the money, and make the major family decisions (see Chapter 7). Economic necessity and the increasing liberation of women from traditional gender roles has brought more and more women into the labor force.

Accompanying these changes has been a substantial increase in the divorce rate and slight increases in the incidence of extramarital sex (Hunt, 1974; National Center for Health Statistics, June, 1983). Most of the people who divorce (5 out of 6 men and 3 out of 4 women) ultimately remarry ("Men Beat Women Back," 1981). This suggests that most people still view marriage as desirable but also that more and more people abandon marriages they find unsatisfactory.

Sex within marriage has changed as well. Married couples now engage in a wider variety of sexual activities (fellatio, cunnilingus, anal stimulation) than did couples of earlier generations (see Chapter 10; Hunt, 1974). Sex is increasingly viewed as something to be enjoyed by both men and women and as a means of improving the emotional quality of marriage rather than as a duty to be performed or a service to be rendered.

Taken together these trends suggest that future marriages may be of shorter duration than in the past. They may, however, be more intimate while they last; there is likely to be an increased emphasis on quality and a decreased emphasis on "til death do us part." Marital sex will be more varied and its quality will be an important factor determining whether the marriage continues or is terminated. As a social institution, however, marriage will endure even though it may take many different forms (Gagnon, 1977; Hunt, 1974).

Homosexual Patterns

The prevalence of homosexual behavior and homosexuality has not increased noticeably over the last several decades and there is little reason to expect increases in the near future (Gagnon, 1977; Hunt, 1974). Similarly, the American public continues to regard homosexuality as sinful and abnormal (see Chapter 11) and probably will do so in the near future.

In at least one way, however, homosexuality has changed rather substantially in recent years. It is more publicly visible today than ever before. Gay activists are making public stands and engaging in social and political battles to establish or maintain laws preventing discrimination on the basis of sexual preference. Some of these efforts have met with failure (Miami, Florida; Wichita, Kansas; and others). But, as people become more open and less concerned about various sexual lifestyles, civil rights legislation in favor of gays seems increasingly likely.

Economic necessity and changing gender roles of men and women may require us to rethink our views of traditional marriage.

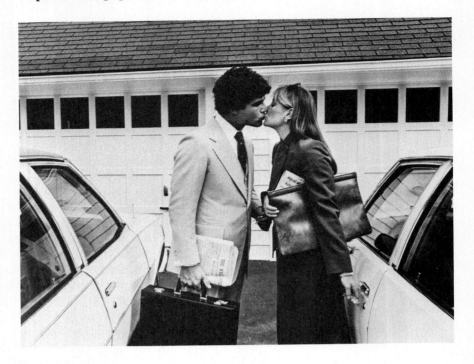

Continuing Concerns

Whatever the sexual agenda for the near future, we most certainly may expect continued struggle with some important issues. One of the most enduring controversies of recent years has been that concerning abortion. Foes of abortion and their supporters are likely to continue their press for Constitutional changes and legislative action to declare the time of conception as the beginning of human life. Abortion then would legally constitute murder. Those who support women's rights to have abortions will counter with arguments that human life cannot be said to begin until a fetus is able to survive outside the mother's body. Ultimately it is probable that the Supreme Court will find it necessary to settle the issue.

The pornography and obscenity debate will continue. Perhaps because it is impossible to do so to the satisfaction of any large majority, the courts will probably be unable in the near future to arrive at an acceptable national definition of obscenity. With all its attendant confusion, regulatory responsibility will remain at the state and local level. Regional inconsistency will continue to be the rule rather than the exception.

Finally, we anticipate that the trend toward overhauling some of our outdated sex laws will continue. Most authorities agree that revisions are sorely needed. This is particularly true where laws regulating the sexual conduct of consenting adults in private are concerned (see Chapter 16; MacNamara & Sagarin, 1977; Slovenko, 1965). Some of these efforts will not be popular but the trend seems well established and unlikely to change.

Glossary

Acquired immune deficiency syndrome (AIDS) A complex of health problems in which victims develop a serious loss of their natural immunity against disease. Thought to be transmitted by a body fluid-borne virus. The majority of AIDS victims are gay males. *439*

Adrenogenital syndrome (AGS) Hermaphroditism in a genetic female because of excess fetal and postnatal production of androgen by the adrenal glands. *180*

Adultery Legal term referring to heterosexual intercourse between unmarried persons, at least one of whom is married to someone else. *495*

Afterbirth The placental and other tissues expelled from the uterus following birth of a child. *73*

Agglutination (coagulation) A test for pregnancy in which the presence of human chorionic gonadotropin (HCG) is tested in the urine of a woman. *68*

Amniotic membrane The fluid-filled sac that forms around the embryo within the uterus. *67*

Anal intercourse Insertion of the penis into the anus. *289*

Analogous Similar in function to another entity. Examples are the penis in males and the vagina in females. *56*

Androgen The term used to refer to a group of hormones known as the "male" sex hormones. Androgen is produced in relatively large quantities by the testes and lesser quantities by the adrenal glands in males and in small quantities by the ovaries and adrenal glands in females. These hormones promote the growth of and maintain the male reproductive and sexual systems. They activate and maintain the sex drive in both sexes. *31*

Androgen-insensitivity syndrome (AIS) Feminization of the genitals of a genetic male due to inability of the male's body to respond to androgen. *183*

Androgynous Having both masculine and feminine characteristics. *208*

Anilingus Oral stimulation of the anus. *289*

Aphrodisiacs Substances meant to directly stimulate or enhance sexual desires. *112*

Areolae Pigmented areas of skin surrounding the nipples of the breasts. *36*

Artificial insemination The artificial introduction of semen into the vagina or uterus for the purpose of inducing fertilization. *67*

Asceticism A doctrine that indulging in bodily and material pleasures interferes with the "higher" spiritual or intellectual values of life. *488*

Autofellatio Self-stimulation of the penis by the mouth. *240*

Axillary hair Underarm hair. *38*

Bartholin's glands Two small glands located on either side of the vaginal entrance. *42*

Bestiality A sexual variation in which a person derives gratification from sexual contacts with nonhuman animals. *375*

Bisexuality   A sexual orientation in which people form identities of themselves as bisexuals and as being sexually attracted to and preferring people of both sexes as sexual partners.   *327*

Blastocyst   The fluid-filled ball of cells that forms around four to five days after fertilization of an ovum and eventually attaches to the lining of the uterus, becoming an embryo.   *66*

Candida albicans   A yeast or fungus that sometimes multiplies out of control in the vagina, causing irritation accompanied by a discharge.   *442*

Carpopedal spasm   Spastic contraction of the hands or feet as a result of intense sexual excitement.   *151*

Castration   Removal of the gonads (testes in males, ovaries in females).   *95*

Cervix   The lower or neck part of the uterus that opens into the vagina.   *45*

Celibacy   The state or practice of abstaining from sexual activity.   *488*

Chancre   The painless open sore or ulceration that is the first symptom of syphilis.   *434*

Chancroid   Sexually transmitted disease characterized by painful chancres on the genitals. Most common in the Far East and tropics.   *438*

Chorion   A membrane that develops around an embryo.   *49*

Chromosomes   Bodies in the nucleus of all cells that contain the genes, or hereditary code.   *30*

Climacterium   The mid-life cessation of ovarian functioning including reductions in estrogen and progesterone production, the end of fertility, and the cessation of menstrual cycling. Usually occurs between the ages of forty-five and fifty.   *54*

Clitoris   A small cylindrical structure located above the vaginal entrance in females; highly sensitive to sexual stimulation.   *42*

Cloning   The reproduction of an organism from a single cell taken from that organism. The resulting individual is genetically identical to the parent individual.   *511*

Coitus   Sexual intercourse between a male and a female in which the penis is inserted into the vagina.   *293*

Companionate love   The affection people feel for those with whom their lives are deeply intertwined.   *450*

Condom   A rubber or gut sheath that is placed over the penis for contraceptive purposes.   *85*

Conception   The fertilization of an ovum by a sperm.   *65*

Contraception   The use of methods, devices, or drugs permitting coitus between a fertile male and fertile female that prevents conception and/or pregnancy.   *73*

Coprophilia   A sexual variation in which a person derives sexual pleasure from feces or defecation.   *384*

Corona   The elevated ridge of tissue of the glans of the penis that is adjacent to the penile shaft.   *56*

Corpora cavernosa   Two cylindrical bodies of erectile tissue that run the length of the penis in the male and the clitoris in the female.   *56*

Corpus luteum   A yellow mass ("yellow body") of cells that develops in the cavity of the ovarian follicle after it releases an ovum at ovulation. The corpus luteum produces and secretes progesterone.   *35*

Corpus spongiosum   The cylindrical mass of erectile tissue running the length of the underside of the penis.   *56*

Culdoscopy   See *Endoscopic sterilization.*

Couvade   Practice in some societies in which the father of a child goes through a ritual sympathetic labor as the mother goes through the actual labor of childbirth.   *479*

Cowper's glands Paired glands that empty into the male urethra just below the prostate. They secrete a mucous substance during sexual arousal that is thought to neutralize the acidity of the urethra. *61*

Cremasteric muscles Muscles in the scrotum that elevate the testes. *58*

Culpotomy Female sterilization method in which the fallopian tubes are surgically severed through an incision in the vagina. *97*

Cunnilingus Oral stimulation of the female genitals. *285*

Culture The shared patterns of belief, thought, speech, and action of a society. *477*

Cystitis Inflammation and irritation of the urinary bladder. *442*

Diaphragm A rubber, cap-shaped contraceptive device that fits over the cervix. *81*

Diethylstilbestrol (DES) Powerful synthetic estrogen used in the "morning-after" pill to prevent pregnancy following unprotected coitus. *77*

Dildo An artificial penis. *244*

Dilation and curettage (D&C) Method of abortion usually used between the eighth and fifteenth weeks of pregnancy in which the cervix is dilated and the fetus is scraped from the uterus using a device called a currete. *100*

Dilation and evacuation (D&E) A vacuum method of abortion usually used between the thirteenth and sixteenth weeks of pregnancy in which the cervix is dilated and the fetus is sucked from the uterus. *100*

Douche To flush out the inside of the vagina with a liquid substance. *85*

Dysmenorrhea Painful menstruation usually experienced as cramping. *53*

Dyspareunia Painful coitus. *409*

Early abortion Vacuum method of abortion used in the first eight weeks of a confirmed pregnancy. *99*

Ectopic pregnancy An "out-of-place" pregnancy in which a fertilized egg implants outside of the uterus, in a fallopian tube, an ovary, or the abdominal wall. *44*

Edema Swelling caused by excessive fluid accumulation in a part of the body. *68*

Ejaculation The expulsion of semen from the penis, usually during orgasm. *156*

Ejaculatory duct The seminal duct passing from the junction of the vasa deferentia and seminal vesicle duct through a portion of the prostate and opening into the prostatic portion of the urethra. *60*

Embryo In humans, the term referring to the unborn from conception to the third month of pregnancy. *30*

Embryo transplantation A procedure in which a developing embryo is removed from the uterus of one woman and transferred to the uterus of a second woman, establishing a pregnancy in the second woman. *511*

Endometrial aspiration Vacuum method of abortion used in the first four to six weeks of a suspected but not confirmed pregnancy. *99*

Endoscopic sterilization Method of female sterilization in which a slender device (endoscope) is inserted through the abdomen (laporoscopy) or through the upper portion of the vagina (culdoscopy) and used to locate and sever the fallopian tubes. *97*

Endocrine glands Glands that secrete chemical substances called hormones directly into the bloodstream. *31*

Endometrium The inner lining of the uterus. *45*

Epididymes Paired coiled tubes attached to the testicles in which sperm are stored, matured, and transported to the vasa deferentia. *59*

Erectile dysfunction The inability of a male to achieve or maintain an erection sufficient for coitus or other desired sexual activities. Formerly called "impotence." *402*

Erection   The stiffening, hardening, and enlargement of the penis or clitoris as a result of vasocongestion during sexual arousal. *147*

Estrogen   The term used to refer to the hormones known as the "female" sex hormones. Estrogen is produced in relatively large quantities by the ovaries and in lesser quantities by the adrenal glands in females and in small quantities by the testes and adrenal glands in males. These hormones promote the growth of and maintain the female reproductive and sexual systems. *31*

Estrus   Recurring periods of sexual receptivity and fertility in nonhuman female mammals. Also called "heat." *110*

Exhibitionism   A sexual variation in which a person derives sexual gratification from exposing his or her genitals to others under socially inappropriate circumstances. *377*

Excitement phase   The first phase of the sexual response cycle. *144*

Fallopian tubes   Tubes extending from the ovaries to the uterus through which ova are conducted. *44*

Fellatio   Oral stimulation of the penis. Slang terms are "blow job," "giving head," and "going down." *285*

Fetishism   A sexual variation in which there is an unusually strong sexual interest in or sexual response to an inanimate object or to a particular body part. *360*

Fetus   In humans, the term referring to the unborn from the third month after conception to birth. *30*

Fimbriae   Fingerlike protrusions from the ends of the fallopian tubes that reach or are close to the ovaries. *44*

Follicles   Small ovarian capsules that contain ova at various stages of maturation. *43*

Follicle-stimulating hormone (FSH)   Pituitary hormone that stimulates the testes to produce sperm and the ovaries to begin the maturation of ova and the production of estrogen. *34*

Follicle-stimulating hormone-releasing factor (FSH-RF)   Substance secreted by the hypothalamus that stimulates the pituitary to release FSH. *35*

Foreskin   See *Prepuce.*

Fornication   Legal term referring to heterosexual intercourse between unmarried people. *494*

Frenulum   The skin tissue on the lower surface of the penis or clitoris that connects to the prepuce or foreskin of the penis or clitoris. *42*

Frottage   A sexual variation in which a person (frotteur) obtains sexual pleasure by rubbing or pressing against others (usually strangers) of the opposite sex. *379*

Fundus   Upper portion of the uterus. *45*

Gay   Term sometimes used to refer to homosexuals. *334*

Gender identity   A person's deep-seated sense of being a male or female. *177*

Gender role   People's views of themselves and others' views of them as masculine or feminine. *177*

Genes   The basic carriers of hereditary codes, contained in the chromosomes. *30*

Genital herpes   Sexually transmitted disease characterized by painful genital sores. Caused by the Herpes Type 2 virus. *436*

Genital tubercle   Primitive prenatal external genital structure that, under the influence of androgen, evolves into part of the penis in males and, in the absence of androgen, evolves into the body and glans of the clitoris in females. *33*

Genital warts *(Condylomata acuminata)*   Warts affecting the genitals. *443*

Germ cells   Reproductive cells—the sperm cells in males and ova, or egg cells, in females. *30*

Gerontophilia   A sexual variation in which a young person is erotically aroused by and prefers elderly persons as sex partners.   *374*

Gigolo   A male prostitute who sells sexual services to women.   *500*

Glans   The tip or head of the penis or clitoris.   *42*

Gonadotropins   Hormones secreted by the anterior pituitary that exert direct effects on the gonads.   *35*

Gonads   The sex glands. Paired glands in males (testes) and females (ovaries) that produce germ cells (sperm, ova) and sex hormones (androgens in males; estrogen and progesterone in females).   *30*

Gonorrhea   One of the most common of the sexually transmitted diseases.   *430*

Gossypol   Male contraceptive pill developed by the Chinese containing derivatives from the cotton plant.   *509*

Grafenberg spot   An area on the anterior vaginal wall that, when stimulated, first produces sensations of a need to urinate then intense sexual arousal. Thought to be associated with urethral glands that secrete fluids that may be expelled ("ejaculated") during orgasm by some women.   *154*

Granuloma inguinale   Rare sexually transmitted disease causing painful blisters around the genital area. Usually found in the tropics.   *438*

Hermaphrodite   An individual whose biological gender is ambiguous because of having a mixture of male and female reproductive structures.   *178*

Heterosexual behaviors   Sexual responses or behaviors directed toward those of the opposite sex.

Heterosexuality   A sexual orientation in which people form identities of themselves as heterosexuals and as being sexually attracted to and preferring opposite-sex people as sexual partners.

Homologous   Similar in structure and origin to another entity. Examples are the scrotum in males and the labia majora in females.   *55*

Homosexual behaviors   Sexual responses or behaviors directed toward others of the same sex.   *323*

Homosexuality   A sexual orientation in which people form identities of themselves as homosexuals and as being sexually attracted to and preferring same-sex people as sexual partners.   *323*

Human Chorionic Gonadotropin (HCG)   A hormone secreted by the chorionic membrane that surrounds an embryo. Its presence is tested for as a sign of pregnancy.   *49*

Humanism   An approach to ethical decision making that places responsibility on the decision maker rather than on absolute rules.   *490*

Hymen   A thin membrane of tissue that rings or partially covers the vaginal opening.   *42*

Hypothalamus   A part of the brain that regulates many body functions.   *36*

Hysterectomy   Surgical removal of the uterus.   *97*

Hysterotomy   A method of abortion in which the fetus is surgically removed through incisions through the abdomen and uterus.   *102*

Incest   Sexual contacts between close relatives (not husband or wife), variously designated by different states and by different societies.   *370*

Incest taboo   A prohibition of matings and sexual liaisons or relations between certain relatives.   *486*

Induced abortion   Deliberate termination of pregnancy in which an embryo or fetus is removed or expelled from the uterus before the fetus is able to survive on its own.   *98*

Inguinal canal   A passage in the male from the abdomen to the scrotum through which the testes normally descend prior to birth.   *58*

Interfemoral intercourse   Sexual activity in which the penis is rubbed between the thighs of the partner.   *329*

Interstitial-cell-stimulating   hormone   (ICSH)   See   *Luteinizing   hormone (LH).*   *35*

Interstitial cells   Cells in the testes that manufacture and secrete male sex hormones (androgen) and very small amounts of estrogen.   *60*

Intrauterine device (IUD)   Small plastic or metal device fitted into the uterus to prevent pregnancy.   *78*

Kegel exercises   Exercises to strengthen the muscles surrounding the vagina.   *417*

Klinefelter's syndrome   A chromosomal anomaly in which an individual has XXY sex chromosomes. Body type is male but the reproductive structures are incompletely masculinized.   *179*

Klismaphilia   A sexual variation in which sexual pleasure is derived from receiving or giving enemas.   *379*

Labia majora   The large, outer, fatty, liplike pads of tissue surrounding the external female genitals.   *42*

Labia minora   The smaller, inner, fatty, liplike pads of tissue surrounding the vaginal and urethral openings in females.   *42*

Labioscrotal swellings   Primitive prenatal external genital structures that, under the influence of androgen, evolve into the scrotum in males and, in the absence of androgen, evolve into the labia majora and mons pubis in females.   *33*

Laminaria   Stick-shaped mass of seaweed which, when inserted into the cervix, expands and causes cervical dilation. Sometimes used as part of abortion procedures.   *99*

Laparoscopy   See *Endoscopic sterilization.*

Laparotomy   Female sterilization method in which the fallopian tubes are surgically severed through small abdominal incisions ("Band-Aid" sterilization).   *97*

Lesbian   Term frequently used to refer to a female homosexual.   *346*

Liaisons   Nonpermanent sexual partnerships or unions motivated primarily by sexual needs.   *485*

LMP   Abbreviation for the date of the first day of the last menstrual period.   *68*

Luteinizing hormone (LH)   Pituitary hormone that stimulates ovulation in the female and the manufacture and release of progesterone from the corpus luteum of the ovary. Called interstitial-cell-stimulating hormone (ICSH) in males, it stimulates the testes to produce androgens.   *35*

Luteinizing hormone–releasing factor (LH-RF)   Substance secreted by the hypothalamus that stimulates the pituitary to release LH.   *36*

Lymphogranuloma venereum   Rare sexually transmitted disease affecting the lymphatic system—usually found in the tropics.   *438*

Masochism   A sexual variation in which sexual pleasure is obtained by receiving pain from a sexual partner.   *382*

Masturbation   Deliberate self-stimulation which is intended to produce sexual arousal.   *230*

Mateships   Relatively permanent sexual, social, and economic unions often recognized legally or religiously, as in marriage.   *485*

Menarche   The first menstrual period.   *38*

Menopause   The cessation of menstrual cycling caused by the cessation of ovarian functioning or climacterium. Usually occurs between the ages of forty-five and fifty. *54*

Menstrual cycle   Periodic changes in the lining of the uterus in preparation for pregnancy if conception occurs, including periodic shedding of portions of the lining during the menstrual period if conception does not occur. Each cycle lasts approximately one month. *38*

Menstrual period   Periodic (approximately monthly) discharge of blood and tissue from the lining of the uterus in the sexually mature, nonmenopausal, nonpregnant female. Also called menstruation or menses. *38*

Mini-Pill   Oral contraceptive pills that contain progestin only. *77*

Monogamous   Mateships involving one man and one woman. *485*

Mons pubis (or mons)   Fatty tissue that lies over the pubic bone and above the vulva in females. *41*

Morning-after pill   See *Diethylstilbestrol*. *77*

Mucosa   A membrane that secretes mucous, a thick slippery fluid. *46*

Müllerian ducts   Embryonic ducts that eventually develop into parts of the female internal reproductive system. In males, the Müllerian ducts degenerate and disappear. *31*

Müllerian inhibiting substance   Substance secreted by the fetal testes in males that suppresses the growth and causes the degeneration of the Müllerian ducts. *31*

Myometrium   The middle muscular layer of the uterus. *46*

Myotonia   Increased muscular tension. *144*

Necrophilia   A rare sexual variation in which a person is sexually attracted to and derives sexual gratification from corpses. *374*

Non-gonococcal urethritis (NGU)   An inflammation of the urethra not caused by gonorrhea. *433*

Nonspecific vaginitis   Inflammations and infections of the vagina not specifically caused by *Candida* or *Trichomonal* organisms. *442*

Nymphomania   A sexual variation in which a woman exhibits an extraordinarily high sex drive. *382*

Obscenity   Legal term used to refer to sexual materials that are offensive according to some standard of decency. *502*

Ophorectomy   Surgical removal of the ovaries. *97*

Orgasm   The peak of sexual arousal and the climactic release of sexual tension. The third phase of the sexual response cycle. *141*

Orgasmic dysfunction   Sexual dysfunction in which a female is unable to reach orgasm even though highly aroused. *406*

Orgasm phase   The third phase of the sexual response cycle during which orgasm occurs. *152*

Orgasmic platform   Term used by Masters and Johnson to refer to the swelling and thickening of the walls of the outer third of the vagina during the plateau phase of the sexual response cycle. *149*

Ova   Female reproductive cells, or eggs. Singular is *ovum*. After fertilization by the male sperm the ovum develops into a new member of the species. *30*

Ovarian cycle   Periodic occurrence in the ovaries of development of a mature ovum, ovulation, and production and secretion of estrogen and progesterone. Each cycle lasts approximately one month. *38*

Ovarian ligaments   Paired ligaments, each of which attaches one ovary to the uterus. *43*

Ovaries   The paired female sex glands that produce ova (eggs) and the hormones estrogen and progesterone. Located in the abdominal cavity. *43*

Ovulation   The release of a mature ovum from the follicle of an ovary. *48*

Ovum transplantation   The removal and transplantation of an ovum from a woman's ovary to a culture dish where it is combined with sperm. The fertilized ovum is then placed in the uterus for implantation. *67*

Parturition   The process of giving birth. *72*

Passionate love   A state of intense affectionate absorption in another person. Also sometimes called "romantic love." *449*

Pedophilia   A sexual variation in which an adult is erotically aroused by and/or derives gratification from sexual contacts with children. *366*

Penile plethysmograph   A device that, when attached to the penis, records changes in penis size. Used as a measure of male sexual arousal. *119*

Penis   The external male organ for copulation and urination. *56*

Perimetrium   The outer fibrous wall of the uterus. *45*

Perineum   The hairless area of skin between the scrotum and anus in males and between the vagina and anus in females. *151*

Pheromone   Airborne hormone like substance that acts as a sexual attractant in some species of animals and insects. *111*

Pill, The   Popular name for oral contraceptives consisting mostly of synthetic estrogens and progesterone. *74*

Pituitary gland   Endocrine gland located at the base of the brain. The anterior (frontal) portion secretes hormones that are important to sexual and reproductive functioning. *35*

Placenta   An organ that forms on the wall of the uterus through which a fetus receives oxygen and nutrients and eliminates waste products—"afterbirth." *49*

Plateau phase   The second phase of the sexual response cycle immediately preceding orgasm. *148*

Polyandrous   Mateships involving one woman and two or more men. *485*

Polygynous   Mateships involving one man and two or more women. *485*

Pornography   Term referring to materials (literature, art, film, etc.) that depict sexuality in a manner presumed to be sexually arousing. *502*

Postnatal   Following birth. *29*

Preejaculatory emission   The mucouslike liquid that sometimes appears at the opening of the penile urethra during the plateau phase of the sexual response cycle. Thought to be secreted by the Cowper's glands. Sometimes contains viable sperm. *152*

Premature ejaculation   A sexual dysfunction in which a male ejaculates too soon for his own and/or his partner's sexual satisfaction. *404*

Premenstrual syndrome   Emotional and/or physical discomfort experienced by some women shortly before menstruation. *52*

Prenatal   Before birth. *29*

Prepuce (foreskin)   The fold of skin that covers the glans of the uncircumcised male penis or the female clitoris. *42*

Progesterone   A hormone produced in females by the ovaries. Present in large quantities during pregnancy. *43*

Progestin   Synthetic progesterone. *75*

Progestin-induced hermaphroditism   Hermaphroditism in a genetic female offspring resulting from administration of progestin to the mother during pregnancy in an attempt to prevent miscarriage. *180*

Prostate   A glandular and muscular organ that surrounds the upper portion of the urethra and the ejaculatory duct in males. Secretions from the prostate make up much of the fluid content of semen.   *60*

Prostitution   The exchange of sexual services for money or other forms of payment.   *500*

Puberty   Period of physical and sexual maturation during which a child becomes capable of sexual reproduction.   *36*

Pubic lice (crabs)   Lice that infest and attach to the pubic hair.   *443*

Pubococcygeus (PC) muscle   Muscle surrounding the vaginal entrance.   *417*

Rape   Coitus performed without the consent of the woman. In forcible rape, force or threat of force is used. In statutory rape the female is too young legally to give consent. Specific definitions vary from state to state.   *384*

Refractory period   A period of time following orgasm during which a person (particularly a male) is not responsive to sexual stimulation.   *143*

Resolution phase   The fourth and last phase of the sexual response cycle during which the body returns to its nonaroused state.   *158*

Retarded ejaculation   A sexual dysfunction in which a male consistently cannot reach orgasm even though highly aroused.   *405*

Rhythm method   General term for birth control methods that involve abstaining from coitus during a woman's fertile period.   *88*

RU-486   Experimental female hormonal contraceptive that blocks the effects of progesterone, preventing successful implantation of a fertilized ovum in the uterine wall.   *78*

Sadism   A sexual variation in which sexual pleasure is obtained by inflicting pain upon a sexual partner.   *382*

Sadomasochism (S&M)   A sexual variation in which sexual pleasure is obtained by inflicting and/or receiving pain. Derived from the words *sadism* and *masochism*.   *382*

Saline abortion   A method of abortion used late in pregnancy (weeks 20 through 24) in which a saline solution is injected into the amniotic sac surrounding the fetus. Abortion usually occurs within 48 hours when the fetus is spontaneously expelled.   *100*

Satyriasis   A sexual variation in which a man exhibits an extraordinarily high sex drive.   *382*

Scrotum   The external sac or pouch of skin and muscles that contains the testes.   *57*

Semen   The fluid ejaculated from the penis during orgasm. In men who are fertile, it contains sperm.   *156*

Seminal vesicles   A pair of glands adjacent to the prostate and opening into the vas deferens in males. The seminal vesicles secrete a portion of the fluid content of semen that nourishes and activates sperm.   *60*

Seminiferous tubules   Coiled tubules in the testes in which sperm are produced.   *59*

Sensate focus   A set of exercises often used in sex therapy designed to heighten a person's or couple's sensual reactions to body stimulation. Also called "pleasuring."   *419*

Sex chromosomes   Chromosomes that carry the genetic codes for sex. Male germ cells (sperm) contain either X or Y sex chromosomes. Female germ cells (ova) contain only X sex chromosomes. The fertilization of an ovum by an X-bearing sperm will result in the conception of a female (XX). The fertilization of an ovum by a Y-bearing sperm will result in the conception of a male (XY).   *30*

Sex flush   The reddish blushlike appearance of the skin that sometimes occurs during sexual arousal.   *147*

Sexual apathy   Sexual dysfunction in which a person experiences little or no sexual desire.   *402*

Sexual dysfunction   A general term referring to problems in which people are unable to function sexually to their own and/or their partner's satisfaction.   *401*

Sexually transmitted disease (STD)   A disease that is contracted and spread primarily through intimate sexual contact. Also called venereal disease.   *429*

Sexual unresponsiveness   Term referring to a female sexual dysfunction in the arousal stage of the desire/arousal/orgasm sequence in which a woman is unable to become sexually aroused as indicated by lack of vaginal lubrication.   *406*

Shaft   Main cylindrical body of the penis or clitoris.   *42*

Situationism   An approach to ethical decision making on the basis of concrete situations and the individuals involved rather than on the basis of absolute rules.   *489*

Society   An enduring, cooperating, self-reproducing group of individuals with organized patterns of interrelationships.   *477*

Sodomy   Ambiguous legal term referring to a variety of sex acts such as anal intercourse, oral-genital contacts, sex relations with animals, and so forth.   *495*

Sperm   The male reproductive cells capable of fertilizing an ovum and thus bringing about conception.   *30*

Spermicide   A substance (foam, cream, jelly) that kills sperm.   *83*

Spermatic cord   A structure connected to each testicle containing the vas deferens and the testicular artery, vein, and nerve.   *58*

Spermatogenesis   The production of sperm.   *59*

Sterilization   A general term for procedures in which people are made incapable (usually permanently) of reproduction.   *91*

Straight   Term sometimes used to refer to heterosexuals.   *345*

Sweating phenomenon   The appearance of drops of lubricating fluid on the walls of the vagina early in the excitement phase of the female sexual response cycle.   *144*

Syphilis   One of the most serious of the sexually transmitted diseases. Primary stage symptoms consist of painless sores appearing on the skin at the site of entry of the causative organism. If untreated, the disease enters a secondary stage in which a rash appears on various parts of the body. A latent stage follows during which no overt symptoms are present. After several months or years late, or tertiary, stage symptoms may appear and the disease may result in death.   *433*

Testes   The male sex glands that produce sperm and androgenic hormones. Located in the scrotum.   *59*

Testosterone   One of the androgen hormones that produce and maintain male sexual characteristics and functioning.   *31*

Toxic shock syndrome (TSS)   A disorder caused by the abnormal growth of the bacterium *Staphylococcus aureus*, thought to be encouraged by tampon use. Symptoms include high fever, diarrhea, headache, and vomiting, and the disorder sometimes leads to death.   *50*

Transsexualism   A condition in which a person's (transsexual) gender identity is at variance with or opposite to his or her biological sex. Sometimes transsexuals seek and obtain sex reassignment, or "sex change," surgery.   *187*

Transvestism   Cross dressing or wearing the clothing of the opposite sex. As a sexual variation, fetishistic transvestism involves wearing the clothing of the opposite sex for the purpose of sexual gratification.   *363*

Tribadism   A form of female homosexual activity in which one woman lies atop the other and the two then thrust their genitals together.   *331*

Trichomonas vaginalis (trichomoniasis) Vaginal infection caused by a parasitic organism. *442*

Trimester A period of three months. Term used to refer to any one of the three time divisions of pregnancy. *68*

Tubal ligation A surgical method of female sterilization in which the fallopian tubes are cut, tied, or cauterized preventing sperm and ova from meeting. *44*

Tumescence Swelling due to congestion with fluids. *145*

Tunica dartos A layer of connective tissue and muscle in the scrotum that tightens and loosens the scrotal skin around the testes. *58*

Turner's syndrome A genetic anomaly in which a person has only an X sex chromosome (XO). Body type is female, ovaries are missing or incompletely developed, and stature is often short. *179*

Urethra The tube through which urine passes from the bladder to the outside of the body. *62*

Urethral folds Primitive prenatal external genital structures that, under the influence of androgen, evolve into part of the penis in males and, in the absence of androgen, evolve into the labia minora in females. *33*

Urethral meatus External opening of the urethra through which urine leaves the body. *56*

Urogenital slit Primitive prenatal external genital structure that, under the influence of androgen, evolves into the penile urethra in males and, in the absence of androgen, evolves into the vestibule of the vulva in females. *33*

Urolagnia A sexual variation in which a person derives sexual pleasure from urine or urination. *384*

Uterus The muscular and glandular pear-shaped organ in the female in which a fetus develops—the womb. *45*

Vacuum curettage Vacuum method of abortion used in the first twelve weeks of a confirmed pregnancy. *99*

Vacuum methods Methods of abortion performed up to the twelfth week of pregnancy in which the embryo or fetus is removed from the uterus by suction through a hollow tube. These include endometrial aspiration, early abortion, vacuum curettage, and dilation and evacuation (D&E). *99*

Vagina The barrel-shaped organ of the female extending from the vulva to the uterus into which the penis is inserted during coitus and through which a baby passes during birth. *45*

Vaginal photoplethysmograph A device that when placed inside the vagina records the volume of blood in the vaginal walls. Used as a measure of female sexual arousal. *131*

Vaginal spermicides Sperm-killing substances placed in the vagina for contraceptive purposes. *83*

Vaginismus A female sexual dysfunction in which strong spastic contractions of the muscles surrounding the vagina make penile-vaginal intercourse impossible. *409*

Vaginitis Inflammation and irritation of the vagina due to infection. *441*

Vasa deferentia The sperm ducts in males leading from the testes to the seminal vesicles. *58*

Vasectomy A surgical method of male sterilization in which the vasa deferentia are severed. *60*

Vasocongestion Congestion or engorgement of body tissues with blood or other fluids. *144*

Venereal disease (VD)   A disease contracted and spread primarily through sexual contact. Aslso called sexually transmitted disease.   *429*

Vestibular bulbs   Bulbs of erectile tissue that surround the vaginal opening and swell during sexual arousal.   *46*

Vestibule   The area surrounding the urethral and vaginal openings.   *38*

Vulva   The collective term for the external female genitals including the mons, clitoris, labia majora, labia minora, and the vaginal and urethral openings.   *41*

Voyeurism   A sexual variation in which a person derives an unusually great amount of sexual pleasure from secretly viewing sexual acts or nudes of the opposite sex.   *376*

Withdrawal (coitus interruptus)   A contraceptive practice in which the male withdraws his penis from the vagina just before ejaculation.   *88*

Wolffian ducts   Embryonic ducts that eventually develop into parts of the male internal reproductive system. In females, the Wolffian ducts degenerate and disappear.   *31*

References

Abarbanel, A. R. (1978). Diagnosis and treatment of coital discomfort. In J. LoPiccolo & L. LoPiccolo (Eds.), *Handbook of sex therapy*. New York: Plenum Press.

Abbot, S., & Love, B. (1972). *Sappho was a right-on woman*. New York: Stein & Day.

Abel, G. G., Barlow, D. H., Blanchard, E. B., & Guild D. (1977). The components of rapists' sexual arousal. *Archives of General Psychiatry, 34*, 895–903.

Abel, G. G., Barlow, D. H., Blanchard, E. B., & Mavissakalian, M. (1975). Measurement of sexual arousal in male homosexuals: Effects of instructions and stimulus modality. *Archives of Sexual Behavior, 4*, 623–629.

Abel, G. G., Blanchard, E. B., & Becker, J. V. (1978). An integrated treatment program for rapists. In R. T. Rada (Ed.), *Clinical aspects of the rapist*. New York: Grune & Stratton.

Abel, G. G., Murphy, W. D., Becker, J. V., & Bitar, A. (1979). Women's vaginal responses during R.E.M. sleep. *Journal of Sex and Marital Therapy, 5*, 5.

Abelson, H., Cohen, R., Heaton, E., & Suder, C. (1971). National survey of public attitudes toward and experience with erotic materials. In *Technical report of the Commission on Obscenity and Pornography* (Vol. 6). Washington, D.C.: U.S. Government Printing Office.

Abrams, R. H. (1943). Residential propinquity as a factor in marriage selection. *American Sociological Review, 8*, 288–294.

Abramson, P. R. (1973). The relationship of the frequency of masturbation to several aspects of personality and behavior. *Journal of Sex Research, 9*, 132–142.

Abramson, P. R., & Mosher, D. L. (1975). Development of a measure of negative attitudes toward masturbation. *Journal of Consulting and Clinical Psychology, 43*, 485–490.

Abramson, P. R., Perry, L. B., Rotblatt, A., Seeley, T. M., & Seeley, D. M. (1981). Negative attitudes toward masturbation and pelvic vasocongestion: A thermographic analysis. *Journal of Research in Personality, 15*, 497–509.

Adams, M. S., & Neel, J. V. (1967). Children of incest. *Pediatrics, 40*, 55–62.

Addiego, F., Belzer, E. G., Comolli, J., Moger, W., Perry, J. D., & Whipple, B. (1981). Female ejaculation: A case study. *Journal of Sex Research, 17*, 13–21.

Adelman, M. R. (1977). A comparison of professionally employed lesbians and heterosexual women on the MMPI. *Archives of Sexual Behavior, 6*, 193–201.

Alan Guttmacher Institute (1981). *Teenage pregnancy: The problem that hasn't gone away*. New York: Alan Guttmacher Institute.

Allgeier, E. R., & Fogel, A. F. (1978). Coital positions and sex roles: Responses to cross-sex behavior in bed. *Journal of Consulting and Clinical Psychology, 46*, 588–589.

Allgeier, E. R., Przbyla, D. P., & Thompson, M. E. (1978). *Planned sin: The influence of sex guilt on premarital sexual and contraceptive behavior*. Unpublished manuscript, State University of New York, Fredonia.

Alston, J. P., & Tucker, F. (1973). The myth of sexual permissiveness. *Journal of Sex Research, 9*, 34–40.

American Law Institute (1962). *Model penal code.* Philadelphia: American Law Institute.

American Psychiatric Association (1980). *Diagnostic and statistical manual of mental disorders* (3rd ed.). Washington, D.C.: American Psychiatric Association.

Amir, M. (1971). *Patterns in forcible rape.* Chicago: University of Chicago Press.

Amir, M. (1972). The role of the victim in sex offenses. In H. Resnik & M. Wolfgang (Eds.), *Sexual behaviors: Social, clinical, and legal aspects.* Boston: Little, Brown.

Amoroso, D. M., Brown, M., Pruesse, M., Ware, E. E., & Pilkey, P. W. (1971). An investigation of behavioral, psychological, and physiological reactions to pornographic stimuli. In *Technical report of the Commission on Obscenity and Pornography* (Vol. 8). Washington, D.C.: U.S. Government Printing Office.

Anchell, M. (1974). *Pornography: A psychiatrist's verdict.* Liguori, Missouri: Liguorian Pamphlets and Books.

And birth control implants for men show promise (1978, September 18). *Sexuality Today*, p. 3.

Ann Landers advises (1976, January 4). *Manhattan Mercury*, Kansas.

Annon, J. S. (1976). *Behavioral treatment of sexual problems.* New York: Harper & Row.

Annual summary for the United States, 1977: Births, deaths, marriages, and divorces (1978, December 7). *Monthly Vital Statistics Report.*

Antill, J. K., & Cunningham, J. D. Self-esteem as a function of masculinity in both sexes. *Journal of Consulting and Clinical Psychology*, 1979, *47*, 783–785.

Appel, F. C. (1970, August). "Just slip this into her drink . . ." *Playboy*, pp. 82–86, 176.

Arafat, I. S., & Cotton, W. L. (1974). Masturbation practices of males and females. *Journal of Sex Research*, *10*, 293–307.

Arafat, I. S., & Yorburg, B. (1973). Drug use and the sexual behavior of college women. *Journal of Sex Research*, *9*, 21–29.

Ard, B.N., Jr. (1974). Premarital sexual experience: A longitudinal study. *Journal of Sex Research*, *10*, 32–39.

Argyle, M. (1967). *The psychology of interpersonal behavior.* Baltimore, Md.: Penguin Books.

Argyle, M. (1975). *Bodily communication.* New York: International Universities Press.

Arkowitz, H. (1977). Measurement and modification in minimal dating behavior. *Progress in behavioral modification* (Vol. 5). New York: Academic Press.

Asayama, S. (1975). Adolescent sex development and adult sex behavior in Japan. *Journal of Sex Research*, *11*, 91–112.

Asayama, S. (1976). Sexual behavior in Japanese students: Comparisons for 1974, 1960, and 1952. *Archives of Sexual Behavior*, *5*, 371–390.

Athanasiou, R. (1972, July). French and American sexuality. *Psychology Today*, pp. 55–56, 86–87.

Athanasiou, R., Oppel, W., Michelson, L., Unger, T., & Yager, M. (1973). Psychiatric sequelae to term birth and induced early and late abortion: A longitudinal study. *Family Planning Perspectives*, *5*, 227–231.

Athanasiou, R., & Sarkin, R. (1974). Premarital sexual behavior and postmarital adjustment. *Archives of Sexual Behavior*, *3*, 207–225.

Athanasiou, R., Shaver, P., & Tavris, C. (1970, July). Sex. *Psychology Today*, pp. 39–52.

Atwood, R. W., & Howell, R. J. (1971). Pupillometric and personality test score differences of female aggressing pedophiliacs and normals. *Psychonomic Science*, *22*, 115–116.

Auerback, A. (1975). Fantasies during marital relations. In H. I. Lief (Ed.), *Medical aspects of human sexuality.* Baltimore: Williams & Wilkins.

Augustine, Saint (1950). The City of God (M. Dods, Trans.). New York: Modern Library. (Originally published after 412 A.D.)

Bain, A. (1868). *Mental and moral science*. London: Longmans, Green.

Baird, D. T., Horton, R., Longcope, C., & Taite, J. F. (1968). Steroid pheromones. *Perspectives in Biology and Medicine, 11*, 384–421.

Baker, M. J. (1974). *The effects in inequity of heterosexual behavior: A test for compensation in inequitable dating relationships*. A thesis submitted in partial fulfillment of the requirements for the degree of Master of Arts, Department of Sociology at the University of Wisconsin-Madison.

Bancroft, J., Jones, W., & Pullan, B. (1966). A simple transducer for measuring penile erection with comments on its use in the treatment of sexual disorders. *Behavior Research and Therapy, 4*, 239–241.

Bandura, A. (1969). *Principles of behavior modification*. New York: Holt, Rinehart & Winston.

Bandura, A. (1977). *Social learning theory*. Englewood Cliffs, N.J.: Prentice-Hall.

Bandura, A., Ross, D., & Ross, S. (1963). Imitation of film-mediated aggressive models. *Journal of Abnormal and Social Psychology, 66*, 3–11.

Barbach, L. G. (1976). *For yourself: The fulfillment of female sexuality*. Garden City, N.Y.: Anchor Books.

Barbaree, H. E., Marshall, W. L., & Lanthier, R. D. (1979). Deviant sexual arousal in rapists. *Behavior Research and Therapy, 17*, 215–222.

Barclay, A. M. (1970). The effect of female aggressiveness on aggressive and sexual fantasies. *Journal of Projective Techniques, 34*, 19–26.

Barclay, A. M. (1971). Information as a defensive control of sexual arousal. *Journal of Personality and Social Psychology, 17*, 244–249. (a)

Barclay, A. M. (1971). Linking sexual and aggressive motives: Contributions of "irrelevant" arousals. *Journal of Personality, 39*, 481–492. (b)

Barclay, A. M. (1973). Sexual fantasies in men and women. *Medical Aspects of Human Sexuality, 7*, 205–216.

Bardwick, J. M. (1971). *Psychology of women*. New York: Harper & Row.

Barlow, D. H., Becker, R., Leitenberg, H., & Agras, W. S. (1970). Mechanical strain gauge recording penile circumference change. *Journal of Applied Behavior Analysis, 3*, 73–76.

Baron, R. A. (1979). Heightened sexual arousal and aggression: An extension to females. *Journal of Research in Personality, 13*, 91–102.

Baron, R. A., & Byrne, D. (1977). *Social psychology: Understanding human interaction* (2nd ed.). Boston: Allyn & Bacon.

Barr, R. F., & Catts, S. V. (1974). Psychiatric opinion and homosexuality. *Journal of Homosexuality, 1*, 213–215.

Barry, H., III, Bacon, M. K., & Child, I. I. (1957). A cross-cultural survey of some sex differences in socialization. *Journal of Abnormal and Social Psychology, 55*, 327–332.

Bart, P. B. (1981). A study of women who both were raped and avoided rape. *Journal of Social Issues, 37*(4), 123–137.

Bartell, G. D. (1971). *Group Sex*. New York: Peter H. Wyden.

Bauman, K. E., & Wilson, R. R. (1974). Sexual behavior of unmarried university students in 1968 and 1972. *Journal of Sex Research, 10*, 327–333.

Bauman, K. E., & Wilson, R. R. (1976). Premarital sexual attitudes of unmarried university students: 1968 vs. 1972. *Archives of Sexual Behavior, 5*(1), 29–37.

Beach, F. A. (Ed.) (1965). *Sex and behavior*. New York: Wiley.

Beach, F. A. (1969, July). It's all in your mind. *Psychology Today*, pp. 33–35, 60.

Beach, F. A. (Ed.) (1977). *Human sexuality in four perspectives*. Baltimore: Johns Hopkins University Press.

Beach, F. A. (1978). Human sexuality in four perspectives. In F. A. Beach (Ed.), *Human sexuality in four perspectives.* Baltimore: Johns Hopkins Press.

Beardslee, D. C., & Fogelson, R. (1958). Sex differences in sexual imagery aroused by musical stimulation. In J. W. Atkinson (Ed.), *Motives in fantasy, action, and society.* Princeton, N.J.: Van Nostrand.

Bebbington, P. E. (1977). Treatment of male sexual deviation by use of a vibrator: Case report. *Archives of Sexual Behavior, 6,* 21–24.

Beigel, H. G. (1953). The meaning of coital postures. *International Journal of Sexology, 4,* 136–143.

Bell, R. R., & Bell, P. L. (1972). Sexual satisfaction among married women. *Medical Aspects of Human Sexuality, 6* (December), 136–144.

Bell, R. R., Turner, S., & Rosen, L. (1975). A multivariate analysis of female extramarital coitus. *Journal of Marriage and the Family, 37,* 375–384.

Bell, A. P., & Weinberg, M. S. (1978). *Homosexualities: A study of diversity among men and women.* New York: Simon & Schuster.

Bell, A. P., Weinberg, M. S., & Hammersmith, S. K. (1981). *Sexual preference: Its development in men and women.* Bloomington: Indiana University Press.

Belsey, E. M., Greer, H. S., Lal, S., Lewis, S. C., & Beard, R. W. (1977). Predictive factors in emotional response to abortion: King's termination study—IV. *Social Science and Medicine, 11,* 71–82.

Belzer, E. G., Jr. (1981). Orgasmic expulsions of women: A review and heuristic inquiry. *Journal of Sex Research, 17,* 1–12.

Bem, S. L. (1974). The measurement of psychological androgyny. *Journal of Consulting and Clinical Psychology, 42,* 155–162.

Bem, S. L. (1976). Probing the promise of androgyny. In A. G. Kaplan & J. P. Bean (Eds.), *Beyond sex-role stereotypes.* Boston: Little, Brown.

Bem, S. L. (1977). On the utility of alternative procedures for assessing psychological androgyny. *Journal of Consulting and Clinical Psychology, 45,* 196–205.

Bem, S. L. (1978). Beyond androgyny: Some presumptuous prescriptions for a liberated sexual identity. In J. Sherman & F. L. Denmark (Eds.), *Psychology of women: Future directions of research.* New York: Psychological Dimensions.

Benditt, J. M. (1980). Current contraceptive research. *Family Planning Perspectives, 12,* 149–155.

Benjamin, H. (1966). *The transsexual phenomenon.* New York: Julian Press.

Benjamin, H. (1967). The transsexual phenomenon. *Transactions of New York Academy of Sciences Series II, 29,* 428–430. (a)

Benjamin, H. (1967). Transvestism and transsexualism in the male and female. *Journal of Sex Research, 3,* 107–127. (b)

Bentler, P. M. (1968). Heterosexual behavior assessment—I. Males. *Behavior Research and Therapy, 6,* 21–25. (a)

Bentler, P. M. (1968). Heterosexual behavior assessment—II. Females. *Behavior Research and Therapy, 6,* 27–30. (b)

Bentler, P. M. (1976). A typology of transsexualism: Gender identity theory and data. *Archives of Sexual Behavior, 5,* 567–584.

Bentler, P. M., & Abramson, P. R. (1981). The science of sex research: Some methodological considerations. *Archives of Sexual Behavior, 10,* 225–251.

Bentler, P. M., & Peeler, W. H., Jr. (1979). Models of female orgasm. *Archives of Sexual Behavior, 8,* 405–423.

Berger, A. S., Gagnon, J. H., & Simon, W. (1971). Pornography: High school and college years. In *Technical report of the Commission on Obscenity and Pornography* (Vol. 9). Washington, D.C.: U.S. Government Printing Office.

Bergler, E. (1947). Analysis of an unusual case of fetishism. *Bulletin of the Menninger Clinic, 2*, 65–67.

Bergler, E. (1948). *Divorce won't help*. New York: Harper & Brothers.

Bermant, G., & Davidson, J. M. (1974). *Biological bases of sexual behavior*. New York: Harper & Row.

Bernard, F. (1975). An enquiry among a group of pedophiles. *Journal of Sex Research, 11*, 242–255.

Bernard, J. (1972). *The sex game*. New York: Atheneum.

Bernard, J. (1973). *The future of marriage*. New York: Bantam.

Bernstein, B. E. (1977). Effect of menstruation on academic performance among college women. *Archives of Sexual Behavior, 6*, 289–296.

Berscheid, E., Dion, K., Walster (Hatfield), E., & Walster, G. W. (1971). Physical attractiveness and dating choice: A test of the matching hypothesis. *Journal of Experimental Social Psychology, 7*, 173–189.

Berscheid, E., & Walster (Hatfield), E. (1974). Physical attractiveness. In L. Berkowitz (Ed.), *Advances in experimental social psychology* (Vol. 7). New York: Academic Press.

Berscheid, E., & Walster (Hatfield), E. (1978). *Interpersonal attraction* (2nd ed.). Reading, Mass.: Addison-Wesley.

Berscheid, E., Walster, E., & Bohrnstedt, G. (1972, July). Body image. *Psychology Today*, 57–66.

Berscheid, E., Walster, E., & Bohrnstedt, G. (1973, November). The body image report. *Psychology Today*, 119–123, 126, 128–131.

Bieber, I., Dain, H. J., Dince, P. R., Drellich, M. G., Grand, H. G., Gundlach, R. H., Kremer, M. W., Rifkin, A. H., Wilbur, C. B., & Bieber, T. B. (1962). *Homosexuality: A psychoanalytical study*. New York: Vintage.

Births, marriages, divorces, and deaths for 1981. (1982, March 30). *Monthly Vital Statistics Report*.

Blair, W. F. (1955). Mating call and stage of speciation in the *Microphyla olivacea–M. carolinensis* complex. *Evolution, 9*, 469–480.

Blau, P. M. (1968). Social exchange. In D. L. Sills (Ed.), *International encyclopedia of the social sciences* (Vol. 7). New York: Macmillan.

Blood, R. O. (1969). *Marriage*. New York: Free Press.

Blumstein, P. W., & Schwartz, P. (1977). Bisexuality: Some social psychological issues. *Journal of Social Issues, 33*(2), 30–45.

Bogen, I. (1974). Attitudes of women who have had abortions. *Journal of Sex Research, 10*, 97–109.

Boggan, E. C., Haft, M., Lister, C., & Rupp, J. P. (1975). *The rights of gay people*. New York: Discus Books.

Boston Women's Health Book Collective (1976). *Our bodies, ourselves* (2nd ed.). New York: Simon & Schuster.

Boszormenyi-Nagy, I., & Spark, G. M. (1973). *Invisible loyalties*. New York: Harper & Row.

Bragonier, J. R. (1976, October). Influence of oral contraception on sexual response. *Medical Aspects of Human Sexuality*, pp. 130–143.

Brannon, R. (1976). The male sex role: Our culture's blueprint of manhood, and what it's done for us lately. In D. David & R. Brannon (Eds.), *The forty-nine percent majority: The male sex role*. Reading, Mass.: Addison-Wesley.

Bremer, J. (1959). *Asexualization*. New York: Macmillan.

Briddell, D. W., & Wilson, G. T. (1976). Effects of alcohol and expectancy set on male sexual arousal. *Journal of Abnormal Psychology, 85*, 225–234.

Broderick, C. B. (1966). Sexual behavior among preadolescents. *Journal of Social Issues, 22*, 6–21.

Broverman, I. K., Vogel, S. R., Broverman, D. M., Clarkson, F. E., & Rosenkrantz, P. W. (1972). Sex role stereotypes: A current appraisal. *Journal of Social Issues, 28*, 59–78.

Brown, D. G. (1966). Female orgasm and sexual inadequacy. In R. Brecher & E. Brecher (Eds.), *An analysis of human sexual response*. New York: Signet.

Brownmiller, S. (1975). *Against our will: Men, women, and rape*. New York: Bantam.

Buhrich, N., & McConaghy, N. (1977). Can fetishism occur in transsexuals? *Archives of Sexual Behavior, 6*, 223–235. (a)

Buhrich, N., & McConaghy, N. (1977). The discrete syndromes of transvestism and transsexualism. *Archives of Sexual Behavior, 6*, 483–495. (b)

Bullough, V. L. (1974). Homosexuality and the medical model. *Journal of Homosexuality, 1*, 99–110.

Bullough, V. L. (1975). Sex and the medical model. *Journal of Sex Research, 11*, 291–303.

Bullough, V. L., & Bullough, B. (1977). *Sin, sickness, and sanity: A history of sexual attitudes*. New York: Garland.

Bunzl, M., & Mullen, S. (1974). A self-report investigation of two types of myotonic response during sexual orgasm. *Journal of Sex Research, 10*, 10–20.

Burgess, A. W., & Holmstrom, L. L. (1974). Rape trauma syndrome. *American Journal of Psychiatry, 131*, 981–986.

Burt, J. J., & Meeks, L. B. (1970). *Education for sexuality*. Philadelphia: Saunders.

Burt, M. R. (1980). Cultural myths and supports for rape. *Journal of Personality and Social Psychology, 35*, 217–230.

Butler, C. A. (1976). New data about female sexual response. *Journal of Sex and Marital Therapy, 2*, 40–46.

Byrne, D. (1974). *An introduction to personality*. Englewood Cliffs, N.J.: Prentice-Hall.

Byrne, D. (1976). The imagery of sex. In J. Money & H. Musaph (Eds.), *Handbook of sexology*. Amsterdam: Excerpta Medica.

Byrne, D. (1977, February). A pregnant pause in the sexual revolution. *Psychology Today*, pp. 67–68.

Byrne, D., & Byrne, L. A. (Eds.) (1977). *Exploring human sexuality*. New York: Thomas Y. Crowell.

Byrne, D., Fisher, W., & DeNinno, J. A. (1975). *Sexual explicitness and thematic content as determinants of the behavioral effects of erotic films*. Unpublished manuscript, Purdue University.

Byrne, D., Fisher, J. D., Lamberth, J., & Mitchell, H. E. (1974). Evaluations of erotica: Facts or feelings? *Journal of Personality and Social Psychology, 29*, 111–116.

Byrne, D., Jazwinski, C., DeNinno, J. A., & Fisher, W. A. (1977). Negative sexual attitudes and contraception. In D. Byrne & L. A. Byrne (Eds.), *Exploring human sexuality*. New York: Thomas Y. Crowell.

Byrne, D., & Lamberth, J. (1971). The effect of erotic stimuli on sex arousal, evaluative responses, and subsequent behavior. In *Technical report of the Commission on Obscenity and Pornography* (Vol. 8). Washington, D.C.: U.S. Government Printing Office.

Byrne, D., & Sheffield, J. (1965). Response to sexually arousing stimuli as a function of repressing and sensitizing defenses. *Journal of Abnormal Psychology, 70*, 114–118.

Carpenter, M. (1979, September 24). Physicians ponder popularity of pregnancy self-test kits. *Medical News*, p. 18.

Carrier, J. M. (1971). Participants in urban Mexican male homosexual encounters. *Archives of Sexual Behavior, 1*, 279–291.

Carrier, J. M. (1977). "Sex-role preference" as an explanatory variable in homosexual behavior. *Archives of Sexual Behavior, 6*, 53–65.

Centers for Disease Control (1977). *Abortion surveillance 1975.* Washington, D.C.: U.S. Government Printing Office.

Centers for Disease Control (1982, October). *Morbidity and Mortality Weekly Report: Annual Summary, 1981.*

Centers for Disease Control (1983, March). AIDS generates attention. *VD Interchange,* pp. 2–5.

Centers, R. (1949). Marital selection and occupational strata. *American Journal of Sociology, 54*, 530–535.

Chiazze, L., Jr., Brayer, F. T., Macisco, J. J., Jr., Parker, M. P., & Duffy, B. J. (1968). The length and variability of the human menstrual cycle. *Journal of the American Medical Association, 203*, 377–380.

Chilton, B. (1972). Psychosexual development in twins. *Journal of Biosocial Science, 4*, 277–286.

Christensen, A., & Arkowitz, H. (1974). Preliminary report on practice dating and feedback as treatment for collge dating problems. *Journal of Counseling Psychology, 21*, 92–95.

Christensen, H. T., & Gregg, C. F. (1970). Changing sex norms in America and Scandinavia. *Journal of Marriage and the Family, 32*, 616–627.

Claim of cure for herpes met with skepticism. (1983, June 24). *Honolulu Star-Bulletin,* p. A–14.

Clark, L., & Lewis, D. (1977). *Rape: The price of coercive sexuality.* Toronto: Women's Press.

Clark, M., & Gastel, B. (1978, August 7). All about that baby. *Newsweek,* pp. 66–71.

Clark, M., Nater, T., & Witherspoon, D. (1982, May 3). Testing a better birth-control pill. *Newsweek,* p. 85.

Clarke, A. C. (1952). An examination of the operation of residential propinquity as a factor in mate selection. *American Sociological Review, 17*, 17–22.

Clemens, L. G. (1967). Effect of stimulus female variation on sexual performance of the male deermouse, *Peromyscus manifulatis. Proceedings of the 75th Annual Convention of the American Psychological Association,* 119–120.

Clopper, R. R., Jr., Adelson, J. M., & Money, J. (1976). Postpubertal psychosexual function in male hypopituitarism without hypogonadotropinism after growth hormone therapy. *Journal of Sex Research, 12*, 14–32.

Coburn, J. (1978, May). Orgasm: Pleasure or tyranny? *Mademoiselle,* pp. 228–229, 265.

Cochran, W. G., Mosteller, F., & Tukey, J. (1954). *Statistical problems of the Kinsey report on sexual behavior in the human male.* Washington, D.C.: American Statistical Association.

Cohen, J., Seghorn, T., & Calmas, W. (1969). Sociometric study of the sex offender. *Journal of Abnormal Psychology, 74*, 249–255.

Coleman, J. C. (1976). *Abnormal psychology and modern life* (5th ed.). Glenview, Ill.: Scott, Foresman and Company.

Comfort, A. (1972). *The joy of sex.* New York: Crown.

Comfort, A. (Ed.). (1974). *More joy.* New York: Crown.

Commission on Obscenity and Pornography. (1970). *Report of the Commission on Obscenity and Pornography.* Washington, D.C.: U.S. Government Printing Office.

Conger, J. J. (1975). Proceedings of the American Psychological Association, Incorporated, for the year of 1974: Minutes of the annual meeting of the Council of Representatives. *American Psychologist, 30*, 620–651.

Constantine, L. L., & Constantine, J. M. (1973). *Group marriage.* New York: Collier Books.

Cook, M., & McHenry, R. (1978). *Nonverbal communication in sexual attraction*. New York: Pergamon Press.

Cosby, B. The regular way. *Playboy*, December 1968, pp. 288–289.

Cosentino, F., & Heilbrun, A. B. (1964). Anxiety correlates of sex-role identity in college students. *Psychological Reports, 14,* 729–730.

Cotton, W. L. (1974). Role-playing substitutions among homosexuals. *Journal of Sex Research, 8,* 310–323.

Crandall, V. J. (1969). Sex differences in expectancy of intellectual and academic reinforcement. In C. P. Smith (Ed.), *Achievement-related motives in children*. New York: Russell Sage Foundation.

Crépault, C., & Couture, M. (1980). Men's erotic fantasies. *Archives of Sexual Behavior, 9,* 565–581.

Croake, J. W., & James, B. (1973). A four year comparison of premarital sexual attitudes. *Journal of Sex Research, 9,* 91–96.

Cross, J. F., & Cross, J. (1971). Age, sex, race and the perception of facial beauty. *Developmental Psychology, 5,* 433–459.

Curran, J. P. (1977). Convergence toward a single sexual standard? In D. Byrne & L. Byrne (Eds.), *Exploring human sexuality*. New York: Crowell.

Curran, J. P., & Lippold, S. (1975). The effects of physical attraction and attitude similarity in dating dyads. *Journal of Personality, 43,* 528–529.

Curran, J. P., Neff, S., & Lippold, S. (1973). Correlates of sexual experience among university students. *Journal of Sex Research, 9,* 124–131.

Cvetkovitch, G., Grote, B., Bjorseth, A., & Sarkissian, J. (1975). On the psychology of adolescents' use of contraceptives. *Journal of Sex Research, 11,* 256–270.

Czaja, J. A., & Bielert, C. (1975). Female rhesus sexual behavior and distance to a male partner: Relation to stage of the menstrual cycle. *Archives of Sexual Behavior, 4,* 583–597.

Dalton, K. (1964). *The premenstrual syndrome*. Springfield, Ill.: Charles C. Thomas.

Dalton, K. (1969). *The menstrual cycle*. New York: Pantheon Books.

Dank, B. M. (1971). Coming out in the gay world. *Psychiatry, 34,* 180–197.

Darwin, C. (1952). The origin of species by means of natural selection. The descent of man and selection in relation to sex. In *Great books of the western world* (Vol. 49: *Darwin*). Chicago: Encyclopedia Britannica. (Originally published in 1871.)

D'Augelli, J. F., & Cross, H. J. (1975). Relationship of sex guilt and moral reasoning to premarital sex in college women and in couples. *Journal of Consulting and Clinical Psychology, 43,* 40–47.

D'Augelli, J. F., & D'Augelli, A. R. (1977). Moral reasoning and premarital sexual behavior: Toward reasoning about relationships. *Journal of Social Issues, 33,* 46–66.

Davenport, W. H. (1965). Sexual patterns and their regulation in a society of the southwest Pacific. In F. A. Beach (Ed.), *Sex and behavior*. New York: Wiley.

Davenport, W. H. (1978). Sex in cross-cultural perspective. In F. A. Beach (Ed.), *Human sexuality in four perspectives*. Baltimore: Johns Hopkins Press.

Davidson, J. M. (1972). Hormones and reproductive behavior. In H. Balin & S. Glasser (Eds.), *Reproductive biology*. Amsterdam: Excerpta Medica.

Davis, K. B. (1929). *Factors in the sex life of 2200 women*. New York: Harper & Row.

Davison, G. G. (1976). Homosexuality: The ethical challenge. *Journal of Consulting and Clinical Psychology, 44,* 157–162.

Dawkins, S., & Taylor, R. (1961). Non-consummation of marriage: A survey of seventy cases. *Lancet, 280,* 1029–1033.

Deaux, K. (1976). *The behavior of women and men*. Belmont, Calif.: Brooks/Cole.

Deaux, K., & Emswiller, T. (1974). Explanations of successful performance on sex-linked tasks: What is skill for the male, is luck for the female. *Journal of Personality and Social Psychology, 29*, 80–85.

Deaux, K., & Farris, E. (in press). Attributing causes for one's own performance: Effects of sex, norms, and outcome. *Journal of Research in Personality.*

de Beauvoir, S. (1952). *The second sex.* New York: Bantam Books.

DeFrancis, V. (1969). *Protecting the child victims of sex crimes committed by adults. Final report.* Denver: American Humane Association, Children's Division.

DeLameter, J., & MacCorquodale, P. (1979). *Premarital sexuality: Ideology, interaction, and behavior.* Madison: University of Wisconsin Press.

DeLora, J. S., & Warren, C. A. B. (1977). *Understanding sexual interaction.* Boston: Houghton Mifflin.

Dement, W. (1964). Experimental dream studies. In *Academy of psychoanalysis: Science and psychoanalysis* (Vol. 7). New York: Grune & Stratton.

Dermer, M., & Pyszczynski, T. A. (1978). Effects of erotica upon men's loving and liking responses for women they love. *Journal of Personality and Social Psychology, 36*, 1302–1309.

Diamant, L. (1970). Premarital sexual behavior, attitudes, and emotional adjustment. *Journal of Social Psychology, 82*, 75–80.

Diamond, M. (1977). Human sexual development: Biological foundations for social development. In F. A. Beach (Ed.), *Human sexuality in four perspectives.* Baltimore: Johns Hopkins University Press.

Diamond, M. (1982). Sexual identity, monozygotic twins reared in discordant sex roles and a BBC follow-up. *Archives of Sexual Behavior, 11*, 181–186.

Dickinson, R. L. (1949). *Atlas of human sex anatomy* (2nd ed.). Baltimore: Williams & Wilkins.

Dickinson, R. L., & Beam, L. (1931). *A thousand marriages. A medical study of sex adjustment.* Baltimore: Williams & Wilkins.

Donnerstein, E., & Berkowitz, L. (1978). Victim reactions in aggressive erotic films as a factor in violence against women. *Journal of Personality and Social Psychology, 41*, 710–724.

Donnerstein, E., & Hallam, J. (1978). Facilitating effects of erotica on aggression against women. *Journal of Personality and Social Psychology, 36*, 1270–1277.

Doty, R. L., Ford, J., Preti, G., & Huggins, G. R. (1975). Changes in the intensity and pleasantness of human vaginal odors during the menstrual cycle. *Science, 190*, 1316–1318.

Downing, G. (1972). *The massage book.* New York: Random House.

Driscoll, J. P. (1971, March-April). Transsexuals. *Trans-action*, pp. 28–31.

Eastman, W. F. (1972). First intercourse. *Sexual Behavior, 2* (March), 22–27.

Edgerton, M. T., Jr., & Meyer, J. K. (1973). Surgical and psychiatric aspects of transsexualism. In C. Horton (Ed.), *Surgery of the external genitalia.* Boston: Little, Brown.

Edwards, J. N. (1973). Extramarital involvement: Fact and theory. *Journal of Sex Research, 9*, 210–224.

Edwards, J. N., & Booth, A. (1974). Sexual behavior in and out of marriage: An assessment of correlates. *Journal of Marriage and the Family, 38* (February), 73–81.

Edwards, J. W. (1976). The concern for health in sexual matters in the "Old Society" and "New Society" in China. *Journal of Sex Research, 12*, 88–103.

Ehrhardt, A. A. (1973). Maternalism in fetal hormonal and related syndromes. In J. Zubin & J. Money (Eds.), *Contemporary sexual behavior.* Baltimore: Johns Hopkins University Press.

Ehrhardt, A. A. (1979, September). *Biological sex differences: A developmental perspective*. Paper presented at the meeting of the American Psychological Association, New York.

Ehrmann, W. (1959). *Premarital dating behavior*. New York: Holt, Rinehart & Winston.

Eichenlaub, J. E. (1961). *The marriage art*. New York: Dell.

Eisenstadt v. *Baird*. 405 U.S. 433 (1971).

Elias, J., & Gebhard, P. (1969). Sexuality and sexual learning in childhood. *Phi Delta Kappan, 50*, 401–405.

Ellis, A. (1961). Frigidity. In A. Ellis & A. Abarbanel (Eds.), *The encyclopedia of sexual behavior* (Vol. 2). New York: Hawthorn Books.

Ellis, H. (1942). *Studies in the psychology of sex* (2 vols.). New York: Random House.

Ellis, L. J., & Bentler, P. M. (1973). Traditional sex-determined role standards and sex stereotypes. *Journal of Personality and Social Psychology, 25*, 28–34.

English, H. B., & English, A. C. (1958). *A comprehensive dictionary of psychological and psychoanalytical terms*. New York: David McKay.

Epstein, A. W. (1975). The fetish object: Phylogenetic considerations. *Archives of Sexual Behavior, 4*, 303–308.

Erikson, E. H. (1964). *Childhood and society* (Rev. ed.). New York: W. W. Norton.

Etaugh, C., & Brown, B. (1975). Perceiving the causes of success and failure of male and female performers. *Developmental Psychology, 11*, 103.

Evans, D. R. (1968). Masturbatory fantasy and sexual deviation. *Behavior Research and Therapy, 6*, 17–19.

Evans, I. M., & Distiller, L. A. (1979). Effects of luteinizing hormone-releasing hormone on sexual arousal in normal men. *Archives of Sexual Behavior, 8*, 385–395.

Exline, R. (1972). Visual interaction: The glances of power and preference. In J. Cole (Ed.), *Nebraska Symposium on Motivation, 1971*. Lincoln, Neb.: University of Nebraska Press.

Eysenck, H. J. (1971). Personality and sexual adjustment. *British Journal of Psychiatry, 118*, 593–608.

Eysenck, H. J. (1972, November). Obscenity—officially speaking. *Penthouse*, pp. 95–102.

Eysenck, H. J. (1974). Personality, premarital sexual permissiveness, and assortative mating. *Journal of Sex Research, 10* (1), 47–51.

Eysenck, H. J. (1976). *Sex and personality*. Austin: University of Texas Press.

Farkas, G. M., & Rosen, R. C. (1976). Effect of alcohol on elicited male sexual response. *Journal of Studies on Alcohol, 37*, 265–272.

Farkas, G. M., Sine, L. F., & Evans, I. M. (1979). The effects of distraction, performance demand, stimulus explicitness, and personality on objective and subjective measures of male sexual arousal. *Behavior Research and Therapy, 17*, 25–32.

Farrell, R. A., & Morrione, T. J. (1974). Social interaction and stereotypic responses to homosexuals. *Archives of Sexual Behavior, 3*, 425–442.

Fasteau, M. (1974). *The male machine*. New York: McGraw-Hill.

Feather, N. T. (1969). Attribution of responsibility and valence of success and failure in relation to initial confidence and task performance. *Journal of Personality and Social Psychology, 13*, 129–144.

Federal Bureau of Investigation. (1981). *Uniform crime reports for the United States—1980*. Washington, D.C.: U.S. Government Printing Office.

Feldman-Summers, S., Gordon, P. E., & Meagher, J. R. (1979). The impact of rape on sexual satisfaction. *Journal of Abnormal Psychology, 88*, 101–105.

Feldman-Summers, S., , & Kiesler, S. B. (1974). Those who are number two try harder: The effect of sex on attributions of causality. *Journal of Personality and Social Psychology, 30*, 846–855.

Ferguson, J. (1975). Spanish fly. In H. I. Lief (Ed.), *Medical aspects of human sexuality*. Baltimore: Williams & Wilkins.

Ferguson, K. D., & Finkler, D. C. (1978). An involvement and overtness measure for lesbians: Its development and relation to anxiety and social Zeitgeist. *Archives of Sexual Behavior, 7*, 211–227.

Ferracuti, F. (1972). Incest between father and daughter. In H. Resnik & E. Wolfgang (Eds.), *Sexual behaviors: Social, clinical, and legal aspects*. Boston: Little, Brown.

Festinger, L. (1951). Architecture and group membership. *Journal of Social Issues, 1,* 152–163.

Festinger, L., Schachter, S., & Back, K. (1950). *Social pressures in informal groups*. New York: Harper & Brothers.

Field, H. S. (1978). Attitudes toward rape: A comparative analysis of police, rapists, crisis counselors, and citizens. *Journal of Personality and Social Psychology, 36*, 156–179.

Finger, F. W. (1975). Changes in sex practices and beliefs of male college students over 30 years. *Journal of Sex Research, 11*, 304–317.

Finkelhor, D. (1974). *Sexually victimized children*. New York: Free Press.

Firestone, S. (1970). *The dialectic of sex*. New York: Morrow Paperbacks.

Fisher, J. D., & Byrne, D. (1976). *Preliminary scaling of 40 erotic slides for sexual arousal and disgust*. Unpublished manuscript, Purdue University.

Fisher, K. (1983, July). Stress: The unseen killer in AIDS. *APA Monitor*, pp. 1, 20–21.

Fisher, S. (1973). *The female orgasm: Psychology, physiology, fantasy*. New York: Basic Books.

Fisher, W. A., Byrne, D., Edmunds, M., Miller, C. T., Kelley, K., & White, L. A. (1979). Psychological and situation-specific correlates of contraceptive behavior among university women. *Journal of Sex Research, 15*, 38–55.

Fisher, W. A., Fisher, J. D., & Byrne, D. (1977). Consumer relations to contraceptive purchasing. *Personality and Social Psychology Bulletin, 3*, 293–296.

Fisher, W. A., Miller, C. T., Byrne, D., & White, L. A. (1978). *Situational and personality determinants of responses to communicating a sexual message*. Unpublished manuscript, Purdue University.

Fleming, M., Steinman, C., & Bocknek, G. (1980). Methodological problems in assessing sex-reassignment surgery: A reply to Meyer and Reter. *Archives of Sexual Behavior, 9*, 451–456.

Fletcher, J. (1966). *Situation ethics*. Philadelphia: Westminster Press.

Ford, C., & Beach, F. A. (1951). *Patterns of sexual behavior*. New York: Harper & Row.

Foster, W. T. (Ed.). (1951). *The social emergency*. Boston: Houghton Mifflin.

Foucault, M. (1978). *The history of sexuality, Vol. 1: An introduction*. New York: Pantheon Books.

Fox, C. A., & Fox, B. (1969). Blood pressure and respiratory patterns during human coitus. *Journal of Reproduction and Fertility, 19*, 405–415.

Fraker, S., Agrest, S., Simons, P. E., Howard, L., Reese, M., & Huck, J. (1978, June 5). Abortion under attack. *Newsweek*, pp. 36–47.

Francoeur, R. T. (1974). The technologies of man-made sex. In R. T. Francoeur & A. K. Francoeur (Eds.), *The future of sexual relations*. Englewood Cliffs, N.J.: Prentice-Hall.

Frank, R. T. (1948). Dyspareunia: The problem of the general practitioner. *Journal of the American Medical Association, 136*, 361–365.

Fraser, A. F. (1968). *Reproductive behavior in ungulates*. London: Academic Press.

Freedman, M. (1975, March). Homosexuals may be healthier than straights. *Psychology Today*, pp. 28–32.

Freeman, E. W. (1978). Abortion: Subjective attitudes and feelings. *Family Planning Perspectives, 10*, 150–155.

Freud, S. (1957–1964). The interpretation of dreams. In J. Strachey (Ed.), *The standard edition of the complete psychological works of Sigmund Freud* (Vols. 4–5). London: Hogarth Press. (Originally published, 1900.)

Freud, S. (1957–1964). Three essays on the theory of sexuality. In J. Strachey (Ed.), *The standard edition of the complete psychological works of Sigmund Freud* (Vol. 7). London: Hogarth Press. (Originally published, 1905.)

Freud, S. (1957–1964). Creative writers and daydreaming. In J. Strachey (Ed.), *The standard edition of the complete psychological works of Sigmund Freud* (Vol. 9). London: Hogarth Press. (Originally published, 1908.)

Freud, S. (1925). Some psychological consequences of the anatomical distinction between the sexes. *International Journal of Psychoanalysis, 8,* 133–142.

Freud, S. (1933). *Collected papers.* London: Hogarth Press and the Institute for Psychoanalysis. (a)

Freud, S. (1933). *New introductory lectures on psychoanalysis.* New York: W. W. Norton. (b)

Freund, K., & Langevin, R. (1976). Bisexuality in homosexual pedophilia. *Archives of Sexual Behavior, 5,* 415–423.

Freund, K., Langevin, R., Wescom, T., & Zajac, A. (1975). Heterosexual interest in homosexual males. *Archives of Sexual Behavior, 4,* 509–518.

Freund, K., McKnight, C. K., Langevin, R., & Cibiri, S. (1972). The female child as a surrogate object. *Archives of Sexual Behavior, 2,* 119–133.

Freund, K., Nagler, E., Langevin, R., Zajac, A., & Steiner, B. (1974). Measuring feminine gender identity in homosexual males. *Archives of Sexual Behavior, 3,* 249–260.

Freund, M., & Davis, J. E. (1973). A follow-up study of the effects of vasectomy on sexual behavior. *Journal of Sex Research, 9,* 241–268.

Friday, N. (1974). *My secret garden: Women's sexual fantasies.* New York: Pocket Books.

Friday, N. (1980). *Men in love.* New York: Delacorte Press.

Friedan, B. (1963). *The feminine mystique.* New York: Norton.

Frieze, I. H. (1974, August). *Changing self-images and sex-role stereotypes in college women.* Paper presented at the meeting of the American Psychology Association, New Orleans.

Frisch, R. F., & Renelle, R. (1970). Height and weight at menarche and a hypothesis of critical body weights and adolescent events. *Science, 169,* 397.

Fromm, E. (1956). *The art of loving.* New York: Harper & Row.

Fuchs, K., Hoch, Z., Paldi, E., Abramovici, H., Brandes, J. M., Timor-Tritsch, I., & Kleinhaus, M. (1978). Hypnodesensitization therapy of vaginismus: In vitro and in vivo methods. In J. LoPiccolo & L. LoPiccolo (Eds.), *Handbook of sex therapy.* New York: Plenum Press.

Furstenberg, F. F. (1976). The social consequences of teenage parenthood. *Family Planning Perspectives, 8,* 148–164.

Gager, N., & Schurr, C. (1976). *Sexual assault: Confronting rape in America.* New York: Grosset & Dunlap.

Gagnon, J. H. (1977). *Human sexualities.* Glenview, Ill.: Scott, Foresman and Company.

Gagnon, J. H., & Simon, W. (1973). *Sexual conduct.* Chicago: Aldine.

Galbraith, G. G., & Mosher, D. L. (1968). Associative sexual responses in relation to sexual arousal, guilt, and external approval contingencies. *Journal of Personality and Social Psychology, 10,* 142–147.

Galbraith, G. G., & Mosher, D. L. (1970). Effects of sex guilt and sexual stimulation on the recall of word associations. *Journal of Consulting and Clinical Psychology, 34,* 67–71.

Gall, M. D. (1969). The relationship between masculinity-femininity and manifest anxiety. *Journal of Clinical Psychology, 25,* 294–295.

Galton, Sir F. (1884). Measurement of character. *Fortnightly Review, 36*, 179–185.

Gawin, F. H. (1978). Pharmacologic enhancement of the erotic: Implications of an expanded definition of aphrodisiacs. *Journal of Sex Research, 14*, 107–117.

Gebhard, P. H. (1965). Situational factors affecting human sexual behavior. In F. A. Beach (Ed.), *Sex and behavior*. New York: Wiley.

Gebhard, P. H. (1966). Factors in marital orgasm. *Journal of Social Issues, 12*, 88–95.

Gebhard, P. H. (1969). Fetishism and sadomasochism. *Science and Psychoanalysis, 15*, 71–80.

Gebhard, P. H. (1971). Premarital coitus among widows and divorcees. In P. Bohannan (Ed.), *Divorce and after*. New York: Anchor Books.

Gebhard, P. H. (1973). Sex differences in sexual response. *Archives of Sexual Behavior, 2*, 201–203.

Gebhard, P. H. (1975). *Mammalian sexual behavior*. Paper presented at the Institute for Sex Research, Bloomington, Indiana. (a)

Gebhard, P. H. (1975, July). *Paraphilias*. Paper presented at the Indiana University Institute for Sex Research, Bloomington, Indiana. (b)

Gebhard, P. H. (1976). The Institute. In M. S. Weinberg (Ed.), *Sex research: Studies from the Kinsey Institute*. New York: Oxford University Press.

Gebhard, P. H., Gagnon, J. H., Pomeroy, W. B., & Christenson, C. V. (1965). *Sex offenders*. New York: Harper & Row.

Geer, J. H., & Fuhr, R. (1976). Cognitive factors in sexual arousal: The role of distraction. *Journal of Consulting and Clinical Psychology, 44*, 238–243.

Geer, J. H., Morokoff, P., & Greenwood, P. (1974). Sexual arousal in women: The development of a measurement device for vaginal blood volume. *Archives of Sexual Behavior, 3*, 559–564.

Geer, J. H., & Quartararo, J. D. (1976). Vaginal blood volume responses during masturbation. *Archives of Sexual Behavior, 5*, 403–413.

Geertz, C. (1960). *The religion of Java*. Chicago: University of Chicago Press.

George, L. K. (1978). The impact of personality in social status factors upon levels of activity and psychological well-being. *Journal of Gerontology, 33*, 840–847.

Gerall, A. A. (1973). Influence of perinatal androgen on reproductive capacity. In J. Zubin & J. Money (Eds.), *Contemporary sexual behavior*. Baltimore: Johns Hopkins University Press.

Gerrard, M. (1977). Sex guilt in abortion patients. *Journal of Consulting and Clinical Psychology, 45*, 708.

Giese, H., & Schmidt, G. (1971). *Studenten-Sexualität*. Reinbek: Rowohlt, 1968. Cited in Eysenck, H. J., Personality and sexual adjustment. *British Journal of Psychiatry, 118*, 593–608.

Glass, C. R., Gottman, J. M., & Shmurak, S. H. (1976). Response acquisition and cognitive self-statement modification approaches to dating skills training. *Journal of Counseling Psychology, 23*, 520–526.

Glick, P. C. (1967, October). Permanence of marriage. *Population Index*.

Goffman, E. (1971). *Relations in public*. London: Penguin Press.

Goldberg, H. (1979). *The new male: From self-destruction to self-care*. New York: William Morrow.

Goldberg, P. (1968). Are women prejudiced against women? *Trans-action, 5*, 28–30.

Goldstein, B. (1976). *Human sexuality*. New York: McGraw-Hill.

Goldstein, M., Kant, H., Judd, L., Rice, C., & Green, R. (1971). Experience with pornography: Rapists, pedophiles, homosexuals, transsexuals, and controls. *Archives of Sexual Behavior, 1*, 1–15.

Golub, S. (1976). The effect of premenstrual anxiety and depression on cognitive function. *Journal of Personality and Social Psychology, 34*, 99–104.

Gonsiorek, J. C. (1977). Psychological adjustment and homosexuality. JSAS *Catalog of Selected Documents in Psychology*, 7, 45. (Ms. No. 1478.)

Goode, W. J. (1959). The theoretical importance of love. *American Sociological Review*, *24*, 38–47.

Gordon, D. C. (1972). *Self-love*. Baltimore: Pelican.

Gordon, M., & Shankweiler, P. J. (1971). Different equals less: Female sexuality in recent marriage manuals. *Journal of Marriage and the Family*, *33*, 459–466.

Gravitz, M. A. (1970). Large scale normal adult base-rates for MMPI "privacy" items: I. Sexual attitudes and experiences. *Journal of General Psychology*, *82*, 153–156.

Gray, S. W. (1957). Masculinity-femininity in relation to anxiety and social acceptance. *Child Development*, *28*, 203–214.

Green, R. (1975). Adults who want to change sex; adolescents who cross-dress; and children called "sissy" and "tomboy." In R. Green (Ed.), *Human sexuality: A health practitioner's text*. Baltimore: Williams & Wilkins.

Green, R., & Money, J. (Eds.) (1969). *Transsexualism and sex reassignment*. Baltimore: Johns Hopkins University Press.

Greenberg, J. S., & Archambault, F. X. (1973). Masturbation, self-esteem, and other variables. *Journal of Sex Research*, *9*, 41–51.

Greene, G., & Greene, C. (1974). *S-M: The last taboo*. New York: Grove Press.

Greene, W. (1971). Personality characteristics of female homosexuals. *Psychological Reports*, *28*, 407–412.

Griffin, S. (1976). Rape: The All-American crime. In S. Gordon & R. W. Libby (Eds.), *Sexuality today—and tomorrow*. North Scituate, Mass.: Duxbury Press.

Griffith, M., & Walker, C. E. (1975). Menstrual cycle phases and personality variables as related to response to erotic stimuli. *Archives of Sexual Behavior*, *4*, 599–603.

Griffitt, W. (1970). Environmental effects on interpersonal affective behavior: Ambient effective temperature and attraction. *Journal of Personality and Social Psychology*, *15*, 240–244.

Griffitt, W. (1973). Response to erotica and the projection of response to erotica in the opposite sex. *Journal of Experimental Research in Personality*, *6*, 330–338.

Griffitt, W. (1975). Sexual experience and sexual responsiveness: Sex differences. *Archives of Sexual Behavior*, *4*, 529–540.

Griffitt, W. (1977). Human sexuality. In M. Wertheimer & L. Rappoport (Eds.), *Psychology and the problems of today*. Glenview, Ill.: Scott, Foresman and Company.

Griffitt, W. (1978, November). *Stereotypes and realities of male and female sexuality*. Paper presented to the Society of Experimental Social Psychology, Princeton.

Griffitt, W. (1979). Sexual stimulation and sociosexual behaviors. In M. Cook & G. Wilson (Eds.), *Love and attraction*. New York: Pergamon Press.

Griffitt, W. (1981). Sexual intimacy in aging marital partners. In J. Marsh & S. Kiesler (Eds.), *Aging: Stability and change in the family*. New York: Academic Press.

Griffitt, W. (1983). Population control through effective contraception. In J. B. Calhoun (Ed.), *Perspectives on adaptation, environment, and population*. New York: Praeger.

Griffitt, W., & Kaiser, D. L. (1978). Affect, sex guilt, gender, and the rewarding-punishing effects of erotic stimuli. *Journal of Personality and Social Psychology*, *36*, 850–858.

Griffitt, W., May, J., & Veitch, R. (1974). Sexual stimulation and interpersonal behavior: Heterosexual evaluative responses, visual behavior, and physical proximity. *Journal of Personality and Social Psychology*, *30*, 367–377.

Griswold v. Connecticut, 381 U.S. 479 (1965).

Groth, A. N., & Birnbaum, H. J. (1978). Adult sexual orientation and attraction to underage persons. *Archives of Sexual Behavior*, *7*, 175–181.

Groth, A. N., & Birnbaum, H. J. (1979). *Men who rape*. New York: Plenum Press.

Haist, M., & Hewitt, J. (1974). The Butch-Fem dichotomy in male homosexual behavior. *Journal of Sex Research, 10*, 68–75.

Hamilton, G. V. (1929). *A research in marriage*. New York: Albert & Charles Boni.

Harford, T. C., Willis, C. H., & Debler, H. L. (1967). Personality correlates of masculinity-femininity. *Psychological Reports, 21*, 881–884.

Hariton, E. B., & Singer, J. L. (1974). Women's fantasies during sexual intercourse: Normative and theoretical implications. *Journal of Consulting and Clinical Psychology, 42*, 313–322.

Harlow, H. F. (1975). Lust, latency and love: Simian secrets of successful sex. *Journal of Sex Research, 11*, 79–90.

Harlow, H. F., & Harlow, M. K. (1965). The affectional systems in behavior of non-human primates. In A. M. Schrier, H. F. Harlow, & F. Stollnitz (Eds.), *Behavior of non-human primates: Modern research trends* (Vol. 2). New York: Academic Press.

Harper, R. A. (1965, May). Overcoming impotence. *Sexology*, pp. 680–682.

Harré, R. (1977). Friendship as an accomplishment. In Steve Duck (Ed.), *Theory and practice in interpersonal attraction*. New York: Academic Press.

Harry, J. (1974). Urbanization and the gay life. *Journal of Sex Research, 10*, 238–247.

Harry, J. (1977). On the validity of typologies of gay males. *Journal of Homosexuality, 2*, 143–152.

Hart, G. (1975). Sexual behavior in a war environment. *Journal of Sex Research, 11*, 218–226.

Hart, G. (1977). *Sexually transmitted diseases*. Burlington, N.C.: Carolina Biological Supply Co.

Hartman, W. E., & Fithian, M. A. (1974). *Treatment of sexual dysfunction*. New York: Jason Aronson.

Hatcher, R. A., Stewart, G. K., Stewart, F., Guest, F., Stratton, P., & Wright, A. H. (1978). *Contraceptive technology, 1978–1979*. New York: Irvington.

Hatcher, R. A., Stewart, G. K., Stewart, F., Guest, F., Stratton, P., & Wright, A. H. (1980). *Contraceptive technology, 1980–1981*. New York: Irvington.

Hatfield, E., Sprecher, S., & Traupmann, J. (1978). Men's and women's reactions to sexually explicit films: A serendipitous finding. *Archives of Sexual Behavior, 7*, 583–592.

Hatfield, E., Traupmann, J., Sprecher, S., Utne, M., & Hay, J. (1982). *Equity and intimate relations: Recent research*. Unpublished manuscript.

Hatfield, E., Utne, M. K., & Traupmann, J. (1979). Equity theory and intimate relationships. In Robert Burgess & Ted L. Huston (Eds.), *Social exchange in developing relationships*. New York: Academic Press.

Hatfield, E., & Walster, G. W. (1978). *A new look at love*. Reading, Mass.: Addison-Wesley.

Hay, J. (1978). *Children's sexuality*. Unpublished manuscript.

Haynes, S. N., & Oziel, L. J. (1976). Homosexuality: Behaviors and attitudes. *Archives of Sexual Behavior, 5*, 283–289.

Hebb, D. O. (1949). *The organization of behavior*. New York: Wiley.

Hedblom, J. H. (1973). Dimensions of lesbian sexual experience. *Archives of Sexual Behavior, 2*, 329–341.

Heer, D. M. (1966). Negro-white marriage in the United States. *Journal of Marriage and the Family, 28*, 262–273.

Heim, N., & Hursch, C. J. (1979). Castration for sex offenders: Treatment or punishment? A review and critique of recent European literature. *Archives of Sexual Behavior, 8*, 281–304.

Heiman, J. R. (1975, April). Women's sexual arousal. *Psychology Today*, pp. 90–94.

Heiman, J. R. (1977). A psychophysiological exploration of sexual arousal patterns in females and males. *Psychophysiology, 14*, 266–274.

Heiman, J. R., LoPiccolo, L., & LoPiccolo, J. (1976). *Becoming orgasmic: A sexual growth program for women*. Englewood Cliffs, N.J.: Prentice-Hall.

Helmreich R. L., Spence, J. T., & Holahan, C. K. (1969). Psychological androgyny and sex role flexibility: A test of two hypotheses. *Journal of Personality and Social Psychology, 37*, 1631–1644.

Henson, C., Rubin, H. B., & Henson, D. E. (1979). Women's sexual arousal concurrently assessed by three genital measures. *Archives of Sexual Behavior, 8*, 459–469.

Henson, D. E., & Rubin, H. B. (1971). Voluntary control of eroticism. *Journal of Applied Behavior Analysis, 4*, 37–44.

Herold, E. S. (1984). *Sexual behavior of Canadian young people*. Markham, Ontario: Fitzhenry and Whiteside.

Herold, E., Mottin, J., & Sabry, Z. (1979). Effect of Vitamin E on human sexual functioning. *Archives of Sexual Behavior, 8*, 397–403.

Hessellund, H. (1976). Masturbation and sexual fantasies in married couples. *Archives of Sexual Behavior, 5*, 133–147.

High, R. W., Rubin, H. B, & Henson, D. (1979). Color as a variable in making an erotic film more arousing. *Archives of Sexual Behavior, 8*, 263–267.

Hirsch, J. (Ed.). (1967). *Behavior—genetic analysis*. New York: McGraw-Hill.

Hite, S. (1976). *The Hite report*. New York: Dell.

Hite, S. (1981). *The Hite report on male sexality*. New York: Alfred A. Knopf.

Hobart, C. W. (1972). Sexual permissiveness in young English and French Canadians. *Journal of Marriage and the Family, 34*, 292–303.

Hoffman, M. (1968). *The gay world: Male homosexuality and the social creation of evil*. New York: Basic Books.

Hoffman, M. (1977). Homosexuality. In F. A. Beach (Ed.), *Human sexuality in four perspectives*. Baltimore: Johns Hopkins University Press.

Hollingshead, A. B. (1950). Cultural factors in the selection of marriage mates. *American Sociological Review, 15*, 619–627.

Hollister, L. (1974). Popularity of amyl nitrite as a sexual stimulant. *Medical Aspects of Human Sexuality, 8*(4), 112.

Holmstrom, L. L., & Burgess, A. W. (1980). Sexual behavior of assailants during reported rapes. *Archives of Sexual Behavior, 9*, 427–439.

Homans, G. C. (1974). *Social behavior: Its elementary forms* (Rev. ed.). New York: Harcourt Brace Jovanovich.

Hooker, E. (1965). An empirical study of some relations between sexual patterns and gender identity in male homosexuals. In J. Money (Ed.), *Sex research: New developments*. New York: Holt, Rinehart, and Winston. (a)

Hooker, E. (1965). Male homosexuals and their "worlds." In J. Marmor (Ed.), *Sexual inversion*. New York: Basic Books. (b)

Hoon, P. W., Wincze, J. P., & Hoon, E. F. (1976). Physiological assessment of sexual arousal in women. *Psychophysiology, 13*, 196–204.

Horner, M. S. (1972). Toward an understanding of achievement-related conflicts in women. *Journal of Social Issues, 28*, 157–175.

Howard, J. J., Reifler, C. B., & Liptzin, M. B. (1971). Effects of exposure to pornography. In *Technical report of the Commission on Obscenity and Pornography* (Vol. 8). Washington, D.C.: U.S. Government Printing Office.

Huey, C. J., Kline-Graber, G., & Graber, B. (1981). Time factors and orgasmic response. *Archives of Sexual Behavior, 10*, 111–118.

Hulka, B. S., Chambless, L. E., Kaufman, D. G., Fowler, W. C., Jr., & Greenberg, B. G. (1982). Protection against endometrial carcinoma by combination-product oral contraceptives. *Journal of the American Medical Association, 247*, 475–477.

Humphreys, L. (1975). *Tearoom trade: Impersonal sex in public places* (2nd ed.). Chicago: Aldine.

Hunt, M. (1969). *The affair*. New York: World Publishing.

Hunt, M. (1974). *Sexual behavior in the 1970's*. Chicago: Playboy Press.

Huntington, G. (1975, July). *Rape and rape investigation*. Paper presented at the Indiana University Institute for Sex Research, Bloomington, Indiana.

Husted, J. R., & Edwards, A. E. (1976). Personality correlates of male sexual arousal and behavior. *Archives of Sexual Behavior, 5*, 149–156.

Huston, T. L. (1973). Ambiguity of acceptance, social desirability and dating choice. *Journal of Experimental Social Psychology, 9*, 32–42.

Iliffe, A. H. (1960). A study of preferences in feminine beauty. *British Journal of Psychology, 51*, 267–273.

Imperato-McGinley, J., Peterson, R. E., Gautie, R. T., & Sturla, E. (1979). Androgens and the evaluation of male gender identity among male pseudo-hermaphrodites with 5∝ reductase deficiency. *New England Journal of Medicine, 300*, 1233–1237.

Istvan, J., & Griffitt, W. (1980). Effects of sexual experience on dating desirability and marriage desirability: An experimental study. *Journal of Marriage and the Family, 42*, 377–385.

Istvan, J., Griffitt, W., & Weidner, G. (1983). Sexual arousal and the polarization of perceived sexual attractiveness. *Basic and Applied Social Psychology, 4*, 307–318.

"J." (1969). *The sensuous woman*. New York: Lyle Stuart.

Jackson, E. D., & Potkay, C. R. (1973). Precollege influences on sexual experiences of coeds. *Journal of Sex Research, 9*, 143–149.

Jacobson, P. H. (1959). *American marriage and divorce*. New York: Rinehart.

James, J., & Meyerding, J. (1978). Early sexual experience as a factor in prostitution. *Archives of Sexual Behavior, 7*, 31–42.

James, W. H. (1974). Marital coital rates, spouses' ages, family size, and social class. *Journal of Sex Research, 10*, 205–218.

Janda, L. H. (1975). Effects of guilt, approachability of examiner, and stimulus relevance upon sexual responses to thematic apperception stimuli. *Journal of Consulting and Clinical Psychology, 43*, 369–374.

Jessor, S., & Jessor, R. (1975). Transition from virginity to nonvirginity among youth: A social-psychological study over time. *Developmental Psychology, 11*, 473–484.

Joe, V. C., & Kostyla, S. (1975). Social attitudes and sexual behaviors of college students. *Journal of Consulting and Clinical Psychology, 43*, 430.

Johnson, A. M. (1953). Factors in the etiology of fixations and symptom choice. *Psychoanalytic Quarterly, 22*, 475–496.

Jones, J. R. (1974). Plasma testosterone concentrations in female transsexuals. In D. R. Laub & P. Gandy (Eds.), *Proceedings of the Second Interdisciplinary Symposium on the Gender Dysphoria Syndrome*. Ann Arbor, Mich.: Edward Brothers.

Jones, K. L., Shainberg, L. W., & Byer, C. O. (1977). *Sex and people*. New York: Harper & Row.

Jones, W. H., Chernovetz, M. E. O'C., & Hansson, R. O. (1968). The enigma of androgyny: Differential implications for males and females? *Journal of Consulting and Clinical Psychology, 46*, 298–313.

Jong, E. (1973). *Fear of flying*. New York: Signet.

Jovanovic, U. J. (1971). The recording of physiological evidence of genital arousal in human males and females. *Archives of Sexual Behavior, 1*, 309–320.

Kaats, G. R., & Davis, K. E. (1970). The dynamics of sexual behavior of college students. *Journal of Marriage and the Family, 32*, 390–399.

Kagan, J. (1958). The concept of identification. *Psychological Review*, *65*, 296–305.

Kagan, J. (1964). Acquisition and significance of sex typing and sex role identity. In M. L. Hoffman & L. W. Hoffman (Eds.), *Review of child development research* (Vol. 1). New York: Russell Sage Foundation.

Kantner, J. F., & Zelnik, M. (1972). Sexual experience of young unmarried women in the United States. *Family Planning Perspectives*, *4*, 9–18.

Kantorowitz, D. A. (1978). Personality and conditioning of tumescence and detumescence. *Behavior Research and Therapy*, *16*, 117–123.

Kaplan, A. G., & Bean, J. P. (Eds.). (1976). *Beyond sex-role stereotypes*. Boston: Little, Brown.

Kaplan, H. S. (1974). *The new sex therapy*. New York: Brunner/Mazel.

Kaplan, H. S. (1979). *Disorders of sexual desire*. New York: Simon & Schuster.

Kaplan, L. J. (1978). *Oneness and separateness: From infant to individual*. New York: Simon & Schuster.

Karacan, I., Williams, R. L., Guerrero, M. W., Salis, P. J., Thornby, J. I., & Hursch, C. J. (1974). Nocturnal penile tumescence and sleep of convicted rapists and other prisoners. *Archives of Sexual Behvior*, *3*, 19–26.

Kassebaum, G. (1972, January). Sex in prison. *Sexual Behavior*, pp. 39–45.

Katchadourian, H. A., & Lunde, D. T. (1975). *Fundamentals of human sexuality*. New York: Holt, Rinehart and Winston.

Katz, A. M., & Hill, R. (1958). Residential propinquity and marital selection: A review of theory, method and fact. *Marriage and Family Living*, *20*, 327–335.

Katzman, M. (1972, February). Early sexual trauma. *Sexual Behavior*, *2*, 13–17.

Kaye, H. E. (1971, April). Lesbian relationships. *Sexual Behavior*, pp. 80–87.

Keen, S. J. (1979). To the editor. *The New England Journal of Medicine*, *301*, 840.

Kegel, A. H. (1952). Sexual functions of the pubococcygeus muscle. *Western Journal of Surgery*, *60*, 521–524.

Kelley, G. (1961). Impotence. In A. Ellis & A. Abarbanel (Eds.), *The encyclopedia of sexual behavior* (Vol. 1). New York: Hawthorn Books.

Kelly, J. A., Furman, W., & Young, V. (1978). Problems associated with the typological measurement of sex roles and androgyny. *Journal of Consulting and Clinical Psychology*, *46*, 1574–1576.

Kennedy, R. (1943). Pre-marital residential propinquity. *American Journal of Sociology*, *48*, 580–584.

Kenny, J. A. (1973). Sexuality of pregnant and breastfeeding women. *Archives of Sexual Behavior*, *2*, 215–229.

Kephart, W. M. (1961). *The family, society, and the individual*. Boston: Houghton Mifflin.

Keyes, D. M., Janzik, H. H., Mayer, K., Eichner, M., & Gupta, D. (1976). L-DOPA effects on sexual behavior: An experimental study. *Journal of Sex Research*, *12*, 117–123.

Kiesler, S. B., & Baral, R. L. (1970). The search for a romantic partner: The effects of self-esteem and physical attractiveness on romantic behavior. In K. J. Gergen & D. Martone (Eds.), *Personality and social behavior*. Reading, Mass.: Addison-Wesley.

Kimmel, D. C. (1978). Adult development and aging: A gay perspective. *Journal of Social Issues*, *34*(3), 113–130.

King, M., & Sobel, D. (1975). Sex on the college campus: Current attitudes and behavior. *Journal of College Student Personnel*, *16*, 205–209.

Kinsey, A., Pomeroy, W., & Martin, C. (1948). *Sexual behavior in the human male*. Philadelphia: Saunders.

Kinsey, A., Pomeroy, W., Martin, C., & Gebhard, P. (1953). *Sexual behavior in the human female*. Philadelphia: Saunders.

Kirk, S. A. (1975). The sex offenses of Blacks and Whites. *Archives of Sexual Behavior*, *4*, 295–302.

Kleitman, N. (1963). *Sleep and wakefulness*. Chicago: University of Chicago Press.

Kline-Graber, G., & Graber, B. (1978). Diagnosis and treatment procedures of pubococcygeal deficiencies in women. In J. LoPiccolo, & L. LoPiccolo (Eds.), *Handbook of sex therapy*. New York: Plenum Press.

Klinger, E. (1971). *Structure and functions of fantasy*. New York: Wiley.

Kohlberg, L. (1969). The cognitive-developmental approach to socialization. In D. A. Goslin (Ed.), *Handbook of socialization theory and research*. Chicago: Rand-McNally.

Kohlenberg, R. J. (1974). Directed masturbation and the treatment of primary orgasmic dysfunction. *Archives of Sexual Behavior, 3*, 349–356.

Kopera, A. A., Maier, R. A., & Johnson, J. E. (1971). *Perception of physical attractiveness: The influence of group interaction and group coaction on ratings of the attractiveness of photographs of women*. Presented at the 79th Annual Convention of the American Psychological Association.

Kopp, M. E. (1933). *Birth control in practice. Analysis of ten thousand case histories of the Birth Control Clinical Research Bureau*. New York: McBride.

Krafft-Ebing, R. V. (1965). *Psychopathia sexualis* (H. E. Wedeck, Trans.). New York: G. P. Putnam's Sons. (Originally published, 1886.)

Kremsdorf, R. B., Holman, M. L., & Laws, D. R. (1980). Orgasmic reconditioning without deviant imagery: A case report with a pedophile. *Behavior Research and Therapy, 18*, 203–207.

Kronhausen, E., & Kronhausen, P. (1964). *Pornography and the law*. New York: Ballantine Books. (a)

Kronhausen, E., & Kronhausen, P. (1964). *The sexually responsive woman*. New York: Ballantine Books. (b)

Kutschinsky, B. (1971). The effect of pornography: A pilot experiment on perception, behavior, and attitudes. In *Technical report of the Commission on Obscenity and Pornography* (Vol. 8). Washington, D.C.: U.S. Government Printing Office.

Landau, B. R. (1976). *Essential human anatomy and physiology*. Glenview, Ill.: Scott, Foresman and Company.

Laner, M. R. (1977). Permanent partner priorities: Gay and straight. *Journal of Homosexuality, 3*, 21–39.

Laner, M. R., & Kamel, G. W. L. (1977). Media mating I: Newspaper "personals" ads of homosexual men. *Journal of Homosexuality, 3*, 149–162.

Langmyhr, G. J. (1976). Varieties of coital positions: Advantages and disadvantages. *Medical Aspects of Human Sexuality, 10* (June), 128–139.

Lavrakas, P. (1975). Female preferences for male physiques. *Journal of Research in Personality, 9*, 324–334.

Laws, D. R. (1980). Treatment of bisexual pedophilia by a biofeedback-assisted self-control procedure. *Behavior Research and Therapy, 18*, 207–211.

Laws, D. R., & Rubin, H. B. (1969). Instructional control of an autonomic sexual response. *Journal of Applied Behavior Analysis, 2*, 93–99.

Lazarus, A. A. (1978). Overcoming sexual inadequacy. In J. LoPiccolo, & L. LoPiccolo (Eds.), *Handbook of sex therapy*. New York: Plenum Press.

LeBarre, H. (1977). *Live alone and be happier than anybody*. (Original Title: *A life of your own*). New York: Popular Library.

Lee, J. A. (1976). Forbidden colors of love: Patterns of gay love and gay liberation. *Journal of Homosexuality, 1*, 401–418.

Lee, J. A. (1977). Going public: A study in the sociology of homosexual liberation. *Journal of Homosexuality, 3*, 49–78.

Lehrman, N. (1970). *Masters and Johnson explained*. Chicago: Playboy Press.

Lennane, K. J., & Lennane, R. J. (1973). Alleged psychogenic disorders in women—A possible manifestation of sexual prejudice. *New England Journal of Medicine, 288*, 288–292.

Leo, J. (1982). The new scarlet letter. *Time*, August 2, pp. 62–66.

Lester, D. (1972). Incest. *Journal of Sex Research*, *8*, 268–285.

Levin, S. M., Barry, S. M., Gambaro, S., Wolfinsohn, L., & Smith, A. (1977). Variations of covert sensitization in the treatment of pedophilic behavior: A case study. *Journal of Consulting and Clinical Psychology*, *45*, 896–907.

Levine, S. (1976). Sex differences in the brain. *Scientific American*, *214*, 84–90.

Levitt, E. E., & Brady, J. P. (1965). Sexual preferences in young adult males and some correlates. *Journal of Clinical Psychology*, *21*, 347–354.

Levitt, E. E., & Hinesley, R. K. (1967). Some factors in the valences of erotic visual stimuli. *Journal of Sex Research*, *3*, 63–68.

Levitt, E. E., & Klassen, A. D. (1973, June). *Public attitudes toward sexual behaviors: The latest investigation of the Institute for Sex Research*. Paper presented at the American Orthopsychiatric Association, New York.

Levitt, E. E., & Klassen, A. D., Jr. (1974). Public attitudes toward homosexuality. *Journal of Homosexuality*, *1*, 29–43.

Lewis, R. A. (1973). Parents and peers: Socialization agents in the coital behavior of young adults. *Journal of Sex Research*, *9*, 156–170.

Lewis, R. A., & Burr, W. R. (1975). Premarital coitus and commitment among college students. *Archives of Sexual Behavior*, *4*, 73–79.

Leznoff, M., & Westley, W. A. (1963). The homosexual community. In H. M. Ruitenbeek (Ed.), *The problem of homosexuality in modern society*. New York: E. P. Dutton.

Lief, H. I. (Ed.). (1975). *Medical aspects of human sexuality*. Baltimore: Williams & Wilkins.

Lief, H. I. (1978, November). Review of "Homosexualities: A study of diversity among men and women" by Bell, A. P., & Weinberg, M. S. *SIECUS Report*, p. 1.

Lincoln, R., Doring-Bradley, B., Lindheim, B., & Cotterill, M. (1977). The Court, the Congress, and the President: Turning back the clock on the pregnant poor. *Family Planning Perspectives*, *9*, 207–214.

Lindzey, G. (1967). Some remarks concerning incest, the incest taboo, and psychoanalytic theory. *American Psychologist*, *22*, 1051–1059.

Lloyd, C. W. (1968). The influence of hormones on human sexual behavior. In *Clinical endocrinology* (Vol. 2). New York: Grune & Stratton.

LoPiccolo, J. (1978). Direct treatment of sexual dysfunction. In J. LoPiccolo & L. LoPiccolo (Eds.), *Handbook of sex therapy*. New York: Plenum Press.

LoPiccolo, J., & Lobitz, C. (1972). The role of masturbation in the treatment of orgasmic dysfunction. *Archives of Sexual Behavior*, *2*, 163–171.

LoPiccolo, J., & LoPiccolo, L. (1978). Impotence as a practical problem. In J. LoPiccolo & L. LoPiccolo (Eds.), *Handbook of sex therapy*. New York: Plenum Press.

Lovelace, L. (1973). *Inside Linda Lovelace*. New York: Pinnacle Books.

Luckey, E. B., & Nass, G. D. (1969). A comparison of sexual attitudes and behavior in an international sample. *Journal of Marriage and the Family*, *31*, 364–379.

Lumby, M. E. (1976). Homophobia: The quest for a valid scale. *Journal of Homosexuality*, *2*, 39–47.

Luschen, M. E., & Pierce, D. M. (1972). Effect of the menstrual cycle on mood and sexual arousability. *Journal of Sex Research*, *8*, 41–47.

Luttge, W. G. (1971). The role of gonadal hormones in the sexual behavior of the rhesus monkey and human: A literature survey. *Archives of Sexual Behavior*, *1*, 61–88.

Lynch, W. A. (1968). *A marriage manual for Catholics*. New York: Pocket Books.

"M." (1971). *The sensuous man*. New York: Lyle Stuart.

Maccoby, E. E. & Jacklin, C. N. (1974). *The psychology of sex differences*. Stanford: Stanford University Press.

MacDonald, A. P., Jr., & Games, R. G. (1974). Some characteristics of those who hold positive and negative attitudes toward homosexuals. *Journal of Homosexuality, 1,* 9–27.

MacDonald, J. M. (1971). *Rape offenders and their victims.* Springfield, Ill.: Charles C. Thomas.

MacDonald, M. L., Lindquist, C. U., Kramer, J. A., McGrath, R. A., & Rhyne, L. L. (1975). Social skills training: Behavior rehearsal in groups and dating skills. *Journal of Counseling Psychology, 22,* 224–231.

MacLean, P. D. (1973). Special award lecture: New findings on brain function and sociosexual behavior. In J. Zubin & J. Money (Eds.), *Contemporary sexual behavior.* Baltimore: Johns Hopkins University Press.

MacNamara, D. E. J., & Sagarin, E. (1977). *Sex, crime, and the law.* New York: Free Press.

Maisch, H. (1972). *Incest.* New York: Stein & Day.

Malamuth, N., & Donnerstein, E. (Eds.) (1984). *Pornography and sexual aggression.* New York: Academic Press.

Malamuth, N. M., Feshback, S., & Jaffe, Y. (1977). Sexual arousal and aggression: Recent experiments and theoretical issues. *Journal of Social Issues, 33,* 110–133.

Malatesta, V. J., Pollack, R. H., Wilbanks, W. H., & Adams, H. E. (1979). Alcohol effects on the orgasmic-ejaculatory response in human males. *Journal of Sex Research, 15,* 101–107.

Maletzky, B. M. (1974). "Assisted" covert sensitization in the treatment of exhibitionism. *Journal of Consulting and Clinical Psychology, 42,* 34–40.

Malinowski, B. (1929). *The sexual life of savages in North-Western Melanesia.* New York: Halcyon House.

Mann, J., Sidman, J., & Starr, S. (1971). Effects of erotic films on the sexual behavior of married couples. In *Technical report of the Commission on Obscenity and Pornography* (Vol. 8). Washington, D.C.: U.S. Government Printing Office.

Mann, T. (1970). The biochemical characteristics of spermatozoa and seminal plasma. In E. Rosenberg et al. (Eds.), *The human testes.* New York: Plenum Press.

Maple, T., Erwin, J., & Mitchell, G. (1974). Sexually aroused self-aggression in a socialized, adult male monkey. *Archives of Sexual Behavior, 3,* 471–475.

Marmor, J. (1971). "Normal" and "deviant" sexual behavior. *Journal of the American Medical Association, 217,* 165–170.

Marshall, D. S. (1972). Sexual behavior on Mangaia. In D. S. Marshall & R. C. Suggs (Eds.), *Human sexual behavior: Variations in the ethnographic spectrum.* Englewood Cliffs, N.J.: Prentice-Hall.

Marshall, D. S., & Suggs, R. C. (Eds.). (1971). *Human sexual behavior.* Englewood Cliffs, N.J.: Prentice-Hall.

Marshall, D. S., & Suggs, R. C. (Eds.). (1972). *Human sexual behavior: Variations in the ethnographic spectrum.* Englewood Cliffs, N.J.: Prentice-Hall.

Marshall, W. L. (1974). A combined treatment approach to the reduction of multiple fetish-related behaviors. *Journal of Consulting and Clinical Psychology, 42,* 613–616.

Martin, D., & Lyon, P. (1972). *Lesbian/woman.* New York: Bantam.

Martinson, F. M. (1976). Eroticism in infancy and childhood. *Journal of Sex Research, 12,* 251–262.

Marx, J. L. (1984). Strong new candidate for AIDS agent. *Science, 224,* May, 475–477.

Maschhoff, T. A., Fanshier, W. E., & Hansen, D. J. (1976). Vasectomy: Its effect upon marital stability. *Journal of Sex Research, 12,* 295–314.

Maslow, A. H., & Mintz, N. L. (1956). Effects of esthetic surroundings: I. Initial effects of three esthetic conditions upon perceiving "energy" and "well-being" in faces. *Journal of Psychology, 41,* 247–254.

Masters, R. E. L. (1962). *Forbidden sexual behavior and morality*. New York: Julian Press.

Masters, W. (1975). *New developments in sex therapy*. Paper presented at the American Psychiatric Association Meetings.

Masters, W. H., & Johnson, V. E. (1965). The sexual response cycles of the human male and female: Comparative anatomy and physiology. In F. A. Beach (Ed.), *Sex and behavior*. New York: Wiley.

Masters, W. H., & Johnson, V. E. (1966). *Human sexual response*. Boston: Little, Brown.

Masters, W. H., & Johnson, V. E. (1970). *Human sexual inadequacy*. Boston: Little, Brown.

Masters, W. H., & Johnson, V. E. (1979). *Homosexuality in perspective*. Boston: Little, Brown.

Masters, W. H., Johnson, V. E., & Kolodny, R. C. (Eds.). (1977). *Ethical issues in sex therapy and research*. Boston: Little, Brown.

Mathis, J. L. (1972). *Clear thinking about sexual deviations*. Chicago: Nelson-Hall.

Maugh, Y. H., III. (1981). "Male pill" blocks sperm enzyme. *Science, 22*, 314.

McArthur, L. Z., & Resko, B. G. The portrayal of men and women in American television commercials. *Journal of Social Psychology*, in press.

McBride, G. (1980). Putting a better cap on the cervix. *Journal of the American Medical Association, 243*, 1617–1618.

McCaghy, C. H. (1971). Child molesting. *Sexual Behavior, 1* (August), 16–24.

McCary, J. L. (1978). *McCary's human sexuality* (3rd ed.). New York: D. Van Nostrand.

McCauley, C., & Swann, C. P. (1978). Male-female differences in sexual fantasy. *Journal of Research in Personality, 12*, 76–86.

McCauley, C., & Swann, C. P. (1980). Sex differences in the frequency and functions of fantasies during sexual activity. *Journal of Research in Personality, 14*, 400–411.

McCauley, E. A., & Ehrhardt, A. A. (1980). Sexual behavior in female transsexuals and lesbians. *Journal of Sex Research, 16*, 202–211.

McClintock, M. (1971). Menstrual synchrony and suppression. *Nature, 229*, 244–245.

McGill, T. E. (1965). Studies of the sexual behavior of male laboratory mice: Effects of genotype, recovery of sex drive, and theory. In F. A. Beach (Ed.), *Sex and behavior*. New York: Wiley.

McGuire, R. J., Carlisle, J. M., & Young, B. G. (1965). Sexual deviations as conditioned behavior: A hypothesis. *Behaviour Research and Therapy, 2*, 185–190.

McGuire, T. F., & Steinhilber, R. M. (1970). Frigidity, the primary female sexual dysfunction. *Medical Aspects of Human Sexuality, 4*, 108–123.

McNeill, J. J. (1976). *The church and the homosexual*. Kansas City: Sheed, Andrews, & McMeel.

McWhirter, D. P., & Mattison, A. M. (1980). Treatment of sexual dysfunction in homosexual male couples. In S. R. Leiblum & L. A. Parvin (Eds.), *Principles and practice of sex therapy*. New York: Guilford Press.

Mead, M. (1969). *Sex and temperament in three primitive societies*. New York: Dell.

Melges, F. T., & Hamburg, D. A. (1977). Psychological effects of hormonal changes in women. In F. A. Beach (Ed.), *Human sexuality in four perspectives*. Baltimore: Johns Hopkins University Press.

Men beat women back to altar. (1981, November 11). United Press International. *Wichita Eagle*.

Messenger, J. C. (1971, February). The lack of the Irish. *Psychology Today*, pp. 41–42, 68.

Messenger, J. C. (1972). Sex and repression in an Irish folk community. In D. S. Marshall & R. C. Suggs (Eds.), *Human sexual behavior: Variations in the ethnographic spectrum*. Englewood Cliffs, N.J.: Prentice-Hall.

Meyer, J. K. (1974). Clinical variants among applicants for sex reassignment. *Archives of Sexual Behavior, 3*, 527–558.

Meyer, J. K., & Reter, D. J. (1979). Sex reassignment. *Archives of General Psychiatry, 36*, 1010–1015.

Michael, R. P., & Keverne, E. B. (1970). A male sex attractant pheromone in rhesus monkey vaginal secretions. *Journal of Endocrinology, 46*, xx–xxi.

Michael, R. P., Keverne, E. B., & Bonsall, R. W. (1971). Pheromones: Isolation of male sex attractants from a female primate. *Science, 172*, 964–966.

Michael, R. P., & Zumpe, D. (1970). Rhythmic changes in the copulatory frequency of rhesus monkeys (*Macaca mulata*) in relation to the menstrual cycle and a comparison with the human cycle. *Journal of Reproduction and Fertility, 21*, 119–201.

Migeon, C. J., Rivarola, M. A., & Forest, M. G. (1968). Studies of androgens in transsexual subjects: Effects of estrogen therapy. *Johns Hopkins Medical Journal, 123*, 128–133.

Miller v. California, 413 U.S. 15, 24 (1973).

Miller, W. R., & Arkowitz, H. Anxiety and perceived causation in social success and failure experiences: Disconfirmation of an attribution hypothesis in two experiments. *Journal of Abnormal Psychology*, in press.

Miller, W. R., & Lief, H. I. (1976). Masturbatory attitudes, knowledge, and experience: Data from the Sex Knowledge and Attitude Test (SKAT). *Archives of Sexual Behavior, 5*, 447–467.

Millham, J., San Miguel, C. L., & Kellog, R. (1976). A factor-analytic conceptualization of attitudes toward male and female homosexuals. *Journal of Homosexuality, 2*, 3–10.

Mirande, A. M., & Hammer, E. L. (1976). Love, sex, permissiveness, and abortion: A test of alternative models. *Archives of Sexual Behavior, 5*, 553–566.

Mischel, W. Sex typing and socialization. (1970). In P. H. Mussen (Ed.), *Carmichael's Manual of Child Psychology* (Vol. 2). New York: Wiley.

Money, J. (1961). Sex hormones and other variables in human eroticism. In W. C. Young (Ed.), *Sex and internal secretions*. Baltimore: Williams & Wilkins.

Money, J. (1971). Prefatory remarks on outcome of sex reassignment in 24 cases of transsexualism. *Archives of Sexual Behavior, 1*, 163–165.

Money, J. (1974). Prenatal hormones and postnatal socialization in gender identity differentiation. In J. K. Cole & R. Dienstbier (Eds.), *Nebraska symposium on motivation*, 1973. Lincoln, Neb.: University of Nebraska Press.

Money, J., & Ehrhardt, A. A. (1972). *Man and woman, boy and girl*. Baltimore: Johns Hopkins University Press.

Money, J., & Mathews, D. (1982). Prenatal exposure to virilizing progestins: An adult follow-up of twelve women. *Archives of Sexual Behavior, 11*, 73–83.

Money, J., Schwartz, M., & Lewis, V. G. Adult erotosexual status and fetal hormonal masculinization and demasculinization: 46, XX congenital virilizing adrenal hyperplasia (CVAH) and 46, XY androgen-insensitivity syndrome (AIS) compared. *Psychoneuroendocrinology*, in press.

Montanelli, D. S., & Hill, K. T. (1969). Children's achievement expectations and performance as function of two consecutive reinforcement experiences, sex of subject and sex of experimenter. *Journal of Personality and Social Psychology, 13*, 115–128.

Monteflores, C., & Schultz, S. J. (1978). Coming out: Similarities and differences for lesbians and gay men. *Journal of Social Issues, 34*, 59–72.

Moos, R. H. (1968). Psychological aspects of oral contraceptives. *Archives of General Psychiatry, 19*, 87–94.

Moos, R. H. (1969). Typology of menstrual cycle symptoms. *American Journal of Obstetrics and Gynecology, 103*, 390–402.

Moos, R. H., Kopell, B. S., Melges, F. T., Yalom, I. D., Lunde, D. T., Clayton, R. B., & Hamberg, D. A. (1969). Fluctuations in symptoms and moods during the menstrual cycle. *Journal of Psychosomatic Research, 13*, 37–44.

Moreault, D., & Follingstad, D. R. (1978). Sexual fantasies of females as a function of sex guilt and experimental response cues. *Journal of Consulting and Clinical Psychology*, *46*, 1385–1393.

Morin, S. F. (1977). Heterosexual bias in psychological research on lesbianism and male homosexuality. *American Psychologist*, *32*, 629–637.

Morin, S. F., & Garfinkle, E. M. (1978). Male homophobia. *Journal of Social Issues*, *34*(1), 29–46.

Morris, J. (1974). *Conundrum*. New York: Harcourt Brace Jovanovich.

Mosher, D. L. (1966). The development and multitrait-multimethod matrix analysis of three measures of three aspects of guilt. *Journal of Consulting Psychology*, *30*, 25–29.

Mosher, D. L. (1968). Measurement of guilt in females by self-report inventories. *Journal of Consulting and Clinical Psychology*, *32*, 690–695.

Mosher, D. L. (1970). *Sex-guilt and reactions to pornographic films*. Paper presented at the meeting of the American Psychological Association, Miami Beach.

Mosher, D. L. (1971). Psychological reactions to pornographic films. In *Technical report of the Commission on Obscenity and Pornography* (Vol. 8). Washington, D.C.: U.S. Government Printing Office.

Mosher, D. L., & Abramson, P. R. (1977). Subjective sexual arousal to films of masturbation. *Journal of Consulting and Clinical Psychology*, *45*, 776–807.

Mosher, D. L., & Cross, H. J. (1971). Sex guilt and premarital sexual experiences in college students. *Journal of Consulting and Clinical Psychology*, *36*, 27–32.

Mosher, D. L., & Greenberg, I. (1969). Females' affective responses to reading erotic literature. *Journal of Consulting and Clinical Psychology*, *33*, 472–477.

Motahar, S. B. (1979, October). *Johns Hopkins Magazine*, p. 60.

Murstein, B. I. (1976). *Who will marry whom?: Theories and research in marital choice*. New York: Springer Publishing.

Murstein, B. I., Goyette, M., & Cerreto, M. (1974). *A theory of the effect of exchange orientation on marriage and friendship*. Unpublished manuscript.

Mussen, P. H. (1962). Long-term consequents of masculinity of interests in adolescence. *Journal of Consulting Psychology*, *26*, 435–440.

Myrick, F. L. (1974). Homosexual types: An empirical investigation. *Journal of Sex Research*, *10*, 226–237.

Napolitane, C., & Pellegrio, V. (1977). *Living and loving after divorce*. New York: Rawson Associates.

National Center for Health Statistics: Advance report, final divorce statistics, 1980. (1983, June). *Monthly Vital Statistics Report*. Vol. 32–No. 3, Supp. DHHS Publ. No. (PHS)83–1120. Public Health Service, Hyattsville, Md.

National Center for Health Statistics. (1976, June 22). NCHS growth charts, 1976. *Vital Statistics Report*. DHEW Pub. No. (HRA) 76–1120. Washington, D.C.: U.S. Government Printing Office.

Nawy, H. (1971). The San Francisco erotic marketplace. In *Technical report of the Commission on Obscenity and Pornography* (Vol. 4). Washington, D.C.: U.S. Government Printing Office.

Nelson, A. (1974). *Personality attributes of female orgasmic consistency (or romance makes you frigid)*. Unpublished M.A. thesis for University of California, Berkeley.

Neubeck, G. (1969). *Extramarital relations*. Englewood Cliffs, N.J.: Prentice-Hall.

Neugarten, B. L., & Kraines, R. J. (1965). "Menopausal symptoms" in women of various ages. *Psychosomatic Medicine*, *28*, 266–273.

New test tube research successful. (1983, July 22). Associated Press. *Manhattan Mercury*, p. A3.

Newcomb, M. D., & Bentler, P. M. (1983). Dimensions of subjective female orgasmic responsiveness. *Journal of Personality and Social Psychology, 44*, 862–873.

Nicholls, J. G. (1975). Causal attributions and other achievement-related cognitions: Effects of task outcome, attainment value and sex. *Journal of Personality and Social Psychology, 31*, 379–389.

Nyberg, K. L. (1976). Sexual aspirations and sexual behaviors among homosexually behaving males and females: The impact of the gay community. *Journal of Homosexuality, 2*, 29–38.

Nyberg, K. L., & Alston, J. P. (1977). Analysis of public attitudes toward homosexual behavior. *Journal of Homosexuality, 2*, 99–107.

O'Connor, J. (1975). Preoccupation with multiple orgasms. In H. I. Lief (Ed.), *Medical aspects of human sexuality*. Baltimore: Williams & Wilkins.

Offir, C. W. (1975, January). Don't take it lying down. *Psychology Today*, p. 73.

Ohlson, E. L., & Wilson, M. (1974). Differentiating female homosexuals from female heterosexuals by use of the MMPI. *Journal of Sex Research, 10*, 308–315.

O'Leary, K. D., & Wilson, G. T. (1975). *Behavior therapy*. Englewood Cliffs, N.J.: Prentice-Hall.

O'Neill, N., & O'Neill, G. (1972). *Open marriage*. New York: M. Evans.

Osborn, C. A., & Pollack, R. H. (1977). The effects of two types of erotic literature on physiological and verbal measures of female sexual arousal. *Journal of Sex Research, 13*, 250–256.

Osofsky, H., & Osofsky, J. (Eds.). (1973). *The abortion experience: Psychological and medical impact*. New York: Harper & Row.

Oswald, I. (1962). Induction of illusory and hallucinatory voices with considerations of behaviour therapy. *Journal of Mental Science, 108*, 196–212.

Packer, H. L. (1968). *The limits of the criminal sanction*. Stanford, Calif.: Stanford University Press.

Paige, K. E. (1973, September). Women learn to sing the menstrual blues. *Psychology Today*, pp. 41–46.

Paige, K. E. (1978, May). The ritual of circumcision. *Human Nature*, pp. 40–48.

Parlee, M. B. (1973). The premenstrual syndrome. *Psychological Bulletin, 80*, 454–465.

Paul VI, Pope. (1968). *On the regulation of birth: Humanae Vitae*. (Encyclical Letter.) Washington, D.C.: United States Catholic Conference.

Pauly, I. B. (1969). Adult manifestations of male transsexualism. In R. Green & J. Money (Eds.), *Transsexualism and sex reassignment*. Baltimore: Johns Hopkins University Press.

Pauly, I. B. (1974). Female transsexualism: Part 1 and Part 2. *Archives of Sexual Behavior, 3*, 487–525.

Peplau, L. A. (1981, March). What homosexuals want in relationships. *Psychology Today*, pp. 28–38.

Peplau, L. A., Cochran, S., Rook, K., & Padesky, C. (1978). Loving women: Attachment and autonomy in lesbian relationships. *Journal of Social Issues, 34*, 7–27.

Perry, J. D., & Whipple, B. (1981). Pelvic muscle strength of female ejaculators: Evidence in support of a new theory of orgasm. *Journal of Sex Research, 17*, 22–39.

Pfeiffer, E., Verwoerdt, A., & Davis, G. C. (1972). Sexual behavior in middle life. *American Journal of Psychiatry, 128*, 1262–1267.

Pheterson, G. I., Kiesler, S. B., & Goldberg, P. A. (1971). Evaluation of the performance of women as a function of their sex, achievement, and personal history. *Journal of Personality and Social Psychology, 19*, 114–118.

Piaget, J. *The psychology of intelligence*. (1950). London: Routledge & Kegan Paul.

Pietropinto, A., & Simenauer, J. (1977). *Beyond the male myth: What women want to know about men's sexuality, a national survey*. New York: Times Books.

Pirke, K. M., Kockott, G., & Dittman, F. (1974). Psychosexual stimulation and plasma testosterone in man. *Archives of Sexual Behavior, 3*, 577–584.

Playboy. (1976, October). What's really happening on campus.

Playboy. (1978, March). The great Playboy sex-aids road test.

Pleck, J. H., & Brannon, R. (1978). Male roles and the male experience. *Journal of Social Issues, 34*, 1–4.

Podell, L., & Perkins, J. C. (1957). A Guttman scale for sexual experience—A methodological note. *Journal of Abnormal and Social Psychology, 54*, 420–422.

Pomeroy, W. B. (1972). *Dr. Kinsey and the Institute for Sex Research*. New York: Harper & Row.

Pomeroy, W. B., & Schaefer, L. C. (1978, May). Beyond the male myth: Two professional views. *SIECUS Report*, pp. 1, 3–4.

Price, J. H. (1981). Update: Toxic shock syndrome. *Journal of School Health, 51*, 143–145.

Pritchard, J. A., & MacDonald, P. C. (1976). *Williams obstetrics* (15th ed.). New York: Appleton-Century-Crofts.

Pritchard, M. (1962). Homosexuality and genetic sex. *Journal of Mental Science, 108*, 616–623.

Przybla, D. P. J., & Byrne, D. (1984). The mediating role of cognitive processes in self-reported sexual arousal. *Journal of Research in Personality, 18*, 54–63.

Quinsey, V. L., Chaplin, T. C., & Carrigan, W. F. (1980). Biofeedback and signaled punishment in the modification of inappropriate sexual age preferences. *Behavior Therapy, 11*, 567–576.

Raboch, J., & Starka, L. (1972). Coital activity of men and the levels of plasmatic testosterone. *Journal of Sex Research, 8*, 219–224.

Rachman, S. (1966). Sexual fetishism: An experimental analogue. *Psychological Record, 16*, 293–296.

Rada, R. T. (1975, March). Alcohol and rape. *Medical Aspects of Human Sexuality*, pp. 48–60.

Rada, R. T. (1978). Classification of the rapist. In R. T. Rada (Ed.), *Clinical aspects of the rapist*. New York: Grune & Stratton.

Rader, C. M. (1977). MMPI profile types of exposers, rapists, and assaulters in a court services population. *Journal of Consulting and Clinical Psychology, 45*, 61–69.

Randall, J. (1969). Preoperative and postoperative states of male and female transsexuals. In R. Green & J. Money (Eds.), *Transsexualism and sex reassignment*. Baltimore: Johns Hopkins University Press.

Rape case reversal angers Utah women. (1978, December 27). *Wichita Eagle* (Associated Press).

Rape: Problems and issues. (1979, September). *Sex and the Law*, pp. 1, 3.

Ray, R. E., & Walker, C. E. (1973). Biographical and self-report correlates of female guilt responses to visual erotic stimuli. *Journal of Consulting and Clinical Psychology, 41*, 93–96.

Razani, J. (1978). Ejaculatory incompetence treated by deconditioning anxiety. In J. LoPiccolo & L. LoPiccolo (Eds.), *Handbook of sex therapy*. New York: Plenum Press.

Reckless, J., & Geiger, N. (1978). Impotence as a practical problem. In J. LoPiccolo & L. LoPiccolo (Eds.), *Handbook of sex therapy*. New York: Plenum Press.

Reik, T. (1944). *A psychologist looks at love*. New York: Farrar & Rinehart.

Reinberg, A., & Lagoguey, M. (1978). Circadian and circannual rhythms in sexual activity and plasma hormones (FSH, LH, testosterone) of five human males. *Archives of Sexual Behavior*, 7, 13–30.

Reiss, B. F., Safer, J., & Yotive, W. (1974). Psychological test data on female homosexuality: A review of the literature. *Journal of Homosexuality*, 1, 71–85.

Reiss, I. L. (1960). *Premarital sexual standards in America*. New York: Free Press.

Reiss, I. L. (1967). *The social context of premarital sexual permissiveness*. New York: Holt, Rinehart, and Winston.

Reiss, I. L. (1968). How and why America's sex standards are changing. *Trans-action*, 5, 26–32.

Reiss, I. L., Anderson, R. E., & Sponaugle, G. C. (1980). A multivariate model of the determinants of extramarital sexual permissiveness. *Journal of Marriage and the Family*, 42, 395–411.

Rettig, S., & Pasamanick, B. (1959). Changes in moral values among college students: A factorial study. *American Sociological Review*, 24, 856–863.

Reversible sterilization. (1979, November 13). *Wichita Eagle*.

Ribal, J. E. (1973). *Learning sex roles*. San Francisco: Canfield Press.

Robbins, M. B., & Jensen, G. D. (1978). Multiple orgasm in males. *Journal of Sex Research*, 14, 21–26.

Robinson, I. E., King, K., & Balswick, J. O. (1972). The premarital sexual revolution among college females. *Family Coordinator*, 21, 189–194.

Robinson, J. P., & Hirsch, P. (1969, October). It's the sound that does it. *Psychology Today*, pp. 42–45.

Robinson, P. (1981, July). What liberated males do. *Psychology Today*, pp. 81–85.

Rodin, J. (1976). Menstruation, reattribution, and competence. *Journal of Personality and Social Psychology*, 33, 345–353.

Roe v. *Wade*. 410 U.S. 113 (1973).

Rogel, M. J. (1978). A critical evaluation of the possibility of higher primate reproductive and sexual pheromones. *Psychological Bulletin*, 85, 810–830.

Rook, K. S., & Hammen, C. L. (1977). A cognitive perspective on the experience of sexual arousal. *Journal of Social Issues*, 33, 7–29.

Rooth, F. G., & Marks, I. M. (1974). Persistent exhibitionism: Short-term response to aversion, self-regulation, and relaxation treatments. *Archives of Sexual Behavior*, 3, 227–248.

Rooth, G. (1973). Exhibitionism outside Europe and America. *Archives of Sexual Behavior*, 2, 351–363.

Rosebury, T. (1971). *Microbes and morals: The strange story of venereal disease*. New York: Viking.

Rosen, D. H. (1974). *Lesbianism: A study of female homosexuality*. Springfield, Ill.: Charles C. Thomas.

Rosenblatt, P. C. (1974). Cross-cultural perspective on attraction. In Ted L. Huston (Ed.), *Foundations of interpersonal attraction*. New York: Academic Press.

Ross, M. W., Rogers, L. J., & McCulloch, H. (1978). Stigma, sex, and society. A new look at gender differentiation and sexual variation. *Journal of Homosexuality*, 3, 315–330.

Rossman, G. P. (1973). Literature on pederasty. *Journal of Sex Research*, 9, 307–312. (a)

Rossman, G. P. (1973, March/April). The pederasts. *Society*, pp. 28–35. (b)

Roth, P. (1967). *Portnoy's complaint*. New York: Random House.

Roth v. *United States*. 354 U.S. 476 (1957).

Royal College of General Practitioners. (1974). *Oral contraceptives and health*. London: Pitman Medical.

Rubin, H. B., Henson, D. E., Falvo, R. E., & High, R. W. (1979). The relationship between men's endogenous levels of testosterone and their penile response to erotic stimuli. *Behavior Research and Therapy*, 17, 305–312.

Rubin, I. (1965). *Sexual life after sixty*. New York: Basic Books.

Rubin, I. (1966). Sex after forty—and after seventy. In R. Brecher & E. Brecher (Eds.), *An analysis of human sexual response*. New York: Signet.

Rubin, J. Z., Provenzano, F. J., & Luria, J. (1974). The eye of the beholder: Parents' views on sex of newborns. *American Journal of Orthopsychiatry, 44,* 512–519.

Rubin, Z. (1970). Measurement of romantic love. *Journal of Personality and Social Psychology, 16,* 265–273.

Rubin, Z. (1973). *Liking and loving: An invitation to social psychology*. New York: Holt, Rinehart and Winston.

Ruff, C. F., Templer, D. I., & Ayers, J. L. (1976). The intelligence of rapists. *Archives of Sexual Behavior, 4,* 327–329.

Rugh, L., & Shettles, L. (1971). *From conception to birth: The drama of life's beginnings*. New York: Harper & Row.

Sachs, D. H., & Duffy, D. G. (1976). Effect of modeling on sexual imagery. *Archives of Sexual Behavior, 5,* 301–311.

Sacred Congregation for the Doctrine of the Faith. (1976, January 16). Declaration on certain questions concerning sexual ethics (English text). *New York Times,* p. 2.

Sagarin, E. (1977). Incest: Problems of definition and frequency. *Journal of Sex Research, 13,* 126–135.

Saghir, M. T., & Robins, E. (1973). *Male and female homosexuality: A comprehensive investigation*. Baltimore: Williams & Wilkins.

Sanday, P. R. (1981). The socio-cultural context of rape: A cross-cultural study. *Journal of Social Issues, 37*(4), 5–27.

Sandford, D. A. (1974). Patterns of sexual arousal in heterosexual males. *Journal of Sex Research, 10,* 150–155.

Schachter, S. (1964). The interaction of cognitive and physiological determinants of emotional state. In Leonard Berkowitz (Ed.), *Advances in experimental social psychology* (Vol. 1). New York: Academic Press, pp. 49–110.

Schaefer, L. C. (1973). *Women and sex*. New York: Pantheon.

Schafer, S. (1976). Sexual and social problems of lesbians. *Journal of Sex Research, 12,* 50–69.

Schafer, S. (1977). Sociosexual behavior in male and female homosexuals: A study in sex differences. *Archives of Sexual Behavior, 6,* 355–364.

Scheer, R., & Golson, B. (1976, November). Playboy interview: Jimmy Carter. *Playboy,* pp. 63–86.

Scheflen, A. E. (1965). Quasi-courtship behavior in psychotherapy. *Psychiatry, 28,* 245–257.

Schill, T., & Chapin, J. (1972). Sex guilt and males' preference for reading erotic magazines. *Journal of Consulting and Clinical Psychology, 39,* 516.

Schmidt, G. (1975). Male-female differences in sexual arousal and behavior during and after exposure to sexually explicit stimuli. *Archives of Sexual Behavior, 4,* 353–364.

Schmidt, G., & Sigusch, V. (1970). Sex differences in responses to psychosexual stimulation by films and slides. *Journal of Sex Research, 6,* 268–283.

Schmidt, G., & Sigusch, V. (1971). Patterns of sexual behavior in West German workers and students. *Journal of Sex Research, 7,* 89–106.

Schmidt, G., & Sigusch, V. (1973). Women's sexual arousal. In J. Zubin & J. Money (Eds.), *Contemporary sexual behavior*. Baltimore: Johns Hopkins University Press.

Schmidt, C., Sigusch, V., & Schafer, S. (1973). Responses to reading erotic stories: Male-female differences. *Archives of Sexual Behavior, 2,* 181–199.

Schofield, C. B. (1979). *Sexually transmitted diseases*. New York: Churchill Livingstone.

Schofield, M. (1965). *The sexual behavior of young people*. Boston: Little, Brown.

Schull, W. J., & Neel, J. V. (1965). *The effects of inbreeding on Japanese children*. New York: Harper & Row.

Schwartz, S. (1973). Effects of sex guilt and sexual arousal on the retention of birth control information. *Journal of Consulting and Clinical Psychology, 41*, 61–64.

Schwartz, S. (1975). Effects of sex guilt on word association responses to double-entendre sexual words. *Journal of Consulting and Clinical Psychology, 43*, 100.

Scientists find a vaccine for herpes victims. (1983, June 13). *Honolulu Star-Bulletin*, p. A-4.

Scoresby, L. (1972). Does sexual experience before marriage help to ensure a better marriage? Answer. *Sexual Behavior, 2* (March), 6–7.

Sears, R. R. (1970). Relation of early socialization experience to self-concepts and gender role in middle childhood. *Child Development, 41*, 267–289.

Selkin, J. (1975, January). Rape. *Psychology Today*, pp. 71–76.

Seman, J. (1956). Premature ejaculation, a new approach. *Southern Medical Journal, 49*, 353–358.

Sevely, J. L., & Bennett, J. W. (1978). Concerning female ejaculation and the female prostate. *Journal of Sex Research, 14*, 1–20.

Shah, F., Zelnik, M., & Kantner, J. F. (1975). Unprotected intercourse among unwed teenagers. *Family Planning Perspectives, 7*, 39–44.

Sherfey, M. J. (1973). *The nature and evolution of female sexuality*. New York: Vintage.

Shope, D. F. (1975). *Interpersonal sexuality*. Philadelphia: Saunders.

Shope, D. F., & Broderick, C. B. (1967). Level of sexual experience and predicted adjustment in marriage. *Journal of Marriage and the Family, 29*, 424–427.

Siegelman, M. (1972). Adjustment of male homosexuals and heterosexuals. *Archives of Sexual Behavior, 2*, 9–25.

Siegelman, M. (1974). Parental background of male homosexuals and heterosexuals. *Archives of Sexual Behavior, 3*, 3–18.

Siegelman, M. (1978). Psychological adjustment of homosexual and heterosexual men: A cross-national replication. *Archives of Sexual Behavior, 7*, 1–11.

Sigusch, V., & Schmidt, G. (1973). Teenage boys and girls in West Germany. *Journal of Sex Research, 9*, 107–123.

Sigusch, V., Schmidt, G., Reinfeld, A., & Wiedemann-Sutor, I. (1970). Psychosexual stimulation: Sex differences. *Journal of Sex Research, 6*, 10–24.

Simon, N., & Senturia, A. (1966). Psychiatric sequelae of abortion. *Archives of General Psychiatry, 15*, 378–389.

Simon, W., Berger, A. S., & Gagnon, J. H. (1972). Beyond anxiety and fantasy: The coital experiences of college youth. *Journal of Youth and Adolescence, 1*, 203–222.

Singer, J. *Androgyny*. (1977). Garden City, N.Y.: Anchor Books.

Singer, J., & Singer, I. (1972). Types of female orgasm. *Journal of Sex Research, 8*, 255–267.

Singer, J. L. (1966). *Daydreaming*. New York: Random House.

Singh, B. K. (1980). Trends in attitudes toward premarital sexual relations. *Journal of Marriage and the Family, 42*, 387–393.

Slovenko, R. (1965). *Sexual behavior and the law*. Springfield, Ill.: Charles C. Thomas.

Smith, R. S. (1976). Voyeurism: A review of literature. *Archives of Sexual Behavior, 5*, 585–608.

Snyder, E. E., & Spreitzer, E. (1976). Attitudes of the aged toward nontraditional sexual behavior. *Archives of Sexual Behavior, 5*, 249–254.

Sokolov, J. J., Harris, R. T., & Hecker, M. R. (1976). Isolation of substances from human vaginal secretions previously shown to be sex attractant pheromones in higher primates. *Archives of Sexual Behavior, 5*, 269–274.

Solnick, R. L., & Birren, J. E. (1977). Age and male erectile responsiveness. *Archives of Sexual Behavior, 6,* 1–9.

Sorensen, R. C. (1973). *Adolescent sexuality in contemporary America (The Sorensen Report).* New York: World Publishing.

Spanier, G. B. (1977). Sources of sex information and premarital sexual behavior. *Journal of Sex Research, 13,* 73–88.

Spanier, G. B., & Cole, C. L. (1975). Mate swapping: Perceptions, value orientations and participation in a Midwestern community. *Archives of Sexual Behavior, 4,* 143–159.

Spence, J. T., & Helmreich, R. (1978). *Masculinity and femininity: Their psychological dimensions, correlates, and antecedents.* Austin: University of Texas Press.

Spengler, A. (1977). Manifest sadomasochism of males: Results of an empirical study. *Archives of Sexual Behavior, 6,* 441–456.

Spitz, C. J., Gold, A. R., & Adams, D. B. (1975). Cognitive and hormonal factors affecting coital frequency. *Archives of Sexual Behavior, 4,* 249–263.

Staples, R. (1973). Male-female sexual variations: Functions of biology or culture. *Journal of Sex Research, 9,* 11–20.

Steele, D. G., & Walker, E. (1974). Male and female differences in reaction to erotic stimuli as related to sexual adjustment. *Archives of Sexual Behavior, 3,* 459–469.

Stein, P. (1975). Singlehood: An alternative to marriage. *The Family Coordinator, 24,* 489–507.

Stephan, W., Berscheid, E., & Walster, E. (1971). Sexual arousal and heterosexual perception. *Journal of Personality and Social Psychology, 20,* 93–101.

Sternglanz, S. H., & Servin, L. A. (1974). Sex role stereotyping in children's television programs. *Developmental Psychology, 10,* 710–715.

Stoller, R. J. (1967). Transvestites' women. *American Journal of Psychiatry, 124,* 333–339.

Stoller, R. J. (1968). *Sex and gender.* New York: Science House.

Stoller, R. J. (1969). Parental influences in male transsexualism. In R. Green & J. Money (Eds.), *Transsexualism and sex reassignment.* Baltimore: Johns Hopkins University Press.

Stoller, R. J. (1977). Sexual deviations. In F. A. Beach (Ed.), *Human sexuality in four perspectives.* Baltimore: Johns Hopkins University Press.

Stone, H. M., & Stone, A. S. (1952). *A marriage manual. A practical guide-book to sex and marriage* (2nd ed.). New York: Simon & Schuster.

Storms, M. D. (1980). Theories of sexual orientation. *Journal of Personality and Social Psychology, 38,* 783–792.

Storms, M. D. (1981). A theory of erotic orientation development. *Psychological Bulletin, 88,* 340–353.

Storr, A. (1964). *Sexual deviation.* Baltimore: Penguin.

Stringer, P., & Grygier, T. (1976). Male homosexuality, psychiatric patient status and psychological masculinity and feminity. *Archives of Sexual Behavior, 5,* 15–27.

Swigert, V. L., Farrell, R. A., & Yoels, W. C. (1976). Sexual homocide: Social, psychological, and legal aspects. *Archives of Sexual Behavior, 5,* 391–401.

Szasz, T. S. (1965). Legal and moral aspects of homosexuality. In J. Marmor (Ed.), *Sexual inversion.* New York: Basic Books.

Tanner, J. M. (1967). Puberty. In A. McLaren (Ed.), *Advances in reproductive physiology* (Vol. 2). New York: Logos Press.

Tavris, C. (1978, February). The Redbook report on male sexuality. *Redbook,* (a)

Tavris, C. (1978, March). The Redbook report on male sexuality. *Redbook,* (b)

Tavris, C., & Offir, C. (1977). *The longest war: Sex differences in perspective.* New York: Harcourt Brace Jovanovich.

Tavris, C., & Sadd, S. (1977). *The Redbook report on female sexuality.* New York: Delacorte Press.

Taylor, G. R. (1970). *Sex in history.* New York: Harper & Row.

Teenage childbearing: United States, 1966–1975. (1977, September 8). *Monthly Vital Statistics Report.*

Terman, L. M. (1938). *Psychological factors in marital happiness.* New York: McGraw-Hill.

Terman, L. M. (1951). Correlates of orgasm adequacy in a group of 556 wives. *Journal of Psychology, 32,* 115–172.

Tesser, A., & Brodie, M. (1971). A note on the evaluation of a "computer date." *Psychonomic Science, 23,* 300.

Thibaut, J. W., & Kelley, H. H. (1959). *The social psychology of groups.* New York: Wiley.

Thielicke, H. (1964). *The ethics of sex.* New York: Harper & Row.

Thomas Aquinas, Saint. (1968). *Summa theologica* (Vol. 43). (T. Gilly, trans.). New York: McGraw-Hill. (Originally published, 1267–73.)

Thompson, N. L., McCandless, B. R., & Strickland, B. R. (1971). Personal adjustment of male and female homosexuals and heterosexuals. *Journal of Abnormal Psychology, 78,* 237–240.

Thompson, N. L., Jr., Schwartz, D. M., McCandless, B. R., & Edwards, D. A. (1973). Parent-child relationships and sexual identity in male and female homosexuals and heterosexuals. *Journal of Consulting and Clinical Psychology, 41,* 120–127.

Tietze, C. (1960). Probability of pregnancy resulting from a single unprotected coitus. *Fertility and Sterility, 11,* 485–488.

Tietze, C. (1974). Human rights in relationship to induced abortion. *Journal of Sex Research, 10,* 89–96.

Tinklenberg, J. R. (1971). Do amphetamines affect sexual function? *Sexual Behavior, 1*(5), 11.

Tolor, A., & DiGrazia, P. V. (1976). Sexual attitudes and behavior patterns during and following pregnancy. *Archives of Sexual Behavior, 5,* 539–551.

Touhey, J. C. (1971). Birth order and virginity. *Psychological Reports, 28,* 894.

Townes, B. D., Ferguson, W. D., & Gillam, S. (1976). Differences in psychological sex, adjustment, and familial influences among homosexual and nonhomosexual populations. *Journal of Homosexuality, 1,* 261–272.

Traupmann, J. (1978). *Equity in intimate relations: An interview study of marriage.* Unpublished Ph.D. dissertation, University of Wisconsin-Madison.

Traupmann, J., & Hatfield, E. (1979, March 22–24). *The impact of intimacy on the mental and physical health of older Americans.* Paper presented at the Workshop on Stability and Change in the Family at Annapolis, Maryland.

Tresemer, D. (1974, March). Fear of success: Popular but unproven. *Psychology Today,* pp. 82–85.

Tsai, M., Feldman-Summers, S., & Edgar, M. (1979). Childhood molestation: Variables related to differential impacts on psychosexual functioning in adult women. *Journal of Abnormal Psychology, 88,* 407–417.

Tsai, M., & Wagner, N. N. (1978). Therapy groups for women sexually molested as children. *Archives of Sexual Behavior, 7,* 417–427.

Tuller, N. R. (1978). Couples: The hidden segment of the gay world. *Journal of Homosexuality, 3,* 331–343.

Twain, M. (1964). The Adventures of Huckleberry Finn. In *The Complete Novels of Mark Twain.* New York: Doubleday. (Originally published, 1884.)

Twentyman, C. T., & McFall, R. M. (1975). Behavioral training of social skills in shy males. *Journal of Consulting and Clinical Psychology, 43,* 384–395.

Two held for sex with children. (1977, February 17). *Austin American-Statesman* (Associated Press).

Udry, J. R. (1974). *The social context of marriage* (3rd ed.). New York: J. B. Lippincott.

Udry, J. R., Bauman, K. E., & Morris, N. M. (1975). Changes in premarital coital experience of recent decade-of-birth cohorts of urban American women. *Journal of Marriage and the Family, 37,* 783–787.

Udry, J. R., & Morris, N. M. (1968). Distribution of coitus in the menstrual cycle. *Nature, 220,* 593–596.

Udry, J. R., Morris, N. M., & Waller, L. (1973). Effect of contraceptive pills on sexual activity in the luteal phase of the human menstrual cycle. *Archives of Sexual Behavior, 2,* 205–214.

Unger, R. K. (1979). *Female and male.* New York: Harper & Row.

Unger, R. K., & Siiter, R. (1974, April). *Sex-role stereotypes: The weight of a "grain of truth."* Paper presented at the meetings of the Eastern Psychological Association, Philadelphia.

U'Ren, M. B. (1971). The image of women in textbooks. In V. Gornics & B. K. Moran (Eds.), *Woman in sexist society: Studies in power and powerlessness.* New York: New American Library.

U.S. Department of Commerce, Bureau of the Census. (1960). *U.S. census of population: 1960.* Subject Reports. Marital Status. Final Report PC (2)—4E, p. 166. Washington, D.C.: U.S. Government Printing Office.

U.S. Department of Commerce, Bureau of the Census. (1971). *Marital status and living arrangements: March 1971.* Current Population Reports, series P-20, no. 225, Washington, D.C.: U.S. Government Printing Office.

Utne, M. K. (1978). *Equity in intimate relations: A test of the theory in marital interaction.* Unpublished Ph.D. dissertation, University of Wisconsin-Madison.

Vance, E. B., & Wagner, N. N. (1976). Written descriptions of orgasm: A study of sex differences. *Archives of Sexual Behavior, 5,* 87–98.

Van de Velde, T. H. (1965). *Ideal marriage.* New York: Random House.

Vatsyayana. (1964). *The Kama Sutra of Vatsyayana: Classic Hindu treatise on love and social conduct* (Sir R. F. Burton, Trans.). New York: E. P. Dutton.

Vener, A. M., & Stewart, C. S. (1974). Adolescent sexual behavior in Middle America revisited: 1970–1973. *Journal of Marriage and the Family, 36,* 728–735.

Volgenau, G. (1978, December 14). Man accuses woman of sex assault. *Wichita Eagle* (Knight-Ridder News Service).

Vonderheide, S. G., & Mosher, D. L. (1981, November). *Relationship of sex guilt and negative attitudes toward masturbation to females' responses to contraceptive imagery.* Paper presented at the Society for the Scientific Study of Sex.

Wagman, M. (1967). Sex differences in types of daydreams. *Journal of Personality and Social Psychology, 7,* 329–332.

Wagner, N. N., Fujita, B. N., & Pion, R. (1973). Sexual behavior in high school: Data on a small sample. *Journal of Sex Research, 9,* 150–155.

Wagner, N., & Solberg, D. (1974). Pregnancy and sexuality. *Medical Aspects of Human Sexuality, 8,* 44–79.

Wallace, D. H., & Wehmer, G. (1972). Evaluation of visual erotica by sexual liberals and conservatives. *Journal of Sex Research, 8,* 147–153.

Walster (Hatfield), E., Aronson, V., Abrahams, D., & Rottman, L. (1966). The importance of physical attractiveness in dating behavior. *Journal of Personality and Social Psychology, 4,* 508–516.

Walster, E., Traupmann, J., & Walster, G. W. (1978). Equity and extramarital sexuality. *Archives of Sexual Behavior, 7,* 127–142.

Walster, E., Walster, G. W., & Berscheid, E. (1978). *Equity: Theory and research.* Boston: Allyn & Bacon.

Warren, C. A. B. (1974). *Identity and community in the gay world*. New York: Wiley.

Warren, C. A. B. (1976). Women among men: Females in the male homosexual community. *Archives of Sexual Behavior, 5*, 157–169.

Waterman, C. K., & Chiauzzi, E. J. (1982). The role of orgasm in male and female sexual enjoyment. *Journal of Sex Research, 18*, 146–159.

Waxenberg, S. E. (1963). Some biological correlates of sexual behavior. In C. Winokur (Ed.), *Determinants of human sexual behavior*. Springfield, Ill.: Charles C. Thomas.

Webb, A. P. (1963). Sex-role preferences and adjustment in early adolescents. *Child Development, 34*, 609–618.

Weiler, S. J. (1981). Aging and sexuality and the myth of decline. In J. Marsh & S. Kiesler (Eds.), *Stability and change in the family*. New York: Academic Press.

Weinberg, M. S. (1970). Homosexual samples: Differences and similarities. *Journal of Sex Research, 6*, 312–325.

Weinberg, M. S., & Williams, C. J. (1975). *Male homosexuals: Their problems and adaptations*. New York: Penguin.

Weinberg, S. K. (1955). *Incest behavior*. New York: Citadel.

Weiner, B., Frieze, I., Kukla, A., Reed, L., Rest, S., & Rosenbaum, R. M. (1971). Perceiving the causes of success and failure. In E. E. Jones & colleagues (Eds.), *Attribution: Perceiving the causes of behavior*. Morristown, N.J.: General Learning Press.

Weis, K., & Borges, S. S. (1973). Victimology and rape: The case of the legitimate victim. *Issues in Criminology, 8*, 71–115.

Weitzman, L. J., Eifler, D., Hokada, E., & Ross, C. (1972). Sex role socialization in picture books for pre-school children. *American Journal of Sociology, 77*, 1125–50.

Werner, H. (1957). The concept of development from a comparative and organismic point of view. In D. B. Harris (Ed.), *The concept of development*. Minneapolis: University of Minnesota Press.

Westoff, C. F. (1974). Coital frequency and contraception. *Family Planning Perspectives, 6* (Summer), 136–141.

Westoff, C., & Bumpass, L. (1973). The revolution in birth control practices of U.S. Roman Catholics. *Science, 179*, 41–44.

Whalen, R. E. (1965). Cyclic changes in hormones and behavior. *Archives of Sexual Behavior, 4*, 313–314.

Whitam, F. L. (1977). Childhood indicators of male homosexuality. *Archives of Sexual Behavior, 6*, 89–96. (a)

Whitam, F. L. (1977). The homosexual role: A reconsideration. *Journal of Sex Research, 13*, 1–11. (b)

White, D. (1981, September). Pursuit of the ultimate aphrodisiac. *Psychology Today*, pp. 9–11.

White, L. A. (1979). Erotica and aggression: The influence of sexual arousal, positive affect, and negative affect on aggressive behavior. *Journal of Personality and Social Psychology, 37*, 591–601.

Wiggins, J. S., Wiggins, N., & Conger, J. C. (1968). Correlates of heterosexual somatic preference. *Journal of Personality and Social Psychology, 10*, 82–90.

Williams, J. H. (1977). *Psychology of women*. New York: W. W. Norton.

Wilson, G. T., & Lawson, D. M. (1978). Expectancies, alcohol, and sexual arousal in women. *Journal of Abnormal Psychology, 87*, 358–367.

Wilson, G. T., Lawson, D. M., & Abrams, D. B. (1978). Effects of alcohol on sexual arousal in male alcoholics. *Journal of Abnormal Psychology, 87*, 609–616.

Wilson, R. (1966). *Feminine forever*. New York: M. Evans.

Wilson, W. C. (1975). The distribution of selected sexual attitudes and behaviors among the adult population of the United States. *Journal of Sex Research, 11*, 46–64.

Wincze, J. P., Hoon, P., & Hoon, E. F. (1977). Sexual arousal in women: A comparison of cognitive and physiological responses by continuous measurement. *Archives of Sexual Behavior, 6*, 121–133.

Witzig, J. S. (1968). The group treatment of male exhibitionists. *American Journal of Psychiatry, 125*, 75–81.

Wolfenden, J., et al. (1956). *Report of the Departmental Committee on Homosexual Offenses and Prostitution*. London: Her Majesty's Stationery Office.

Wolff, C. (1971). *Love between women*. New York: Harper & Row.

Wolpe, J. (1966). *The practice of behavior therapy*. New York: Pergamon Press.

Womack, W. (1975, July). *Incest*. Paper presented at the Institute for Sex Research, Indiana University.

Women on Words and Images. (1972). Dick and Jane as victims: Sex stereotyping in children's readers. In *Women on words and images*. Princeton, N.J.

Woody, R. H. (1973). Integrated aversion therapy and psychotherapy: Two sexual deviation case studies. *Journal of Sex Research, 9*, 313–324.

Wortman, C. (1978, December). *Psychological reactions to victimization*. Paper presented at Kansas State University, Manhattan.

Yates, A. (1978). *Sex without shame*. New York: Morrow.

Young, W. C., Goy, R. W., & Phoenix, C. H. (1964). Hormones and sexual behavior. *Science, 143*, 212–218.

Young, W. C., Goy, R. W., & Phoenix, C. H. (1965). Hormones and sexual behavior. In J. Money (Ed.), *Sex research: New developments*. New York: Holt, Rinehart, and Winston.

Zajonc, R. R. (1968). Attitudinal effects of mere exposure. *Journal of Personality and Social Psychology, 9*, Monograph Supplement, 1–29.

Zelnik, M., & Kantner, J. F. (1977). Sexual and contraceptive experience of young unmarried women in the United States, 1976 and 1971. *Family Planning Perspectives, 9*, 55–71.

Ziegler, F. J. (1971, July). Male sterilization. *Sexual Behavior*, pp. 71–73.

Ziel, H. K., & Finkle, W. D. (1975). Increased risk of endometrial carcinoma among users of conjugated estrogens. *New England Journal of Medicine, 293*, 1167–1170.

Zilbergeld, B. (1978). *Male sexuality: A guide to sexual fulfillment*. Boston: Little, Brown.

Zilbergeld, B., & Evans, M. (1980, August). The inadequacy of Masters and Johnson. *Psychology Today*.

Zillman, D. (1971). Excitation transfer in communication-mediated aggressive behavior. *Journal of Experimental Social Psychology, 7*, 419–434.

Zimbardo, P. G. (1977). *Shyness: What it is, what to do about it*. Reading, Mass.: Addison-Wesley.

Zimmerman, M. K. (1977). *Passage through abortion: The personal and social reality of women's experiences*. New York: Praeger.

Zitrin, A., Dement, W. C., & Barchas, J. D. (1973). Brain serotonin and male sexual behavior. In J. Zubin & J. Money (Eds.), *Contemporary sexual behavior*. Baltimore: Johns Hopkins Press.

Zuckerman, M. (1973). Scales for sex experience for males and females. *Journal of Consulting and Clinical Psychology, 41*, 27–29.

Zuckerman, M., Tushup, R., & Finner, S. (1976). Sexual attitudes and experience: Attitude and personality correlates and changes produced by a course in sexuality. *Journal of Consulting and Clinical Psychology, 44*, 7–19.

Zuckerman, M., & Wheeler, L. (1975). To dispel fantasies about the fantasy based measure of fear and success. *Psychological Bulletin, 82*, 932–946.

Acknowledgments

Photos

Page
5   Brown Brothers
8   Jean Francois Allaux
14   Photo by Dellenback. Courtesy of the Kinsey Institute for Research in Sex, Gender & Reproduction, Inc., Indiana University
16   © Joel Gordon 1981
20   Courtesy Reproductive Biology Research Foundation St. Louis
71   Mary Ellen Mark/Archive Pictures Inc.
114 Diana Olson Rasche
116 Jerry Howard/Positive Images
123 Vito Palmisano
135 Charles Gatewood
181, 184   J. Money and A. Ehrhardt; *Man and Woman, Boy and Girl*; Johns Hopkins University Press
188 Derek Bayes, *Life* Magazine © 1961 Time Inc.
189 Bruno de Hamel
190 Gender Dysphoria Program, Inc.
196 © Bettye Lane
199 Tom McCarthy/Hillstrom Stock Photo
210 Sherry Ewaskowitz/Hillstrom Stock Photo
210 Abigail Heyman/Archive Pictures Inc.
220 William Burlingham
220 Scott, Foresman photo
225 © Bill Binzen
254 Jerry Howard/Positive Images
259 © Michael Hayman/Click/Chicago Ltd.
281 Mark Antman/The Image Works
315 © Meg Gerken/Click/Chicago Ltd.
328 Sydney freelance/Gamma-Liaison
341 © Bettye Lane
353 Alex Webb/Magnum Photos
364 © Bettye Lane
378 Jean C. Pigozzi/Archive Pictures Inc.
385 © Joel Gordon 1981
393 Robin Schwartz/International Stock Photo
400 Jean-Claude Lejeune
408 UPI

420   Alan Carey/The Image Works
430   American Society for Social Hygiene 1926
432–437   Centers for Disease Control, Atlanta, GA 30333
441   © Bettye Lane
443   Centers for Disease Control, Atlanta, GA 30333
452   © Ulrike Welsch
456   Eugene Richards/Magnum Photos
458   Arnold J. Saxe
472   Ellis Herwig/Stock, Boston
483   Mark Antman/The Image Works
492   Vicki Lawrence/Stock, Boston
501   Steve Smith/Gamma-Liaison
510   Louise Gubb/Gamma-Liaison
514   Robin Schwartz/International Stock Photo

Figures, Tables, and Quotations

p. 50   Fig. 2–11   From *Essential Human Anatomy and Physiology*, 2nd edition, by Barbara R. Landau. Copyright © 1976, 1980 by Scott, Foresman and Company.

p. 53   Table   Made up of data from "Menstruating, Reattribution and Competence" by J. Rodin in *Journal of Personality and Social Psychology*, Vol. 33, 1976. Copyright © 1976 by the American Psychological Association. Reprinted by permission of the author.

p. 66   Fig. 3–1   From *Essential Human Anatomy and Physiology*, 2nd edition, by Barbara R. Landau. Copyright © 1976, 1980 by Scott, Foresman and Company.

pp. 74, 89, 90   Tables 3–1, 3–2, Fig. 3–10   From *Contraceptive Technology 1978–1979* by Robert A. Hatcher et al. Copyright © 1978 by Irvington Publishers, Inc., New York. Reprinted by permission.

p. 107   Quotation from Ann Landers, *Chicago Sun-Times*, Sept. 28, 1976. Copyright © 1976 by the Field Newspaper Syndicate. Reprinted by permission.

p. 118   Fig. 4–1   Based on data from "Sexual Experience and Sexual Responsiveness: Sex Differences" by William Griffitt in *Archives of Sexual Behavior*, Vol. 4, 1975. Copyright © 1975 by Plenum Publishing Corporation. Reprinted by permission.

p. 119   Fig. 4–2   From "Cognitive Factors in Sexual Arousal" by J. H. Geer and R. Fuhr in *Journal of Consulting and Clinical Psychology*, Vol. 44, 1976, p. 241. Copyright © 1976 by the American Psychological Association. Reprinted by permission of the author.

p. 126   Table 4–2   From "Heterosexual Behavior Assessment—I. Males" and "Heterosexual Behavior Assessment—II. Females" by Peter M. Bentler in *Behavior Research and Therapy*, Vol. 6, 1968. Copyright © 1968 by Pergamon Press, Ltd. Reprinted by permission of Pergamon Press and the author.

p. 127   Fig. 4–3   From "Preliminary Scaling of 40 Erotic Slides for Sexual Arousal and Disgust" by J. D. Fisher and D. Byrne. Reprinted by permission of Donn Byrne.

p. 133   Quotation   From "Responses to Reading Erotic Stories: Male-Female Differences" by Gunter Schmidt, Volkmar Sigusch and Siegrid Schaefer in *Archives of Sexual Behavior*, Vol. 2, No. 3, 1973. Copyright © 1973 by Plenum Publishing Corporation. Reprinted by permission.

p. 143   Fig. 5–1   From "The Sexual Response Cycles of the Human Male and Human Female Comparative Anatomy and Physiology" by William H. Masters and Virginia E. Johnson in *Sex and Behavior*, edited by Frank A. Beach. Copyright © 1965 by John Wiley & Sons, Inc. Reprinted by permission of Frank A. Beach.

p. 169   "Sex of Orgasm Questionnaire" from "Written Descriptions of Orgasm: A Study of Sex Differences" by Ellen Belle Vance and Nathaniel N. Wagner in *Archives of Sexual Behavior*, Vol. 5, No. 1, 1976. Copyright © 1976 by Plenum Publishing Corporation. Reprinted by permission.

p. 173   Table 5–1   From *The Female Orgasm: Psychology, Physiology, Fantasy* by Seymour Fisher. Copyright © 1973 by Basic Books, Inc., Publishers. Reprinted by permission of Basic Books, Inc. and Penguin Books Ltd.

p. 183   Table 6–1   From *Man and Woman, Boy and Girl* by John Money and Anke A. Ehrhardt. Copyright © 1972 by The Johns Hopkins University Press. Reprinted by permission of The Johns Hopkins University Press and John Money.

p. 200   Table 7–1   Based on data from *The Psychology of Sex Differences* by Eleanor Emmons Maccoby and Carol Nagy Jacklin. Copyright © 1974 by the Board of Trustees of the Leland Stanford Junior University. Reprinted by permission of Stanford University Press.

p. 170   Fig. 5–7   Based on data from *Sexual Behavior in the Human Male*, 1948 and *Sexual Behavior in the Human Female*, 1953 by Alfred C. Kinsey et al. Reprinted by permission of The Kinsey Institute for Research in Sex, Gender and Reproduction.

pp. 202–3   Table   Summarized from "Sex Role Stereotypes: A Current Appraisal" by I. K. Broverman, S. R. Vogel, D. M. Broverman, F. E. Clarkson and P. S. Rosenkrantz in *Journal of Social Issues*, Vol. 28, No. 2, 1972. Copyright © 1972 by The Society for the Psychological Study of Social Issues. Reprinted by permission.

p. 209   Table 7–2   Reproduced by special permission of the Publisher, Consulting Psychologists Press, Inc., Palo Alto, California 94306, from *The Bem Sex Role Inventory* by Sandra Bem, Ph.D. Copyright © 1978. Further reproduction is prohibited without the Publisher's consent.

p. 217   Fig. 8–1   Based on data from *Sexual Behavior in the Human Male*, 1948 by Alfred C. Kinsey et al. Reprinted by permission of The Kinsey Institute for Research in Sex, Gender and Reproduction.

p. 227   Table 8–2   Made up of data from "Women's Fantasies During Sexual Intercourse: Normative and Theoretical Implications" by E. B. Hariton and J. L. Singer in *Journal of Consulting and Clinical Psychology*, Vol. 42, 1974. Copyright © 1974 by the American Psychological Association. Reprinted by permission of the author.

p. 231   Fig. 8–2   Based on data from *Sexual Behavior in the Human Male*, 1948 and *Sexual Behavior in the Human Female*, 1953 by Alfred C. Kinsey et al. Reprinted by permission of The Kinsey Institute for Research in Sex, Gender and Reproduction.

p. 234   Quotation from Ann Landers, *Chicago Sun-Times*, Dec. 16, 1976. Copyright © 1976 by the Field Newspaper Syndicate. Reprinted by permission.

p. 238   Fig. 8–3   Based on data from *Sexual Behavior in the Human Female*, 1953 by Alfred C. Kinsey et al. Reprinted by permission of The Kinsey Institute for Research in Sex, Gender and Reproduction.

p. 242   Figure   Based on data from "Directed Masturbation and the Treatment of Primary Orgasmic Dysfunction" by Robert J. Kohlenberg in *Archives of Sexual Behavior*, Vol. 3, 1974. Copyright © 1974 by Plenum Publishing Corporation. Reprinted by permission.

pp. 251, 253, 255, 261   Fig. 9–1, Table 9–1, Figs. 9–2, 9–3   Based on data from *Sexual Behavior in the Human Male*, 1948 and *Sexual Behavior in the Human Female*, 1953 by Alfred C. Kinsey et al. Reprinted by permission of The Kinsey Institute for Research in Sex, Gender and Reproduction.

p. 265   Table 9–2   From "Social Attitudes and Sexual Behaviors of College Students" by V. C. Joe and S. Kostyla in *Journal of Consulting and Clinical Psychology*, Vol. 43, 1975, p. 430. Copyright © 1975 by the American Psychological Association. Adapted by permission of the author.

p. 293   Fig. 10–1   From *Human Sex Anatomy* by Robert Latou Dickinson. Copyright 1949 by The Williams & Wilkins Company, Baltimore, Maryland. Reprinted by permission.

pp. 303, 306, 406–7, 408, 411   Quotations reprinted with permission of Macmillan Publishing Company from *The Hite Report* by Shere Hite. Copyright © 1976 by Shere Hite.

p. 327   Table 11–1   Based on data from *Sexual Behavior in the Human Male*, 1948 and *Sexual Behavior in the Human Female*, 1953 by Alfred C. Kinsey et al. Reprinted by permission of The Kinsey Institute for Research in Sex, Gender and Reproduction.

p. 335   Table 11–4   Made up of data from *Homosexualities: A Study of Diversity Among Men and Women* by Alan P. Bell and Martin S. Weinberg. Copyright © 1978 by Alan P. Bell and Martin S. Weinberg. Reprinted by permission of Simon & Schuster, Inc. and Mitchell Beazley Limited.

p. 345   Table   From "Media Mating I: Newspaper 'Personals' Ads of Homosexual Men" by M. R. Laner and G. W. L. Kamel in *Journal of Homosexuality*, Vol. 3, 1977, pp. 149–162. Copyright © 1977 by the Haworth Press Inc. All rights reserved. Reprinted by permission.

pp. 365, 367, 378–79   Quotations from "Sexual Deviation" by Robert J. Stoller in *Human Sexuality in Four Perspectives* edited by Frank A. Beach. Copyright © 1976, 1977 by The Johns Hopkins University Press. Reprinted by permission.

pp. 368, 369   Quotations from "Adult Sexual Orientation and Attraction to Underage Persons" by A. N. Groth and H. J. Birnbaum in *Archives of Sexual Behavior*, Vol. 7, 1978. Copyright © 1978 by Plenum Publishing Corporation. Reprinted by permission.

p. 375   Quotation from Ann Landers, *Chicago Sun-Times*, Jan. 4, 1976. Copyright © 1976 by The Field Newspaper Syndicate. Reprinted by permission.

p. 381   Excerpts and table from "Assisted Covert Sensitization in the Treatment of Exhibitionism" by Barry M. Maletzky in *Journal of Consulting and Clinical Psychology*, February 1974. Copyright © 1974 by the American Psychological Association. Reprinted/ Adapted by permission of the publisher and author.

p. 384   Table 12–1   Based on data from "Manifest Sadomasochism of Males; Results of an Empirical Study" by A. Spengler in *Archives of Sexual Behavior*, Vol. 6, 1977. Copyright © 1977 by Plenum Publishing Corporation. Reprinted by permission.

p. 415   Table 13–1   From *Sexual Behavior in the 1970s* by Morton Hunt. Copyright © 1974 by Morton Hunt. Reprinted by permission of Lescher & Lescher, Ltd.

p. 464   Table 15–1   From *Patterns of Sexual Behavior*, Table 5, page 88 by Clellan S. Ford and Frank A. Beach. Copyright 1951 by Clellan Stearns Ford and Frank Ambrose Beach. Copyright © 1979 by Frank Ambrose Beach. Reprinted by permission of Harper & Row. Publishers, Inc.

p. 466   Fig. 15–1   From "Correlates of Heterosexual Somatic Preference" by J. S. Wiggins, N. Wiggins and J. C. Conger in *Journal of Personality and Social Psychology*, Vol. 10, 1968. Copyright © 1968 by the American Psychological Association. Reprinted by permission of the author.

p. 467   Fig. 15–2   From "Female Preferences for Male Physiques" by Paul J. Lavrakas in *Journal of Research in Personality*, Vol. 9, 1975. Copyright © 1975 by Academic Press, Inc. Reprinted by permission of the author.

p. 469   Table 15–2   Based on data from *Shyness: What it is, What to do about it* by Philip G. Zimbardo. Copyright © 1977. Reprinted by permission of Addison-Wesley Publishing Company, Reading, Massachusetts.

Name Index

Subject Index